Managing Child Nutrition Programs

Leadership for Excellence

Josephine Martin, PhD, RD

Martha T. Conklin, PhD, RD

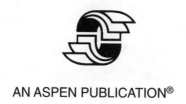

AN ASPEN PUBLICATION®

Managing Child Nutrition Programs

Leadership for Excellence

Josephine Martin, PhD, RD
President, The Josephine Martin Group
Decatur, Georgia
Adjunct Professor, Department of Nutrition
Georgia State University
Atlanta, Georgia

Martha T. Conklin, PhD, RD
Senior Research Professor, Nutrition and Food Systems
Director, Applied Research Division
National Food Service Management Institute
The University of Southern Mississippi
Hattiesburg, Mississippi

AN ASPEN PUBLICATION®
Aspen Publishers, Inc.
Gaithersburg, Maryland
1999

The author has made every effort to ensure the accuracy of the information herein. However, appropriate information sources should be consulted, especially for new or unfamiliar procedures. It is the responsibility of every practitioner to evaluate the appropriateness of a particular opinion in the context of actual clinical situations and with due considerations to new developments. The author, editors, and the publisher cannot be held responsible for any typographical or other errors found in this book.

Aspen Publishers, Inc., is not affiliated with the American Society of Parenteral and Enteral Nutrition.

Library of Congress Cataloging-in-Publication Data
Managing child nutrition programs : leadership for excellence /
[edited by] Josephine Martin, Martha Conklin.
p.   cm.
Includes bibliographical references and index.
ISBN 0-8342-0917-9
1. School children—Food—United States—Administration.
2. School children—United States—Nutrition—Administration.
I. Martin, Josephine, Ph.D.   II. Conklin, Martha, Ph.D.
LB3479.U54M26   1999
371.7′16—dc21   99-13065
                                                                          CIP

Orders: (800) 638-8437
Customer Service: (800) 234-1660

About Aspen Publishers • For more than 35 years, Aspen has been a leading professional publisher in a variety of disciplines. Aspen's vast information resources are available in both print and electronic formats. We are committed to providing the highest quality information available in the most appropriate format for our customers. Visit Aspen's Internet site for more information resources, directories, articles, and a searchable version of Aspen's full catalog, including the most recent publications: **http://www.aspenpublishers.com**
Aspen Publishers, Inc. • The hallmark of quality in publishing
Member of the worldwide Wolters Kluwer group.

Editorial Services: Lenda Hill
Library of Congress Catalog Card Number: 99-13065
ISBN: 0-8342-0917-9

Printed in the United States of America

1   2   3   4   5

Table of Contents

List of Contributors

Sally R. Anger, MS
Nutrition Programs Supervisor
CES Nutrition Consultant
North Carolina Cooperative Extension Service
Washington, North Carolina

Gertrude B. Applebaum, BS
Vice President
inTEAM Associates, Inc.
Corpus Christi, Texas

Janet Beer, RD, LD
Food Service Director
Tigard-Tualatin School District
Tigard, Oregon

Mary Begalle, RD
State Director
Food & Nutrition Service
Minnesota Department of Children,
    Families and Learning
St. Paul, Minnesota

Betty Bender, MS, RD, LD
Consultant
Nicholasville, Kentucky

John Bennett, MA
President
John Bennett Creative Services for Child
    Nutrition Professionals, Inc.
Phoenix, Maryland

Nena P. Bratianu, MEd
Consultant
S.E. Food & Nutrition Associates, Inc.
Atlanta, Georgia

Dorothy Caldwell, MS, RD
Special Assistant to the Under Secretary
Food, Nutrition and Consumer Services, USDA
Alexandria, Virginia
Formerly State Director of Child Nutrition
Arkansas Department of Education

Deborah H. Carr, MS, RD
Research Associate
National Food Service Management Institute
Applied Research Division
The University of Southern Mississippi
Hattiesburg, Mississippi

Tami J. Cline, MS, RD
Director of Nutrition Services
National Dairy Council
Rosemont, Illinois

Martha T. Conklin, PhD, RD
Senior Research Professor
Nutrition and Food Systems
Director, Applied Research Division
National Food Service Management Institute
The University of Southern Mississippi
Hattiesburg, Mississippi

Evelina Cross, PhD, LDN, RD
Professor
School of Human Ecology
Louisiana State University
Baton Rouge, Louisiana

Harriet Deel, EdD
Retired State Director of Child Nutrition
West Virginia Department of Education
Charleston, West Virginia

Tab Forgac, MS, RD, LD
Vice President, Nutrition and Marketing
National Dairy Council
Rosemont, Illinois

Barbara Gilbert, MS, RD
Assistant Director of Finance for Food Service
Dekalb County School System
Decatur, Georgia

Ruth Gordon, MEd, RD
Education Program Manager
Nutrition Education and Training Program
School & Community Nutrition
Georgia Department of Education
Atlanta, Georgia

Mary B. Gregoire, PhD, RD
Chair
Department of Hotel, Restaurant, & Institution
    Management
Iowa State University
Ames, Iowa

Jane Gullett, RD
Oregon Department of Education
Child Nutrition Program Specialist
Salem, Oregon

Marlene Gunn, MS, RD
Consultant
Corinth, Mississippi

Annette Bomar Hopgood, MEd, LD
Director
School & Community Nutrition
Georgia Department of Education
Atlanta, Georgia

Janet W. Horsley, MPH, RD, CSP
Project Coordinator-MCH-LEND Program
Virginia Institute for Developmental
    Disabilities
Virginia Commonwealth University
Richmond, Virginia

Gail M. Johnson, MS, RD, CNP
Director of Child Nutrition Program
East Baton Rouge Parish
Baton Rouge, Louisiana

Elaine Keaton, RD
Director
School Nutrition Programs
Albuquerque Public Schools
Albuquerque, New Mexico

Helene Kent, MS, RD
Director, Women's Health Section
Colorado Department of Public Health and
    Environment
Denver, Colorado

Nadine Mann, PhD, RD,
Assistant Director
Child Nutrition Program
East Baton Rouge Parish School System
Baton Rouge, Louisiana

Amanda Dew Manning, MS, MPA
President
Amanda Dew Manning & Associates, Inc.
Arlington, Virginia

Josephine Martin, PhD, RD, LD
President, The Josephine Martin Group
Decatur, Georgia
Adjunct Professor, Department of Nutrition
Georgia State University
Atlanta, Georgia

Penny McConnell, MS, RD
Director
Office of Food and Nutrition Services
Fairfax County Public Schools
Springfield, Virginia

Carol McLeod, RD, LD
Food Service Director
Newberg Public Schools
Newberg, Oregon

Karen Merrill, MS, RD
Consultant
Albuquerque, New Mexico

Mary Kay Meyer, PhD, RD
Research Scientist
Division of Applied Research
National Food Service Management Institute
University of Southern Mississippi
Hattiesburg, Mississippi

Melanie Moentmann, MBA, RD
Director, School Nutrition Programs
Independence Public Schools
Independence, Missouri

Mary Nix, MEd
Consultant
Kennesaw, Georgia

Charlotte B. Oakley, PhD, RD, FADA
Associate Professor
School of Human Sciences
Mississippi State University
Starkville, Mississippi
Formerly Food and Nutrition Specialist
National Food Service Management Institute
University of Mississippi

Dorothy Pannell-Martin, BS, MA
President
inTEAM Associates, Inc.
Alexandria, Virginia

Jennifer J. Parenteau, RD
Child Nutrition Program Specialist
Oregon Department of Education
Salem, Oregon

Sara Clemen Parks, PhD, RD
Associate Dean
Outreach, Cooperative Extension, and
    International Programs
College of Health and Human Development
Pennsylvania State University
University Park, Pennsylvania

Jeanette C. Phillips, EdD
Consultant
Oxford, Mississippi

Julia Sanders
Manager
Huntington High School Food Service
Huntington, West Virginia

Jean B. Shaw
Consultant
Annandale, Virginia

Wanda L. Shockey, MEd, RD
Director, Child Nutrition Unit
Arkansas Department of Education
Little Rock, Arkansas

Shelly G. Terry, MS
Chief, Nutrition and Transportation Services
Maryland Department of Education
Columbia, Maryland

Preface

Every day over 50 million children attend schools and child care facilities where they have need for their bodies and minds to be nourished. Child nutrition programs (CNPs) provide an infrastructure for meeting those needs. The philosophical foundations for child nutrition programs were laid in the 1920s and 1930s by school food and nutrition professionals. They articulated a need to have healthful meals accessible to all children and to link the cafeteria and the classroom in order for children to relate nutrition knowledge learned in the classroom with the food served in the cafeteria. This early philosophy was confirmed in legislation with the passage of the National School Lunch Act of 1946 and the Child Nutrition Act of 1966. The pioneers recognized a need for building an infrastructure based on sound nutrition and nutrition education. Using sound financial management principles they operated a not for profit business in the school setting. The legislative foundation emerged from knowledge acquired in World Wars I and II about the physical conditions of young people who could not meet requirements for the draft and the success of temporary feeding programs during the depression. The philosophical basis was further delineated by the War on Poverty, which spawned legislation ensuring that all children would have access to healthful meals.

Since its beginning in the 1930s, the program has grown in every direction—from one meal a day during the school year to breakfast, lunch, and after-school snacks—from school year to year round, from school age to preschool through high school and even adult care programs. The Nutrition Education and Training Program has been added to enhance the link among the cafeteria, the classroom, and the community. The National Food Service Management Institute (NFSMI) was established to conduct applied research and education and to disseminate information to improve the quality and cost effectiveness of programs. Team Nutrition funds support nutrition education, training, and marketing efforts.

The purpose of the programs is clear; the scope of programs is complex. *Managing Child Nutrition Programs: Leadership for Excellence* is designed to accent strategic program areas and the need for strategic thinking, planning, and research as a vehicle for achieving and sustaining program excellence. Although the need for and philosophy of the programs were established many years ago, practically everything else about the program has changed. The world is faced with rapid expansion of information and technological and social changes that will have a massive impact on the way programs are managed in the future and the customers served. Managing programs requires personnel willing to update their knowledge and skills continually to meet the challenges of change.

Rapid program expansion necessitates the recruitment of new professionals to meet the program's growth needs and to fill the positions of seasoned professionals who have guided the program during the last quarter of a century. *Managing Child Nutrition Programs: Leadership for Excellence* is written to underscore the need for program standards and competent personnel to provide leadership for continuous program improvement. The American School Food Service Association's *Keys to Excellence* and the NFSMI competencies for school food and nutrition program directors provide a consistent thread throughout the book as a constant reminder of the need for program standards, assessment, and competent personnel. Each chapter identifies the relationship of these two resources to achieving the programs envisioned.

Managing Child Nutrition Programs: Leadership for Excellence is designed for use by school food and nutrition professionals at the state and district level and by school administrators. The book was conceived as a resource to help CNP professionals develop innovative and comprehensive child nutrition programs. It also can be used by college and university professors and graduate students either as a text or supplemental resource for courses included in dietetics or hotel and restaurant curricula. The book will also be useful as a reference for dietitians and food service managers exploring school food and nutrition programs as a new career opportunity and as a source for them to meet professional education requirements for certification and/or registration. With the anticipated growth of the program, there will be a continuing need for students to consider child nutrition programs as a viable career option.

The book is not intended as a basic text in any of the management areas of food service. For most chapters, it is assumed that persons using the book have some basic knowledge of food service operations and management. *Managing Child Nutrition Programs* will help the director of federally assisted programs achieve excellence in outcomes. Its focus is on the integration of food and nutrition services and food service management, which is an underlying tenet of federally assisted child nutrition programs.

A distinguishing characteristic of the book is that it is a coordinated effort of professionals who contributed chapters and case studies. The book contains 27 chapters and 16 case studies written by 38 professionals selected for their competence in a specific program area. The authors come from private consulting, academia, state agencies, and local school districts. A case study prepared by a practicing professional describing a successful approach to solving a specific problem supports each theoretically based chapter. Communication, leadership, and decision making are three basic competencies woven throughout the chapters. They provide basic linkages for integration and coordination of program activities essential for effective management.

Chapters in *Managing Child Nutrition Programs* are grouped into the four program areas identified in *Keys to Excellence:* Administration, Nutrition, Operations, and Communications and Marketing. In addition, there are introductory and concluding sections. This book will be a valuable resource for directors to use in developing an improvement plan to implement actions identified by using *Keys to Excellence* to assess program needs; reviewing and revising performance standards for quality control; updating knowledge and stimulating professional development.

Managing Child Nutrition Programs: Leadership for Excellence provides a blueprint for designing programs of the future. Just as a blueprint for any structure contains only the vision, fulfillment is dependent upon the leaders of the future.

Josephine Martin, PhD, RD
Martha T. Conklin, PhD, RD

Acknowledgments

We want to recognize the colleagues and organizations who have helped and supported us in the development of this book: the National Food Service Management Institute, particularly the Executive Director, Jane Logan, Deborah Carr, Jerry Cater, Laurel Lambert, Mary Kay Meyer, and Brenda Whiddon at the Applied Research Division, and Charlotte Oakley at the Education Division; Dorothy Caldwell, Special Assistant for Nutrition and Nutrition Education, Office of the Under Secretary for Food, Nutrition and Consumer Services, U.S. Department of Agriculture who was part of our writing team when the book was first conceived; Barbara Borchow, Executive Director, American School Food Service Association; Jane Boudreaux, Interim Dean of Health and Human Sciences, The University of Southern Mississippi; Ann Raymond, professional journalist and editor who made many suggestions for clarifying thoughts in the chapters; Thelma G. Flanagan, a first generation child nutrition leader whose vision had a major influence on the development of child nutrition programs and whose history *School Food Services* was a major source for chapters 1 and 2; Richard Dengrove at the Food and Nutrition Service library who provided valuable historical information; Joe Richardson from the Congressional Research Service who supplied legislative summaries and Jean Y. Jones of the Congressional Research Service whose valuable historical data filled many missing gaps; Carol Bloomquist, computer documentation specialist, and Kevin Martin and Ron Fread whose help on Sunday afternoons made it possible to get copies to the publisher in an organized manner.

Most importantly, we thank the chapter and case study contributors who have shared their expertise in child nutrition. They are the ones who have provided the essence of leadership for excellence as they have described their walks through the journey of managing child nutrition programs.

A special thanks goes to Margaret Simko, Robert Wood Johnson Medical School, whose vision and foresight led Aspen Publishers to suggest we develop this book and show support and encouragement throughout the entire process was an inspiration that kept us moving toward the goal; and to Sara Parks, Pennsylvania State University, for her futuristic thinking and encouragement for us to undertake this project that documents the vital role child nutrition professionals play each day in the lives of children. We are also grateful to the editorial services staff at Aspen—in particular Mary Anne Langdon, for her patience in working with us and for giving encouragement for the completion of the book, and to Lenda Hill for the thoroughness of copyediting the manuscript, to the permissions staff of Laureece Woodson, and the marketing expertise of Joyce Meals.

Finally, we wish to acknowledge the support and encouragement of our families and special friends who have waited endless hours as we have committed time to the book . . . and, yes, a special thanks to Cindy Lou!

Foreword

This is a book about leadership, about the future, and about nurturing our nation's children both physically and intellectually. *Managing Child Nutrition Programs: Leadership for Excellence* is about more than surviving the new millennium. It is about the leadership needed to assure quality child nutrition programs and how the need for excellence in these programs has changed over time. To fully reap the benefits of good nutrition, children must have access to good food and nutrition information and to responsible practitioners who manage food and nutrition programs in this country's primary and secondary schools.

Managing Child Nutrition Programs: Leadership for Excellence is a book placed in the context of a rich history—a legacy of feeding children and of improving individual lives over time. The leadership and traditions of over a half-century have brought child nutrition programs in the forefront as we approach the next century.

Martin and Conklin, the book's two authors, are well qualified to provide the "past, present, and future" perspectives on quality standards for child nutrition programs, as well as to discuss leadership qualities needed for these programs to survive and to thrive into the future. I know of no one who has read or researched more widely in the management of child nutrition programs than these two authors. They have been in more schools—have researched and consulted—more than anyone else I know. Consequently, they have a comprehensive, direct contact with the reality of child nutrition programs which supplement their research. They are also devotees of my own definition of leadership—about shaping the future. Thus, whenever I have wanted to discover current wisdom about leadership or quality in child nutrition programs, I have asked myself, "What are Martin and Conklin thinking and saying?" And whenever I find myself disagreeing with them, I know my perspectives are at odds with current and accepted wisdom.

This leads me to several thoughts about *Managing Child Nutrition Programs: Leadership for Excellence*. First, why is the book necessary? The authors detail some contemporary issues that point to program challenges exacerbated by environmental changes reflecting the need for transformational leadership at every level of the program: expanded programs to reach a wider audience and to be operated year-round; declining participation of the paying student; shortages of well-qualified individuals to fill increasing job vacancies in child nutrition management positions; increased recognition through research of the relationship among academic performance, classroom attendance and behavior, and healthy eating habits of students; and societal demands that programs provide nutritious meals and nutrition education while remaining solvent as a business within the local school district. I agree that these are significant issues and I also agree that leaders can create new circumstances and can reshape programs to address these issues. This book provides not only the "trials and triumphs" of child nutrition programs, but also the tools to keep them "on track for the future." Thus, the war has not, in my opinion, been lost as far as quality is concerned. The chapter on nutrition integrity is a particularly important contribution to defining quality standards; it sets the stage for ensuring our future.

Second, I agree that child nutrition programs must improve to meet the challenges of the highly competitive marketplace facing managers in our nation's school system. Peter Drucker, a leading futurist on management issues, has described the challenge of continuous change very dramatically; he has said, "rarely has an institution (a profession), a leadership group, faced as demanding, as challenging, as exciting a test as the one that leading in turbulent times now poses." Similarly, managers of child nutrition programs must understand the strategies needed to address the challenges presented by the rapidly changing environments they face in their daily operations. A first step is to understand the role that the food service operation plays as a healthy eating and nutrition laboratory, which is well-defined in the chapters "Educating Beyond the Plate: The Cafeteria–Classroom Connection," and "Menu Planning to Develop Healthy Eating Patterns." I was also pleased to see the chapter on "Nutrition Management for Children with Special Food and Nutrition Needs."

Third, I agree that the journey to improved quality requires leadership in all aspects of child nutrition program operations: understanding the role of public policy and the legislation underlying the programs, nutrition standards, designing and implementing menus based on consumer needs and wants, managing employees for outstanding customer service, developing food production and procurement systems aimed at producing cost-effective healthful meals, and assuring school environments conducive to healthy and socially appropriate behaviors are all important dimensions leading to and maintaining quality standards. This book addresses each of these issues in a comprehensive and innovative manner. The theory and the practical examples provided in the case studies accompanying each content area should help readers to improve or to understand their performance. I also agree that some of the early attempted reforms in quality standards, while important steps to the future, have not always been successful in meeting the needs of children or their families.

Fourth, the authors have included four chapters on marketing and communications. Marketing helps us to understand the needs and wants of our programs' key stakeholders, it provides a framework for analyzing trends impacting our audience and the role food plays in developing healthy lifestyles, and it guides strategic planning needed to assure the future of child nutrition programs. With the accelerated rate of change in today's society, it is a tool managers use to be prepared for the eventuality of competing with food operations anytime or anywhere. To compete in the future managers must create a sensing organization that constantly monitors, queries, verifies, tries, and innovates. The organizations best equipped for the twenty-first century are those who can develop market plans to position, and re-position, child nutrition programs within the broader context of the nation's educational system. Similarly, the book's chapters on communication and community relations certainly provide significant advice and strategies needed to be persuasive in selling the importance food and eating are to a child's well-being.

Finally, I was particularly pleased to see the authors' chapter on "Dreams and Deeds for the Millennium." There is no one better prepared than Josephine Martin to bring us the historical perspective or to lead us into the future. The leadership and guidance provided by Josephine has shaped the profession for almost four decades and for many years to come. Today, her influence continues as she shares her expertise with the profession as a dietetic educator. She has been diligent in challenging each of us in our quest for quality; she has taught us the journey goes beyond economic survival, and that we must care about our nation's children. This book represents a new venue for

Josephine Martin to extend her vision of quality child nutrition programs to others in school administration and allied health.

It is difficult for me to realize that Martha Conklin has also been a leader and an advocate for leadership in child nutrition programs for almost a quarter of a century. She has brought her interest in cost-effectiveness analysis to the child nutrition arena. She has given meaning to the term "applied research" in child nutrition programs, providing strategies and tools for identifying new ways of looking at and doing those things necessary to keep young people and school food and nutrition employees engaged in meaningful ways. Her insights into the challenges of accomplishing goals through people will surely bring us miles closer to having the school food and nutrition program be an integral part of the total school day. Her ability to ask the right questions, to identify the important research agendas, and to contribute her own views have opened new ways of thinking about quality. She has helped with her research leadership to develop the discipline underlying the child nutrition profession and the management of child nutrition operatives.

This book, in many respects, is an unusual book—it is about a personal journey of the authors and the 38 colleagues they have invited to contribute along the way. They have reminded us of the programs' philosophical foundations articulated by professional leaders and members of Congress more than a half decade ago . . . philosophical foundations that have stood the test of time and will take us into the new millennium. It reflects the values and standards of this country's leading child nutrition experts. In the words of George Bernard Shaw, "we are made wise not by the recollections of our past, but by the responsibilities for our future." For me, this book represents a journey taken on behalf of all of us who are wrestling with the profound changes in our society and the leadership needed to assure child nutrition program survival into the 21st century. Nothing will change in the future without fundamentally new ways of thinking. This is the real work of leadership and this book is a good place to begin the journey.

Sara Clemen Parks, RD, PhD
President
The American Dietetic Association
1993–1994
Associate Dean
Outreach, Cooperative Extension
and International Programs
College of Health and Human
Development
Pennsylvania State University
University Park, Pennsylvania

PART I

Introduction

CHAPTER 1

Perspectives on Managing Child Nutrition Programs

Josephine Martin

We are made wise not by the recollections of our past, but by the responsibility for our future.

—George Bernard Shaw

OUTLINE

- Introduction: Managing for Long-Term Success
    Purpose and Objectives
- Moving toward Excellence through Leadership
- Leadership: A Function of Management
- Uniqueness of Child Nutrition Programs
- Multifaceted Purpose of School Food and Nutrition Programs
    Nutrition Service To Meet School Day Nutrition Needs of All Children
    Integral Component of the Comprehensive Health Program
    Resource for the Instructional Program
    Nutrition Center for the School Community
    Nonprofit Business Operated for the Benefit of the School District
- Perspectives on Managing Child Nutrition Programs
- A Systems Approach to Managing Child Nutrition Programs
    Managing the System for Excellence
- Summary

INTRODUCTION: MANAGING FOR LONG-TERM SUCCESS

Tomorrow is another day in child nutrition. Not the day that we experienced yesterday, or today. It is another day that will reflect the myriad events that occurred before the clock struck midnight and events that are happening now. In managing child nutrition programs for long-term success, school food and nutrition professionals need to be constantly aware of changes occurring in the environment and the potential impact they may have on the program and the way it is managed.

Change in our society and the need for looking at a new way to manage are realities. Leaders of the nation's top corporations recognize that change is necessary in order to survive. Former IBM President Thomas Watson said that if an organization is to meet the challenge of a changing world, it must be prepared to change everything about itself except its basic beliefs and values. Watson recognized the importance of resources, organizational structure, timing, and innovation. "But," he said, "they are transcended by how strongly the people in the organization believe in its basic precepts and how faithfully they carry them out."[1(p280)] The basic philosophy of the child nutrition programs was defined in The National School Lunch Act (NSLA) of 1946, was reinforced in The Child Nutrition Act of 1966, and was further refined when the Nutrition Education and Training Amendment was passed in 1977 (Exhibit 1–1). Prior to the provision of federal funding for the programs, pioneers in academia and practice had outlined beliefs and concepts that formed the philosophical foundation for child nutrition programs. That philosophy simply stated the following:

- All children should have access to healthful meals and supplements when they are under the care of the school or other institutional setting.
- The nutrition program should be structured in the school setting to help children develop healthy food habits for a lifetime.

- The program should be operated on sound business principles and practices.

Caldwell and colleagues[2] list three essential functions of a school food and nutrition program. These include the following:

1. Access to a variety of nutritious, culturally appropriate foods that promote growth and development, pleasure in healthy eating, and long-term health, as well as prevent school day hunger and its consequent lack of attention to learning tasks
2. Nutrition education that empowers students to select and enjoy healthful food and physical activity
3. Screening, assessment, counseling, and referral for nutrition problems by qualified individuals and the provision of modified meals for students with special needs

Child nutrition programs exist in schools and other child care institutions to achieve these purposes, and program directors would wisely use these as a yardstick for measuring management effectiveness. The system for delivering these services at the school district level varies and is best when customized to meet the needs of the community served. For long-term success, the program must be viewed as an integral part of the school program. Throughout this book, the school food and nutrition professional will be urged to manage the program to help achieve educational and health objectives and to recognize that success depends upon a collaborative effort as described by Dr. E. Neige Todhunter a half-century ago. Figure 1–1 graphically shows the relationship of the school food and nutrition program to the school, home, community, and the child.

Managing a child nutrition program is a complex task, regardless of its size or scope, whether at the national, state, or district level. Even if the world were standing still, it would be complex. Many factors affect decision making and emphasize the complexity of the man-

Exhibit 1–1 Synopsis of Congressional Policy

The National School Lunch Act of 1946

It is declared to be the policy of Congress, as a measure of national security, to safeguard the health and well-being of the nation's children . . . to assist states in providing nonprofit school lunch programs

The Child Nutrition Act of 1966

In recognition of the demonstrated relationship between food and good nutrition and the capacity of children to develop and learn, it is the policy of Congress as a measure of national security to strengthen and expand food service program

Section 19: Nutrition Education and Training (1977)
Congress finds that:

- proper nutrition of nation's children is a matter of highest priority,
- the lack of understanding and relationship of good nutrition to health can lead to rejection of food and plate waste,
- many food service personnel lack training in nutrition, nutrition education, and food service management skills,
- many classroom teachers lack training in the fundamentals of nutrition and nutrition education,
- parents have a significant influence on children's eating habits and many lack sound nutritional knowledge, and
- there is a need for children to learn about nutrition and how it affects their lives

Food Service Management Institute (1990)

PL 101-147 (1989) authorized funds for a food service management institute to carry out activities to improve the general operation and quality of food service programs authorized by the NSLA and the Child Nutrition Act. Activities include applied research, education and training, and information dissemination.

Healthy Meals for Americans Act (1994)

Healthy Meals for Americans Act requires the implementation of the nutrition principles of the Dietary Guidelines for Americans in school meals.

Source: Reprinted from *National School Lunch Act of 1946*, Public Law 79-396, Stat. 281, Section 2 and the *Child Nutrition Act of 1966.*

agement task. Some of these include synchronizing all parts of the system to keep the program running effectively; responding to the number and types of personnel that make up the school team and their needs; keeping the internal and external stakeholders involved in program functions, goals, needs, and successes; coping with the competition within and without the system; and balancing what may be perceived as dichotomies, the program's function as a nutrition program to meet school day nutri-

tion needs of children and operating a food service program that in many instances must be self-supporting. The director in the new millennium will not see these as dichotomies, but will manage the food service program to meet children's needs and be cost effective.

The world is not standing still; changes are occurring in every facet of the child nutrition enterprise that affect the way it is managed. Just a few of the changes that critically affect programs include

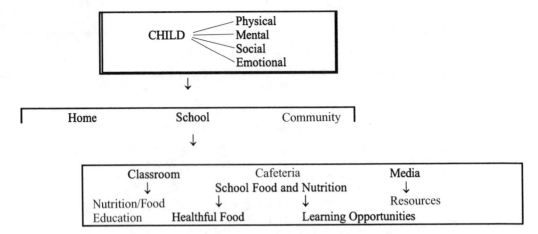

Figure 1–1 School Food and Nutrition: Integral Part of Education. *Source:* Reprinted with permission from E. A. Martin, *Roberts Nutrition Work with Children*, 4th ed., p. 454, © 1978, University of Chicago Press.

- what is happening in the production, processing, and distribution of food
- changes occurring in the educational system
- the strategies employed to keep all students engaged in the education process
- the availability of technology and its implication for every facet of the program from student decision making to operational support
- demographics of the work force and the sensitivity of these programs to fluctuations in the economy at the local, state, and national level
- the steadily increasing competition; the information /communication flow
- most important, the changing nature and needs of the customer

To bring the impact of these changes even closer to the program, think about

- managing seamless programs
- organizing and staffing for an expanded school day that requires breakfast, lunch, after-school snacks, and possibly evening meals; year-round schools
- implementing universal breakfast programs

- incorporating the school food and nutrition program into the comprehensive health program
- making child nutrition programs an integral part of the community social services system

Thinking about how to manage child nutrition programs for excellence in the future requires visionary leadership.

Child nutrition programs are big business and present many challenging management opportunities. In 1998, the federal budget for child nutrition programs exceeded 5 billion dollars, and nearly 95,000 schools participated in the lunch program and 31,000 in the breakfast programs. Every day in 1998, 26.1 million children ate a reimbursable school lunch and 6.1 million children had a school breakfast.[3] Accounting for school meals is not as simple as counting total numbers; they must be accounted for as free, reduced-price, or paid; and there must be a nutritional accounting to see that meals are meeting the goals of the Dietary Guidelines for Americans and the recommended dietary allowances (RDA). While the national numbers are staggering, the numbers in an average-sized school district of 2,800 children would reflect a budget of nearly

$125,000 per month, serving 50,000 meals per month. The child nutrition program is the largest business in some communities. Changes in the environment affect the program, regardless of its size or scope—whether at the national, state, or local level.

Changes are pervasive throughout the program and are happening at an accelerated speed. The child nutrition program director seeking excellence must be prepared to anticipate the changes,[4] and respond with greater speed, more agility, and more flexibility[5] by devising alternatives and implementing strategies that keep the food and nutrition needs of children at the center of the program's focus. Getting on the fast track for managing child nutrition programs for long-term success is an

---

TALES OF TWO MARYS

For several years there has been lots of talk about school vouchers, home schooling, schools without doors, and alternative approaches for high-risk students, including the disruptive, the dropout, etc. Mary Won, food service director, has heard all this talk, but it didn't seem to have an impact on the school food and nutrition program until one day when 25 percent of the student enrollment had been placed in alternative educational programs. Mary Won panicked—the food orders had been placed, the personnel hired, and yet the potential meal service reduced 25 percent. The loss in dollars blinded Mary Won to the need for children to have healthful meals regardless of where they were having class.

Mary Tou also had heard the talk about school vouchers, home schooling, schools without doors, and alternative schools. Each time she heard one of the projected ideas, she put on her "thinking

cap." If kids are home at noon, how will they be fed? What could we do to create a "box home-lunch"? Sitting with the school nutrition team, they brainstormed and a bunch of wonderful ideas emerged. "That's it," said Mary, "we will have a box home-lunch." She still had to think about the alternative school where kids didn't have a set school day, but came to class at will. Creative team thinking produced ideas that were presented to the administrators, who helped make the decision about the food service in the school. Consequently, Mary Tou neither lost participation nor her shirt. In fact, more kids were having school-prepared meals than ever! Thinking out of the box helped Mary Tou and her team keep kids eating healthful meals, regardless of where they were meeting class.

Source: Originally appeared in May 1998 issue of THE FUTURIST. Used with permission from the World Future Society, 7910 Woodmont Avenue, Suite 450, Bethesda, Maryland 20814. 301/656-8274. http://www.wfs.org>.

---

essential step in providing leadership for excellence.

Mary Tou was thinking productively; that is, she was asking, "How many different ways can we look at this problem?" "How can we rethink the way we see it?" Instead of looking at the past as a solution to a new problem, the future demands that we think "out of the box."[6]

If you always think the way you've always thought, you'll always get what you've always gotten. *The Futurist,* May 1998.

Purpose and Objectives

The purpose of the chapter is to help school food and nutrition program directors, potential directors, graduate students, and school administrators develop a conceptual framework for managing cost-effective child nutrition programs in a dynamic environment for long-term success.

The objectives for the chapter are as follows:

- Discuss the characteristics of excellence as a force in managing for long-term success.
- Discuss the need for visionary leadership in managing child nutrition programs.
- Describe the uniqueness of the child nutrition program,.
- Describe the multifaceted nature of child nutrition programs.
- Discuss perspectives on managing programs.
- Present and discuss a systems approach to managing child nutrition programs.

MOVING TOWARD EXCELLENCE THROUGH LEADERSHIP

> Excellence not only implies competence, it implies a striving for the highest standards in every phase of life. Understanding the complexities in our society is essential for anyone concerned with excellence.[7(pp159–160)]

Progress made in the twentieth century in child nutrition programs has been phenomenal, as described in Chapter 2. There are many pockets of excellence in the 95,000 schools participating in child nutrition programs, excellence to be identified and emulated. However, excellence in the 1990s may be viewed as mediocrity in the decades ahead. Excellence in child nutrition programs is evolutionary. It doesn't happen instantly and it doesn't remain stable.

In the pockets of excellence, whether we see them in the area of nutrition education, the procurement operation, or personnel training and standards, or whether we see them at the national, state, or local level, some things always stand out. Common threads weave their way through excellent programs. Mescon and Mescon[8] identify three *A*s that exist where there is program excellence: *attitude, aggressiveness,* and *appearance.* We may choose to refer to these three as commitment, assertiveness, and image. Regardless of the words chosen to describe it, excellence is a way of thinking, a mind-set, based on a set of beliefs, a vision, and an *attitude* say Mescon and Mescon. Directors seeking excellence in child nutrition have a commitment to program values and belief in their own ability to achieve those values. They know that focusing the child nutrition program on meeting the child's health and education needs is the right thing to do. When the director's unwavering belief and commitment to program values is communicated throughout the organization, the commitment becomes contagious. When the entire team throughout the organization is focused on the goal, they will see it accomplished. The first essential ingredient for excellence is *attitude* or commitment.

The second *A* essential for excellence is *aggressiveness,* say Mescon and Mescon, or we may choose to use the word *assertiveness.* Use of the term in relation to achieving excellence may require a paradigm shift to change the connotation from negative to positive. Being aggressive means being willing to step out, to speak up for the program; to think out of the box, to take some risks as necessary to move the program forward. Directors need to put a positive spin on aggressiveness as a requirement for excellence. School food and nutrition programs operate in a highly competitive environment inside and outside the educational system.

Being complacent about the place of school food and nutrition as a part of the education environment can open doors to competition unheard of to date. Aggressive food and nutrition program directors imagine what customers might want 10 years from now, what sorts of foods will be available, and what the educational environment will be. Unless school food and nutrition professionals are making this type of reassessment of their programs, they may be overtaken on the road to the future.[9] To deal effectively with competition, the program director at all levels must step out and speak up for program values and needs. Directors must constantly assess the program in terms of its contribution to achieving educational goals today, but also the needs of the future. In the absence of an aggressive approach to maintain a competitive advantage and to seek positive consideration for child nutrition programs at all levels, the programs could easily be placed on the bottom rung of the decision-making ladder.

Numerous factors compete for program success. At the school district level, competition includes time in the school day; space in the building, funds in the budget; and even such things as band uniforms, computers, and classroom parties. Nontraditional sources of competition will emerge as contenders for the child's time and money. School food and nutrition professionals are challenged to think about two sets of questions that may help to identify the need to be aggressive in speaking out for the program.[9(p18)]

Facing a Competitive Future

Now	Five years from now
• Who are your customers today?	• Who will your customers be in five to ten years?
• How do you reach your customers today?	• How will you reach your customers in the future?
• What is your current competition?	• What will your competition be in five years?
• What do you consider to be the basis for your competitive advantage today?	• What will be the basis for your competitive advantage in the future?
• What makes the school food and nutrition program unique in your setting?	• What services, skills, and capabilities will make the school food and nutrition program unique in five years?
• Could your customers get the same meals in another food service establishment?	• Why will your customers seek the school food and nutrition program as "the place to be" in the future?
• Is your price equal to or better than your customer would pay in another setting?	• How will you maintain quality and service within a price the customers can afford?
• What are your sources of revenue today?	• How will you generate new sources of revenue?
• Is nutrition education an integral part of your program today?	• What will you do to have nutrition education expanded to reach all students?
• Is the cafeteria environment conducive to a positive social experience?	• What will you do to make the meal experience a positive time for the customer.

Source: Reprinted by permission of Harvard Business School Press. From *Competing for the Future* by G. Hamel and C.K. Prahad. Boston, MA. 1994, pp. 17–18. Copyright © 1994 by the President and Fellows of Harvard College, all rights reserved.

According to Hamel and Prahalad,[9] leaders should have a reasonably detailed set of answers to the questions in the second column. They also indicate that, unless the answers are substantially different from the ones in the first column, an organization may not expect to remain a market leader or to have a competitive advantage for that market. Leadership in a market must be reinvented. While the primary market will continue to be school-age children, that is probably the end of where the sameness begins. Children will be different, education will be different, food will be different, and expectations for the program will be different.

The third *A* Mescon and Mescon[10] identified as essential for excellence is *appearance*, or image. Leadership for excellence recognizes that an effective child nutrition program has a positive image. Image is more than a public relations campaign or a marketing program. It embraces everything about the child nutrition program apparent to human senses, including

- ambiance of the cafeteria and its location in the school plant
- the way food looks and is served
- appearance and competence of the entire school food and nutrition team
- recognition by the board of education or in the federal budget
- inclusion as a partner in decision making for the organization
- the appearance of materials and services provided from the state or federal level

Concerted efforts by the United States Department of Agriculture (USDA)–Food and Nutrition Service (FNS), American School Food Service Association (ASFSA), and state agencies to polish the program's image have paid dividends. The image of child nutrition programs was enhanced by congressional action directing that program meals meet the nutrition goals of the Dietary Guidelines for Americans,[11] by the Goals 2000: Educate America Act,[12] identifying nutrition as an important factor in learning readiness, and by the coordinated health program including nutrition

as one of the eight areas of health. Team Nutrition and Training materials prepared by the USDA and state agencies present a new image and new program expectations. Another image enhancement occurred when the Secretary of Agriculture elevated the position responsible for these programs to "an undersecretary in the Department of Agriculture." This was a highly visible, image-producing decision. Attitude, aggressiveness, and appearance—three *A*s for excellence.

Leadership for excellence is reflected in the action of every member of the team. Child nutrition programs cannot achieve excellence unless personnel at every level of the organization accept the need for high standards of performance and strive to achieve those. Gardner gave the example that a missile could blow up on its launching pad because the designer was incompetent or because the mechanic who adjusted the last valve was incompetent.[13] The same is true for the child nutrition program. The school food and nutrition program may fail to meet nutrition goals because the menus were not adequate, or it may fail to meet its goals because the person preparing the vegetables did not follow the standardized recipe regarding amount of seasoning. Excellent directors are needed and so are excellent food service assistants. By and large neither the director not the assistants succeed unless the attitude of excellence permeates the entire operation.

ASFSA's *Keys to Excellence* identifies program expectations.[14] Achieving excellence is contingent upon all members throughout the organization understanding and supporting the expectations through practice. This requires competent personnel,[15,16] for directing the program; for managing, preparing, and serving healthful meals; and for developing the program as a nutrition laboratory.

Peters and Waterman[17] made an extensive study to identify management attributes that characterize excellent and innovative companies. They identified innovation as a concept that defines a truly excellent manager and described eight attributes of excellence identified in the most successful companies. These have been adapted to describe successful child nutrition programs.

- *Preference for action*. The innovative child nutrition program focuses on creating a work environment where decisions can be made at the lowest possible level. A flexible organization and an empowered team are needed to respond to the frequency of change in the school food and nutrition programs.
- *Freedom to take risks*. Leaders exist at all levels in the innovative child nutrition organization. Creativity is encouraged and taking risk is a positive attribute. Team members are rewarded for solving problems. Keeping the status quo, doing business as usual, or staying with those things that brought success in the past is no longer enough to keep the program viable. The greatest success will come from daring to take risks—to be pioneers, to use imagination, and think "out of the box."
- *Focus on the customer*. Excellent child nutrition programs stay close to their internal and external customers. They listen to their needs, conduct satisfaction surveys, have an advisory council, talk with them in the cafeteria, and attend their meetings. The innovative director creates ways to keep the program customer focused.
- *People first*. Quality and productivity are in the hands of the people at the school site, in the back office, or on the delivery truck. Every member of the team is viewed as a source of ideas and not just a pair of hands. Productivity is achieved where there is respect for every individual in the organization. The innovative organization has an outcome-based training plan for personnel, sets reasonable and clear expectations for their performance, and makes them feel that they are contributing to the organization by being responsible for their functional area.

- *Basic values*. Success begins with knowing and adhering to a set of values. Quality, service, sanitation/safety, and meeting children's needs are child nutrition program values. The innovative leader maintains focus on these values.
- *Distinctive competence*. Knowing what to do and how to do it characterizes the excellent director. Doing those things that we do best is an adage to keep in mind whether we are running a major corporation or a school food and nutrition program. Focus is vital in managing programs. Diversifying the program with activities that fit neither the mission of the program nor the competence of personnel is an indication of loss of focus. Biolos states that focus is at the core of a sound strategic position in the market. The following were adapted from his questions to relate to focus in managing child nutrition programs.[18] Questions for the school food and nutrition professional to think about:

1. *How can school food and nutrition programs lose their focus?* The most common answer to this question is the pressure to increase revenue or to increase student participation at all costs. This may be a reaction to proposed legislation, revised policy, or simply inertia. It is possible to increase revenue by expanding offerings without regard to the nutrition mission. Increased student participation in the reimbursable program may result from branded foods or school-prepared foods not consistent with the Dietary Guidelines for Americans and even with an improper focus on the offer versus serve provision.

2. *What is the mission of the school food and nutrition program?* The director should be able to answer this question in a few words. Those few words should be known to the entire school food and nutrition team and become the measuring stick used to determine whether a new idea, food, or activity fits the mission.

3. *Is the program strategy focused on the mission?* A positive answer to this question will reveal that all activities support the program's mission, which is different from the competitor's activities.

4. *Do your customers know the focus of the school food and nutrition program?* The focus is communicated through the way the program is marketed. This may be through a formal marketing plan or the informal marketing that takes place. The manager/director can determine whether the customers know and understand the focus by conducting surveys, involving students in selecting foods to be purchased for the menu, talking with customers informally, doing key informant interviews with individual teachers and students, or conducting focus groups. In identifying your customer base, keep in mind that administrators are very important customers who may not understand the program focus. Chapter 19 describes effective marketing strategies.

5. *Do you need to reinvent your program to stay focused?* When the same jargon becomes ordinary with overuse, a new approach may be necessary. This could involve the cafeteria ambiance, the logo, the menu presentation, or many other ideas that would keep the program focused. Leaders focus on reinventing their programs to keep them fresh and focused on their customers of today. Staying on target, or focused, takes discipline, hard choices, and clarity of purpose. Directors that keep the program on target usually end up better than their competitors, both in terms of nutrition integrity and financially sound programs. It's a challenge, but worth the effort.

- *Minimal management and labor.* Keeping the organization simple is important. Maintaining a high-performance workplace is dependent on competent personnel and organization. Personnel costs consume a major portion of the budget. Creative staffing, maximizing labor hours and responsibility, and using technology as a support system are keys to goal achievement. The innovative director seeks different ways of doing things and eliminates unnecessary tasks. Building a work culture that believes in simplifying the work is the key to doing more with less and to doing it better and more quickly.

- Decision making pushed downward. Allowing for decisions to be made at the lowest level supports excellence. However, standards are an important prerequisite to any decision making. They should be focused on the organization's core values. A decision-making process should assure consideration of all options consistent with core values. Being able to distinguish between decisions that should be made at the director level and those that could be made at the site is essential to shared decision making. A team approach to identifying decisions that can be made at the school level will project support of site-based management. Standards and requirements should be understood and shared at all levels of the organization. When the team is pulling in the same direction, self-management and empowerment take on value and meaning for all personnel.

Managing to sustain excellence in program management requires constant innovation that results in renewed and refreshing approaches. Just as innovative companies are especially adroit at continually responding to change of any sort in their environment, innovative child nutrition programs have strategies for responding to changes in the environment.[19]

Finally, Peters and Waterman concluded that successful companies get where they are because there is a strong leader in charge. Company cultures and shared values are inherent in successful companies. Even after the leadership torch has passed from a Thomas Watson or another such leader, the company cultures and shared values persist. Examples of child nutrition program excellence exist in every region—at the state, district, and school level, where precedents were set many years ago and continue even though the original leaders have long been gone. True leaders evoke leadership at all levels of the organization and promote excellence in every activity, whether that is clearing the tables or directing the nutrition education program. Excellence is self-perpetuating. It is a process and not a single event.

LEADERSHIP: A FUNCTION OF MANAGEMENT

Excellence in child nutrition programs requires leadership as an integral function of management.[20] Leadership is broader than management. Management of child nutrition programs includes planning, organizing, motivating or directing, and controlling. Warren Bennis[21] distinguishes between managing and leading. He defines managing as doing things right and leading as doing the right things (right). The director has a range of leadership behaviors available for managing the program. These behaviors range from being very controlling and autocratic to being able to release a high degree of control. In deciding how to lead, school food and nutrition professionals must be aware of forces that have an impact on their behavior. They must

- understand themselves, the individuals, and the group with whom they work
- the organization and the environment in which they work
- be able to assess the level of the staff and their readiness for being functioning members of a team or to be self-managers

Most directors and managers would like to have empowered personnel who are self-managers; however, in reality, not every director or every staff person is ready or comfortable with this style of management. Effective leaders are sensitive to the situation and know how and when to modify their style. If direction is in order, they direct; if the people are ready for considerable freedom, they provide such freedom. The director who prefers the more participative style of leadership will provide opportunities to (1) raise the level of employee motivation, (2) increase the readiness of staff to change, (3) improve the quality of managerial decisions, (4) enhance teamwork, and (5) develop new skills.[22]

There is hardly an activity in the school food and nutrition program director's day that does not involve one of the management functions, and there is hardly an activity that could not be looked at from the perspective of leading.

In identifying the need and initiating contact to work with special education and instructional services, Linda was fulfilling a leadership role. She is acting assertively or, using the word of Mescon and Mescon,[23] aggressively, to develop the program's potential for meeting children's needs. She is stepping out front to collaborate with other leaders in the school district.

A leader's unique role is to move the organization forward. Programs operate in a dynamic society; they cannot stand still. They move forward or fall back. Nanus[24] indicates that visionary leadership is essential for moving an organization forward. Visionary leadership begins with a vision of a desired future that acts as a signpost, pointing the way to help people understand the program and where it intends to go.

Nolan et al.[25] suggest that managers need to do more downboard thinking as chess players do. While concentrating on present moves, the manager must be thinking downboard to know how environmental factors will affect the program. They indicate that downboard thinking is necessary for developing a strategy for dealing with events in the environment and in managing and monitoring implementation of that strategy. A more comprehensive discussion of leadership is included in Chapter 5. A brief

---

Recipe for Successful Visionary Leadership

Ingredients	Method
• Vision • Communication • Shared purpose • Empowered people • Appropriate organizational change • Strategic thinking	1. Add communication to stated vision to achieve shared purpose. 2. To shared purpose, add empowered people, appropriate organizational change, and strategic thinking. 3. Blend to optimize the mixture.

Source: Adapted with permission from Burt Nanus, *Visionary Leadership*, p. 156, © 1992, Jossey-Bass Inc., Publishers.

LOOKING AT LINDA

Linda, the new food and nutrition program director of the Rock City School District, came on board April 1. The school district has 17 schools with on-site preparation. All schools participate in the National School Lunch Program (NSLP) and all schools have breakfast programs. Lunch participation in the district is 78 percent, with elementary schools serving 85 percent and secondary schools an average of 65 percent. The financial condition of the district is reasonably good. The district has an operating balance of three and one-half months. It is a suburban school district with only 28 percent free and reduced-price meals. Some of the schools are in dire need of new equipment.

The district has a new superintendent, who came from another state. The school district has a lot of site-based management. Principals in the district have much autonomy, and managers have dual reporting responsibility; for some tasks they report to the principal and for other tasks to the food and nutrition program director.

Linda observes that nutrition education in the school district has been included in lesson plans at the discretion of the classroom teacher. She has not observed any accommodation for children with disabilities in her school visits. When she asks about this, she gets the reply, "That's taken care of by special education," or about nutrition education, "The curriculum specialist for the district works with teachers on the curriculum." Linda makes a note to call the special education coordinator and the instructional specialist in the central office to make appointments by July 1 to explore ways of collaborating with the special education and instructional services to meet the needs of children with disabilities and integrate nutrition education into the instructional program. She also asks the administrative assistant to secure copies of the USDA Instruction on serving children with disabilities and copies of the Centers for Disease Control and Prevention (CDC) guidelines for involving the program in comprehensive health. She realizes the need to take her colleagues some resource material and to make these contacts prior to planning preschool in-service.

discussion of leadership as a management function is included in this chapter to emphasize the importance of leadership in moving the program forward.

UNIQUENESS OF CHILD NUTRITION PROGRAMS

Child nutrition programs are different from other institutional food services in a variety of ways. Understanding the uniqueness of child nutrition programs is necessary for the school food and nutrition professional to manage them effectively.

- Child nutrition programs serve a specific segment of the population, children up to the age of 21. The primary purpose for the program is to serve children who are in an educational or child care setting during a specific period of time. This affects program management because children, unlike adults, are in the process of forming food habits for their lifetime. Not only the food, but the way it is served will influence their food practices. Children are not little adults; they are learners. Everything that happens to them during the school day should provide a positive learning experience. Children have distinct physical, social, and emotional needs that managers should understand and consider in developing customer-focused programs.
- *All children in the school should have access to the school food and nutrition program.* Management systems have to be in place to ensure that programs are available and children have access. This involves assurance that children will be served without discrimination, that meal periods are adequate to provide time for children to eat and that space is available for seating; and, finally, that service in the cafeteria is organized for speed and effectiveness for them to select, receive, and eat food. As a general rule, the school food and nutrition professional is one of the few school leaders who has an opportunity to serve every child in school every day of the year. However, this cannot happen unless appropriate management systems are in place.
- *The program has a dual role of combining comprehensive nutrition service for children with food service management focusing on promoting a healthy population.* School nutrition is one of eight areas of a comprehensive school health program.[26] The school food and nutrition professional has an opportunity to develop and manage the program to have the cafeteria function as a laboratory for practicing healthy food behaviors. The school has children for an entire school year, or several years. This provides an opportunity for the practice of school food and nutrition professionals to have an impact on long-time food behaviors. Healthful foods, nutrition messages, and daily practice in selecting healthful meals positions the cafeteria as a learning laboratory. The school serves a community-based population, and opportunities are available to work with parents to ensure consistent messages and reinforcement of the lessons from the cafeteria. In many school districts, at least half the revenue for the program must come from sales of meals.

Although the program's primary goal is to make healthful meals available to all children, it is a nonprofit food service and must be cost effective. Sound business and management principles used in any cost-effective program are applicable in school food service. Spears reviews research related to a service profit chain model that shows that profit is linked with customer retention, which is a byproduct of customer satisfaction.[27] School food and nutrition professionals' primary focus is on serving all children healthful meals, and on meeting their responsibility for generating enough revenue to meet budget requirements.

- *The program framework is set by federal and state policy, and funding is a coopera-*

tive effort of federal, state, and local government. Unlike some other cooperatively financed programs that could be discontinued if funds were significantly reduced or eliminated, school attendance is required and children will always have need for food during the school day. Changes in the political or economic environment could diminish revenue for the program since a large portion is received from public funds that are subject to the annual appropriation or tax-levying process. Although permanent legislation and funding structures exist for most programs, this does not preclude changes being made in program standards or funding by Congress, state legislatures, and local school boards. School food and nutrition professionals cognizant of political and economic circumstances that have potential impact on programs strategically plan for program stability. Being politically savvy and assuming an advocate role is essential to building sustainable programs.

- *Part of the federal financial support is made available through government-donated commodities.* A basic purpose of school food and nutrition programs stated in Section 2 of the NSLA is to "encourage the domestic consumption of nutritious agricultural commodities."[28] This policy is translated into a requirement for schools to utilize donated foods to the extent possible, and it is further supported by an authorizing provision for funding a guaranteed level of commodities for distribution to schools. Government-donated commodities comprise approximately 20 percent of the food used in schools each year. With passage of the Healthy Meals for Americans Act, the quality of donated foods has been improved to the extent practicable, to be consistent with the Dietary Guidelines for Americans. Donated commodities for schools are not viewed as "nice to have" but as an integral financial resource that makes it possible to operate

financially effective programs. While legislation provides assurance of the value of commodities to be received during any one year, there is no assurance of the specific items to be received, or the time of delivery. Menu planning and procurement systems must have sufficient flexibility to use the foods effectively when delivered. Effective use of commodities is necessary in school food and nutrition programs. School food and nutrition programs are recognized by the agricultural community as a major market for food. Commodities are closely tied to funding provisions and political support for child nutrition programs.

- *Managing child nutrition programs provides an opportunity and challenge for school food and nutrition professionals to combine their talents of food service manager, community nutritionist with focus on children, and nutrition educator.* Very few positions in the field of nutrition and food service management require this combination of talent to the same degree as school food and nutrition programs. As previously noted, the program provides an opportunity for the professional to become an educator and advocate in support of children's needs while pursuing the challenge of managing a large-scale business. The same management skills are needed to manage the operational areas of the system, manage the nutrition and nutrition education services, marketing, and communication parts of the system. The school food and nutrition program provides an exciting career option to the person with strong management skills and a special commitment to children.

- *The child nutrition program is the only part of comprehensive health that is expected to be self-supporting.* This creates a challenge for school food and nutrition professionals to be creative and innovative in managing the food service to parallel customers' wants with their nutritional needs. Communicating with and understanding students and their needs is a prerequisite to effective program management. The program must respond to their emotional and social needs as well as to their physical needs for food. School food and nutrition professionals recognize that customer satisfaction drives customer retention, which drives program financial effectiveness. To achieve a program that is self-supporting, they operate programs to achieve efficiency and effectiveness.[29]

- *Strategies for implementing nutrition objectives often face competition within the school for time, money, and space.* Although most institutional food service operations face competition for customers, there is at least one issue that makes it unique in school food and nutrition programs. The school food and nutrition program has a twofold purpose, to provide healthful meals that contribute to the health and well-being of children and to help them develop healthy food behaviors. School food and nutrition programs exist in schools to help achieve educational objectives. If children are not participating in the program, its purpose cannot be achieved. Just as the classroom teacher needs the child on task to achieve classroom objectives, school food and nutrition professionals need students eating healthful meals to achieve nutrition objectives. Participation is higher when there is less competition for money, appetite, and time. Students value lunchtime for socializing. If the time or seating space in the cafeteria infringes on this need, they may choose another option for using the time. Another forceful competitor is the student's money. If other foods are available, at the school store or as a school activity fund-raising project, the customer may choose those for multiple reasons, including time, money, space, and the need to socialize.

MULTIFACETED PURPOSE OF SCHOOL FOOD AND NUTRITION PROGRAMS

The school food and nutrition program has the potential of serving at least five major purposes in the school community.

Nutrition Service To Meet School Day Nutrition Needs of All Children

The primary purpose of the school food and nutrition program is to meet the nutrition needs of all children during the time they are under the supervision of the school or child-care facility. Programs available to help achieve this goal include school breakfast, school lunch, and after-school snacks, meals for children in day-care homes and child-care centers; and the Summer Food Service Program. To achieve this primary goal requires an understanding of the interrelatedness of every part of the food service system, beginning with menu planning and ending with service of meals to children. The author of Chapter 4 provides a comprehensive discussion of the meaning of nutrition integrity in school food and nutrition programs and the authors of Chapters 11 and 12 describe ways of meeting nutrition needs of preschool children with disabilities and other preschoolers.

Integral Component of the Comprehensive Health Program

Second, school nutrition is identified as one of the eight components of the Comprehensive School Health Program. The school food and nutrition program is the laboratory for students to practice nutrition lessons learned in the classroom. It provides an opportunity for them to practice positive eating behaviors and reinforces classroom nutrition messages and positive practices learned in the home. Children's food habits are shaped by a variety of influences, and the school cannot be held solely responsible.[30] Simply learning classroom lessons alone is probably not enough to affect changes in their eating behaviors and neither is just offering nutritious meals. It takes the school, home, and community working together to ensure positive food behaviors. The school food and nutrition program serves as a resource to the classroom in a variety of ways by giving demonstrations, planning tasting parties, providing information, and arranging field trips. There is evidence that dietary behaviors tend to stay constant over time, and poor eating habits established in childhood tend to persist through adulthood.

Nutrition education should be developmental and sequential, beginning in early childhood so that students develop healthy dietary habits and an understanding of the influence of nutrition on health.[31] As a component of the comprehensive health program, the goal of the school food and nutrition program is to maximize each child's education and health potential for a lifetime.[32] Contemporary studies[33] relating to the development of healthy food habits recognizes the role of the school nutrition program as a component of a health promotion and prevention model.

Traditionally knowledge-based studies did not take into account the multiple factors involved in developing healthy eating behaviors. While those studies reported increased knowledge about food and nutrition, there was no evidence of behavior change. More recently nutrition education programs and studies are incorporating the multicomponent prevention model, beginning in elementary school and extending to high school and use the school nutrition program as a part of the model to promote the intake of a varied diet within the context of the Dietary Guidelines for Americans. From these studies it appears that eating habits are influenced by the interaction between students and their social and physical environment, not simply by knowledge of the healthfulness of food. This recognition of an important role for the school food and nutrition program opens doors for the school food and nutrition director to further develop the program as a laboratory for health promotion

and prevention programs. Ways to develop the program as an integral component of school health are discussed in Chapter 9.

Resource for the Instructional Program

Third, the school food and nutrition program is a resource to the instructional program. Through a multidisciplinary approach, the program can be used as a resource not only in health, but in social studies, language arts, mathematics, computer technology, and the sciences. In an Oregon school, the business mathematics class was given major managerial responsibility for the program. School food and nutrition programs offer opportunities for meaningful experiences in many areas of the curriculum. School food and nutrition is unique in that its purpose is primarily to provide nutritious meals that customers enjoy. The school meal experience should be structured as a laboratory where students learn to enjoy a variety of healthful foods and learn the relationship of food to achieving their personal goals.

The nutrition education function should be an integral part of the job description and workday for the manager and director. Developing a strategy to make this happen may require changes in management practices and staffing schedules. One food and nutrition program director has solved the problem by counting only four of the manager's eight hours when calculating meals per labor hour. This allows the manager four hours each day for nutrition education, marketing activities, community relations, and bookkeeping.

Nutrition Center for the School Community

Fourth, the school food and nutrition program is a nutrition center for the school community. Federal food assistance programs provide a continuum of nutrition services, beginning with the Supplemental Program for Women, Infants, and Children (WIC) program and ending with a Nutrition Program for the Elderly. The school has an opportunity to be a coordinating link for all these programs as many recipients are directly linked with the school. By supporting and providing a consistent nutrition message for program recipients, the school could have a major influence on community health. Simplifying social services within a community would benefit recipients and reduce administrative costs for the community. One function of the school food and nutrition program identified by Marx and colleagues[2] was screening, assessment, counseling, and referral for nutrition problems. Achieving this important step in the nutritional health of children will require coordinated efforts of social services, public health, and education. Building alliances with the community is described in Chapter 22.

Nonprofit Business Operated for the Benefit of the School District

Fifth, the school food and nutrition program is a nonprofit business operated for the benefit of the educational enterprise. As far back as the 1920s, school lunch pioneers recognized a need for the school food and nutrition professionals to have expertise and commitment to nutrition, to have social vision, and also to be competent in the area of business management.[34] Key achievement four from the *Keys to Excellence* identifies standards for financial management[35] and functional area three of the directors' competencies identifies competencies needed by directors to achieve effective business management.[36] As previously noted, even in the small school district the school food and nutrition program may be one of the largest businesses in the community and may be one of the largest employers in the school district. Its purpose is to serve the educational enterprise. It not only meets school day nutrition needs of students, it serves other purposes for the school by

- allowing for a more efficient school day, enabling customized meal breaks and a shorter school day

- serving as a motivator for getting children to school on time and in some instances for keeping children in school
- providing energy needed for students to learn and supporting improved classroom performance including test scores
- giving time for students and teachers to have space and social opportunities
- involving the community in the school

Although the school food and nutrition program exists to meet an educational purpose, it must also be cost effective. This requires the use of sound financial and business practices just as if it were a profit-making food service. The profit in school food is better meals for the customer. Any excess revenues over expenses should be used for program improvements and renewals. As a tax-supported enterprise, the community looks to the school food and nutrition program to operate both efficiently and effectively. The authors of Chapter 7 describe ways of making the program financially sound and accountable.

PERSPECTIVES ON MANAGING CHILD NUTRITION PROGRAMS

Managing child nutrition programs begins with a clearly identified vision and set of objectives. Programs should be managed to ensure

- accessibility to all children
- acceptability of appealing meals to customers
- accountability (nutritional and financial)

The program is not unique in needing to be managed. All organizations need managing, regardless of their size or purpose. It's a way of making sure that all the important things get done.[37] (An organization is defined as a group of people working together in a structured and coordinated way to accomplish goals.[38])

The child nutrition program is unique among educational and food service systems. It is multifaceted, and management could be viewed from the perspective of any one of its multiple functions. However, to accomplish the program's basic purpose of being a catalyst for "safeguarding the health and well-being of the nation's children," it must be managed to accomplish all of its multiple facets. To achieve its goals within the educational system, the child nutrition program is a food delivery system, a curriculum laboratory, a not-for-profit business, an integral part of a community network for healthy people, an advocate for healthful meals and nutrition education for all children, and an adult education center.

Understanding management and organization is prerequisite to an effective operation. Just about everybody agrees on what management is, but many stop short when it comes to knowing how to manage. They agree that management is *a set of functions* (planning, organizing, directing or motivating, leading and controlling) directed at an organization's resources (people, funds, food and supplies, facilities and time) for achieving goals effectively and efficiently.[39] And they agree that it is *a process* whereby these unrelated resources are used to accomplish program objectives. The director is aware that forces both inside and outside the system are constantly affecting the program. The question faced by the school food and nutrition program director is "How can I manage this multifaceted program to accomplish the objectives?"

A SYSTEMS APPROACH TO MANAGING CHILD NUTRITION PROGRAMS

A systems approach to managing the multifaceted child nutrition program supports both effectiveness and efficiency. Child nutrition programs may be viewed best as a system of mutually dependent variables. Questions to be answered in looking at it as a system include the following:

- What are the strategic parts of the system?
- What is the nature of their interrelatedness and mutual dependency?

- What are the main processes in the system that link the parts together and facilitate their working together?
- What are the outcomes desired of the system as a whole and of each of its parts?[40]

A major goal of this chapter is to provide a conceptual framework for managing child nutrition programs at the state or district level using a systems approach. A conceptual framework provides a structure for organizing the program, a way of looking at the program holistically, and a process for managing to see that all parts of the program are functioning and synchronized.[41,42] A systems approach provides a pattern of thinking, a process for analyzing issues, and making decisions, and finally, a management style. The framework identifies the parts or subsystems, how they function independently and how they interact.

A systems approach has three characteristics.

1. It is an interrelated set of interacting components. Every system has a purpose and each of its parts should contribute to that purpose.
2. Every system is part of a still larger system. The school food and nutrition system is part of the educational system.
3. Systems are complex, and a change in one variable will affect change in others.[43]

Using a systems approach in managing child nutrition programs helps the director see all the critical variables, their constraints, and their reactions on each other. A systems approach provides a framework for keeping the many facets of the program operating synergistically. The five basic concepts of Luchsinger and Dock[44] further clarify the systems approach.

1. Systems are designed to accomplish objectives.
2. The parts or subsystems have an established arrangement.
3. Interrelationships exist among the subsystems or parts.

4. The flow of resources through the system is important.
5. The organization's objectives are more important than the subsystems.

A systems approach to managing child nutrition programs is shown in Figure 1–2. Program objectives drive the systems approach and are shown in the center of the model. A system has three distinct parts—input (of resources), transformation, and output.[45] The parts of a system are as stated.

- Input of resources required for administering and implementing the program.
- Transformation includes processing or turning resources into products, services, or information. Three processes are involved in transforming resources into outcomes. These are administration and implementation, management functions, and linking processes.
- Outcomes identify the results desired of the system.

In addition to these three parts, the system consists of controls, feedback, and forces in the external environment. Controls and evaluation are included in this model as a part of administrative processes. Management functions (planning, organizing, directing/motivating, leading, and controlling) and linking processes (communications, decision making, and balance) drive resource use and determine how the program will be administered and implemented. Social, political, and economic forces both inside and outside the school system have an impact on program management and outcomes.

Input

Input of resources includes all resources required to produce desired output and meet program objectives. Resources are fiscal (all funds from federal, state, and local sources), facilities and equipment, people (labor and skill), food and supplies (purchased and USDA–donated foods), and time.

Transformation

Transformation, the second part of the systems approach, includes administration and implementation processes, managerial functions, and linking processes. Managerial functions and linking processes are used to perform administrative and implementation processes simultaneously, and to some extent independently.

Administration and Implementation. Administrative processes include the following, which occur in the central office in most school districts.

- *Planning and evaluation:* Assessment, strategic planning, setting objectives, developing standing and single-use plans
- *Environmental scans*: Systematic scans of[46]:
  1. macroenvironment (technology, social, economic, and political factors)
  2. the industry environment (food production, processing, packaging, marketing)
  3. the competitive environment (competitor profiles, market segmentation patterns, research and development trends, and potential new competitors)
  4. customer environment, including listening to feedback from the community
  5. education environment (trends and issues in administration and instruction, policies and funding)
- *Rules, policies, and regulations*: The basis for setting standards and monitoring performance. Include policies, procedures, standards, guidelines and schedules that are consistent with mission, vision, and objectives. Monitored controls are essential for quality programs
- *Financial management*: Budgeting, accounting, records, reports
- *Technology*: Applications related to menu planning and food systems management, point of service, procurement and inventory control, human resources, free and reduced-price meal policy, sanitation and safety

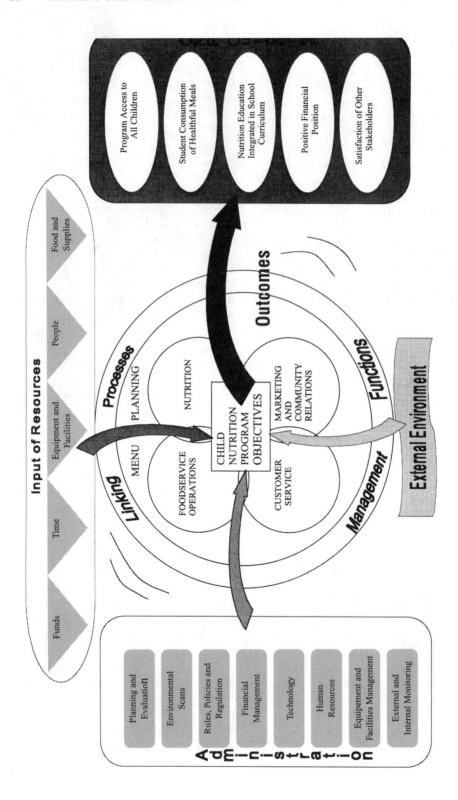

Figure 1–2 A Systems Approach to Managing Child Nutrition Programs

- *Equipment and facilities management*: Design and layout, maintenance, purchase; sanitation and safety
- *Human resources*: Setting and implementing standards and controls; all activities related to recruitment, retention, training, monitoring, mentoring, and coaching personnel
- *Procurement*: Purchasing system, distribution, specifications, descriptions, selection, distribution and coordination
- *External and internal monitoring*: Audits, management reviews, program assessments, coordinated review effort (CRE), accreditation.
- *Facilitating*: Assisting employees to help maximize their skills

Implementation, shown in the circle of the model, includes all activities that occur at the school (site of preparation and service to customers). This may be referred to as the technical and educational core of the program. The four parts, or subsystems of the implementation process, are shown in the circle (see Figure 1–2). These parts, which function as separate subsystems, use resources to carry out activities necessary to meet program goals. Although the subsystems function somewhat independently in carrying out their purpose, they are interactive and interrelated. The menu has an impact on all the subsystems. It is the most critical point of control in the implementation process. The menu is the basis for quality, productivity, cost control, customer acceptability, and nutrition integrity. It also initiates the food manufacturing cycle of procurement, preparation, sanitation, and service systems. Subsystems of the implementation process include the following:

- *Food service operations:*
  1. Purchasing or requisitioning food and supplies, including receipt of food and inventory control, preparation, sanitation and safety, and distribution and service
  2. Implementing program requirements related to all aspects of free and reduced-price meal policies including eligibility and accountability.
  3. Supervising implementation of operational processes
  4. Coordinating operational processes with central office
  5. Performing food cost analyses, forecasting and modifying menus
- *Nutrition services, including nutrition education*: Managing the menu including planning, analysis, preparation and services, coordinating food service activities with the comprehensive school health program, collaborating with instructional staff to achieve multidisciplinary nutrition education, assessing program needs, ensuring nutrition integrity and customer satisfaction, and providing nutrition and program information to students
- *Customer service*: Implementing free and reduced-price meal policy, meeting needs of children with disabilities or special needs and working with special education to have needs identified; conducting customer satisfaction surveys and focus groups involving students, parents, and teachers; working with student advisory groups; nurturing positive relations with parents and teachers; systematic communication with school administrators; maintaining an empowered school food and nutrition team; building positive student-staff relationships
- *Marketing and community relations*: Developing and implementing a plan to market the program to students, parents, decision makers and the community; developing program advocacy through a child nutrition alliance; building partnerships to support a continuum of nutrition services within the school community; being an advocate for school nutrition as an integral part of the comprehensive health program

Management Functions. Management functions include planning, organizing, directing/motivating, and leading and controlling. These tasks are to be performed for each activity and may be used as a "to do" list when initiating a new task. The management tasks perform a framework for school food and nutrition professionals to use when working independently or as a team leader.

School food and nutrition professionals who practice a participative management style will use a team approach to carry out the management functions. By working with and through the team, objectives are determined, standards or expectations are set, and responsibility is accepted. The director supports the team by seeing that resources are provided and giving technical support and feedback to support the team manager. Standards and program requirements are understood and used by the project manager to evaluate and control outcomes. For example, the training team plans a systemwide training activity, organizes the plan, secures resources (including instructor/facilities), communicates with personnel, provides leadership in conducting training, and follows up to see that training skills were developed and are being implemented.

Linking Processes. Linking processes include decision making, communication, and balance. They are used to determine and connect management functions and resources to achieve program objectives.

- Decision making requires choosing a course of action from two or more alternatives. This suggests that school food and nutrition professionals have skills necessary to make appropriate choices. Some decisions may be made independently and some with a group process. The use of an appropriate technique, whether involving the group or making an independent decision, is essential to choosing the best alternative. New management theories support decisions being made at the lowest possible level in the organization. Shared decision making is

conducive to self-management and empowerment. Spears indicates that decision making is sometimes referred to as the essence of management because practically every action the director takes involves a decision.[47]

- Communication may be the director's most important skill. Effective management is dependent on working with and through people. Communication links the school food and nutrition program with the school, community, decision makers, and public in general. Decision making and communication connect the management functions.

- Balance refers to the ability of the director to maintain organizational stability. School food and nutrition professionals know how to maintain stability amid a lot of anxiety. Balance simply means recognizing and dealing with realities. During the early 1980s there was considerable discussion of eliminating federal assistance for paying children. In many instances, schools developed alternative meal systems without regard to nutrition objectives and in some instances schools actually dropped the NSLP. The decision to drop the program may have been made out of fear of losing federal support. However, the Congress did not eliminate funds for paying children. Balance means that alternatives are considered consistent with program objectives even in times of stress. Another simple example is maintaining balance between offering only foods that children request, such as french fries and burgers, and meeting program standards for serving foods with less fat.

Outcomes

Five outcomes of an effective and efficient child nutrition program are as follows.

1. Program access to all children. Meals are available and accessible to children. At least four areas are included in acces-

sibility.[48] The four areas include the following:

- *Setting:* Nutritionally adequate meals are available to all children during the school day. Participation in the National School Lunch Program, the breakfast program and the after-school snack program allows schools to offer healthful meals and food choices to all children regardless of their families' socioeconomic level. Federal reimbursement and effective management make it possible for meal prices to be within reach of the majority of children who do not qualify for free or reduced-price meals. The school participates in the programs offered under the NSLA of 1946 and The Child Nutrition Act of 1966.The school or child-care facility offers breakfast, lunch, and after-school snacks. The cafeteria environment supports healthy meal habits.
- *Resources:* Access means that children have adequate resources to buy the meal or qualify for a free or reduced-price meal or snack. There is no overt discrimination of children who qualify for free or reduced-meals either in the application process or at the point of service. Adequate seating space is available to accommodate all children served at a specific meal period either in the main dining area or another site on the school campus.
- *Time:* Meal periods are scheduled, and service is managed to allow children adequate time for eating after being served.
- *Quality:* Quality issues include nutritive value, appearance and other sensory factors, student-staff relations, and sanitation and safety. Quality food is not distinguishable from quality service in the mind of the customer.

2. Consumption of healthful meals. If the customers consume healthful meals, that is evidence of satisfaction and practice of healthy food behaviors. The ultimate outcome would be that children incorporate similar behavior in their food practice in other settings and in their adult lives.

3. Nutrition education and services integrated into the curriculum. Sequential and multidisciplinary nutrition education coordinated with comprehensive school health and use of the cafeteria as a learning laboratory provide evidence of a program that is an integral part of education. The ultimate outcome would be that children understand the contribution of food and nutrition to a healthy life-style and practice healthy food behaviors.

4. Positive financial position. An organization that achieves program objectives, is effectively managed, and uses sound financial and accounting practices in all subsystems also achieves a positive financial position consistent with the policies of the organization. The ultimate outcome would be financial integrity reflecting stewardship of public monies.

5. Satisfaction of other stakeholders. Support for child nutrition program policies, budgets, facilities, and personnel is evidence of stakeholder satisfaction. Empowered and self-managed school food and nutrition professionals and instructional personnel collaborating with the school food and nutrition team reflect satisfaction of internal stakeholders. The ultimate outcome would be that child nutrition programs would be an integral part of the educational program and available to all children as an educational benefit. The school food and nutrition program may be the most underused instructional laboratory in the entire school setting. An understanding

of its potential should be a challenge to future leaders to manage it as a nutrition education program and operate it as a business.

Managing the System for Excellence

Earlier in the chapter management was defined in two ways: working with and through people and managing processes. The conceptual framework identifies the processes to be managed and shows interrelationships of parts of the system. A schematic does not show human interrelationships. Leadership for excellence requires positive interpersonal skills in working with the team and understanding the limits of formal authority. School food and nutrition professionals desiring an empowered, self-managed team recognize the value of being accepted as part of the team. This acceptance authority is powerful in achieving long-term success. Program success reflects a committed school food and nutrition team and a "boss" who understands and supports the program. Understanding the need for a shared vision and shared ownership will influence the leadership style chosen by the school food and nutrition professional in managing the system for excellence.

> The standard of quality is now so high that unless you have an empowered work force and a spirit of partnership with all stakeholders, you can't compete, whether you work in the private sector, public sector, or social sector.[49]

An important part of the management process that is sometimes overlooked is the need to manage the environment in which the team works. This means managing relationships of the school food and nutrition team with other groups inside and outside the school system. It also indicates that the director should be scanning the environment to make sure that objectives are appropriate, clearly understood by the team, and support a high-productivity workplace.[50]

SUMMARY

Long-term success implies a quest for excellence in child nutrition programs and the need for visionary leadership. The leader for tomorrow will share a vision of what the program should be—to achieve the goal of providing all children access to healthful meals and foods and opportunities for developing healthy food behaviors. That visionary leader will also have the ability to manage the program to achieve nutrition goals and operate it as a business enterprise. School food and nutrition leaders of today are building that future. Today's actions influence tomorrow's success.

The future is uncertain. However, there are several things we know for sure. We know that children will need to have their nutritional needs met wherever they are under the care of the school or child-care facility; we know that change is certain; and we know that programs will operate in an even more competitive environment. Managing within this environment requires competent leaders with vision. When Wayne Gretsky, hockey star, was asked for the key to his success, he replied that he always skated to where he thought the puck would be. That's vision. Directors must lead to their vision, and be willing to change everything about the program except its basic beliefs. That is managing for long-term success.

> To begin with the end in mind means to start with a clear understanding of your destination. It means to know where you're going so that you better understand where you are now and so that the steps you take are always in the right direction.
> *Source:* Stephen Covey, *The Seven Habits of Highly Effective People.*[51(p98)]

Managing for long-term success in child nutrition programs begins with the end in mind and builds programs toward that end. The attributes of excellence identified by Mescon and Mescon[52] should influence the director's philosophy and style of management. Leadership propels programs forward, and this means that the director is willing to take risks to keep the program relevant for the customers to be served. This requires continuous reinvention of the program. The eight characteristics adapted from those identified by Peters and Waterman[53] are useful concepts to keep in mind in managing for long-term success.

Finally, long-term success is dependent on the school food and nutrition professionals having a conceptual framework and using a systems approach for managing the program. The ability to see all the parts and their interrelationships and identify resources needed as they relate to program outcomes, will be a guide for managing to ensure long-term success. Within this one chapter, it was possible to include only a small amount of information needed for using a systems approach to managing. For additional information on management, including emerging management practices, use the references listed at the end of this chapter, read professional journals, and use the vast resources of the Internet, NFSMI, and the Food and Nutrition Information Center at the National Agricultural Library.

This chapter has described the complexity of the multifaceted child nutrition program and suggested a conceptual framework for managing the program. Uniqueness of the child nutrition program presents insights into needs to be considered for long-term success. The conceptual framework provides school food and nutrition professionals at the state or district level, graduate students, potential directors, and school administrators a holistic view of the management and leadership needs of the program. Beginning with the end in mind is the key to leadership for excellence.

We are what we repeatedly do. Excellence, then, is not an act, but a habit.

—Aristotle
Nichomachean Ethics, 350 B.C.

REFERENCES

1. T. Watson, *A Business and Its Beliefs* (New York: McGraw-Hill, 1963), 280.
2. E. Marx et al., eds., *Health Is Academic* (New York: Teachers College Press, 1998), 195–197.
3. U.S. Dept. of Agriculture, *Program Information Data*, Food and Nutrition Service (Arlington, VA: USDA, March 1998).
4. W. Burkan, "Developing Your Wide-Angle Vision," *The Futurist* 32, (March 1998):35–38.
5. P. Pritchett, *Culture Shift* (Dallas, TX: Pritchett Publishing Co., 1993).
6. M. Michalko, "Thinking Like a Genius," *The Futurist* 32, no. 4 (1998):21–25.
7. J. Gardner, *Excellence*. (New York: Harper & Row, 1961), 159–160.
8. T. Mescon and M. Mescon, "The Evolution of Excellence," *Sky Magazine*, July 1983, 74–80.
9. G. Hamel and CK Prahalad, *Competing for the Future* (Boston: Harvard Business School Press, 1994), 17–18.
10. Mescon and Mescon, "Evolution of Excellence," 74–80.
11. Public Law 103-448, Healthy Meals for Americans Act, Section 18 (1994).
12. Public Law 103-227, Educate America Act (1994).
13. Gardner, *Excellence*, 131.
14. American School Food Service Association, *Keys to Excellence: Standards of Practice for Nutrition Integrity* (Alexandria, VA: 1995).
15. D. Carr et al., eds., *Competencies, Knowledge and Skills of Effective District School Nutrition Directors/Supervisors* (University, MS: National Food Service Management Institute [NFSMI], 1996).
16. NFSMI, *Competencies, Knowledge, and Skills Required of Effective School Nutrition Managers* (University, MS: 1995).
17. T. Peters and R. Waterman Jr., *In Search of Excellence: Lessons from America's Best Run Companies* (New York: Harper & Row, 1982).
18. J. Biolos, "Why Focus Is Vital . . . and How To Achieve It, *Harvard Business Review Newsletter*, July 1997. Hbsp.harvard.edu/frames/groups/newsletters/jul97.
19. Peters and Waterman, *In Search of Excellence*, 12.
20. M. Spears, *Foodservice Organizations: A Managerial and Systems Approach*, 3rd ed. (Englewood Cliffs, NJ: Prentice Hall, 1995), 43.

21. W. Bennis, *On Becoming a Leader* (Reading, MA: Addison-Wesley Publishing Co., 1989).

22. R. Tannenbaum and W. Schmidt, "How To Choose a Leadership Pattern," *Harvard Business Review: Business Classics* (1991): 115–124.

23. Mescon and Mescon, "Evolution of Excellence," 74–80.

24. B. Nanus, *Visionary Leadership* (San Francisco: Jossey-Bass, 1992), 9.

25. T. Nolan et al., *Plan or Die! 10 Keys to Organizational Success* (San Diego, CA: Pfeiffer & Co, 1993), 51.

26. Centers for Disease Control and Prevention, Guidelines for School Health Programs To Promote Lifelong Healthy Eating," *Morbidity and Mortality Weekly Report* 45, no. RR-9 (1996): 1–41.

27. Spears, *Foodservice Organizations,* 514.

28. Public Law 79-396. The National School Lunch Act, Stat 281, Section 2 (1946).

29. Spears, *Foodservice Organizations,* 59.

30. Marx et al., *Health Is Academic,* 197.

31. E. Martin, *Nutrition Education in Action* (New York: Holt, Rinehart and Winston, 1963), 72.

32. Institute of Medicine. *Schools and Health. Our Nation's Investment* (Washington, DC: National Academy Press, 1997).

33. American Dietetic Association, "Position of the ADA: Dietary guidance for healthy children ages 2 to 11 years," *Journal of the American Dietetic Association* 99, no. 1 (1999): 93–101.

34. E. Smedley, *The School Lunch,* (Philadelphia: Emma Smedley, 1930): 191.

35. ASFSA, *Keys to Excellence,* 4–5.

36. Carr et al., *Competencies,* 63.

37. R.E. Allen, *Winnie-the-Pooh on Management.* (New York: Dutton, 1994): 2–4.

38. P. Schoderbek, *Management Systems,* 2nd ed. (New York: John Wiley & Sons, 1971): 59.

39. Spears, *Foodservice Organizations,* 59.

40. H. Koontz and C. O'Donnell, *Principles of Management: An Analysis of Managerial Functions (*New York: McGraw-Hill, 1972): 12–14, 44.

41. Spears, *Food Service Organizations,* 53.

42. Schoderbek, *Management Systems,* 322.

43. Koontz and O'Donnell, *Principles of Management,* 44.

44. V. Luchsinger and B. Dock, *The Systems Approach: A Primer* (Dubuque, IA: Kendall and Hunt, 1976).

45. Schoderbek, *Management Systems,* 325.

46. J.W. Pfeiffer et al., *Shaping Strategic Planning* (San Diego, CA: Scott, Foresman & Co., 1990), 135–140.

47. Spears, *Foodservice Organizations,* 585.

48. J. Martin, "Child Nutrition and the World Food Summit," *CNI Nutrition Week* 26, no. 46. (1996): 5.

49. S. Covey. Three Roles of the Leader in the New Paradigm. In *The Leaders of the Future,* edited by F. Hesselbein, M. Goldsmith, and R. Beckhard. The Drucker Foundation. (San Francisco: Jossey-Bass, 1996), 156.

50. Harvard Newsletter. *What You Must Learn to Become a Manager: An Interview with Linda Hill.* Http://www.hbsp.harvard.edu. 1998: 1

51. S. Covey, *The Seven Habits of Highly Effective People* (New York: Simon & Schuster, 1989).

52. Mescon and Mescon, "Evolution of Excellence," 74–80.

53. Peters and Waterman, *In Search of Excellence.*

CHAPTER 2

History of Child Nutrition Programs

Josephine Martin

Those who cannot remember the past are doomed to repeat it.

—Santayana

OUTLINE

- Introduction: A Historical Perspective
- The Formative Years: Before 1944
  - The Twentieth Century
  - The 1930s
- The Benchmark Years: 1945–1960
  - The National School Lunch Act of 1946
- Challenges and New Directions: The 1960s
  - The Child Nutrition Act of 1966
- Triumphs and Trials: The 1970s
- Trials and Triumphs: The 1980s
- On Track for the Future: The 1990s
- Summary

INTRODUCTION: A HISTORICAL PERSPECTIVE

What is child nutrition and how has it become what it is today? More importantly, where is it going? To answer these questions requires a look into the past—a look at the social and economic conditions that influenced the development of the program, at the leaders who had the wisdom to commit to writing a vision of the future, at practitioners who practiced what they preached, at those who began with the end in mind, at movers and shakers who were not afraid to risk being wrong for the sake of their beliefs, at the important role of partnerships. A look at the past is an organizational scan to identify who we are and where we have come from; only then can we determine where the child nutrition programs may be headed.

The purpose of this chapter is to look at the past as a means of understanding the present and shaping the future. As this chapter unfolds, you will see how policy and legislation are made and the importance of school food and nutrition leaders accepting responsibility for helping to shape program direction. This is achieved by being active at the federal, state, and local level in activities that lead to positive policies. Although this chapter deals primarily with national policy and legislation, the principles for understanding and influencing policy are similar at all levels of government.

Albrecht[1] describes this process of looking at the past as historicizing, or developing an understanding of how the enterprise became what it is today.

For school food and nutrition leaders responsible for managing child nutrition programs and providing leadership for excellence, an understanding of how the child nutrition program became what it is today will provide a common starting point in shaping the future. Looking at the past will help to build a common frame of reference and a shared sense of the history of child nutrition. It will help students and professionals who are new to the field of child nutrition management under-

> *"Historicizing . . . a process of examining the history of a business enterprise to establish a perspective for considering its possibilities for success in the future."*
>
> Reprinted from THE NORTHBOUND TRAIN. Copyright © 1994 Karl Albrecht. Reprinted by permission of AMACOM, a division of American Management Association International, New York, NY. All rights reserved. http://www.amanet.org.

stand the relationship of social and economic events to how the programs developed. More importantly, it will provide the reader a pattern of looking at the environment as a means of understanding the past, managing the present, and shaping the future.

As child nutrition leaders you will be shaping the future. You will be asking such questions as,

- How did the program develop from a welfare program in the 1930s to an educational program for all children?
- How were the program standards established?
- Why did Congress specify that all meals would meet nutrition standards?
- Why did the National School Lunch Act (NSLA) emerge from the Senate Agriculture Committee and not from an education committee?
- Why are donated foods an integral part of the program funding?
- Why can't it be an all-cash program?
- Why didn't the Congress include nutrition education and training in the original bill?
- How did the program grow from just school lunch to all-day, all-year food service programs?
- What is the relationship between child nutrition programs and all other food assistance programs?
- What is my responsibility for helping to shape the future? These and many others

are questions will come to mind as you establish your vision and your plans for the future. We look at the past to get direction for the future. A study of the past helps to identify persistent issues that can lead to strategies for success in achieving program improvements.

Of one thing the child nutrition leader can be sure—change. As we review program development, note changes, and face issues, it is worth remembering that society changed much faster in the last decade of the twentieth century than in the first 90 years, and that information is proliferating at an incomprehensible pace. Futurists tell us we can expect the pace of change to be even more accelerated in the future. Recognizing the speed of change, the school food and nutrition professional is aware that programs of the future must be different and must look different, because the customers will be different and programs must be managed differently. While change in the way of doing things is inevitable and essential, it is equally important that the philosophy underpinning these programs be the foundation upon which changes are made. Tom Watson,[2] former president of IBM, stated that he believed that if an organization is to meet the challenge of a changing world, it must be prepared to change everything about itself except those basic beliefs as it moves through corporate life. In this chapter and in the book much emphasis is given to values and beliefs related to program management. If you accept the Watson premise, then you must safeguard the basic beliefs that form the programs' foundation by building an organizational structure that preserves those beliefs, and yet reflects a contemporary approach to managing and operating a customer-driven child nutrition program.

Thelma Flanagan[3] observed that any study of school lunch history, as revealed in publications from 1904 until 1972, shows that most early program philosophies, concepts, and goals were sound, and most leaders were professionally trained and dedicated. Flanagan also noted that many things that are considered innovative today were advocated and practiced even before federal and state governments became involved in the program. As the reader looks through the history of child nutrition programs and reflects on the triumphs and trials, it will become clear that great progress has been made. The child nutrition leaders have always faced challenges and have made progress in spite of problems such as political pressures, state laws, meal schedules, competitive foods, personnel, or finance.

This chapter is about the past, but it is also about the future. Examining history helps uncover when and how the program foundation was laid. It is about public policy and how policy is made. The child nutrition program is at the center of public policy. Children do not vote and need advocates for public policy that support their needs. An understanding of how actions in one area result in consequences in another will help understand the public policy process. As the history unfolds, it will be quite a revelation to some to learn that pioneers advocated for the comprehensive program that has emerged through the twentieth century.

The objectives of the chapter are to

- describe the development of child nutrition programs in the twentieth century
- discuss the impact of social, political, and economic forces in the environment on program development
- describe the basic beliefs and philosophical and conceptual bases that have shaped child nutrition programs
- challenge the school food and nutrition professional to take ownership of the traditions and philosophies that provide the program foundation

> Examining history helps uncover root principles, cause-and-effect relationships, and insight into dynamics, trajectories, and consequences. It is easy and dangerous to ignore history or casually revise it. . . .
>
> *Source:* Rosabeth Moss Kanter, *The Futurist*, August–September 1998, p 43.

THE FORMATIVE YEARS: BEFORE 1944

School feeding is not a twentieth century invention. It's at least 200 years old. According to Flanagan,[3] school feeding started in Munich in 1790 when Count Rumford established a soup kitchen for unemployed workmen and invited hungry schoolchildren to eat. The French opened canteens in 1849, and Victor Hugo started school feeding in England in 1865 by serving meals in his house to children attending a nearby school. And in America, the Children's Aid Society of New York City initiated the first school feeding program in 1853. This organization started vocational schools for the poor and served free meals to the children who attended. In Philadelphia, the Starr Center Association provided penny lunches in several schools in poor districts of Philadelphia in 1894. As the history of school food and nutrition programs is reviewed, the reader will note the leadership role of the Philadelphia city schools in child nutrition throughout the twentieth century.

The real beginning of school feeding in America began in Boston in 1894. Under the leadership of Ellen H. Richards, the Boston School Committee approved a resolution "that only such food as was approved by them should be sold in the city school houses." While the concept of satellite schools may be thought of as a development of the twentieth century, Mrs. Richards prepared foods in the New England Central Kitchen and transported them in baskets to 15 high schools in Boston. Programs were also operating in other cities before the turn of the century. The Cleveland, Ohio, schools arranged with a concessionaire as early as 1893 to deliver baskets to students, and in 1899 the Horace Mann School of Teachers College, Columbia University, served children attending the experimental school. Some Minnesota schools were serving lunches before 1900, and Connecticut began its first program in New Haven in 1904.

Most of these early programs were motivated by charity. Even then there were visionaries who saw the program as more than a feeding program. At the Children's Aid Society the goal was to feed vagrant children in hopes that it would cause them to seek instruction in industry and in mental training. And in Boston, Ellen Richards said of children who received lunches, "They are more attentive and interested in the lessons during the last hour of the morning and the result in their recitations gives the proof."[4(p5)]

The Twentieth Century

Two books were published in the early part of the twentieth century that focused public attention on the social consequences of undernourishment. *Poverty,* written by Robert Hunter, described the economic and social effects of poverty. It pointed out that children in a weak physical and mental state resulting from poverty learned little or nothing at school.[5] Spargo's *The Bitter Cry of the Children*[6] was the second book to be written on the same theme. He estimated that the United States had several million undernourished children and noted that Europe had attacked the problem of malnutrition through school feeding programs.

Child feeding programs had their greatest growth in the large industrial cities and were more often offered as a convenience rather than as making a difference in children's physical and mental performance. The earliest recorded school board support for school feeding occurred in New York City. When the superintendent of schools observed that children were spending their lunch money on items bought from pushcarts and other street vendors, he urged the school officials to provide nourishing meals for all schools. An unconvinced school board approved the establishment of lunches for two elementary schools as a pilot program in 1903. The pilot was to determine whether a three-cent lunch could be planned to meet one-fourth of the child's food needs and still be self-supporting. After two years of operation, the New York Board of Education gave permission to expand the program to other schools. The board agreed to supply space, equipment, and utilities, but the cost of food and service was to be covered by student revenues. At about the same time, programs were implemented in Chicago and St. Louis. However, it was determined in St. Louis that it was illegal to spend public funds for the purchase of food, and the school feeding program was turned over to a voluntary society called The Penny Lunch Association.

By 1913 school lunch programs were operating in 30 cities in 14 states. Most of these programs were in the hands of volunteer parent groups and interested civic organizations. In some places the programs were operated by private concessionaires. These profit-making organizations did not show much interest in working with teachers in planning meals and coordinating the feeding experience with classroom instruction. School administrators were beginning to take note of the value of the feeding program to a child's school behavior, and a trend was developing for school authorities to assume responsibility for the operation of the program.[7] The role of nutrition in a child's educational performance continues to be a major concern of the administrator who has a holistic view of the curriculum.

Lunch at school was a necessity in rural schools, since most of the children were bused to school. Often the lunch was prepared in the classroom by the teacher, with children bringing food from home and having it warmed at school. With the assistance of the federal-state extension service, schools often had garden projects. A 1919 report from the extension service indicated that nearly 72,000 children in 2,930 schools in the United States were receiving hot lunches as a result of home demonstration projects.

Lunches didn't just happen. There were many pioneers who made it happen. Among these were several . . . that would be called visionaries. These include Emma Smedley, director of the Philadelphia school lunch program and author of *The School Lunch*, first published in 1920[8] and revised in 1930. Smed-

ley described an ideal school lunch program that reflected basic concepts and philosophies that continue to guide the development of an integrated program. Mary de Garmo Bryan, a former American Dietetic Association (ADA) president and the third American School Food Service Association (ASFSA) president, was a professor of institutional management at Teachers College, Columbia University. The influence of her teaching was reflected not only by the practice of students who studied with her and implemented the philosophy and practice learned under her guidance in their home states but also by the basic beliefs laid down in *The School Cafeteria*.[9] This book was widely used as a reference and text to guide philosophy and practice nationwide. Dr. Bryan was influential in providing support for the basic philosophy and language contained in the National School Lunch Act (NSLA) of 1946. Thelma Flanagan's career in school lunch began with the Works Progress Administration (WPA) and transitioned into the Florida Department of Education as director of Florida's school food service program. She was the fourth president of ASFSA. Her influence was widely felt in four areas: (1) as a charter member of the ASFSA, she advocated for the development of professional personnel standards and training; (2) as a first-generation state director, she influenced the development of the program standards published by the Southern States Work Conference, which had a major impact on programs in the 14 participating states and in the nation; (3) as a state program director, she promoted the need for a systematic financial management system that allowed local school districts maximum flexibility in program management; and (4) she recognized the necessity of partnerships with allied organizations, such as the Association of School Business Officials and the chief state school officers in achieving program goals. Dr. Neige Todhunter, a former ADA president, instigated some of the earliest personnel workshops at the University of Alabama and, even more importantly, described the five-star program. She called this partnership of principal, parent, teacher, food service personnel, and students working together on shared goals the path to success. The last visionary to be included in this list of pioneers and visionaries is Ethel Austin Martin, who outlined a plan for teachers in a book, *Nutrition Education in Action*,[10] published in1963. Martin's practical experience emerged from an illustrious career in nutrition education with the National Dairy Council, one of the earliest industry supporters of nutrition education practices and materials.

Emma Smedley's story of the Philadelphia school lunch program was told in *The School Lunch*.[11] She described a basic philosophy of program management and identified characteristics of an ideal lunch program. The Philadelphia Board of Education officially assumed responsibility for the school lunch program in 1910, the first large school district to make the commitment. Prior to 1910, the program was operated either by volunteers or concessionaires. Dr. Cheesman A. Herrick, who was principal of the William Penn High School in 1909, is credited with accomplishing the transfer of responsibilities for operation and support of the lunch program to the Philadelphia School Board.[12] The impetus came from a group of students who protested against the lunchroom's being operated by a concessionaire. Dr. Herrick requested that the board establish a system to ensure that lunches served would be based upon sound principles of nutrition and to require that the program be under the direction of a home economics graduate. The board granted his request on an experimental basis and on the condition that the program would be self-supporting. Within a year the experiment had proven successful and the foundation was laid for school lunch programs in Philadelphia to be a responsibility of the board. Philadelphia's program grew. By 1922 it was considered a special branch of the educational system, and in 1925 the director was given greater authority to manage the financial aspects of the program.

The school lunch program expanded rapidly throughout the United States during the 1920s. Some programs were developed through state-sponsored activities, and many programs emerged from community activity. The School Lunch Improvement Association under the direction of the South Carolina Department of Education was active in developing programs on a community basis.[13] Los Angeles was serving 20,000 children daily and food was sold at cost or below cost. Children who could not pay were served free. Chicago probably had the most extensive program, as it served lunches in all schools in the city.

Smedley stated, "The beneficial results to the children who received wholesome food provided by reliable agencies, and the general focusing of public attention on the subject of malnutrition in children, gradually awakened school boards to the fact that feeding was a legitimate part of the educational plan. From a mere standpoint of economics vast sums of money were being wasted through the inability of many children to assimilate knowledge on an empty or discomforted stomach."[14(p5)] She continued, "Nothing has given greater impetus to school feeding than the glaring defects of many of the boys examined for the draft in 1917. It was proven at that time that if we are to expect a sturdy nation, the function of our schools must be extended to the care of bodies as well as minds."

The first accounts of the impact of physical deficiencies and malnutrition relating to the ability of young men in military service goes back to World War I. This concern reached nutrition researchers, including Dr. Mary Schwartz Rose and Dr. Lydia Roberts. Martin[15] indicated that World War II reawakened the country to the need for a well-fed, physically fit population. The growth of the school lunch program in the 1920s most likely reflected an awareness of problems in World War I in which large numbers of young men were unable to fight because of physical deficiencies related to malnutrition. This awareness also found its way into the research laboratories of nutritionists seeking ways to alleviate malnutrition.

School lunch facilities in the 1920s were simple. Flanagan included a little poem in her history which describes the facility situation of the era.

> *Sing a song of Hot Lunch, potatoes on to boil*
> *Four and twenty minutes, on our blue flame oil*
> *Makes them nice and creamy, serve them while they're hot;*
> *Don't you think that such a dish would help an awful lot?*[16]

Source: Reprinted with permission from T. Flanagan, School Food Services, in *Education in the States: National Education Association*, p. 557, © 1972, National Education Association.

With limited space in the school building, the lunchroom was often started in the basement and occasionally in the attic of the school. Equipment considered necessary included the blue flame oven, a double boiler, a large kettle with cover, baking pan, and tea kettle. Although there were some central kitchens, many schools had their own kitchens. In 1926 W.S. Ford wrote a doctoral dissertation entitled *Some Administrative Problems of the High School Cafeteria.* In his study he found that the only equipment available in all the schools reviewed were a cook's table and a range. He concluded that implementing cafeteria-style service resulted in increased participation, which in turn made the program cost effective.

Many of these feeding programs had sound goals and were concerned with nutrition. Undoubtedly the most comprehensive statement of goals was recorded by Emma Smedley, who described a two-fold aim of school lunch: "to meet the food requirements of the child, helping to lay a foundation for physical vigor upon which the structure of mental training can be effectively built; and to serve as an educational factor, instilling wise food habits, offering an opportunity for lessons in courtesy and consideration and providing a laboratory for the prac-

tical demonstration of allied subjects of study."[17(p5)] Emma Smedley described an ideal school lunch plan[18] and also identified the characteristics of a quality program. Words chosen by Smedley to describe the ideal lunch plan are visionary and yet reflect the period in which she lived. Most of the concepts that she included in the ideal plan (Exhibit 2–1) are currently part of the national child nutrition program. Editorial notes in brackets indicate how closely the development of the program has paralleled the plan she described.

Smedley also indicated other program qualities that have implications for directors managing contemporary school food and nutrition programs. She indicated that a program must

- represent an ideal in food selection, preparation, and cleanliness, thus subtly implanting in the child's mind a liking for good food properly served, and a distaste for any other kind
- be considered as an opportunity to give the child practice in making choices and buying; they should gain valuable lessons in how to buy for value, develop self-restraint in buying, and accept responsibility for selecting quality food; they may also gain an understanding of the factors that enter into the selling price of the food
- be the responsibility of the school authorities to conduct the operation, rather than some outside organization
- be recognized as a vast operation that provides professional opportunities for trained cafeteria managers or school dietitians; the manager should have the same rank as a teacher of home economics[19]

The reader is advised to compare the Smedley description of the ideal with the policies outlined by Mary de Garmo Bryan in 1936,[20] the NSLA in 1946, and by ASFSA in *Keys to Excellence: Standards of Practice for Nutrition Integrity.*[21] At the time Smedley and Bryan articulated the program vision, there was neither federal nor state money allocated for school feeding. This vision for the program should be

Exhibit 2–1 The Ideal School Lunch Plan

The ideal school lunch plan provides for the food needs of every child who comes within the school system, during the time they are under school supervision. The lunch program should make available to every child either one meal a day, breakfast or lunch; or supply wholesome food to supplement the lunch from home or other source. It should provide for all children including those with special nutrition needs and in extended day programs. The nutrition service should reach all children, with prices low enough to be within reach of the majority of pupils and yet uphold standards of quality and service. For those children who are unable to pay for meals, special provision should be made. If our educational system is to be effective in promoting improved quality of life, children from poor homes must receive the benefits of school nutrition service. Programs should be administered in such a way that no child is discriminated against. [Note: Accomplished with PL 91-248, 1970]

The program should be closely linked with the work of the classroom and operated in cooperation with medical and health services. [Comprehensive health identifies nutrition services as one of the eight basic areas.] *It is one of the most effective links between the school and the home . . . and it provides a great opportunity for children of different cultures to learn about America and its culture. Food is a common denominator regardless of nationality and school menus should offer ethnic choices as a means of accommodating children with different ethnic background and providing American children opportunities to learn about other cultures.* [Our globalized society makes this Smedley concept even more timely. Ethnic meals have become one of the more popular choices in school meals in the 1990s.]

It should be considered both as a business and one with a social aspect. The person in charge should have business training, scientific knowledge of foods, and social vision. The director should understand both the business and broad educational aspects of the program. [The National Food Service Management Institute (NFSMI) competencies identified for managers and directors indicate the need for competencies in both nutrition education and school food service management.]

Space and equipment should be provided by the school board as for any other school activity. The program should be operated as a department of the board and should be uniform in all schools with standardized equipment, service and prices. It should provide adequate kitchen and dining space for the enrollment and the dining area should be light and airy. [Policies and standards adopted by the Southern States Work Conference (SSWC) in 1947 reflected this philosophy, which is an integral part of the operating philosophy today.]

The program of the future may meet community needs by selling food to working mothers of school children.

Source: Data from E. Smedley, The History of Child Nutrition Programs, *The School Lunch,* pp. 7–16, 24 and 189–194, © 1930.

a driving force in standards for programs regardless of funding sources.

The basic principles articulated by Smedley have been transmitted through the years in a variety of documents, including basic beliefs contained in the SSWC bulletin published in 1967. The principles laid down by pioneers have been a driving force in program development. Although the ideal has not been fully achieved, it provides a conceptual framework for programs of the future and a challenge for school food and nutrition leaders seeking program excellence.

There was a recognized need for standards to guide the types of meals offered children in these rapidly developing school lunch programs. The United States Department of Agriculture (USDA) defined the first national standards for school lunches in the 1920s. USDA defined the important elements of a child's diet as milk, supplemented by other protein-rich foods, bread or cereal food in other forms; butter or other foods containing fat; vegetables; and fruits and sweets. In New York City and Arizona an attempt was made to provide children with one-third of their daily needs based on volume of foods, since average daily requirements of vitamins were unknown at that time.

National groups were beginning to take some ownership of childhood hunger and malnutrition and became involved in helping to solve the problem. The National Congress of Parents and Teachers (PTA) was an early partner in advocating for school lunch in the educational system. American agriculture was also preparing for a role in the future development of the school lunch program. At least three states had passed state laws pertaining to school lunch before 1925. Missouri's school lunch law, which passed in 1921, was the first. Connecticut's school lunch law was passed in 1923, and Ohio passed a school lunch law in 1925.

The 1930s

The 1930s did not come in silently. Two major national events in the 1930s dramatically influenced the development of the national school lunch program. The first was the Great Depression that occurred when the stock market crashed in 1929, and the second was World War II.

Impact of the Great Depression

The development of the school lunch program during the Great Depression addressed three national needs: it provided food for underfed and hungry children, work for hundreds of unemployed persons, and an outlet for the huge surplus of commodities. Surplus corn was burned for fuel while hunger among the nation's schoolchildren posed an overwhelming social problem. Classroom teachers used their own money to feed children. Benevolent organizations such as the American Red Cross and The American Friends Service Committee fed children in many areas of the country. The PTA volunteered with labor and food. Some states allocated money. States also experienced inadequate funds.

The federal government became active in school lunch programs during the 1930s. During this decade agricultural surpluses that could not be sold in the normal channels were accumulated. It was imperative that an outlet be found for the surplus that would be considered socially desirable and yet not in conflict with the economic structure.[22] One of the most obvious needs and outlets for this food was the children of the nation, many of whom were malnourished to the point of physical and mental deterioration.

The first federal aid for school lunch was provided through the Reconstruction Finance Corporation and went to Missouri in 1933.[23] The Civil Works Administration and the Federal Emergency Relief Administration provided some financial assistance for labor employed in the school lunch program from 1932 to 1934. Up to this time, the serving of meals at school had been a service maintained primarily for high school students and as a fundraising enterprise for schools and concessionaires. Little attention had been given to the nutrition needs of the students either in preparing meals or in making them available to all children, whether or not the child was able to pay the charge.

Franklin D. Roosevelt had promised the American people a New Deal. Shortly after he became President in 1935, several new programs, including the WPA, were established. The WPA provided the first substantial contribution for school lunch from federal sources. The WPA was created to provide work for needy persons on public works projects. Since there were needy women in nearly every city, town, and rural community in America, the school lunch program became a ready outlet for their employment.

Each state had a supervisor of the WPA lunch program and a supporting staff of district and local school lunch supervisors. This staff visited the individual schools to give technical assistance. The supervisory staff generally had special knowledge and abilities in food service. Menus, recipes, and manuals developed by the WPA staff helped local cooks and helpers in the performance of their duties. This supervisory assistance and the manuals helped to improve the quality of meals served as well as set standards for equipment, personnel, sanitation, and safety. Site-based WPA employees were expected to have two to five days of pre-service training and to continue training after employment. A staffing formula determined the number of persons to be employed at a site.

Meal prices were kept very low, since most of the labor was provided by WPA. No charge was made to needy children, and no discrimination was to be shown to those who received free meals. Reports reflect the rapid growth of the program. By March 1941, WPA lunch programs were in operation in all states, the District of Columbia, and Puerto Rico, with 23,160 schools serving an average of nearly two million lunches daily and employing 64,298 persons. Another federal agency, The National Youth Association (NYA), which began in 1935, provided job training for unemployed youth and part-time work for needy students. These NYA employees supplied assistance in the lunch program as part-time employees.[24,25]

Congress enacted Public Law 320 in 1935 in an effort to increase consumption of agricultural products. Under Section 32 of the Agricultural Adjustment Act, direct purchase of surplus farm products to be distributed to needy families and nonprofit school lunch programs was begun. Schools received six million pounds of commodities in fiscal year 1936. Commodities were allocated on the basis of the number of children certified as needy or undernourished. Then as now, there was grumbling about the commodities. Some of the foods were unfamiliar. Thelma Flanagan relates the story of one mountain-area school lunch manager who said about fresh grapefruit, "I've biled 'em and fried 'em, and they ain't fitten to eat yet. But just give me a little time, and I'll find a way to make the children like em." The attitude behind that determined expression was the spirit of school lunch per-

sonnel, regardless of the handicaps and difficulties, they worked with teachers to encourage children to try such new foods as herring roe, olives, and bread made with wheat flour.

Thus the pattern was set for the future national school lunch program. Ironically, it was a pattern in which the agriculture industry and USDA, rather than education, would be most influential in securing federal aid and in promoting the national school lunch program. The WPA and the Commodity Distribution Program gave roots to the modern-day school lunch program. It served two basic economic purposes: providing employment in local communities and increasing the consumption of agricultural products; it also served a social purpose: meeting the food needs of children during the school day. The late Lawrence Cremin, professor emeritus, Columbia University, told students always to be aware that every piece of federal legislation passed had a basic economic purpose. He noted that it may also provide a social purpose, but the reason for most congressional action is its impact on the economy.[26]

By 1937, 15 states had passed laws authorizing local school boards to operate lunch programs. The laws generally authorized the serving of meals at cost and usually provided for food only; however, four states made provisions for needy children. These states were Missouri, Wisconsin, Vermont, and Indiana. A Georgia ruling by the attorney general in 1937 stated that school funds could not be used for school lunch since it was not an educational purpose.[27] The growth of the program nationwide was consistent, rising from 3,839 schools and 342,031 children in March 1937; in March 1945, more than six million children in 43,959 schools participated in federally assisted school lunch programs.

Before leaving the 1930s there is a need to review the influence of another pioneer and visionary in academia who strengthened the foundation for program and personnel standards. Dr. Mary de Garmo Bryan, a World War I dietitian and former ADA president, had observed firsthand the physical conditions of troops in the war. After the war she became a professor of institutional management at Teachers College, Columbia University. Dr. Bryan knew the work of Emma Smedley in Philadelphia and the school lunch program in New York City. Students came from many states to study with Dr. Bryan and earn a graduate degree. In the course in school lunch management, an integral part of the graduate curriculum, she taught the beliefs and principles articulated by Smedley. She used the New York City Schools as the laboratory for students to practice the skills learned in class. Upon graduation these Teachers College graduates incorporated the beliefs and principles in practice as school food and nutrition program directors. And the philosophy was spread throughout the country. The philosophy and operational practices advocated by both Dr. Bryan and Emma Smedley preceded any federal funding and even minimal state funding for the programs. Now, as then, school food and nutrition professionals should base programs on student and educational needs rather than on the source of financing. Just as in the 1990s movie *Field of Dreams,* if you build a solid program, "they will come."

In 1936, Dr. Bryan's beliefs, principles and operational guidelines were published in *The School Cafeteria.*[28] The book embraced the philosophy of Mary Swartz Rose: "The expensive machinery of education is wasted when it operates on a mind listless from hunger or befogged by indigestible food."[29(pvii)] In defining the purpose of the school lunch program, Dr. Bryan traced its evolution from its beginning as a charity program, its development as a convenience for students, and finally its status as an indispensable part of the health and teaching programs for all children. The program continues to serve this threefold child-focused purpose. It is from this philosophy that *The School Cafeteria*'s wisdom emerges. Dr. Bryan taught students that the type of management, qualifications of personnel, financial policies, kinds and prices of foods served, and use of the

cafeteria as a teaching center should be guided by the philosophy that it is an indispensable part of the health and teaching program for all children.[30] N.L. Englehardt of Teachers College said of *The School Cafeteria* that it provides "a vision for the future." Dr. Bryan[31] outlined a fourfold role of school lunch in the educational program.

1. It is a source of nourishing food which helps to combat malnutrition and hunger and helps maintain the health and vigor essential to the success of the teaching program.
2. It is a center for the teaching of proper food selection and of good health habits.
3. It provides an opportunity for correlating classroom teaching with interests and experiences of children which center around food.
4. It is a way of engaging the community in the work of the school and of providing some nutrition education to parents through this outlet.

Exhibit 2–2 contains a summary of basic beliefs regarding the school lunch program that are summarized from *The School Cafeteria.*[32] The influence of Emma Smedley is reflected in the philosophy promulgated by Dr. Bryan. As the program developed in the 1930s and 1940s Dr. Bryan's influence was most visible as she contributed to the philosophy and concepts contained in the NSLA, served as president of ADA and later of ASFSA.

As the calendar's pages turned to the decade of the 1940s, the school lunch program was growing rapidly under the WPA. The growth of the program from 1939 to 1942 was phenomenal. The 1941–1942 school year became the peak year under the WPA in student participation and in the use of commodities. WPA and NYA provided support for labor and USDA provided food valued at $21 million. By February 1942, 92,916 schools nationwide were participating in the program serving six million children daily.[33] Dr. Bryan's students were

Exhibit 2–2 Basic Beliefs: *The School Cafeteria*

Basic Beliefs: The School Cafeteria

1. The school feeding program is part of the health program. It is difficult for a child to have an adequate diet if his noon meal is inadequate.
2. There is a relationship between the child's nutritive status and scholastic achievement.
3. Every child in school through the noon hour should have at least one meal.
4. There is a need for special feeding of some children.
5. The school lunch program should be used in teaching health.
6. The school should have a system for letting children know when their lunches are nutritionally adequate.
7. High standards of quality and preparation for all items offered must be maintained.
8. Demonstration plates visually show children an adequate and attractive meal.
9. Signage helps children understand food values and meal costs.
10. Cafeteria may be used for vocational training in food service management.
11. Adequate time should be allowed for children to eat.
12. The cafeteria can be used for social experiences.
13. The noon lunch offers an opportunity to teach table manners; an occasional sit-down meal for this purpose is suggested.
14. There should be plans to correlate classroom teaching with cafeteria experiences.
15. A tour of the school kitchen can be a field trip for young children.
16. The art department can use the cafeteria to display student artwork and the business education department will find many opportunities in school lunch operations for students to practice their skills.
17. Menus are sent home to parents.
18. Parents and students are involved in identifying food preferences and planning menus.
19. There seems to be no reason for retaining the commercial concessionaire.
20. The cafeteria is built and equipped by public funds as part of the school plant.
21. School feeding is a function of the board of education and should be managed by the board and not some outside group.
22. The director is appointed by the superintendent, who sees that procedures are established for the proper business administration and who, by the careful selection of a well trained director, safeguards the educational aspects of school feeding.
23. School managers are recommended by the director and are responsible to her or him for food service operation. They should work closely with principals for ways to use the cafeteria for other educational uses, cooperate with teaching staff, and participate in all school activities.
24. Managers should be as well trained as the classroom teacher. Persons trained in home economics are the most logical persons for management positions. Technical qualifications are not enough. The manager must be able to work with people, like people, have a scientific attitude, and have an appreciation of the social significance of his or her work.
25. Records are essential to good business and accounting procedures.
26. The menu should always be planned in consideration of the child's food needs for an entire day, the food habits of the community, the amount of money available for the meal and equipment available for preparation, and to provide variety and attractive food.
27. Lunch is expected to furnish one-fourth to one-third of the calories, protein, minerals, and vitamins required during the day. Children should have at least one cup of milk at noon.
28. Choices will be provided for all the food categories of the menu.

---

continues

Exhibit 2–2 continued

29. Parents are encouraged to include vegetables in the lunch from home.
30. Menus should consider the aesthetics of color, appearance, texture, and flavor.
31. The aim is to establish through the use of school funds a lunch that meets the need of the individual school and to make sure that each child at school receives the lunch.
32. The success of the lunchroom depends upon the intelligent cooperation of parents and teachers.

Source: Data from M. Bryan, *The School Cafeteria*, pp. 15–349, © 1936, F.S. Crofts & Co.

finding their niches as directors in Louisiana, Washington, Massachusetts, Florida, and many other states across the nation and as instructors in academia. *The School Cafeteria* was used as a reference by food and nutrition program directors and as a textbook in universities across America.

A few states began supporting and contributing limited funds for the program. In 1942, Utah enacted a unique bill that placed a 4 percent tax on wines and liquors to provide revenue to be distributed to local school districts based on the number of meals served. South Carolina's School Lunch Act, passed in 1943, was designed to continue and expand the lunch program in the public schools—and to provide for the supervision and promotion of school lunches in the state. In that year, South Carolina ranked first in the United States both in the number of schools with school lunch programs and in the number of lunches served. There were 188,000 students having meals each day in South Carolina's 1,524 schools. The legislature appropriated funds to provide one supervisor for each county in the state.

The West Virginia Department of Education had published a curriculum guide in 1938 entitled *The Hot Lunch at School: A Manual of Suggestions for Teachers.*[34] This guide proposed that if educational possibilities are fully explored, school lunch might be used to achieve some of the large aims of all public school education. Dr. E. Neige Todhunter at the University of Alabama emphasized the school's responsibility for helping the child develop good food habits by saying, "the selection of adequate meals should become a habit just as training has made speaking, reading, and writing possible without conscious effort."[35(p7)]

Meanwhile, the U.S. Office of Education published a bulletin entitled, *Making School Lunches Educational.*[36] In the foreword, John W. Studebaker, Commissioner of Education, stated, "It is coming to be widely recognized that an adequate noon meal is indispensable if pupils are to be well nourished, and that only well-nourished pupils are able to derive maximum benefits from the opportunities provided by the school." In a second paragraph, he said, "Little has been said concerning the importance of the school lunch as a learning experience for boys and girls. . . . In some schools the lunchroom is a laboratory in which pupils learn the best ways of solving some of their basic problems in healthful living and citizenship. It is only an economical use of school resources to see that the educational potentialities of the school lunch are realized in every school." Valuable resources were identified to support the use of the school lunch program for educational purposes, including a 226-page manual published in 1942 by the Ohio Dietetic Association entitled *Manual for Managers of Rural and Other Small School Lunchrooms.*

In 1940, a nonprofit self-financed organization, the SSWC was founded under the auspices of state departments of education and state educational associations with support from land-grant colleges and universities. Its purpose was to study educational problems in the 13 participating southern states. In 1945, the SSWC sponsored a three-year study of school lunch operations, including its place in the curriculum, impact on children's health, and method of financing SSWC workshop participants represented major stakeholders in the school lunch program, including superintendents, state agency school lunch staff, instructional personnel, local food and nutrition program directors and managers, and representatives from USDA. This early collaborative planning a- mong all stakeholders in the program undoubtedly influenced the rapid growth of programs in the southern states. The outcome of the project was publication of a bulletin that contained beliefs and standards for program management. The bulletin *School Lunch Policies and Standards* was first published in 1947 and revised in 1953 and 1967.[37] With regard to financing, the SSWC recommended that at least the cost of supervision, labor, and facilities be provided from tax funds. The SSWC executive group approved three projects to study school lunch after the original study in 1945. From these collaborative efforts school lunch policies and standards were identified that influenced the development of programs in the nation but nowhere was the influence greater evidenced than in the states that participated in the SSWC.

Impact of World War II

The Selective Service figures gave impetus to the need for improving food consumption of young people. These figures indicated that one-third of all men rejected for military service were physically unfit because of nutritional deficiencies. Even more alarming was the report to Congress by Selective Service Director Lewis Hershey stating that the United State suffered 155,000 casualties as a result of malnutrition. Surgeon General Thomas Parran's statement to Congress that "We are wasting money trying to educate children with half-starved bodies" was a stimulus for the advancement of the school lunch program. The first effort to provide federal funds for the school lunch program was made by Representative Jerry Voorhis of California in 1942. Although the bill did not pass, it served as a fore-runner for many bills to be offered between 1944 and 1946.[38]

World War II had a positive impact on the nation's economy. As defense industries provided work for thousands of people, many women joined the work force for the first time and the need for WPA employment declined. WPA was closed in the early part of 1943, and labor supplied to the schools was eliminated. The war also required huge supplies of food to support the U.S. Armed Forces and Allied armies, and this soon drained off the surplus that had been provided to schools. The shortage of gasoline and problems in distribution made it almost impossible to distribute food to schools. While the war had a positive impact on the economy, its impact on school lunch programs was initially negative as WPA was eliminated; however, it was turned into a positive as reflected in subsequent action of the Congress. Another impact that the war had on school lunch was food rationing. The two major organizations focusing on school lunch programs, The National School Cafeteria Association and the Food Service Directors Conference, urged the Office of Price Administration (OPA) to remove child feeding projects from the restaurant classification and set ration allowances that would make it possible for schools to furnish approximately one-third of the child's daily nutritive requirements at the noon meal. In January 1944 OPA announced that a plan had been worked out. By April 1944, the number of schools with lunch programs had declined to 34,064 and student participation had dropped to five million meals daily.[39] That was the bottoming out of the program; there was not to be another decline for many years.

When WPA was phased out, there was a large outcry of support for the continuation of the school lunch program. School administrators testified to Congress on the impact of the program on learning and attendance, nutrition leaders testified to its value in helping improve nutritional status of children, and agricultural leaders recognized the value of the program to the local farm economy. The 78th Congress in

July 1943 enacted Public Law 129 authorizing the use of 50 million dollars of Section 32 funds for maintaining the lunch and milk programs for the 1943–1944 school year. The new program was administered by the U.S. War Food Administration, which provided funds to reimburse meals. The federal dollars were to be used to help purchase food and could not be used for labor or other purposes.[40]

Another controversy that emerged with the close of the WPA concerned the designation of a state agency to administer the program. Because of the program's success in health, education, and agriculture, several state agencies were vying for administration. When the issue emerged at a regional meeting being held in Georgia, the state school superintendent called Georgia Senator Richard Russell, chairman of the U.S. Senate Agriculture Committee, for a decision. Shortly thereafter, Senator Russell called with the answer that the state educational agency would be the administering agency. Many of the WPA state supervisors became the first state school lunch directors. Some of the first state directors were Thelma Flanagan, Florida; Lucille T. Watson, Georgia; Ruth Powell, Arkansas; Martha Bonar, West Virginia; John Stalker, Massachusetts; W.H. Garrison, South Carolina; Rodney Ashby, Utah; Wade Bash, Ohio; Edith Blakely, Connecticut; Earl Langop, Missouri; Ruth Cutler, New Hampshire; Gordon Gunderson, Wisconsin, and Jim Hemphil, California.

Federal funds were provided for the school years 1944–1945 and 1945–1946. Authority to use the funds was extended to child care centers. The 1945–1946 authorization contained a provision that funds used for child care would be no more than 2 percent of the funds. The requirements for receiving federal aid were as follows:

- Meals must meet one-third of the daily dietary allowance for 10- to 12-year-old children.
- Schools must maintain accurate records of cost of food and report food purchases to the state.

- Federal cash payments could not exceed the cost of food used for the program.
- Total payments could not exceed the amount provided for food purchases from all sources.

The program grew rapidly, and Congress provided a supplemental appropriation of $7.5 million in December 1945. By April 1946, 45,119 schools were participating in the program, serving 6.7 million children daily, an increase of 11 thousand schools and about 1.5 million children over the 1943–1944 school year.[41]

The Quest for a Permanent School Lunch Program

A joint committee of the National School Cafeteria Association and the Food Service Directors Conference was formed in April 1944. It was called The Committee To Obtain the Support of Congress for a Nationwide School Lunch Program. The committee distributed a statement to 30,000 schools seeking support for a program to feed the hungry, to be a means of ensuring the physical vigor of America's youth, and to meet the "imperative needs of our country" in times of danger.[42] World War II ended in 1945. Men came home; they reestablished themselves in the workplace or enrolled in schools and colleges under the GI Bill of Rights. The women who had gone to work during the war continued to work, many while their husbands completed their education. Nine bills were introduced by Congress proposing the establishment of a permanent school lunch program. Similar bills were considered in the House of Representatives and by the Senate. Congressman John W. Flannagan (VA), Chairman of the Committee on Agriculture in the House, and Senator Richard B. Russell (GA), Chairman of the Committee on Agriculture in the Senate, were the two primary managers for the bills. The proposal contained two titles or two parts; one provided a permanent school lunch program to be administered by the state educational agency and the second title proposed providing funds for nutrition education, training, and equipment. At the national level Title I was to be administered by USDA and Title II was to be administered by the Office of Education. In spite of overwhelming Congressional support for permanent legislation, the debate extended over a two-year period. Some members argued that the program had been operating successfully for 11 years without permanent legislation, and a small minority simply opposed the program.

Committee hearings were held in the first session of the 79th Congress and HR 3370 was reported out. Persons testifying included Surgeon General Paran, the Presidents of the General Federation of Women's Clubs and the National Conference of Parents and Teachers, the Legislative chairman of the National Education Association; USDA's Chief of Food Distribution; Maryland's State School Lunch Director Gertrude Bowie; representatives of state home economics supervisors; and Frank Washman, Chicago's school lunch director. Among those testifying in Senate committee hearings were Georgia's state school lunch director, Lucille T. Watson, who was asked by Senator Russell to testify; Massachusetts' John Stalker; and Dr. Mary de Garmo Bryan. During the two years of debate many local and national organizations actively lobbied for passage of a bill. The Congressional Record lists names of 32 national groups that endorsed the bill and asked for its enactment. Groups included most if not all the farm groups; those interested in the welfare of children, such as the PTA; professional groups including the NEA and ADA; and all major educational, medical, civic, and labor groups.

A review of the debate from the Congressional Records for 1945–1946 provides valuable insights into the rationale that Congress used in establishing the school lunch program on a permanent basis. One interesting statement that appeared in a Senate Agriculture Committee Report has great significance as it deals with national policy related to food service and nutrition for children. It states: *"A discussion of social and political policy involving the welfare and freedom of our citizens and the proper separation of functions between national government, state government, local government, and the family properly begins when we have assured ourselves of a citizenry sound in body and mind, and no argument on policy can possibly precede this consideration. We conclude that federal assistance should be given—to the states who would administer the programs."*

The report further identified the objectives of federal assistance to school lunch programs:

- To stimulate and to help make it possible for all schools to make a nutritious noon lunch available at cost to all children, and at less than cost to those who need such lunches but are unable to pay the full cost.
- To assist the schools in improving the health and physical development of schoolchildren by helping to prevent underfeeding and malnutrition.
- To help the states provide practical situations through which children can be taught to select and eat balanced diets and to practice habits of sound nutrition both in school and at home.
- To aid in improving existing school lunch programs, expanding them where necessary, and establishing new ones, to the end that the ways and means available for improving and stabilizing the farm markets will be increased.[43]

After extensive hearings in committees of both the Senate and the House of Representatives, the bills were debated on the floor of both bodies. Some quotes from congressional members are included here to illustrate the intensity of support, issues discussed, and concerns. These statements also reflect the scope of support both geographically and politically. Then, as now, it was a goal of Congress that this program should have bipartisan support, that children should never become pawns in the political arena.

Regarding responsibility for the program, Mr. Granger, Utah, stated: *"One of the greatest educational factors to come out of the war is the discovery that a balanced diet can contribute to the health of an individual . . . to improve the physical standards of the youth of this nation, it is in my opinion, the responsibility of government."*[44(p1461)]

And the pervasive issue of states' rights as related to responsibility for education was discussed by Mr. Harless, Arizona: *"If it is a matter of states' rights or children's rights, I am on the side of children's rights,"* and *"This bill will make the school lunch program an integral part of our school system."*[44(p1465)] Some Congressmen feared that federal dollars would go to children who didn't need the lunch. Mr. Sabath, Illinois, replied: *"I would just a little rather know that a few children got the help who did not need it, than to know that many children who needed the help could not have it."*[44(p1465)] In regard to making the program available to all children, Mr. Harless stated: *"It is essential for the national defense of our country that all of the youth of the nation be properly fed. It is not only necessary for the national defense, but it is necessary for peacetime operations, that the children of this nation be given good, wholesome food; that they be given a diet that will mature their bodies and make it possible for them to acquire a complete education."*[44(p1465)]

The understanding that Congress had of the opportunity inherent in the school lunch program for children to learn to eat a variety of food at school that would impact their families' food habits and buying practices was incredible and provided almost universal support for Title II of the proposed bill. Mr. Pace, Georgia, said: *"And it is good for them when they leave the schools to have some understanding and appreciation of what a balanced diet means to the human body."*[44(p1464)] And Mr. Flannagan, Virginia: *"Those who shout hallelujah for states' rights at the expense of the children are more than willing to accept federal aid to maintain the health of their hogs and cattle."*

There were other concerns and issues debated, including the fear this would become a federal program. Mr. Hope, California, stated, *"This bill requires the use of existing state agencies. It is different from the present program that is almost altogether a federal program clear down to the local level, but here we use the state and the local educational set-up."*[44(p1466)] Mr. Cannon of Missouri: *Even in homes of . . . high economic standards children frequently . . . fail to eat properly and the charts of the school lunch program show an immediate gain when hot meals are available. In providing meals we are . . . producing a sturdier generation . . . and securing his/her scholarship.*[44(p1466)] Mr. Hope commented on hearing from all the leading farm organizations in support of this bill, then stated: *"Why is it in the interests of the farmers of this country to have legislation of this kind? The answer is obvious. It will help agriculture because its point is to promote better nutrition, a better understanding of food values, and a greater consumption of farm products in this country."*[44(p1469)] And Mr. Voorhis, California: *"Unless Congress passes this legislation, it is not possible to tie in the worthwhile purposes of a school lunch program with the proper purposes of the agricultural program of the nation."*[44(p1471)] From these statements by members of Congress, the reader can see that the program was viewed as a viable means of sup-

---

Mr. Chelf, Kentucky: *"I am for the bill, because I know full well that with this program—a smile will replace an unhappy expression of a child—a red rose color will supplant a pale or 'pallored' look, and health will rule out an emaciated, undernourished condition of our school children. America owes this to our youth."*[44(p1461)]

porting the agricultural interests of the country. It is important that school food and nutrition leaders shaping the programs of the future continue to keep members of Congress apprised of the important role it has in supporting the agriculture and food industry in states and local communities.

The house debate on the proposed bill to establish a permanent school lunch program continued into 1946. Mr. Sabath, Illinois, told the House, *"Remember poor nutrition is not confined altogether to the poorer families. Oftimes children in the families of wealth, while given plenty of food of its kind, are given the wrong kind of food, and suffer from malnutrition."*[44(p1464)]

Other concerns were discussed:

- Can parochial schools participate?
- Will the sale of soft drinks, candy, or gum on school premises be affected?
- How will we protect poor children from discrimination?
- If we include nutrition education, will the U.S. Department of Education run it like a federal program?
- How can we keep this a local program?
- Why do we need a permanent program? It's been a success for the 10 years it's been in operation.
- How much will states be required to match the federal money?

The proposed bill had two titles: Title I would provide a permanent school lunch program; Title II would provide a program of nutrition education, training, and equipment assistance. There was almost unanimous support for the concept of providing training and education. However, some members of Congress feared that Title II administered nationally by the Office of Education would interfere with the states' prerogative and responsibility for education and that a federal agency would attempt to prescribe education needs of a state. Ultimately Title II was stricken from proposed bills because of this jurisdictional battle over responsibility for education. The bill passed

the House of Representatives on February 21, 1946.

The Senate debated the bill on February 26, 1946. Senator Russell, Georgia, stated:

> *This bill provides for legislative standards to let schools of the nation know where they stand with respect to the program; heretofore, there have been schools which have hesitated to install school-lunch programs because they were year-to-year . . . and in my opinion, this has been one of the most helpful ones [programs] which has been inaugurated and promises to contribute more to the cause of public education in these United States than has any other policy which has been adopted since the creation of free public schools. . . . I have found that what the children have learned in school concerning the preparation of food in the school and the value of various foods, was carried home to their parents. In some cases schoolchildren were able to educate their own parents as to a better use of food, and as to the nutritive values of various food. . . . The bill protects the rights of all children of this nation of whatever race, color, or creed.*[45(p1610)]

Senator Allen Ellender, Lousiana; Senator Richard Russell, Georgia; and Senator George Aiken, Vermont, were three of the most ardent supporters in the Senate for passage of the bill. In an eloquent speech, Senator Ellender outlined six reasons for passing the legislation:

1. Children attend school on a more regular basis when they are well nourished.
2. Children progress better in their studies.
3. School consolidation requires that many children be transported to school, leaving home very early and getting home late, which makes for a very long day.

4. With World War II many women joined the work force and are no longer home to make lunches for their children.
5. It will provide opportunities for much-needed instruction in nutrition and applied economics.
6. It will make lunches available to all children.

He concluded his remarks upon introducing his version of the bill as follows:

The program to date has been put into effect through the leadership and vision of school officials, socially minded parents, and public service organizations. There is much evidence that aid from the Federal Treasury has given great impetus to this development. . . . The time has come to enact sound and permanent legislation to the end that all children, and especially those most in need of it, shall be assured of the benefits of this important service.[46]

Some members of Congress were concerned that USDA would bypass states and go directly to local systems, as had been reportedly done in at least one state. That fear was quickly allayed by showing that the funds would be sent to the states and the program would be administered by the state educational agency where there was one. Senator Aiken, Vermont: *"The health of our children is the last thing with which we should deal in a miserly manner. I do not see that we can put a dollar value on the health of boys and girls in the schools of this country regardless of the state in which they live. . . . As a school director during a 15-year period, I know for a fact that a child that has enough to eat and has the right things to eat is definitely a better student than a child that goes to school with little of the proper food to eat."*[47(p1625)]

Bessie Brooks West,[48(p1698)] president of the ADA, urged the Senate to provide for strong coordination between education and agriculture in administering the bill. A resolution signed by participants attending a national school lunch conference in Chicago on February 9, 1946, was sent to Congress urging favorable action on the bill. The conference was sponsored by the two organizations, The National School Cafeteria Association and the Food Service Directors Conference, that were to merge a few months later and become the American School Food Service Association. Conference participants included representatives of state departments of education, nutritionists, parent organizations, and farm and civic groups from 32 states.

After extensive debate the Senate passed a bill that was slightly different from the House bill. The conference committee of the House and Senate was held May 20. The Conference Committee Report on H.R. 3370 was accepted by the House of Representatives on May 23, 1946,[49] and by the Senate on May 24, 1946.[50]

A bipartisan trio of Senators, Senator Ellender (Democrat), Senator Aiken (Republican), and Senator Russell (Democrat), strongly advocated passage of the bill. However, Senator Russell of Georgia is known as the "father of the school lunch program," for it was his bill that was adopted by Congress and signed by the president on June 4, 1946.[51]

President Harry S Truman's signature established the school lunch program on a permanent basis. Upon signing the National School Lunch Act, Public Law 396, President Truman said, *"Today, as I sign The National School Lunch Act, I feel that the Congress has acted with great wisdom in providing the basis for strengthening the nation through better nutrition for our schoolchildren . . . I hope that all state and local authorities will cooperate fully . . . in establishing the cooperative school lunch in every possible community."*

As noted by Flanagan, the years from 1930 to 1945 can be characterized as a period of state and national awareness of the importance of school lunch to the health and education of children and to the agricultural community.

THE BENCHMARK YEARS: 1945–1960

The National School Lunch Act of 1946

Section 2 of the National School Lunch Act, which has not been changed since its passage in 1946, defines the Act's purpose and is the basis for national policy:

> It is hereby declared to be the policy of Congress, as a measure of national security, to safeguard the health and well-being of the nation's children and to encourage the domestic consumption of nutritious agricultural commodities and other food, by assisting the States, through grants-in-aid and other means, in providing an adequate supply of food and other facilities for the establishment, maintenance, operation and expansion of nonprofit school lunch programs.[52]

Provisions of NSLA

The act brought the federal government into permanent partnership with states and local school districts. As noted in the statement of policy, the assistance to states would primarily be in the form of grants-in-aid. Funds would be appropriated annually and distributed to the states on the basis of the number of children between the ages of 5 and 17, inclusively, and the need for assistance in the state as indicated by the per capita income. This meant that states with a lower per capita income would receive a greater proportion of the federal funds than states whose per capita income was equal to or greater than the national average. The rate of reimbursement for all meals during the 1946–1947 school year was nine cents.

Public Law 396 was a simple bill with fewer than five pages. The NSLA contained 11 sections when passed in 1946; after reauthorization in 1996, it contained 27 sections. Practitioners generally refer to the parts of the NSLA by section. A brief description of the sections of the NSLA will give the reader an overview

of how philosophy and debate are translated into law.

- Section 4 provided general cash assistance to be apportioned to states on the basis of number of children enrolled and the state's per capita income. The general cash assistance, known as Section 4 funds, was to be paid to schools on the basis of the number of meals served by type (A, B, or C). During the first year of operation, the rate of reimbursement was begun at nine cents per lunch. With program growth this rate had dwindled to as little as two cents per lunch in some states by 1960. For 25 years, the only cash available to schools was the Section 4 funds, which were paid for all meals.
- Section 5 provided that $10 million of the appropriation could be used by states for purchasing equipment that would be used in storing, preparing, or serving food.
- Section 6 authorized funds for USDA administrative costs and for direct purchase of food for distribution to the schools to help them meet nutrition standards. Entitlement commodities are purchased with funds authorized in this section.
- Section 7 required that federal funds be matched from funds within the states beginning with a dollar-for-dollar match and progressing to a three-to-one match from sources within the state by 1956. Because of concern expressed by some states that state dollars would not be provided, the USDA allowed the matching requirement to be met by counting funds from all non–federal sources, including payments from children and adults for meals. The cost or value of land could not be used for matching purposes. Congress was critical of this interpretation that allowed matching from children's payments. Report No. 450 on the Agricultural Appropriation Bill for fiscal year 1948 stated: "The committee believes that the States should by direct appropriations match the money provided by

the Federal Government."[53] The USDA retained its liberal interpretation and did not emphasize the need for states to provide tax money to match the federal money. From 1946 until 1975, the states were required to match all meals. The law was changed in 1975 to require the 3 to 1 match only for meals served to non-needy students.

- Section 8 restricted the use of federal funds to purposes associated with securing and handling food.
- Section 9 of the act contained three major provisions: First, it required that lunches served by the schools would meet minimum nutritional requirements based on tested nutritional research. The Secretary of Agriculture prescribed three types of lunches, designated as Type A, Type B, and Type C, as shown in Exhibit 2–3. Schools were allowed to serve Type A and Type B meals without milk; however, the reimbursement rate was reduced two cents for each meal when milk was not served.[54]

The second provision of Section 9 required that meals would be served without cost to children determined to be unable to pay and prescribed a restriction prohibiting any type of segregation or discrimination against children because of their inability to pay. The third provision of this section related to schools using commodities distributed by USDA.

- Section 11 described requirements for records and reporting and for oversight by federal government.

Another major provision of the NSLA was the establishment of the federal-state partnership. Under the WPA and the War Food Administration, the federal government worked directly with local entities. The NSLA made it perfectly clear that the role of the secretary of agriculture was to define state responsibility, establish national standards, and maintain general supervision, but the state educational agency was responsible for program administration within the state.[55] Senator Allen Ellender (LA) was the most ardent advocate that responsibility for this program be shared and for as long as he remained in the Senate, he attributed the program's success to the federal, state, and local partnership.

Exhibit 2–3 Meal Patterns for the National School Lunch Program (1946)

The Type A meal pattern based on one-third of the daily food requirement of a 10- to 12-year-old child, would contain

1. one-half pint of whole milk (meeting minimum butterfat and sanitation requirements of state and local laws) as a beverage
2. two ounces of fresh or processed meat or poultry, of cooked or canned fish, or cheese; or one-half cup cooked dry beans, peas, or soybeans; or four tablespoons of peanut butter; or one egg
3. six ounces of raw, cooked, or canned vegetables and/or fruit
4. one portion of bread, muffins, or other hot bread made of whole-grain or enriched flour
5. two teaspoons of butter or fortified margarine

The Type B meal pattern met the same specification for bread and milk and half the portion in the other groups.

The Type C meal pattern consisted of one-half pint whole milk, which could supplement lunches children brought from home.

Source: Adapted with permission from J. Caton, *The History of the American School Food Service Association: A Pinch of Love*, p. 112, © 1990, American School Food Service Association.

School food and nutrition leaders of the present and the future should seek ways to maintain this shared responsibility by federal, state, and local authorities. With technological advancements and the ease of information flow, it will be a greater challenge to keep all three levels of government in proper perspective. As history reflects, school food and nutrition programs began with a grass-roots effort and this grass-roots effort has been the driver to present-day success. Federal assistance for the programs is a major resource needed to support the state program as a means of helping to provide quality nutrition services for children in local communities. Program leaders must decide how to use technology in ways to advance the program's mission. Keeping the program focus as close to the children served as possible is essential for program excellence The most effective programs for children will occur when state and local authorities claim ownership and use national standards and federal funds to support state and local needs.

Upon passage of the NSLA, the states were confronted with the problem of legally administering the program. Several states passed legislation authorizing the establishment of school lunch programs. For most states this was not necessary, as state and local participation in the program was voluntary.

The NSLA required states to enter into a written agreement with the secretary of agriculture

- concerning the receipt and disbursement of funds and foods received for distribution
- providing for supervision of the program in all schools to ensure compliance with the provisions of the NSLA Act and regulations and directives issued by the secretary

Local school boards were required to enter into an agreement with the state and agree for the schools to do the following:

- Serve lunches meeting the minimum nutritional requirements established by the secretary.
- Serve meals without cost or at reduced cost to children who were determined by local school authorities to be unable to pay the full cost of the lunch, and not to segregate or discriminate against such children in any way.
- Operate the program on a nonprofit basis.
- Use as far as practicable the commodities declared by the secretary to be in abundance, and to utilize commodities distributed by the secretary.
- Maintain proper records of all receipts and expenditures and submit reports to the state agency as required.

In those states where it was not legal for the state education agency to administer the program in private and parochial schools, a provision was included to allow for a proportionate share of the funds to be allocated to another agency to do so.

Beginning Implementation at the State Level

Anecdotal evidence was shared by some state agency staff of the trials and challenges encountered in communicating information to local school authorities and getting programs

Nothing is more important in our national life than the welfare of our children, and proper nourishment comes first in attaining this welfare. . . . To you who carry out the program locally falls the crucial job of seeing to it that we build well for the future.—Harry S Truman, October 22, 1946.

Courtesy of Harry S. Truman. Prepared statement read at the First National Conference of State School Lunchroom Officials sponsored by the U.S. Department of Agriculture in 1946 in Washington, D.C.

under way by the beginning of the school year. Driving from county to county in midsummer explaining program operating procedures was a trying ordeal. State agency staff members were accompanied by USDA staff as they visited superintendents and board members in thousands of counties to explain the new law.

In October 1946, USDA called the First National Conference of State School Lunchroom Officials in Washington, DC. The purpose of the meeting was to interpret the NSLA and develop a common understanding of standards and procedures.[56] One of the speakers at that conference was Agnes E. Meyer, special writer on national welfare for *The Washington Post* (later she became the publisher).[57] She challenged the state leaders to be innovative in developing programs. She characterized the birth of the national school lunch program as follows: *"It is laughable to remember how we stumbled into the school lunch program. Surely God looks after our poor blundering democracy, and helps us to do the right thing, even though for the wrong reasons. When the farm organizations realized that cattle and pigs could not consume their surplus, they remembered that there are some 24 million youngsters in the schools. What couldn't that many hungry kids do to a surplus, given the chance."* [57(p33)] But Agnes Meyer did not stop there. She saw the future for child nutrition programs that had been described earlier by Emma Smedley: *"What we must aim for is the gradual evolution toward a free hot midday meal for every child, at least in the nursery and grammar schools. It should be provided in the same spirit in which we now provide each child with free textbooks."* And she continued, *"It will take time to achieve free lunches in nursery and grammar schools. Since the human animal learns quickest through necessity, it will in all likelihood take the bitter lesson of another depression. Of course, if we used our intelligence we would organize a free school lunch program as soon a possible as a defense against the social and economic maladjustments of depression."* [57(p34)]

American School Food Service Association Formed

ASFSA was officially organized October 11, 1946. It was a national organization formed from the merger of the Food Service Directors Conference and the National School Cafeteria Association. The newly formed organization was initially called the Food Service Directors Association. Two months later, when the first newsletter was released, it became the School Food Service Association. Officers were president, Constance Hart of Rochester, New York; president-elect, Betsy Curtis, Ohio; treasurer, L. A. Wiles, Michigan; and secretary, Thelma Flanagan, Florida. Flanagan's active influence in developing the school food service profession spanned four decades, and still today, the foundation she laid lives in program standards and operations and in the persons she mentored.[58] The purpose of ASFSA was to promote the expansion, educational use, and improvement of school food service programs and to further the professional growth of the members. Conventions and newsletters were planned to provide opportunities for professional development for members, including networking. The national association and its state affiliates, as they were formed, placed great emphasis on personnel training, improving meal quality, and job performance standards. Since 1960, ASFSA has provided for the coordination of member initiatives in support of safeguarding and expanding federal assistance for child nutrition programs.

The First Year's Operation

By the close of the 1946–1947 school year,[59] all states, as well as the District of Columbia, Puerto Rico, and the Virgin Islands had established programs under the NSLA. It is estimated that approximately six million children participated in the program that first year. More than 100 million of the total lunches served were served at no cost to children. Once the program was in operation, it was obvious that less than half the needed federal money was available. Trying to forecast the number of lunches to be served and set a reimbursement rate that would stretch funds over the entire year without the aid of a computer was little short of a nightmare. Congress provided a supplemental appropriation to get schools through the year. Some states, including Utah, New York, Illinois, Rhode Island, and South Carolina, made substantial contributions through tax levies. But by and large the financial gap was filled by children's payments. Then as now children's payments provided a substantial portion of the program costs and used to meet federal matching requirements for school lunch.

Schools relied heavily on the donated foods to supply valuable food products to supplement the purchased foods. States received funds for the purchase of equipment, which proved to be a challenge. They had not identified equipment needs and were not familiar with manufacturers or suppliers. State agencies and local districts were unprepared to use equipment funds. Since many mistakes were made in the use of funds, Congress did not again provide equipment funds until 1966. While the authorization for non–food assistance was in the NSLA for a number of years, it was not funded. The Child Nutrition Act of 1966 again authorized some funds, and this provision was strengthened in 1970 when the non–food assistance program was authorized by Public Law 91-248. The authorization for funds was eliminated as part of the 1981 Budget Reconciliation Act.

Training Programs Initiated

State agencies and local school districts were faced with the task of employing and training personnel to fill positions at the state, district, and local level. *School Lunch Policies and Standards,* the bulletin published by SSWC described job responsibilities for personnel at all levels, including the school principal. It also contained a recommendation that all school lunch personnel should be employed in the same manner and on the same basis as other school personnel, and that they be trained for the service they were to render.[60] Workshops were sponsored by states and the federal government. Colleges and universities were encouraged to help train personnel. Many colleges and universities in cooperation with state agencies offered workshops on campus during the summer. For many women, coming to the college-based workshop was a first trip away from home for a week. The educational level of personnel varied from the person with some college training to one who could hardly read and write. Workshops were also conducted in the school districts. State agency staff spent the entire summer in training personnel. *The School Cafeteria* was widely used as a resource in all areas of program management and operation, including personnel, purchasing, equipment, and menu planning. The first ASFSA convention in Dallas in the summer of 1947 offered some training opportunities on a national basis.

Financing and Staffing: Major Concerns

The SSWC recommended that combined tax funds cover as a minimum the non–food costs of the program, plus all free lunch costs, so that paying pupils would be charged only for food costs. And Dr. R. L. Johns, a University of Florida professor and nationally recognized leader in school finance, in addressing the 1947 ASFSA convention, said, "It would seem reasonable to recommend that states provide for the financing of at least the nonfood costs of the school lunch program." He compared the food to the consumable supplies children use in the classroom. Would then, it not seem reasonable for the child's food to be treated as a consumable supply if the school lunch is an educational experience?[61] The rapid growth of the school lunch program made it difficult to set and implement standards for supervisory personnel. Therefore, in 1948 the ADA, the American Home Economics Association, and the ASFSA formed a joint committee for developing standards for personnel.[62] The standards established by this committee recommended that

- state directors hold a master's degree or equivalent, including graduate courses in institutional management, community nutrition, principles of supervision, public school administration, and curriculum development; it also recommended that they have five years experience in school lunch management or supervision or four years experience plus a year of directed training or experience in food, nutrition, and institutional management
- system level supervisors have a minimum of a bachelor's degree with three years experience in quantity food production
- managers have a bachelor's degree and two years experience as an assistant to the manager of a large school lunch operation
- the cost of supervision, labor, and facilities should be financed from the same sources as other school costs

Training had been offered on a regional basis even before the NSLA was passed. The General Education Board, a national group organized to provide financial support for the improvement of education, provided a grant that helped finance a southeast regional workshop at the Florida State College for Women in 1944 and a second one at The University of Georgia in 1945. (The SSWC received support from General Education Board.) In July 1949, a national workshop for state-level personnel was held at Iowa State College, cosponsored by USDA, Iowa State College, U.S. Office of Education, and the Millers' National Federation. Thirty-two supervisors attended this graduate-level course centered around developing recommendations and procedures related to the educational program, program planning, research, supervision, training, and equipment and facilities. The recommendations developed at this workshop influenced program development throughout the nation.[63] Some state agencies were actively setting personnel standards. In 1947, the Florida Board of Education autho-

rized school lunch certificates for persons with a degree. The Georgia Board of Education set as a minimum a home economics degree for state agency personnel and recommended the same for school district personnel. Louisiana was among the first states to establish professional criteria for parish-level personnel. During these benchmark years, state associations were affiliating with ASFSA, and more training opportunities were being developed in the states. State agencies had developed procedures for reviewing programs and providing technical assistance. Federal personnel began to withdraw from oversight of local programs.

THE WAY THINGS WERE

A page from the ledger of the Union County, SC, schools notes that a Christmas dinner in 1950 consisted of ham; sweet potato soufflé, English peas, cranberry sauce, apples (no charge), roll, ginger cookies, milk. Help cost was $21.65, utilities were $2.00, and paper goods $3.00. The cost per meal was 31.8 cents. Meal combinations for the 1950–1951 year in Union County were not too different from 1998 menus. The menus generally contained at least three or four fruits and /or vegetables. But there was a definite difference in food preparation. On one day, the ledger indicated that the menu consisted of dry lima beans, turnip greens, beets, corn muffin, and apple pie. The production record indicated that nine bags of lima beans were cooked with two pounds of fatback, and nine cans of turnip greens with two pounds of fatback; the apple pie had three pounds of shortening and four pounds of oleomargarine.

Source: Data from J. Martin and the Supervisor of Union County Schools, Union County, South Carolina, and a 1950 ledger maintained by a school lunch manager.

By 1950, more and more educators were seeing the program as an integral part of the total education program. It was said to be as necessary as a library to building a well-rounded curriculum and as important to education as algebra.[64] Support for nutrition education came from industry leaders such as the National Dairy Council, National Livestock and Meat Board, and General Mills. The University of Georgia received a General Mills Grant to develop a movie that was called *The School That Learned to Eat*. School gardens and nutrition education programs were operable in many schools.

USDA initiated a national study in response to the concern about the adequacy of the Type A Lunch Pattern. Buford High School in Lancaster County, South Carolina, was one of 15 schools selected to participate in the study. A history of the South Carolina school lunch program notes that participating schools were required to keep accurate records of all foods served, including plate waste, and uncooked and cooked weights. The primary purpose of the study was to determine the amounts of various food items required by children of different ages and sexes.[65]

The organizational partners who supported the passage of the NSLA continued to exert their influence; now the influence was directed at program quality and standards. Of major concern in the early days of the NSLA, as now, was the sale of foods of minimal nutritional value in competition with school meals. The American Medical Association, the American Dental Association, ASFSA, the Association of School Business Officials and the PTA issued statements disapproving the sale of carbonated beverages by schools. The Council on Food and Nutrition of the American Medical Association went on record as opposing the sale and distribution of confections and soft drinks in school lunchrooms.

There were administrative difficulties. State agencies requested USDA to reduce the reporting requirements. At the request of the chief state school officers,[66] USDA appointed an advisory committee in 1953 to help formulate policies, rules, and regulations regarding administration of the program. The report of the advisory committee asked USDA to allocate as much of the appropriation in cash as possible. With more children participating, the reimbursement rate had dropped from 8.7 cents in 1947 to less than 5 cents in 1954; in the meantime, the cost of producing a meal had increased. The advisory group concluded that there was almost no follow-up on their recommendations.

Two events occurred in 1954 that had a significant impact on school lunch. First, Congress authorized the Special Milk Program, which not only met a need for children who brought lunches from home, it also removed milk surplus from the market. The special milk program also provided extra milk for children participating in the lunch program. The second event that had a national impact on school lunch and on all of education was the case of *Brown versus Topeka*, regarding the Topeka, Kansas, school board decision to prohibit a black student from attending a white school. The courts ruled in favor of the black student, beginning the end of separate schools for white and black students. As more and more black families chose to have their children attend schools nearer their homes, school enrollments in those schools increased and there was a need to expand school lunch programs.

Russia's launching of Sputnik, the first rocket, in 1957 created a national concern for improving the quality of education in America for all children. Congress responded to this widespread need to improve the teaching of math and science in public and private elementary and secondary schools by passing The National Defense Education Act. Although the impact on school lunch was indirect, it was nevertheless there. Hungry children couldn't learn.

USDA reviewed and adapted the meal pattern as the National Research Council made changes in recommended dietary allowances. One of the first notable changes to promote improved quality was the recommendation that a vitamin A–rich food be included in the menu at least twice weekly and that a vitamin C–rich food be included daily. Three changes were made in the menu pattern in 1958, including requirements that (1) the fruit and vegetable component be met with two or more vegetables or fruits or a combination of both, and the allowance that full-strength fruit or vegetable juice could be counted as meeting not more than one-fourth cup of this requirement; (2) protein-rich foods be served in the main dish and no more than one other item; and (3) made adjustments in portion sizes for various age groups.[67] The school lunch menu most often resembled the "blue plate special" in the early years of the NSLA. However, several societal events occurred in the 1960s that would change the pattern of meal planning. McDonalds and the Golden Arches came into being, resulting in schools considering more choices and particularly offering hamburgers and french fries. Then pizza became a near staple in the American diet. These two changes in the commercial food world, along with widespread access to media influence, necessitated that program managers consider offering more choices to accommodate students' preferences. These decisions were often made with little regard to the nutrient composition of the offerings beyond the traditional meal.

Networks, Partners, and Advocates

Although extensive emphasis has been given to networking and partnerships in the 1990s, the reader should note that the school food and nutrition programs have had extensive networks of partners since the beginning of the program. As a matter of fact, it was the stakeholders who provided the leadership and advocacy for the program before there was an association of school food and nutrition personnel. It has often been said that parent groups were the initiators of food at school. During the debates in the 1940s, the PTA was a major supporter and advocate. The ADA and the American Home Economics Association were professional groups advocating for the program.

One of the strongest supporters and voices for school lunch was the chief state school officers (CSSO), generally known as state school superintendents or commissioners. Dr. Edgar Fuller was executive secretary for the CSSO and a voice for the programs both with the executive and legislative branches in Washington.

In September 1956, ASFSA issued a report card of sorts on the first decade of operation under the National School Lunch Program (NSLP).[68] By that time ASFSA had a national office in Denver and had employed Dr. John Perryman as the executive director who had a major role in program development, including its image, over the next two decades. The report card described the progress made as seen by Dr. Edgar Fuller, executive secretary of the CSSO association, and most state school food service directors. Many states had experienced phenomenal growth both in number of participating schools and in number of meals served, while some states could not initiate programs for lack of facilities. Although Georgia was not allowed to use school funds for school lunch operations, the Georgia General Assembly passed a massive school construction program in 1950, which included provisions for school lunch facilities in every new school building. Other states, including North Dakota, New Hampshire, and Wisconsin, provided facilities in all or nearly all new buildings. The state building programs moved school lunch from the basement to a prominent place in the school building. The ASFSA report showed great progress in the states in developing and conducting statewide training programs. Kansas reported that 86 percent of the school food and nutrition personnel attended state-sponsored training, and South Dakota required attendance of cooks at college short courses.

Not a lot of progress was made in the area of state financing. Many state agency personnel believed, with Congress, that USDA had erred in allowing children's payments to be counted as matching funds. They believed that the one big chance school lunch had to get state tax dollars had been lost with that decision. However, some states were successful in getting state funds appropriated. The Massachusetts state legislature guaranteed nine cents reimbursement for each lunch by providing state supplements to the NSLP Section 4 money. South Carolina provided 50 cents per child in average daily attendance to local schools in addition to providing a supervisor in each county. Other states making significant state tax contributions included California, Hawaii, Louisiana, New York, and Utah. Since 1949, Louisiana has been a leader in state funding for the program. Governor Huey Long promoted a free lunch program for children.

The report card indicated that a number of states were collaborating with instructional personnel to incorporate nutrition education into the classroom and to use the cafeteria as a laboratory. Several states published guides such as New York's *Let's Teach Nutrition* and Florida's *Growing through School Lunch Experiences*. The progress of the first decade was summarized by a statement from Ohio that indicated that progress made in one decade with the NSLP would have taken 50 years if each state had acted independently.

ASFSA's legislative committee was fervent in its efforts to secure increased appropriations from Section 4 funds and USDA commodities, but with minimum success. Increased numbers of meals served without an increase in appropriations meant that schools were receiving less reimbursement per meal. In some states the reimbursement dropped as low as two cents per lunch. Creative approaches were used in states to determine rates of reimbursement as a means of encouraging participation and also to find ways to apply the funds to the schools making the greatest effort to provide a quality program. In Georgia an advisory group of superintendents, principals, and school food and nutrition leaders working with the state agency developed a reimbursement formula that considered number and percentage participation, percentage free, sale price, availability of competitive foods, and cash balances. School records were reviewed and rates as-

signed on a school-by-school basis. Some states also used a formula for sending the funds to the school districts for allocation to the schools. This early period of school lunch program growth provided benchmarks for measuring program outcomes and for examining strategies used to achieve the growth.

CHALLENGES AND NEW DIRECTIONS: THE 1960S

To the disappointment of national and state leaders, USDA did not follow up on recommendations made by the School Lunch Advisory Committee in 1958, which addressed long-range needs. Again, the CSSO under the direction of Dr. Fuller took action and asked USDA to pursue the recommendations of the advisory committee and seek a revision in the NSLA for presentation to Congress in 1960. Since USDA did not respond to this request, the CSSO drafted a bill to revise the NSLA, which was introduced in the U.S. House of Representatives.[69] In testifying before a Congressional committee, Dr. Fuller spoke to the need for revision in the apportionment formula and pointed out that states with the highest student participation were paying the lowest reimbursement rates and, conversely, those states with lowest student participation were able to pay the highest rates. He also spoke to the need for state agency administrative funds to support program expansion and growth, reminding Congress that other federal programs, including the National Defense Education Act and Vocational Education Act, provided for state administration. The USDA opposed the bill.

In the meantime state and local education agencies provided training on a regular basis. Many of the state agency efforts were conducted in cooperation with state universities. There was a persistent question regarding the impact of training on program operations. Does it make a difference in the quality of operations? Are the most effective training strategies being used? USDA's Southeast Regional

Office and the Florida Department of Education developed a bulletin, *Evaluation of School Lunch Training*. The bulletin was distributed nationally by USDA and focused on evaluation before, during, and after training.

The year was 1962. There was a new president in the White House and a new perspective on the needs of this country. Many positive changes occurred in the decade, along with many trials. Several of President John Kennedy's goals were to have long-lasting effects on the child nutrition program. America's efforts to match Russia's launch of Sputnik in 1957 was reflected in President Kennedy's goal to put a man on the moon in the 1960s. Secretary of Agriculture Orville Freeman used this goal as a launching pad to issue the statement, "never let it be said of America in the sixties, that it put a man on the moon and failed to put food in the mouths of hungry children." A bill to amend the NSLA that contained the elements of the CSSO proposals had the support of the Kennedy Administration and of many groups, including the CSSO, ASFSA, the American Parents Committee, PTA, and state school food service directors. In Congressional hearings, Secretary of Agriculture Orville Freeman and USDA's school lunch program administrator supported the bill. It addressed two major concerns: (1) to have a more appropriate formula for apportioning money to the states and (2) to have supplemental funding for meals served to needy children. The bill also addressed the need for state administrative funds. Georgia's state school superintendent and the newly appointed state director visited Senator Russell in his Georgia office to explain the value of the proposed changes to Georgia schools. Since Georgia had a program in every school and had a high participation rate, the schools were receiving less than three cents per lunch.

Congress approved the legislation and Public Law 87-823 was signed by President John Kennedy on October 15, 1962. This was the first substantive change to the NSLA since it was enacted in 1946, and it began a new era in school lunch. The act amended Section 4 and added a new Section 11. The amendment to Section 4 provided that funds would be apportioned on the basis of (1) the participation rate for the state and (2) the assistance need rate for the state. It also added language that, contingent upon adequate appropriations, no state would receive less than five cents per lunch, with a range up to nine cents for states with lowest per capita income.

The new Section 11 provided for supplemental funds to be paid for meals served in needy schools. It required that the following criteria be considered in determining schools to receive supplemental funds: (1) economic condition of the school area, (2) need for free/reduced meals, (3) percentage free/reduced meals served, (4) lunch price compared with other schools in the state, and (5) need for additional assistance. The assistance resulting from this legislation was in the form of special commodities, and the program was called the Special Commodity Assistance Program (SCAP).[70] Section 11 support was not made in cash payments until 1966 and then it was limited to needy schools.

A new war was launched in America—the War on Poverty. With this, national awareness of hunger and malnutrition gained momentum in the 1960s. A 1962 USDA study indicated that nine million children attended schools without a lunch program. As a means of focusing national attention on school lunch, National School Lunch Week was established by a Joint Resolution of Congress, October 9, 1962. The resolution designated the seven-day period beginning the second Sunday in October each year to be observed with appropriate ceremonies and activities.[71] Speaking at ASFSA's annual convention in 1963, the assistant secretary of agriculture spoke to the need for program expansion.

Early in the Kennedy Administration Bud Wilkinson, Oklahoma's former football coach, was named the nation's first physical fitness coordinator. He linked exercise and fitness inextricably with nutrition when he made the statement, "It is possible to be well-nourished and not physically fit, but it is not possible to be physically fit without being well-nourished." Wilkinson's statement citing nutrition as an integral part of physical fitness sent a dramatic message around the nation.

The meal pattern was modified to reflect current research. With revision of the recommended dietary allowance in 1963, USDA expanded meal pattern requirements to and recommendations include iron-rich foods in school meals. A major issue emerged from the U.S. Grocers' Association, which expressed concern over potential competition with local markets when government distributed food to schools. It also cited the high cost of such a program.[72] The commodity issue was to become a persistent one that Congress would deal with many times in subsequent years.

The decade of the 1960s was a time of trial. The president was assassinated. In support of President Lyndon Johnson's goals for The Great Society and continuing the War on Poverty, Congress passed the Civil Rights Act. With increased emphasis on both civil rights and the plight of the poor, Congress passed the Elementary and Secondary Education Act (ESEA) in 1965. The ESEA was administered by the department of education. Both acts had a major impact on school lunch. The ESEA provided funds for strengthening state departments of education (Title V) and for helping local school districts expand and strengthen programs in schools with high concentrations of educationally deprived children (Title I).

School food and nutrition leaders working on an SSWC project had outlined ways to use ESEA funds effectively for free lunches, nutrition education, equipment, starting breakfast programs, and state agency staffing. When the new federal funds arrived in the states, school food service offices applied for funds based on the SSWC plans—and millions of dollars were available for these justified purposes. This extensive support from ESEA was short-lived.

By the next appropriation, the instructional people in schools asked for the money to be used for purposes related to classroom instruction, attendance, and compensatory education. A ruling was handed down that Title I was not to be used for school food and nutrition purposes.[73] Prior to the ruling, many states and districts had budgeted ESEA funds to supplement NSLA funds. An analysis of 500 Title I projects indicated that more than 100 used funds to provide for breakfasts or expanded school lunch programs. Some state agencies budgeted Title I administrative funds for nutrition education.[74]

Congress heard an outcry from across the nation when ESEA funds were no longer available to support feeding programs for children. An iron-clad bond emerged among partners at the local, state, and national level in support of funds for feeding children. Stories were heard of children raiding dumpsters on weekends for food, of children taking part of their school meal home for younger siblings, of the emaciated appearance of children who came to school without food and went home without food, of the many times a teacher or principal would carry a sick or disruptive child to the cafeteria in the morning for a glass of milk and piece of toast. These were but a few of the heart-rending tales that Congress members were told in hearings, letters, and back-home visits.

The ESEA had set a precedent. Hungry children had been fed, and this had made a difference. Schools had used funds effectively for child nutrition purposes; superintendents, nutritionists, social workers, and health officials reported to Congress the value of breakfasts and lunch in getting children to school on time and keeping them on task in the classroom. Success stories were reported from teachers and superintendents. A South Georgia superintendent reported that prior to starting the Title I breakfast program, some children from low-income families never got to school on time. After the breakfast program began, children were at school by 6:30 AM, waiting on the doorstep for breakfast when he arrived. Many public interest groups began working at the community level as well as in Washington advocating increased child nutrition programs.

All of this gave impetus to the need for expanded programs and additional funds for feeding children. The fiscal year 1966 Appropriations Act provided the first monies to fund Section 11 (NSLA), the special assistance provision that had been added in 1962.[75] When President Johnson submitted his proposal for the Child Nutrition Act to Congress, he indicated that many children do not have the 25 cents to buy lunch and many attend schools that lack facilities.

The Child Nutrition Act of 1966

The Child Nutrition Act was passed in 1966.[76] In its Declaration of Purpose, Congress stated:

In recognition of the demonstrated relationship between food and good nutrition and the capacity of children to develop and learn, based on the years of cumulative successful experience under the NSLP with its significant contributions in the field of applied nutrition research, it is hereby declared to be the policy of Congress that these efforts shall be extended, expanded, and strengthened . . . as a measure to safeguard the health and well-being of the Nation's children, and to encourage the domestic consumption of agricultural and other foods by assisting States . . . to meet more effectively the nutritional needs of children.

The Child Nutrition Act authorized

- a pilot breakfast program for two years to help close the nutrition gap for needy children or for children who travel long distances by bus

- the special milk program for three years
- non–food assistance (equipment) on a three-to-one matching basis for the purpose of extending lunch and breakfast programs
- state administrative expense funds to support state expansion efforts
- the USDA as the federal agency for administering all school food service programs

Basic requirements for the breakfast program paralleled those for school lunch. The meal would be based on sound nutrition standards, the program would be nonprofit, there would be no discrimination between paying and nonpaying children, and the school would be responsible for maintaining accurate records and reports. The meal pattern for the breakfast program was established by USDA to provide at least one-fourth of the recommended daily allowance (RDA). The meal pattern included one-half pint fluid, whole milk, served as a beverage or on cereal; one-half cup of fruit or full-strength fruit or vegetable juice; one slice of whole-grain or enriched bread, rolls, or muffins; or three-fourths cup of whole-grain or enriched cereal. It was suggested that the breakfast include protein-rich foods as often as practical.

With the escalation of the Vietnam War, there was not enough money to fund the Child Nutrition Act fully, but a beginning was made with an appropriation of $7.5 million for breakfasts and $12 million for non–food assistance. There were several obstacles facing breakfast program expansion. Some administrators were reluctant to expand breakfast at the expense of lunch; others were getting money from a combination of the Economic Opportunity Act (EOA) and Title I funds at higher rates than the Child Nutrition Act provided; in many instances there were philosophical barriers regarding the role of the breakfast program in school and the responsibility of parents to provide breakfast, and in other places the primary barrier was bus schedules.

In some places the principal barrier was school food service personnel. When food service personnel in a school in South Carolina were told that a breakfast program would be operated during the next school term, the entire staff resigned with the exception of one person. The director faced the new school term with a new program and an entirely new staff, and she proudly told of the way the new staff pitched in and the school had a great year.

School food and nutrition leaders were confronted with many operational issues related to program expansion, including staffing, escalating meal costs, food management companies, state funding, competitive foods, personnel training, and standards. States were making progress in developing personnel standards and in providing training. Some examples of training programs for school-based personnel are included to describe the diversity of approaches to training. In Georgia, a comprehensive training program for managers was established in cooperation with vocational education, and in Mississippi a certification program was implemented in connection with its training program and a requirement for new managers' training. South Dakota's training program had been ongoing on university campuses since the 1940s, and California had a collaborative relationship with universities for a formal training for food service personnel. (See Chapter 4 for additional information on training.)

States were also making progress in getting certification for food service directors based on standards similar to those established by the Joint Committee in the late 1940s. Florida established a certificate for food service directors in the early 1950s. Louisiana was another leader in establishing professional requirements for food service directors and in state funding. The Georgia certification for directors was recommended by the Teacher Education Council and established by the state board of education in 1965. Many state agencies were silent on requirements for the food service director, and the position was often filled by principals, business managers, and managers who had achieved the position because of success at the school level.

Two reports provide a picture of the school food and nutrition program after two decades of operating under the NSLA[77] USDA reports indicated that 71,000 schools participated in the lunch program in fiscal year 1967 and that free and reduced-price meals accounted for only 11 percent of the total meals served. The average rate of reimbursement was 4.5 cents, and the meal cost was 48 cents.

ASFSA prepared another report card of school lunch operations in 1967, which was compiled from a survey in which 37 states participated. The findings were as follows:

- Only 11 states had certification plans, with 12 states requiring the state director to have a master's degree.
- Personnel training was a shared responsibility, with 20 states conducting training and 14 states sharing responsibility with higher education.
- State and local tax contributions varied widely, with 15 states appropriating from 1 to 50 cents per child per year and seven states appropriating over $5 per child per year.
- Only five reporting states did not use Title I (ESEA) funds to supplement NSLP funds. These funds were used for labor, food, reduction of lunch prices, equipment, breakfast programs, and system-level supervision.
- States were proactive in making program improvements, including preparing training courses, developing bulletins, and promoting breakfast programs; nine states were involved in research studies.
- Sixteen states were processing claims electronically, and several states were involved in computer programs for planning menus, nutrient analysis, and production records.
- There was a nationwide trend toward centralization of purchasing, record keeping, and menu planning.

• Georgia had initiated a comprehensive computerized claims payment process and a management information system in 1965.

The War on Poverty had awakened the nation to the need for attention to the nutritional welfare of children. If education goals were to be realized, a healthy and productive citizenry achieved, and health care costs controlled, the basic nutrition needs of children had to be addressed. From 1966 to 1968 many significant events took place, among them four nationwide studies.

1. USDA sponsored a study by the Wisconsin Alumni Research Foundation on the nutritive content of school lunches. The study consisted of chemical analysis of 6,000 meals in 300 randomly selected schools. The study showed that meals were generally meeting the nutritional goal of one-third of a child's daily food needs.[78]
2. USDA conducted a study of the food consumption of households during the spring of 1965.[79] The study revealed that U.S. diets had deteriorated since the last parallel study in the previous decade. The findings gave impetus to a national effort directed by Secretary of Agriculture Orville Freeman to make a comprehensive effort for a nationwide nutrition education program. Secretary Freeman directed that priority be directed toward children and young families. State school lunch agencies were directed to be proactive in developing coordinated nutrition education programs and determining the extent of still-unmet school day nutrition need in schools. The local school district was expected to determine need, expand and strengthen programs, and initiate breakfast programs, all directed toward meeting total school day nutrition needs of children.
3. The Committee on School Lunch Participation,[80] a broad-based group of five women's groups conducted a study of the school lunch program with a goal of full participation of children from low-income families. The findings reported in *Their Daily Bread* and at a national press conference included inadequate funding at all levels, pupil sale prices too high, large numbers of unreached students, and the sense of defeat and dissatisfaction felt by school food and nutrition personnel. The Committee reported negative attitudes relating to many aspects of the program, including commodities, the welfare stigma, and lack of parental responsibility. The study set as a goal the establishment of a universal free program and recommended the following: an effort to reduce sale price to 20 cents, a federal reimbursement rate of 11 cents per meal, that children's payments not be counted as matching money, that commodity level and quality be stabilized, a uniform method for determining need be established, that special assistance (Section 11) rates be high enough to enable schools to reach all needy pupils, and, finally, that incentive grants be available to encourage and advocate development of comprehensive school food and nutrition programs.
4. USDA conducted a study in 1968, Operation Metropolitan, to determine the extent and adequacy of programs in cities of 250,000 or more. This study gave impetus to providing funding for major cities to build centralized food preparation facilities that would allow distribution of meals to schools in the inner cities.[81]

School food and nutrition leaders at every level of ASFSA were mobilized and energized in support of program expansion. The state directors' section of ASFSA held a postconvention workshop in August 1967 following the annual national conference. This two-day workshop allowed time for the state directors to explore common needs and develop strategies for working together. For many state directors, this was the first time for a national meeting, as USDA meetings were held on a regional basis. The meeting was planned by the regional representatives of the state directors' section, which had been meeting regularly at a time that coincided with ASFSA's legislative committee. The state directors' section was analyzing needs and providing information to the legislative committee through its chairperson.

USDA called a national meeting of state school food service directors in 1968 for the first time in 22 years. Rodney Leonard, administrator of USDA's consumer and marketing service, which had oversight responsibility for school food and nutrition programs, indicated that the impetus for this workshop was his participation in a southeast area brainstorming retreat held in Sapphire, NC, in 1967. The retreat convinced him of the need for state directors to share ideas and work with USDA officials to develop long-range goals and plans mutually for school food service and nutrition education. From this national workshop, four committees were appointed to explore various needs: (1) ways of reaching needy children; (2) federal-state administration, requirements, and policies; (3) financial needs and problems; and (4) nutrition education and personnel training. Each committee made recommendations for consideration by USDA. One major outcome was a collaborative effort by USDA and land-grant colleges to hold a series of five workshops for school food service directors and supervisors. The first workshop was held at The University of Tennessee in 1969.

During the 1960s, ASFSA and the Association of School Business Officials (ASBO) collaborated in preparing several publications, including *School Food Purchasing Guide, The School Food Service Director,* and *A Guide for Financing School Food Service Programs.* ASBO's school food service committee was expected to produce a bulletin on a periodic basis. Thelma Flanagan and Irene Ponti of Connecticut, along with John Perryman, were influential in developing the partnership with ASBO. A number of school food and nutrition leaders became Registered School Business Officials (RSBO), a professional registration begun by ASBO in 1964.

An issue that had been discussed since the 1950s was the role of food management companies in school food service operations. With the clearly stated legislative intent that only nonprofit food service programs would be eligible for federal assistance, it appeared that legislation would be necessary to allow school districts that contracted with management companies to continue receiving federal assistance. In the late 1960s a bill was introduced and rejected that would have allowed school districts contracting with management companies to receive federal funding. However, USDA issued a rule that allowed food management companies to contract with school food authorities for the operation of certain aspects of school food programs contingent upon the contracts meeting federal and state requirements.[82]

Amid the many studies and recommendations was the strong need identified for nutrition programs for young children in day-care homes and child-care centers and for school-age children during the time school was not in session. One of the heart-rending stories of this era came from a classroom teacher in southeast Georgia who was telling her students goodbye at the end of the school term and wishing them a happy summer, when one of her young students looked up at her with tears in his eyes and said, "But where am I going to get my something to eat?" This message was repeated thousands of times throughout the nation. Leaving children without food for three months was cruel. In response, Congress amended the NSLA in 1968 to create the special food service program for children. Pilot projects were authorized to provide (1) a full-year food program for children in day care and (2) a summer food program. Other provisions included an allowance for the special dietary needs of students, an extension of the school breakfast program, and provision of state administrative funds for the child care, summer and section 11 programs.[83]

In response to the outpouring requests of community action groups, advocates, and the research community, Congress approved formation of the Senate Select Committee on Nutrition and Human Needs to explore the issue of hunger and nutrition. Perhaps as much as any other single force, the Select Committee brought credibility to the issue as it heard testimony from all walks of life that presented problems, described needs, and proposed solutions. The bipartisan committee was composed of seven senators, including George McGovern (SD), chair; Edward Kennedy (MA); Hubert Humphrey (MN); Patrick Leahy (VT); Edward Zorinsky (NE); Charles Percy (IL); Robert Dole (KS); and Richard Schweiker (PA). The committee gathered and reported information that in many instances was used to support proposed legislation or was drafted into proposals by appropriate committees of the Senate. The committee heard from academia, community advocates, educators, health and nutrition professionals, the public, school food and nutrition personnel, and the medical community. One of the many accomplishments of the Select Committee was creating national awareness of the relationship between nutrition and chronic disease, which ultimately led to the establishment of Dietary Guidelines for America.

The School Cafeteria was the basic reference on school lunch from 1936 until the 1960s, when two textbooks were written. *School Food Centers*, coauthored by Ruth Heckler and N. L. George, Assistant Superintendent in Oklahoma City Public Schools, published in 1960, focused on administrative aspects. *The School Lunch,* written by Marion Cronan, was published in 1962 and presented a more holistic approach to school lunch operations. *The School Lunch* was used extensively as a reference in program operations and for training for many years. In 1975, Dorothy Van Egmond Panell authored *School Foodservice*

Management, which filled a needed gap as a reference for food service directors, and in 1986 Mary Nix and Jay Caton published *I Can Manage* as a practical guide in managing at the school site.

ASFSA's Advocacy Role Established

No record of the 1960s would be complete without including at least three more events. As pressure mounted on Congress to provide for meals and nutrition education for children, members of Congress looked to ASFSA for information to confirm the need and provide an operational framework for program growth. Among leaders in the House of Representatives was the Honorable Carl Perkins (KY), chairman of the Education and Labor Committee, who had a major influence on child nutrition program legislation throughout the 1970s. In 1968, Congressman Perkins requested Dr. Perryman of ASFSA to bring a panel of school food and nutrition leaders to testify before his committee on the needs in their states. The panel was composed of representatives from New Mexico, Massachusetts, Missouri, North Carolina, Georgia, and Florida. The hearing was scheduled during the Poor People's March on Washington, when thousands came to the city and camped on the grounds of government buildings. While the ASFSA panel was testifying at the meeting of the Education and Labor Committee, the sound of marching footsteps was heard coming through the doors in the rear of the room. From the corners of their eyes with their faces focused on the committee, the panel could see a group of the poor people entering to hear the testimony. As Mr. Perkins asked panel members: "Do you have hungry children in your state?" "Could you use extra funds?" "Would you promote more breakfast programs?" "How many hungry children are out there?" the panelists were answering questions to the best of their knowledge. Panel members gave him an estimated number of needy children in their states. Then he asked, "What will it take to feed all the children?" (One panel member recalled, "At one point during the hearing, I felt a gentle tap on my shoulder and looked around. There stood a woman from Americus at my shoulder, and she whispered, 'I'm so glad to know that we have people who care about our children and are working to see that they are fed.' After the hearing I was invited to Tent City to have a meal with the Georgia group.") As the hearing closed, Mr. Perkins asked the panel if schools could use $100 million to feed kids . . . and in unison the heads gave affirmative nods. To which the Chairman responded, "Would someone please say something, the court recording machine doesn't record nods?" Then he asked Dr. Perryman to provide data within a week to reflect the number of needy children by state. That's how the first $100 million for feeding needy kids came to be. Prior to that appropriation, small amounts of money had been given. Equally important was the recognition that ASFSA would become part of a major network to seek adequate legislation and funding for child nutrition programs. Responsibility for solutions to the issue of hunger was to be shared by many groups working for a common cause.

The second major event in these last years of the 1960s was the role of the media in publicizing the issue of hunger. One of the most dramatic events was a CBS documentary, *Hunger in America*. Cameras traveled from East Coast to West Coast, from rural area to inner city, from the deserts to the sea, pointing out that pockets of poverty exist throughout the nation. Robert Coles and Al Clayton compiled a book of photographs with text entitled *Still Hungry in America*.[84] A number of other books chronicled the issue of hunger in America, including *Hunger USA*,[85] *Let Them Eat Promises*,[86] and *The School Lunchroom: Time of Trial*.[87] These media events enhanced national awareness of the extent of need and aroused in the American people a higher level of commitment to ending hunger.

ASFSA was becoming more proactive and gaining greater recognition as a major partner in the quest for adequate legislation and funding of nutrition programs. ASFSA invited leaders from 14 organizations, including doctors, dentists, teachers, school administrators, parents, health-related organizations, the restaurant industry, USDA, and public interest groups to attend a two-day meeting in Washington to craft a blueprint for child nutrition programs. The major agenda was to address the question Congressman Perkins had proposed, "What will it take to feed all of America's children?" This networking conference produced a commitment from the participating organizations and a nine-point Blueprint for Action, (Exhibit 2–4).

The Blueprint formed the agenda for a 1969 planning conference in Dearborn, MI that involved more than 100 school food service leaders. From the Dearborn conference, a *legislative initiative* emerged that would transform funding of child nutrition programs, a *professional development* outreach that would include member certification, a *nutrition education* effort that actively involved students, and a *public relations* initiative. The report, The Doctrine of Dearborn, defined ASFSA's major initiatives for at least seven years. The Dearborn conference was ASFSA's second planning conference, the first having been held in 1962. The value of member buy-in achieved through joint planning and open discussion resulted in phenomenal successes achieved in the 1970s.[88]

As the Vietnam war escalated, more national focus was given to the war effort and the controversy surrounding America's role in the war. Richard M. Nixon was elected president in 1969. Early in his administration he sent a message to Congress describing the need for overhauling and coordinating food assistance programs. He announced a number of provisions that would shape the program's future[89]:

- The establishment of the Food and Nutrition Service in the USDA with the exclusive concern to be administration of the federal food programs
- A plan to coordinate all services related to food and nutrition under the auspices of the federal government

Exhibit 2–4 ASFSA's Blueprint for Action

- A universal school food service free to every student
- A nutrition education program based in the classroom and tied to the lunchroom
- A professional development program for those entering the child nutrition field and those already in it
- A commitment to use the latest technology for improving school food service products, preparation, and delivery to students
- An expanded role for research and evaluation as a basis for improving all programs
- Using schools and their food service operations to serve a larger clientele; the school as a community center had far-reaching implications for being a major force in the war against hunger
- A three-phased timetable that by 1980 would provide full meal service at school with no charge to any child, and the money to pay for that service
- A public information program that was well-defined and supported by organizations concerned with children's welfare

Source: Adapted with permission from J. Caton, *The History of the American School Food Service Association: A Pinch of Love*, pp. 248–249, © 1990, American School Food Service Association.

- A special supplemental food program for women, infants, and children
- A plan to expand and coordinate the food stamp and commodity distribution program to provide family food assistance
- A call for a White House conference with extensive private sector involvement for improving the food available to Americans

Finally, in the closing paragraph of his message to Congress, Nixon stated: *"But the moment is at hand to put an end to hunger in America itself for all time."*

On June 11, 1969, President Nixon appointed Dr. Jean Mayer as special consultant to the president in charge of organizing the White House conference on food, nutrition, and health in December 1969. Between June and December, state committees were organized to identify, study, and analyze state needs and report these to the task force. Invitations to attend the White House conference were sent to a cross-section of leaders in academia, medicine, public health, the nutrition community, food industry advocates, school food and nutrition professional associations, and social service and civic groups. About 3,000 persons

attended the conference. National task forces were appointed to develop recommendations in six major areas, with 26 task forces serving as subcommittees to these panels. John Perryman (ASFSA), Marion Cronan (MA), and Thelma Flanagan (FL) were among the school food and nutrition leaders tapped for panels.

The report of the White House conference was delivered to President Nixon on December 20, 1969. The conference report contained recommendations related to all phases of child nutrition programs. Two of the more significant ones called for free breakfasts and lunches for all of the nation's schoolchildren and the establishment of a national nutrition education initiative that would permeate all levels of government and reach the child in effective ways. The report of the White House conference on food, nutrition, and health is worthy of review as school food and nutrition leaders seek program excellence.

The War on Poverty spawned almost as many programs as the Great Depression. The EOA initiated the Head Start program for preschoolers. When it was discovered that the diets of many Head Start children were nutritionally deficient, a working relationship was established between USDA and EOA to extend the child nutrition program benefits to preschool children. (See Chapter 11 for more discussion of the Head Start program.)

In December 1969, The Children's Foundation sponsored a meeting in Chicago of 60 lawyers to look at legal remedies to expand program access to more children. At that meeting, Dr. Bruno Bettelheim, a distinguished child psychologist, spoke about the impact of food delivery on the child's physical and emotional well-being. His comments gave emphasis to another dimension of the child nutrition programs; the manner in which food is delivered to children. He stated: "How one is being fed, and how one eats, has a larger impact on the personality than any other human experience."[90] The impact of the Bettleheim speech has placed focus on the eating environment as a critical factor in meeting children's needs.

Congress was bombarded with calls for the expansion of the school breakfast program. Georgia's Senator Herman Talmadge responded to his constituents by asking that a tour of schools be arranged, beginning in middle Georgia and ending in Atlanta, for him to view the need for and value of breakfast programs. He wanted to observe programs and talk with principals and teachers. At the conclusion of the two-day tour, he advised the state director that he would introduce a bill to strengthen and expand the school food and nutrition program. The bill that he sponsored was enacted in 1970 as Public Law 91-248, which revolutionized school food and nutrition programs by building on the proud history of the past and incorporating provisions to ensure that all children would have access to healthful meals during the school day. The bill authorized all schools serving free and reduced-price lunches to receive special assistance funds, established uniform national guidelines to determine eligibility for the free and reduced-price meal program, changed state matching requirements for the lunch program, authorized funds for nutritional training and surveys, created the National Advisory Council on Child Nutrition and provided the secretary with authority to issue regulations concerning competitive foods in schools.

Although the nation achieved the goal of having a man on the moon in the 1960s, it had not achieved the goal of meeting all the nutrition needs of school children.

TRIUMPHS AND TRIALS: THE 1970S

Public Law 91-248 was the first of 16 laws to be enacted between 1970 and 1979 that would directly affect child nutrition programs. The decade of the 1970s was a time when the meaning of involvement, action, and sharing responsibility was crystal clear. It was a time when school food and nutrition leaders as well as all nutrition advocates were on the offense. By the end of the decade that stature was to change. For the most part, the 1970s were rewarding for program advocates. With rapid program expansion throughout the nation, school districts employed scores of well-trained personnel to jump-start programs, to oversee building central kitchens, to retrofit an existing facility planned to serve only one meal and a few children, to develop training programs, and to facilitate nutrition education.

Large numbers of personnel were employed in school food and nutrition programs to staff new and expanded programs, which created a need for increased training. Many persons, competent in other areas of food service or nutrition, did not have previous program experience or an understanding of the school food and nutrition programs. State agencies, ASFSA, and vocational schools expanded training. Under the leadership of ASFSA president, Louise Sublette, a certification program was developed that provided a career ladder in school food and nutrition programs.

Along with the advocacy for new and expanded programs came congressional requests for hard data on program costs. Up to this time each state had its own procedures for program accounting and record keeping consistent with meeting federal reporting requirements. Some states included indirect costs in calculating meal prices, others did not; some included the value of donated foods in meal costs, others did not. There was no way to compare meal costs since no standard was available for meal cost accounting. From this need, USDA funded a research project in the early 1970s to investigate financial aspects of the school food and nutrition program. Thelma Flanagan and Dr. Bob Garvue, of Florida State University, conducted this study, which was part of a much larger study, looking at all of education. The aim of the school food service portion of the study was to gather data that would lead to a uniform system of accounting and record keeping. This would result in states having comparable and accurate data to meet congressional requests.[91] ASFSA members were aggressively promoting a Universal School Lunch Program.[92] If this goal was to be realized, it was imperative for states to provide Congress with accurate and comparable data to establish a funding base for programs.

Many forces were operable at the national, state, and local level leveraging program expansion. The actions of community service groups such as the Community Nutrition Institute, the Children's Foundation, Food Research and Action Committee, and Public Voice were visible not only in Washington but in states and local communities; legal actions were brought against local school boards for failure to respond to the hunger and nutrition needs of children; the ASFSA, ADA, and other professional groups established communication networks for reaching all members of Congress. Labor unions and church groups were partners in the massive effort to secure adequate food and nutrition programs for the nation.

The report of the White House conference was used by ASFSA, along with the doctrine of Dearborn to map a national legislative strategy. The ASFSA theme for 1970 was "feed them all." Between 1971 and 1974 at least four bills were introduced for a universal food service program. Leaders in this effort included Congessman Perkins and Senators Humphrey

and McGovern. Bills were introduced in the Senate and in the House of Representatives for universal school lunch. The response to such an effort was confronted with the words "it costs too much."

The Budget Improvement Act of 1974

Congress determined a need for improved management of the budget process in the 1970s and passed the Budget Improvement Act, which had a profound impact on school food and nutrition programs. Since 1946, for budget purposes, school lunch program funds had been categorized as education. Under the Budget Improvement Act, child nutrition funds were no longer classified under the category of education, but were placed in the income security (welfare) category. The reclassification of school food and nutrition funds for budget purposes gave rise to questions about the use of Section 4 funds (general assistance) for paying children. This question was to be debated many times by Congress during the next two decades.

The debate over the role of Section 4 came sooner than expected. In 1975 President Gerald Ford proposed that states be given a block grant for child nutrition programs with a flat appropriation. Dr. John Perryman wrote in the January 1976 *School Foodservice Journal* after defeat of the proposal and passage of a positive bill in 1975 that "it is quite apparent that he [President Ford] anticipated providing no federal assistance whatsoever for the paying child."[93]

ASFSA and ADA initiated national legislative workshops for the purpose of training members in the area of public policy and legislation. ASFSA's first legislative workshop, held in 1972 with about 100 persons attending, has continued to grow. The 1998 legislative action conference (LAC) had an attendance in excess of 600 persons. Learning the art of communicating with members of Congress, of recognizing the important role of congressional staff, of understanding the issues, of comprehending the significance of timing in the legislative process were but a few of the education sessions at each conference. The legislative issues were thoroughly discussed prior to members going "on the hill" for congressional visits. Many groups arrange meetings with their state delegation to explain the status and needs of programs in their states. At least one congressional committee hearing was generally scheduled during the time of the LAC. The banquet honored a member of Congress who had had a significant impact on child nutrition program legislation. One such memorable banquet was in 1977 when ASFSA honored Senator Hubert Humphrey for his leadership for child nutrition programs. He was introduced by Dr. Jean Meyer, who served as task force chair for the 1969 White House conference.

Senator Humphrey, having completed chemotherapy for a malignancy that was to claim his life very soon, told the group that Congress would probably pass a nutrition education bill that year. And he said that they would not pass it for the right reasons; they would pass it because they would realize that the high cost of health care could be reduced if people would adopt healthy eating habits. He indicated that Congress had not put a price on the suffering caused by chronic disease, or the impact of chemotherapy on the body, but they would finally come to the conclusion that this nation could not afford the luxury of poor food habits. His comments could be summarized with the phrase, chronic disease has pediatric beginnings and geriatric endings.

As the 1970s progressed, the nation was faced with internal strife and economic concerns. President Nixon resigned after the Watergate hearings and Gerald Ford became president. The Middle East oil crisis had an economic impact on the United States that was felt by individuals and institutions. Inflation escalated with the crisis, and budget deficits increased. Congressional concern began to shift to budget deficits and inefficiencies. An energy shortage emerged. The federally assisted child nutrition programs, having been highly visible

in the media for a decade, came under attack for waste. A media blitz resulted that focused on the amount of food wasted in schools. From this evolved congressional debate about the amount of food wasted in school programs and eventually the amendments that created offer verse serve (OVS) in 1975. More information about OVS is included in Chapter 3.

Under ASFSA's leadership state school food and nutrition leaders were interacting regularly with congressional leaders. Sam Vanneman, ASFSA's Washington representative, provided daily reports from Congress; Louise Frolich, ASFSA's liaison with state directors and the legislative committee, reviewed the *Congressional Record* almost daily and transmitted summaries to state and national school food and nutrition legislative leaders. When a problem appeared to be looming on the horizon with a pending bill, a call would go out for a legislative fly-in. Members would fly into Washington for a day to help their congressional delegation understand the meaning of the issue to their states. One such fly-in was called in 1975 after President Ford vetoed a bill. About 150 members flew in for a briefing prior to contacting Congress. One congressman told his delegation that he trusted President Ford's judgment regarding the needs of the country more than that of school food and nutrition personnel. The state legislative leader, in leaving his office after thanking him for the visit, quietly said to him, "Mr. Congressman, when you say your prayers tonight, I hope you will seek guidance about how you will vote tomorrow." The next day the House of Representatives as usual opened with prayer. The chaplain began "Give us this day our daily bread" and proceeded with the prayer. When the call came for voting, anxious school food and nutrition leaders sitting in the gallery watched as their congressmen voted. That reluctant congressman waited until almost all votes had been cast, before finally pulling the yes lever to override the veto. The veto was overridden by a vote of 397 to 18 in the House and by 79 to 12 in the Senate.[94]

Several hundred school food and nutrition leaders met in Vail, Colorado, in the fall of 1976 to plan directions for the future. That meeting represented a new beginning for the ASFSA. A plan emerged that charted ASFSA direction for five years. An extremely significant event at this meeting was the resignation of the executive director, John Perryman. His political science background and superlative communication skills had conveyed a positive image of school food and nutrition programs. These unique qualities had been used to communicate the vision of child nutrition programs that had been verbalized by Mary de Garmo Bryan and Emma Smedley a half-century earlier. His resignation left a large gap in the center. Filling the vacant position was not easy.

A peanut farmer from southern Georgia was elected president of the United States and ASFSA's president was from northern Georgia. Hunger issues had been a major concern of both President Carter and Martin in working on state issues in Georgia. However, the national budget deficit was growing and inflation was escalating when Jimmy Carter became president. There was a national cry to reduce the size of federal spending, to get the budget back in balance. The school lunch program was characterized by some as a "sacred cow" that no one would dare touch with cuts. Therefore, as a means of offering up cuts for the budget in the late 1970s, USDA proposed a cut in Section 4 funds that was accepted by Congress in 1980. Several years later the USDA official proposing this cut indicated that it was offered because he was sure it would not be accepted, but it was. And this began a half-dozen years of struggle to maintain the gains realized in the 1960s and the 1970s. This environmental scan of the 1970s helps explain the rapid development of child nutrition programs in the 1970s.

A quick review of the triumphs of the 1970s, including the 19 bills that amended or modified the National School Lunch Act of 1946 and/or The Child Nutrition Act of 1966, demonstrate the power of partnerships focused on a common goal. An active and energized cadre of school food and nutrition persons worked diligently to meet the rapid pace of program growth, which involved keeping abreast of the bills introduced, providing testimony to congressional committees, and implementing the new legislation at the state and local level. Although each of the 19 laws passed was assigned a number that was preceded by the number of the congressional session, it was an amendment to one of the two umbrella laws that provide for the child nutrition programs.

As previously noted, the first substantive change to the NSLA did not happen for 15 years after its passage in 1946. In contrast, each of the 19 bills passed in the 1970s contained substantive changes. New programs were created and existing programs authorized by the NSLA and/or The Child Nutrition Act were modified; most were modified several times. Amid all these changes, the basic policy was not altered. From year to year, programs were modified to extend provisions or make improvements. The provisions in these 19 bills related to Section 4 and Section 11 funding, competitive foods, commodities, nutrition education, the breakfast program, the summer program, the child care program, provisions for free and reduced-price meals, the women, infants, and children (WIC) program, non–food assistance, and the special milk program. Following is a summary of changes by program area.

Public Law 91-248: the 248th bill passed in the 91st session of Congress. This law amended various sections of the National School Lunch Act of 1946 and the Child Nutrition Act of 1966. Senator Talmadge, chairman of the Senate Committee on Agriculture, Forestry and Nutrition, referred to it as the act that reformed the school lunch program.

Performance Funding for Meals and Commodities

A major accomplishment of the 1970s was a shift away from a capped appropriation and establishment of performance funding for lunches and breakfasts. With performance funding, schools were guaranteed a rate of reimbursement for the school year by meal type. Special assistance funds were authorized for free and reduced-price meals. Prior to the shift to performance funding, the appropriation level was based on the number of meals served the preceding year. With rapid increases in all categories of meals, funds would run out before the end of the school year. Congress would sometimes pass a supplemental appropriation to make up for the shortfall; however, that was not a certainty.

Another funding issue addressed was the reimbursement level for each meal by category. General assistance (Section 4) funds were provided for all meals, and special assistance (Section 11) funds provided an additional amount for free and reduced-price meals. Legislation provided for all rates to be adjusted semiannually for inflation. When the economic crisis occurred, Congress reduced the requirement for adjustment of rates to an annual basis.

Several of the new provisions related to reduced-price meals. In 1973, for the first time, Congress set special assistance rates for free lunches and specified that the reduced-price rate would be 10 cents less than the free lunch rate. In 1978, the reimbursement rate for reduced-price lunches was lowered by 10 cents, by setting it at 20 cents less than the free rate. However, an allowance was made for states that charged less than 20 cents for reduced-price meals to receive an additional reimbursement amount. Especially needy provisions were provided for both the school lunch and the school breakfast programs. In 1973, performance funding was applied to the breakfast program and in 1974 the commodity program was given entitlement status with annual adjustments for inflation.

Uniform Guidelines for Free and Reduced-Price Meals

In 1970, Public Law 91-248 made sure that children from low-income families, regardless of the school they attended, would have access to free or reduced-price meals. Congress directed the secretary of agriculture to develop uniform national guidelines for determining eligibility for free and reduced-price meals. Prior to this legislation, special assistance (Section 11) funds were targeted to schools with a high percentage of economically needy children, and each school district determined criteria for free and reduced-price eligibility.

In 1971, Public Law 92-32 established a provision for eligibility for free lunches to be based on a family income equal to 100 percent of the Census Bureau's poverty income level. Then, in 1972, Public Law 92-433 gave states the option of increasing the eligibility level for free lunches up to 25 percent above the income guidelines and reduced-price lunches up to 50 percent above the guideline, and a year later raised the optional eligibility for reduced-price lunches to 75 percent above the income guideline. In 1975, Public Law 94-105 expanded the eligibility for reduced-price meals to 95 percent above the guidelines. This provision was contained in the bill that President Ford vetoed when the veto was rejected by Congress. In 1978, Public Law 95-627 raised the income eligibility cutoff level from 100 to 125 percent of the USDA poverty guidelines.

National Advisory Council

Public Law 91-248 provided for the establishment of a National Advisory Council. The Council members were appointed by the secretary to advise USDA's Food and Nutrition Service on matters related to program implementation and to collaborate on regulatory concerns and legislative needs. The Council members consisted of child nutrition practitioners, industry representatives, school board members, and the public. The Council's first report was delivered to President Nixon in the Oval Office. Authorization for the council was eliminated with the Budget Reconciliation Act of 1981.

Authorization To Control the Sale of Competitive Foods

Foods sold in competition with school meals had been an issue since the 1940s. In the absence of a USDA regulation concerning the sale of foods and beverages in competition with school meals, each state and/or local school district was left to handle the problem by policy or regulation. In 1970, 1972, and 1977, Congress addressed the issue of competitive foods. In 1970 a provision contained in Public Law 91-248 gave the secretary authority to issue a regulation concerning competitive foods. Upon USDA's issuance of the regulation, the soft drink bottlers' association and other industry representatives concerned about the regulation received a court ruling that the secretary had exceeded his authority by restricting the sale of foods and beverages in schools. In 1972, Public Law 92-433 prohibited the secretary from prescribing regulations prohibiting the sale of competitive foods. In 1977, Public Law 95-166 restored to the secretary the authority to approve the types of competitive foods sold during the time of food service in schools. USDA ultimately issued another rule that defined foods of minimal nutritional value and restricted the sale of foods and beverages in the food service area during the meal period. The rule is extremely weak, as the definition of location is determined by the school and in many places is not enforced. This flurry of bills in the Congress relating to competitive foods reflects the intensity of the issue. The most positive control for the sale of foods and beverages in competition with the school nutrition program will emerge from the state or local community. Several states, including Mississippi, have state board–approved policies that prohibit the sale of

foods and beverages in competition with school meals. Many school districts have strong policies that protect the integrity of foods offered at school.

Special Milk Program Made Permanent

The special milk program was made permanent in 1970.[95] It was begun in 1954 and operated on a year-to-year basis until 1966, when it was authorized under the Child Nutrition Act of 1966. Public Law 93-150 amended the milk program in 1973 so that children eligible for a free lunch would also be eligible for additional free milk. In 1974, a provision was added that established a minimum rate of reimbursement of five cents for each half-pint of milk served in the special milk program with a second provision that the rate would be adjusted annually for inflation. In 1975, eligibility for participation in the special milk program was expanded to include Puerto Rico, the Virgin Islands, American Samoa, and the Trust Territory of the Pacific Islands. The effects of the economic crisis and inflation were beginning to be felt in nutrition programs. In 1977, Public Law 95-166 identified limited conditions under which children could get free milk.

Nutrition Training and Surveys

Public Law 91-248 authorized funding for nutrition training and surveys. States could apply for funding for these special projects. In 1975, USDA was authorized to make grants to states for nutrition education.

School Breakfast Program Made Permanent in 1975

In 1971, Public Law 92-153 extended the School Breakfast Program through fiscal year 1973. The legislation also provided that the secretary's guidelines for determining eligibility for free and reduced-price meals would be used for it as well as for lunch. Minimum rates of reimbursement for breakfasts were set in 1973 for the three categories of meals and for severe need. The reduced-price rate was five cents less than the free rate. Provision was included that rates would be adjusted for inflation. Authorization was provided in 1973 to extend the breakfast program through fiscal year 1975 when Public Law 94-105 gave it permanent status in 1975. The severe need rate for the breakfast program was increased in 1977.

The Summer Food Service Program Established as a Separate Program

In 1971, Public Law 92-35 authorized additional funds for the summer program. The initial appropriation provided insufficient funds to cover the number of lunches served. The summer program was experiencing rapid growth. The program was extended several times in the 1970s. Public Law 94-105 made the summer program and the child care program into two separate programs. It was extended in 1977 through fiscal year 1980, and changes were made to prevent fraud and abuse in the program. The summer food service program had not been permanently authorized in 1997. A request was made in 1998 for the program to be reauthorized.

The Child Care Food Program Established and Made Permanent in 1978

Public Law 92-433 (1972) extended the special food service program, which included child care through fiscal year 1975. The child care food program was created in 1975 apart from the summer food program. Rates for the child care program were authorized at the same level as in the school lunch program. Public Law 95-627 (1978) made the child care food program permanent and substantially revised it by providing a three-tier system of meal reimbursements based on the income groups of children in day-care centers and providing separate payment rates for meals served in family or group day-care homes.

Commodity Program Funded

In 1973, Public Law 93-13 required the secretary to grant cash in lieu of commodities to states when the USDA was unable to provide at least 90 percent of the commodities promised at the beginning of the year. The department was experiencing difficulty getting commodities delivered to schools in a timely manner. Shipments were delivered as late as May, and schools had to pay summer storage costs. For at least two years, the department provided for some cash in lieu as a means of providing funding stability in the schools. Public law 93-326 (1974) established a guaranteed level of commodity assistance to be adjusted annually, thus putting commodity value on same basis as cash reimbursement. Another law was passed in 1974 (Public Law 93-347), which extended the use of Section 32 funds for purchasing commodities through 1977. Because of the uncertainty of commodity delivery and its future there was talk of discontinuing the commodity program. Kansas was the only state that actually phased out the program. Public Law 94-105 (1975) contained special provisions for states that had phased out the commodity program by June 30, 1974, to get cash in lieu of commodities. Since that time Kansas has received cash in lieu of entitlement commodities. However, the state is eligible to receive bonus commodities. Again in 1977, a provision was included in Public Law 95-166 to extend to the USDA authority to purchase commodities to meet commitments.

The commodity issue was unstable. Many school districts, particularly those with central food-preparation facilities or those using ready-prepared foods were requesting cash in lieu of commodities. The 1977 amendments required USDA to conduct a study of cash in lieu of commodities as a response to the need from school districts. Some parts of the food industry also joined in the request that the program be cashed out. Proponents of the commodity program recognized the importance of the child nutrition programs to the agricultural economy. One of the basic program purposes as stated in the NSLA declaration of policy is to increase the consumption of nutritious agricultural commodities. The issue of commodities was possibly the most controversial issue among members of the school food and nutrition profession. Legislation was enacted in the 1980s to permit a limited number of school districts to participate in community alternatives.

Special Supplemental Food Program for Women, Infants, and Children Established

The WIC program was initially authorized in 1972 under Section 17 of the Child Nutrition Act of 1966 and has been reauthorized every four years since its beginning. The legislation contained provisions that required documentation of its progress. The WIC program, unlike the school programs, required that qualified personnel be employed and that an evaluation component be included. Because of this required evaluation, the WIC program has been able to document its impact on reducing infant mortality and low birth weights. Since it was not given permanent status, the WIC program must be considered for reauthorization every four years. Funding for the program is appropriated annually and is capped. In many instances funding is inadequate to meet the identified need of states. For more information about WIC, see Chapter 3.

Nutrition Education and Training Program Established

Beginning with the debates in 1945 and continuing with debates leading up to the passage of the Child Nutrition Act and extending into the 1970s, efforts were made to have funding for nutrition education and training. The ASFSA, ADA, and the Society for Nutrition Education advocated to secure nutrition educa-

tion included in the legislation. The first breakthrough came in 1970 with Public Law 91-248, which authorized funds for nutritional training and surveys and allowed for a small amount of state-allocated funds to be used for this purpose. As evidence mounted from hearings in the Senate select committee on hunger and malnutrition relating chronic disease and nutrition, renewed efforts were made to secure nutrition education and training funds. Public Law 94-105 (1975) authorized the secretary to make cash grants to state agencies to conduct nutrition education projects.

The Five-State Nutrition Education project was an example of projects funded with this provision. Five states in the southeast region applied for a grant to develop a nutrition education training program. The five states included Alabama, Florida, Georgia, Mississippi, and Tennessee. The project was designed to develop a competency-based team approach to nutrition education for school food service managers and elementary school teachers of grades three to five. The project provided a five-day workshop for teachers and managers to develop collaboratively a nutrition education plan for their schools. Three follow-up days were provided for each of the state teams. This project demonstrated the value of state collaboration on projects and, even more important, defined an effective process for making the school food service program a laboratory for nutrition education by using a team approach to training managers and teachers.

The Middle East oil crisis had created a national concern regarding conservation of energy and avoidance of waste. This concern was felt by school food service as media focused on school food and nutrition programs. As noted by the preamble to the Nutrition Education and Training (NET) program, there was recognition that waste in school programs was associated with lack of personnel training and also lack of nutrition education where children learn to eat healthful foods. Finally, 39 years after passage of the NSLA, Public Law 95-166

(1977) was enacted, which authorized funding for the NET program. Unlike other child nutrition programs that make no mention of personnel to manage programs, a nutrition education specialist was recommended for coordination of programs.

The preamble to the NET program in Section 19 of the Child Nutrition Act of 1966 succinctly outlines a conceptual framework and rationale for managing a child nutrition and nutrition education program. It states the following:

- •. The proper nutrition of the nation's children is a matter of highest priority.
- • The lack of understanding of the principles of good nutrition and their relationship to health can contribute to a child's rejection of highly nutritious foods and consequent plate waste in school food service operations.
- • Many school food and nutrition personnel have not had adequate training in food service management skills and principles.
- • Many teachers and school food service operators have not had adequate training in the fundamentals of nutrition or how to convey this information so as to motivate children to practice sound eating habits.
- • Parents exert a significant influence on children in the development of nutritional habits, and lack of nutritional knowledge on the part of parents can have detrimental effects on children's nutritional development.
- • There is a need to create opportunities for children to learn about the importance of the principles of good nutrition in their daily lives and how these principles are applied in the school cafeteria.

NET funding was authorized at 50 cents per child enrolled and was contingent upon a state plan. States received funding at this level in fiscal years 1978 and 1979 and then it was reduced. The NET program funding was provided as a grant to states. It was the only federal money allotted to states for meeting state needs for training and nutrition education. The NET program is the smallest of the child nutrition programs; however, it has been difficult to maintain on a stable basis. Although there is strong advocacy for the program and congressional support for the concept, keeping it funded continues to be an issue. Part of the difficulty in maintaining funding may be attributed to the variety of ways that it has been administered in the states. Unlike the school lunch and breakfast program, states have discretion in how and where it is administered. In some states the program is administered in the health department; in others, in the instructional department of education; and in the majority it is in the child nutrition program. It has generally been most effective when administered as an integral part of the school food and nutrition program. The issue of funds for the NET has been pervasive since 1979 even though a strong advocacy is in place.

The 1970s were a time of many triumphs and some trials. In 1975, President Gerald Ford proposed to replace the child nutrition programs with a block grant. This proposal was defeated; however, it would appear again in the 1980s and again in the 1990s. The 1975 proposal was the first attempt to modify the program's nutrition purpose for all children to a welfare program to reach only the needy.

This overview of the legislative issues and the frequency of their modification in the 1970s provides insight into the fragile nature of any legislation. It also creates an awareness of the importance of school food and nutrition professionals' understanding and being involved in the legislative process.

For each of the 19 bills passed in the 1970s multiple hearings were held in the Senate and in the House. Generally, one or more school food and nutrition professionals and SFS partners would present testimony at each hearing. ASFSA members were in constant contact with their congressional delegations, and ASFSA was actively partnering with other advocates in support of child nutrition issues. The trials encountered signaled challenges to be confronted in the 1980s. The 1970s provided opportunities for many child nutrition professionals and their partners to develop public policy skills that would be extremely helpful in the 1980s and 1990s as major threats to the programs were proposed.

TRIALS AND TRIUMPHS: THE 1980S

The decade of the 1980s could be characterized as the best of times and the worst of times. It was the best of times because congressional support for the programs was at an all-time high, tremendous success had been achieved in getting programs approved and funded, and many partnerships and networks were established in support of child nutrition programs. The ASFSA had a vision for the future of the programs, and the school food and nutrition community was energized, motivated, organized, and competent to deal with issues that were to emerge.

Jimmy Carter was president in 1980 and faced with escalating deficits and an Iranian hostage crisis. It was the worst of times because interest rates were soaring and the American public was asking for controls to be placed on federal spending, which was perceived to be at the center of escalating inflation. The impact of this crisis on child nutrition programs was reflected in Public Law 96-499 (1980), known as the Omnibus Reconciliation Act of 1980, which resulted in a $400 million reduction in child nutrition program funding. The following reductions were made[96]:

- income eligibility criteria reduced by using Office of Management and Budget (OMB) poverty guideline instead of USDA guideline and substituting a standard deduction for special hardship deduction
- school lunch reimbursement rates lowered by four and one-half cents for both cash and commodity assistance
- extra reduced-price reimbursement eliminated for states charging less than maximum allowed charge

- child care food supplement rate reduced by three cents
- annual for semiannual inflation adjustment substituted for all meal reimbursement rates
- subsidy for paid milk served in schools with meal service programs frozen at five cents per half-pint
- meal reimbursements for most summer food programs limited to two meals per day
- nutrition education and training authorization reduced to $15 million per year

On the plus side, the summer food program, WIC, NET, state administrative expense, and commodity distribution programs were reauthorized through 1984.

Ronald Reagan was elected president in 1980. The ASFSA held its third major planning conference in Williamsburg, VA. From this conference emerged a five-year plan that set ASFSA's direction for promoting program expansion and quality improvements. Some plans were sidetracked as the Reagan Administration aggressively moved to reduce the national deficit and the size of government by cutting federal programs and spending.

School food and nutrition leaders under the guidance of ASFSA's leadership mounted a campaign to save the programs. Marshall Matz, who had joined ASFSA's legislative team in 1979 as Washington representative, helped develop an effective strategy to defend child nutrition programs from proposals to have them cut, eliminated, or block granted. ASFSA's legislative network became even more sophisticated; Focus 435, a strategy to have a school food and nutrition contact with every member of the House of Representatives, was implemented.

Despite all the efforts by child nutrition advocates, another Omnibus Reconciliation Act was passed in 1981 (Public Law 97-35). This time the cuts were even deeper. Child nutrition funding was reduced by $1.4 billion or approximately 25 percent. Among the changes: another lowering of the income eligibility criteria for reduced-price meals from 195 percent of the OMB poverty guideline to 185 percent; a substantial reduction in school lunch and breakfast cash reimbursement rates and commodity assistance; allowable charges for reduced-price lunches raised from 20 cents to 40 cents and for reduced-price breakfasts from 10 cents to 30 cents. The bill also excluded private schools charging tuition in excess of $1,500 per year from participating in any child nutrition program, prohibited participation in the special milk program of any school offering meal service, changed the method of paying reimbursement for child care centers, and reduced the number of meals that could be reimbursed in the centers. The act limited the summer food program by changing criteria for sponsorship. It ended the food service equipment program and lowered funding authority for the NET program to $5 million per year.[97]

The impact of these cuts was nearly disastrous. Student participation in the school lunch program declined from 26 million in 1980 to 24 million per day. The uncertainty of funding combined with the cuts created turmoil in schools. A large number of schools dropped the NSLP. Many others, while maintaining the NSLP, expanded the à la carte offerings as a means of generating revenue to offset program cuts. In many of these schools, the NSLP was perceived as a welfare program where only poor children ate the NSLP meal. The à la carte program in many instances had the effect of a being a food service in competition with the NSLP. The à la carte offerings were often based on student preferences without regard to the nutritional needs of students.

Congress authorized a pilot program for a limited number of school districts to test the concept of receiving cash in lieu of commodities beginning in 1982. This pilot program was extended many times. It is not unusual for pilot programs to become almost permanent as authorization continues to be extended. From 1981 through 1988 the Reagan administration proposed curtailing food assistance sharply, and to shift the burden of federal support to the states and private charities. Measures were introduced each year to reduce the programs even more. Some of the measures proposed included eliminating Section 4 funding for paid meals; others proposed providing a block grant to the states and allowing states to determine how the funds would be used; others simply proposed block grants with an appropriated amount for school meals, thereby eliminating performance funding. One of the more draconian measures was the proposal to allow catsup to be counted as a vegetable.

While the 1981 cuts were detrimental, they were sufficient to provide child nutrition advocates with an even greater determination to maintain the programs for all children. Even Congress seemed to feel that these programs had taken more than their share of cuts in 1981. ASFSA's defense in the 1980s was as effective as its offense had been in the 1970s. The efforts of the administration failed because by midway in the first Reagan term, a national consensus had emerged that federal nutrition programs were essential community resources and that no community could cope with hunger on its own. Congress refused to limit federal support for school lunch and breakfast programs for children from low-income families.[98]

By midterm in the Reagan years there appeared to be some release of the determination to change the nature of the programs to welfare programs. Another child nutrition bill was not passed until 1986, when expiring programs, including NET, SAE, WIC, the commodity distribution program, and the Summer Food Service Program, were reauthorized through 1989.[99] As previously noted, some programs are permanently authorized and others must be considered for reauthorization every four years. The NSLP, the School Breakfast Program, and the Child and Adult Care Food Program (CACFP) are permanently authorized, which means that Congress does not have to take any action on these programs.

However, it does not preclude Congress from changing the programs in any way it desires. This was most evident in 1996 when Congress, through the Welfare Reform Act, changed the NET program authorization from permanent with mandated funding to discretionary.

The 1986 amendments also provided automatic eligibility for free meals to children in households receiving food stamps or approved for Aid to Families with Dependent Children (AFDC), where the AFDC eligibility did not exceed 130 percent of the federal poverty guidelines. It restored the provision that allowed private schools with tuition in excess of $1500 to participate in the programs. This legislation made many substantive changes to the child nutrition program that either clarified or modified existing programs.

There were no more major reductions in the programs. According to a report from the Congressional Research Service, The National Defense Reauthorization Act for 1987 included essentially the same provisions for child nutrition as the 1986 amendments. This backup legislation was approved by Congress as a means of protecting the amendments in the event of a presidential veto.

Public law 100-71 (1987) made provision to restore some of the programs eliminated earlier and to provide for appropriations to cover funding shortfalls in the program. As another election year was near, it was not unexpected to see some lessening of the draconian measures that had been taken earlier in the 1980s. Public Law 100-327 (1988), the Commodity Distribution and Reform Act, provided measures that responded to concerns of school food and nutrition personnel regarding the quality of commodities being purchased for programs. This legislation provided (1) for an advisory council to report its findings and recommendations annually to the secretary of agriculture and to the authorizing committees of the Senate and the House and (2) a comprehensive set of requirements for the secretary to follow to reform all aspects of the commodity distribution program. From these requirements the USDA overhauled the quality of commodities and the system used to make products program-friendly.

As an integral part of the ongoing concern regarding commodity distribution, Congress authorized some school districts to test two different methods of commodity support, including cash in lieu and the commodity letter of credit on a pilot basis. The authority to continue these programs was extended through 1990,[100] and again extended in 1994 to 1998 and extended once more in 1998 until 2003. As noted, it is not unusual for Congress to continue pilot programs once they have been initiated.

Two laws were passed in 1987 that had an impact on child nutrition programs. The NSLA was amended to permit adult day-care centers to receive reimbursement under the child care food program. The growing numbers of homeless persons, including children, prompted Congress to establish the Stewart B. McKinney Homeless Assistance Act.

As the cloud over the child nutrition programs seemed to have passed, ASFSA's desire to resume an offense was discussed. The questions was, "What can ASFSA propose that would have a positive impact on programs and wouldn't cost much money?" The nation was still trying to recover from the economic catastrophies of the early 1980s, including the salvaging of savings and loans institutions. ASFSA had been through another five-year planning conference and established an agenda for the last part of the decade. One item that had been on the agenda since 1976 and the Vail conference was a need for a food service management institute. In 1987, ASFSA asked Congress to approve a feasibility study to determine the need for a food service management institute. Congress approved $50,000 for a feasibility study to look at the need for establishing an institute in Mississippi. The study was conducted and submitted to Congress supporting an institute. Despite the USDA's response to the study report, which noted that sufficient research, training, and education were being conducted without such an institute. Congress authorized the institute in 1989 and funded it in 1990. (1991 fiscal year appropriations.)

Between 1988 and 1990, Congress enacted a number of measures restoring or strengthening child nutrition. George Bush was inaugurated as U.S. president in 1989. Although the budget deficit continued to be a burning issue with Congress and the American people, the nation seemed to have once again turned attention to needs of people rather than total concentration on reducing the size of government.

The School Breakfast Program

Public Law 100-135 (1988) added three cents to the school breakfast rate and Public Law 101-147 (1989) provided start-up money to assist schools in getting breakfast programs under way.

Child Care Food and Adult Care Program

Public Law 100-135 added three cents to the breakfast rate in child care centers and authorization for an additional meal to be offered. In 1989, authorization was provided for certain schools to claim reimbursement under the school lunch program for snacks served in after school care programs. Public Law 101-147 renamed the program the CACFP and authorized several demonstration projects.

Summer Food Service Program (SFSP)

Public Law 100-135 restored participation in SFSP to colleges and universities offering sports programs for youth, and authorized some demonstration projects related to sponsorship.

Reauthorized Programs

Public Law 101-147 reauthorized the following programs: State Administrative Expense, WIC, and the Commodity Program.

School Lunch Program

Public Law 101-135 modified requirements for the meal application by requiring the addition of a social security number of an adult member of the household and made provisions for testing alternatives for meal counting requirements. Public Law 101-147 required schools to offer low fat milk as an option. It also required USDA to develop and publish, *Nutrition Guidance for Child Nutrition programs*, for use in the school lunch and breakfast, CACFP, and summer food programs.

Food Service Management Institute

The NFSMI was authorized under Section 21 of the NSLA in 1989 (Pub.L. 101-147),[101] funded in fiscal year 1991, and given permanent authorization in 1994. The institute is unique in that its purpose is to support improved operations in federally assisted food and nutrition a programs through applied research, education, and training and to serve as a clearinghouse for studies, materials, and findings. For more information about NFSMI, see Chapter 3.

ON TRACK FOR THE FUTURE: THE 1990S

Turning the corner into the 1990s appeared to offer promise of a less traumatic time for child nutrition programs than the first half of the 1980s. Although the issue of the federal deficit was still on the minds of congressional members and the American people, for the moment, there seemed to be less threat of program reductions. Concern was growing for the number of homeless people and the need to provide for them, especially the young children who were in homeless shelters. Demonstration projects were authorized to determine effective ways to help homeless preschool children.

There was continuing concern about how to structure the commodity program so that it could best meet the needs of contemporary school food and nutrition programs. Since the beginning of federal support for school lunch programs in the 1930s, technological advancements in food processing, changes in the labor market, food delivery systems, and health and education programs had created a demand for changes in the quality of food, its form, and the method of delivery. Public Law 101-124 provided for a study of the bonus commodities being delivered.

At least three events of the early 1990s had a major impact on the direction that programs were to take. *Healthy People 2000,* the health objectives of the nation with specific objectives for child nutrition programs, was a major force in linking child nutrition programs to health. The Revised Dietary Guidelines for Americans and the Food Guide Pyramid were products that supported the nation's health objectives. The second event was the adoption of the educational goals by the nation's governors, which linked nutrition to learning readiness. In 1994, Congress formally adopted *Goals 2000* as an integral part of the Educate America Act (Pub.L. 103-227). The third event emerged from ASFSA, which defined nutrition integrity at its 1989 five-year planning conference and made it a cornerstone for school programs.

Since the early 1970s ASFSA had advocated for a universal school feeding program. And in the early 1990s two needs emerged that gave stimulus to that goal. States and local districts

---

UNIVERSAL FEEDING—
THE SCHOOL DISTRICT OF
PHILADELPHIA

During the 1990–1991 school year, the USDA initially approved a three-year pilot program that allowed all students to participate in the universal feeding program (UFP). Unlike the regular programs, schools are not required to take meal applications to determine a child's eligibility, and no children pay for their

---

meals. The pilot program has been extended through June 30, 2000.

The program is designed to increase student participation in breakfast and lunch and to eliminate burdensome paperwork. Paperwork was reduced by eliminating meal applications, tickets, and eligibility lists. Major benefits derived from the UFP was the removal of the stigma that goes with identifying children who receive free and/or reduced-price meals and providing relief to administration.

Some examples of the impact that the UFP has had are as follows:

- Of the students enrolled in UFP schools, 66.5% participated in the lunch program compared with 41% in non–UFP schools.
- Of students enrolled in UFP schools, 25.7% participated in the breakfast program compared with 12.9% enrolled in non–UFP schools.
- The UFP saves school administrators an estimated 24,000 hours annually by eliminating the need to review and process free and reduced-price meal applications.
- The elimination of meal tickets or rosters saves cafeteria workers an estimated 19,000 hours annually.

The UFP has proven to be very successful and has received positive responses from parents, children, administrators, and the community.[102]

Source: Courtesy of P. Schmid, *Universal Feeding—The School District of Philadelphia,* unpublished article, 1998, Philadelphia, Pennsylvania.

---

voiced concern to Congress about the amount of paperwork required. In response, Congress authorized two or more pilot programs to reduce paperwork and increase participation.[102] Generally, these pilots were referred to as pilot universal school food service programs. The Philadelphia school district was selected to conduct one of the pilot programs. From the 1920s with Emma Smedley, Philadelphia continues to be a leader in the program.

In 1992 the nation elected Bill Clinton as president. As Governor of Arkansas, Clinton had been a proponent of improving education and a national leader in having the governors adopt the national education goals. Both he and Mrs. Clinton were longtime advocates for expanded and improved services for children. Therefore, it was no surprise to have education and children topping a list of their priorities.

From the beginning of the Clinton administration, school meal quality became a major issue. USDA held hearings across the nation about the school meals program, which resulted in a report to Congress. In 1994 Congress passed the Healthy Meals for Americans Act, amendments to the NSLA.[103] These comprehensive amendments required implementation of the Dietary Guidelines in school meals, provided for improvements in the commodity program, and directed the USDA to provide technical assistance and training to help improve the program. In support of these requirements, Congress appropriated $20 million for nutrition education and public information and training of parents, teachers, and personnel. USDA's rules for implementing the requirements gave states and school districts flexibility in the process of implementation. (See Chapter 10 for more information about regulatory provisions related to meal options.)

The process used to achieve a focus on nutritional quality of school food and nutrition programs created some controversy. However, for the first time in NSLA's history the focus was on the quality of meals offered. Funds were appropriated for developing a comprehensive information, education, and training program for all school food and nutrition program stakeholders. *Team Nutrition*, the name

chosen for the project, incorporated the essential elements of a marketing and education program needed to create public awareness of the relationship between nutrition and health, and nutrition and learning. Literally thousands of schools joined the *Team Nutrition* initiative.

The tide had a momentary turn. The 1994 general election had a massive impact on the way the nation is governed. There was a Democrat in the White House; however, both houses of the Congress had Republican majorities. National concern regarding the state of the economy and the size of the budget deficit were priority issues with both the executive and the legislative branches of government. The Republican majority devised a Contract with America—a plan for downsizing government and getting the budget deficit under control. The Speaker of the House of Representatives set as a goal to have the Contract with America adopted in the first 100 days of the session. The Contract proposed to refocus school meals programs by eliminating all support for paying children and appropriating money through block grants to states where the governor of each state would determine the distribution of funds for food assistance programs. ASFSA, under the leadership of President Vivian Pilant, and its child nutrition partners mobilized forces that effectively defeated most of the measures relating to child nutrition programs.

The following material is condensed from an article by Karolyn Schuster that originally appeared in the May 1998 issue of *Food Management Magazine*.[104]

With the threat of a refocused program over, school food and nutrition members resumed their efforts to implement the directives of the Healthy Meals for Children Act. In 1996, Congress passed a small bill indicating that school districts could use any reasonable approach to meal planning as long as the nutrition goals of the Dietary Guidelines for Americans were achieved.[105]

Another first in the long and successful history of the NSLP was achieved in 1997. President Clinton appointed Shirley Watkins, for-

The most resounding success of Vivian Pilant's year-long term as ASFSA President centered on an unexpected challenge—federal block grants, and a completely unexpected challenger—Newt Gingrich. . . . Many in school food service saw this as the most threatening period in the 50-year history of the school lunch program. As initially conceived, the Contract would have dismantled the federal school nutrition program and replaced it with a state-administered systems of block grant funding. In the worst case scenario, the national program delivering 32 million meals a day to the nation's students would have been gone. The federal standards for monitoring food quality and meal components would have been obsolete. The publicly released proposals in the fall of 1994 were an open declaration of war.

School food and nutrition professionals were briefed, rehearsed, equipped with media talking points, and sent out to preach their message that school meals were an intrinsic and valuable part of the education system and not an adjunct of the welfare program. ASFSA had never before mobilized its 65,000 members so quickly, or completely. They were everywhere, buttonholing local congressional representatives, writing letters, rallying teachers and parents, courting the media.

ASFSA sent a Call to Action letter to 19,000 school food directors to reinforce the seriousness of the threat. Documents were produced that spelled out the effect of the proposal on each state . . . how much funding would be lost, how many children would lose access to school meals. Realizing that many directors could not take a position because of the politics involved, the letter stated "this is what these proposals are going to do to the school meal program in your state. If you can't speak out yourself, get this information to someone who can."

The mobilization, orchestrated by Pilant and Marshall Matz, longtime legislative counsel to ASFSA, with the support of ASFSA staff and other association leaders produced incredible results. ASFSA Past President, Gene White, now retired as California's state director, volunteered her time to be in Washington to help lead the defense against program obliteration. Between February 20 and March 31, ASFSA collected 1,143 news clippings on the block grant proposals. School lunch became a rallying cry for a wide variety of political and social interests opposed to various contract provisions. The slogan *Hungry Children Can't Learn* crystallized the opposition.

When the last Contract motion was defeated and the last vote taken, the national school breakfast and lunch programs had survived. Congressman Newt Gingrich, the Speaker of the House, wounded by the defeat, vowed publicly that he would not let himself be "school lunched" again.

Source: The following material is condensed from an article by Karolyn Schuster that originally appeared in the May, 1998 issue of *Food Management Magazine,* and is adapted with permission. Copyright 1998 by Penton Media Company.

mer director of Memphis, Tennessee's school food and nutrition program, as USDA's Undersecretary of Agriculture for Food, Nutrition, and Consumer Services. Federally assisted food and nutrition programs for the first time would be directed by an undersecretary who understands the programs and their politics, and one whose vision is focused on children.

The 1998 Reauthorization

Reauthorization of programs that have not been given permanent status by Congress must be considered every four years. During the reauthorization period, it is not unusual for congress to review all programs, even those permanently authorized, and make changes. Sometimes the changes strengthen the programs, and sometimes they do not. New provisions are much easier to achieve when legislation is proposed by the executive branch. For a number of years there were no such proposals. However, the executive office proposed legislative changes in 1998. The ASFSA also identified proposals that were considered by Congress.

The influence of these proposals was reflected in the legislation approved by the 105th Congress. Expiring programs were reauthorized through 2003.[106] New programs were authorized expanding after-school snacks to complement congressional goals for after-school care, pilot programs were authorized for universal breakfast programs in a limited number of elementary schools, and seamless nutrition programs were authorized as a means of reducing paperwork. Pilot programs previously authorized, including the universal lunch programs and the commodity programs, were extended through 2003. Recent national concern about the safety of our food system prompted the funding for a food safety program including training and inspections for federally assisted food programs. The prevailing practice in Congress is to require offsetting legislation to cover any new programs. This provision is called PAYGO.

Child nutrition professionals have sharpened their legislative skills during the last half-century. They have been proactive in identifying program needs and helping their congressional delegations understand the value of programs to their states and communities. They have been successful in efforts to sustain and improve programs in times of tri-

als; the trials endured have strengthened their understanding of public policy and how it is made. School food and nutrition professionals are ready for action in the new millennium that will move the programs farther along the continuum of the ideal lunch program that Emma Smedley articulated many years ago.

SUMMARY

As child nutrition program leaders look to the future, the outlook is bright. Networks are in place, and coalitions are working together to see that the progress is sustained and to see that programs continue to be expanded until there is assurance that all children will have nutritional security.

Child nutrition programs are positioned at the center of the nation's efforts to improve health, education, and nutrition for children. Programs of the future, as in the past, will face trials and triumphs A mobilized cadre of school food and nutrition professionals focused on the goal will overcome the trials. The foundation is laid for achieving the ideal program envisioned by the pioneers "that all children will have access to healthy meals, provided in an attractive environment, served by caring, well-trained personnel and will grow through this experience to have healthy food habits for a lifetime."[107]

Undersecretary Shirley Watkins, delivering the Carl Perkins Memorial Lecture, shared her vision of the future with members attending the 1998 ASFSA Annual National Conference in New Orleans, LA. She said:

> Carl Perkins knew what we needed to do, and he had the courage and the vision to articulate and enable the establishment of child nutrition as a centerpiece of American education philosophy. We as nutrition professionals need to clarify our thinking, enhance our capabilities, and enrich

our own experience to make sure that we remain true to what he expected of us. As I envision the future, it will look like this

- Where we are a nutrition business
- Where we have support from all segments of our big community
- Where schools have nutrition standards that are valued as part of the learning environment
- Where children are taught in every classroom about nutrition
- Where all children begin their day with a breakfast and ready to learn

- Where kids eat their meals in a kid-friendly atmosphere
- Where nutritious snacks are available for the children during after-school enrichment
- Where we have a seamless program with up-to-date information to market our business
- Where the agriculture community provides the best commodities to supplement purchased foods

And that nutrition education, training and marketing are funded as integral parts of the nutrition enterprise."[108(p7)]

REFERENCES

1. K. Albrecht, *The Northbound Train* (Washington, DC: AMACOM, 1994).

2. T. Watson, *A Business and Its Beliefs* (New York: McGraw-Hill, 1963), 4–6.

3. T. Flanagan "School Food Services," in *Education in the States* (Washington, DC: National Education Association, 1972); 557–565.

4. M. Bryan, *The School Cafeteria* (New York: F.S. Crofts & Co., 1936).

5. R. Hunter, *Poverty* (New York: Macmillan Co., 1906), 119–122.

6. J. Spargo, *The Bitter Cry of Children* (New York: Macmillan Co., 1906).

7. Flanagan, "School Food Services," 559.

8. E. Smedley, *The School Lunch* (Philadelphia: Emma Smedley, 1930).

9. Bryan, *The School Cafeteria.*

10. A.E. Martin, *Nutrition Education in Action*, New York: Holt, Rinehart, Winston: 1963.

11. E. Smedley, *The School Lunch*, 13–16.

12. G. Gunderson, *The National School Lunch Program: Background and Development* (Washington, DC: Food and Nutrition Service, USDA, 1971).

13. K. Gaston, *Statements of History of School Food Service Programs in South Carolina: 1971.* Unpublished documents (Columbia, SC: SC Department of Education).

14. Smedley, *The School Lunch*, 5.

15. E. Martin, *Roberts' Nutrition Work With Children* (Chicago: University of Chicago Press, 1954).

16. Flanagan, "School Food Services," 559.

17. Smedley, *The School Lunch*, 5.

18. Smedley, *The School Lunch*, 189–194.

19. Smedley, *The School Lunch*, 191–194.

20. Bryan, *The School Cafeteria.*

21. American School Food Service Association, *Keys to Excellence: Standards of Practice for Nutrition Integrity* (Alexandria, VA: 1995).

22. Report No. 553 to accompany S. 962, Providing Assistance to the States in the Establishment, Maintenance, Operation, and Expansion of School-Lunch Programs, July 28, 1945, U.S. Senate.

23. Flanagan, "School Food Services," 561.

24. Flanagan, "School Food Services," 562.

25. Gunderson, *National School Lunch Program*, 13.

26. L. Cremin, *The History of Education.* Unpublished class notes (New York: Teacher's College, 1959).

27. Unpublished letter from Attorney General to State School Superintendent, M.D. Collins (Atlanta, GA: 1937).

28. Bryan, *The School Cafeteria.*

29. Bryan, *The School Cafeteria,* vii.

30. Bryan, *The School Cafeteria,* xvi.

31. Bryan, *The School Cafeteria,* 15.

32. Bryan, *The School Cafeteria,* 15–349.

33. Gunderson, *The National School Lunch Program*, 15.

34. West Virginia Department of Education, *The Hot Lunch at School: A Manual of Suggestions for Teachers* (Charleston, SC: State Department of Education, 1938), 8.

35. E.N. Todhunter, *Everyday Nutrition for School Children* (Auburn, AL: Extension Division, University of Alabama, 1945), 7.

36. U.S. Office of Education, *Making School Lunches Educational.* Nutrition Education Series, Pamphlet # 2 (Washington, DC: 1944).

37. T. Flanagan et al., *School Food Service Policies and Standards* (Tallahassee, FL: Southern States Work Conference, 1967).

38. Flanagan, "School Food Services," 563–564.

39. Gunderson, *National School Lunch Program*, 13.

40. Gunderson, *National School Lunch Program*, 14.

41. Gunderson, 14.

42. Flanagan, "School Food Services," 565.

43. Report No. 553 to accompany S. 962.

44. *Congressional Record*, February 19, 1946.

45. *Congressional Record*, February 26, 1946.

46. *Congressional Record*, S 503, February 8, 1945.

47. *Congressional Record*, February 26, 1946.

48. *Congressional Record*, February 27, 1946.

49. *Congressional Record*, May 23, 1946, 5527.

50. *Congressional Record*, May 24, 1946, 5602.

51. Flanagan, "School Food Services," 566.

52. Public Law 79-396, Stat 281, Sect 2, 1946.

53. House Committee on Appropriations, *Department of Agriculture Appropriation Bill, Fiscal Year 1948. House Report 450* (Washington, DC: U.S. Congress, 1947).

54. J. Caton, *The History of the American School Food Service Association: A Pinch of Love* (Arlington, VA: American School Food Service Association, 1990).

55. Public Law 79-396.

56. Flanagan, "School Food Services," 557–565.

57. "Recommended Standards for the Selection of Personnel Responsible for the Supervision and Management of the School Lunch Program," *School Food Service News*, January/February 1949, 33–34.

58. Caton, *History of the American Food Service Association*, 91–92.

59. Flanagan, "School Food Services," 569.

60. Flanagan et al., *School Food Service Policies and Standards*.

61. Flanagan, "School Food Services."

62. "Recommended Standards for the Selection of Personnel."

63. Flanagan, "School Food Services."

64. Flanagan, "School Food Services," 572.

65. Gaston, *Statements of History of School Food Service Programs*.

66. Flanagan, "School Food Services," 573.

67. Flanagan, "School Food Services," 577.

68. Flanagan, "School Food Services," 574.

69. Flanagan, "School Food Services," 575–576.

70. Gunderson, *The National School Lunch Program*.

71. Public Law 87-780, 76 Stat., October 9, 1962.

72. Flanagan, "School Food Services," 577.

73. Flanagan, "School Food Services."

74. Flanagan, "School Food Services," 580.

75. Public Law 89-136, 80 Stat., 1966.

76. Public Law 89-642, 80 Stat., 1966, 885–890.

77. Flanagan, "School Food Services," 587–589.

78. Consumer Research Service, *Study on Nutritive Content of Type A School Lunches* USDA: 1967. Hyattsville, Maryland.

79. Consumer Research Service, *Food Consumption of Households in the United States: Report No. 1: Household Food Consumption Survey 1965–1966* (Washington, DC: Spring 1965).

80. Committee on School Lunch Participation, Jean Fairfax, Chair, *Their Daily Bread: A Study of the National School Lunch Program* (Atlanta, GA: McNully-Rudd Printing Service, 1968).

81. Flanagan, "School Food Services," 583.

82. Caton, *History of the American School Food Service Association*, 226.

83. Public Law 90-302, 82 Stat. 117, Section 3, 1968.

84. R. Coles and A. Clayton, *Still Hungry in America* (New York: World Publishing Co., 1969).

85. *Hunger, U.S.A: A Report by the Citizens' Board of Inquiry into Hunger and Malnutrition in the United States* (Washington, DC: New Community Press, 1968).

86. N. Kotz, *Let Them Eat Promises:* The Politics of Hunger in America (Englewood Cliffs, NJ: Prentice-Hall, 1969).

87. B. Bard, *The School Lunchroom: Time of Trial* (New York: John Wiley & Sons, 1968).

88. Caton, *History of the American School Food Service Association*, 221–227.

89. *White House Conference on Food, Nutrition, and Health: Final Report* (Washington, DC: Superintendent of Documents, 1969).

90. B. Bettleheim, *Food to Nurture the Mind* (Washington, DC: The Children's Foundation, 1969).

91. Flanagan, "School Food Services."

92. Caton, *History of the American Food Service Association*, 249, 267.

93. J. Block, "The Bloc Grant." *School Foodservice Journal*, January 1976, 15–17.

94. *The Atlanta Constitution*, "Congress Overrides Nutrition Bill Veto," Washington (UPI), October 8, 1975.

95. Public Law 91-295. 1970.

96. J. Jones, *Federal Domestic Food Assistance Legislative Chronology, 1935–1992* (Washington, DC: The Library of Congress, Supt of Documents, November 30, 1992), 18.

97. Jones, *Federal Domestic Food Assistance*, 18.

98. R. Leonard, "Another Half-Loaf," *Food Management*, March 1989, 32.

99. Public Law 99-591, Amendments to the NSLA and the Child Nutrition Act, 1986.

100. Public Law 99-237, 1985.

101. Jones, *Federal Domestic Food Assistance*, 34.

102. P. Schmid, Unpublished article included with permission, July 1998, Section 9.

103. Public Law 103-448, Section 18, 1994.

104. K. Schuster, "Silver Visions: Vivian Pilant," *Food Management Magazine*, May 1998, 54–57.

105. Public Law 104-149, 1996.

106. Public Law 105-336, 1998.

107. J. Martin, "Child Nutrition Program Legislation," *Topics in Clinical Nutrition,* #9, no. 4 (1994): 9–19.

108. S. Watkins, *Carl Perkins Memorial Lecture.* Presented at the American School Food Service Association Annual Conference, New Orleans, LA, July 14, 1998.

CHAPTER 3

Overview of Federal Child Nutrition Legislation

Josephine Martin

OUTLINE

INTRODUCTION

The goal of this overview is to describe the purpose and provide brief descriptions of 10 child nutrition programs. It will also serve as a ready reference for school food and nutrition professionals. Programs included in this overview will be those with special emphasis on nutrition needs of preschool and school-age children. The National School Lunch Act of 1946 and the Child Nutrition Act of 1966 provide authorization, as well as policy, for specific program requirements and funding provisions for the programs. Any overview of legislation is time sensitive and reflects the status of programs at a given time. This overview reflects status in 1998. Because legislation is dynamic and subject to change with each session of Congress, school food and nutrition professionals need to adopt a systematic process for updating their knowledge. The Internet provides the capability for immediate access to current laws, rules, and regulations.

The description of each of the 10 programs includes program structure, purpose, authorization, state agency administration, target population, and basic funding/benefit structure. Although programs have their own purpose and structure, they emerge from the same basic policies, and have been authorized over a long period of time. A description of the following programs is included: the National School Lunch Program (NSLP); school breakfast; child care (renamed Child and Adult Care Food Program [CACFP] in 1978 to include adult day-care centers); summer food service; commodity assistance; special milk; the special Supplemental Food Program for Women, Infants, and Children (WIC); Nutrition Education and Training (NET); state administrative expenses (SAE); and commodity supplemental food program (CSFP). Cash or commodity assistance is provided to schools or other qualifying institutions that offer meal services or milk to children. The legislation also provides

funding for state and local costs of operating some programs. In 1989, Congress authorized the establishment of a food service management institute and provided funding in fiscal year 1991. Authorization for the programs is provided in the National School Lunch Act of 1946 (NSLA), the Child Nutrition Act (CNA) of 1966, and the Agriculture and Consumer Protection Act of 1973, and funding is made available under agricultural appropriations laws.[2]

School food and nutrition leaders managing for excellence will develop strategies to coordinate child nutrition programs with other food assistance programs in the community to help ensure consistent service and messages. Community nutritionists and school food and nutrition professionals working with any of these programs should emphasize the continuum of nutrition services they provide. The awareness of a continuum of services will underscore the need for collaborative effort at all levels to help program recipients learn how to make healthful food choices. The nation will move more closely to this goal when communities are collaborating to deliver consistent nutrition messages to program recipients.

Objectives for the Chapter

- Provide a framework for viewing the federal food assistance programs as a continuum of nutrition services for all age groups.
- Discuss administration and organization of the programs at the federal, state, and local level.
- Identify programs authorized by the NSLA and by the CNA of 1966.
- Present an overview of 10 federally assisted child nutrition programs .
- Describe the basic policy that supports the development of all programs.

Administration and Organization of Programs

Programs are administered at the federal level by the Food and Nutrition Service (FNS), U.S. Department of Agriculture (USDA) under the direction of the Undersecretary for Food, Nutrition, and Consumer Services. The state agency administering the programs varies among the states. With the exception of New Jersey, all public school lunch and school breakfast programs are administered by state educational agencies. Administration of the CACFP varies among the states. At the local level, school programs are administered by the district board of education. In many instances the school board also administers the CACFP and the Summer Food Service Program (SFSP). Through the NSLA and the CNA of 1966, school meals programs are established administratively and philosophically to benefit children's health, education, and the agricultural economy. The ultimate success of these programs depends on a cooperative and collaborative relationship among local, state, and federal authorities for program management (Figure 3–1).

Generally, the child nutrition programs are administered by a designated state agency and are required to meet both state and federal requirements. As a minimum, the federal mandates must be adhered to; however, states are permitted to be more restrictive unless prohibited by federal law. For this reason, school food and nutrition professionals should always seek interpretations from their responsible state agency.

At the local level, the school board's responsibility for child nutrition programs is comparable to that for all other parts of the educational system. The school board, or its designee (usually the superintendent) agrees to accept responsibility for the child nutrition programs administered by the district.

A Continuum of Services

A broad perspective of federal food assistance is cited to challenge school food and nutrition professionals to view child nutrition programs as part of a continuum of nutrition services, beginning with attention to the youngest of our population and continuing throughout the lifetime (Figure 3–2).

The federal food assistance programs, with their goals to reach people at risk, provide an opportunity at the national, state, and school community level to reinforce and build seamlessly on each other.[3] The wave of the future is to use a multidisciplinary approach in managing broad social issues, including food and nutrition programs. Sharing responsibility with community resources will help the school food and nutrition leader achieve program goals and will give the community shared ownership of the programs.

> The destiny of our nation depends upon how well we care for three groups of our citizens: children in the dawn of life, the handicapped in the shadows of life, and the elderly in the sunset of life. How well we care for them is a bellwether of our conscience as a nation . . . and this will determine our destiny.
> —The late Hubert H. Humphrey, Senator from Minnesota

Viewing child nutrition programs as an integral part of the nation's food security system poignantly identifies the congressional commitment to meeting food and nutrition needs of the American people. Food security as defined by the World Food Summit (1996) is *when all people at all times have physical and economic access to sufficient food to meet their dietary needs for a productive and healthy life.*[4] In addition to the child nutrition programs, other federal food assistance programs include the food stamp program, elderly nutrition pro-

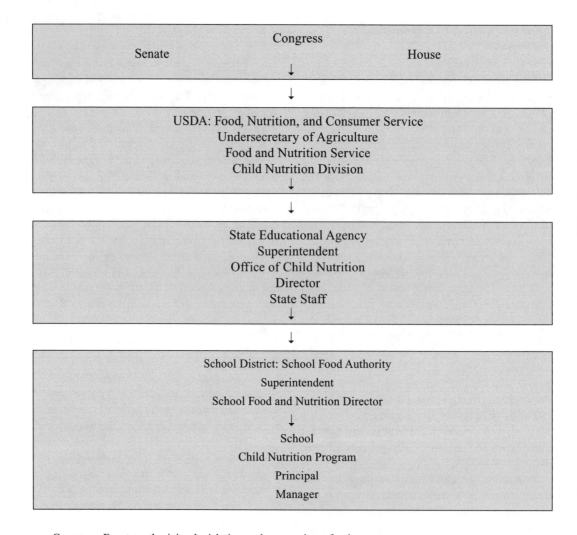

Congress: Enacts authorizing legislation and appropriates funds.

USDA: Sets policy; prepares rules and regulations; administers policies: promotes outreach; provides oversight and leadership; provides payments to states; monitoring and audits; technical support; administers programs; conducts analysis and evaluation.

State Agency: Administers programs consistent with state and federal laws; interprets federal regulations; provides leadership: sets state policy and standards; provides technical support and assistance; makes payments and financial management; evaluates programs.

School Food Authority: Sets local policy; administers programs consistent with federal, state, and local requirements; sets standards and monitors program operations; provides technical support and assistance; coordinates programs operation; establishes and monitors controls; markets program; coordinates nutrition program within the instructional and business areas of the district.

School: Operates programs to fulfill mission of reaching children with healthful meals.

Figure 3–1 Organization and Administration Child Nutrition Programs

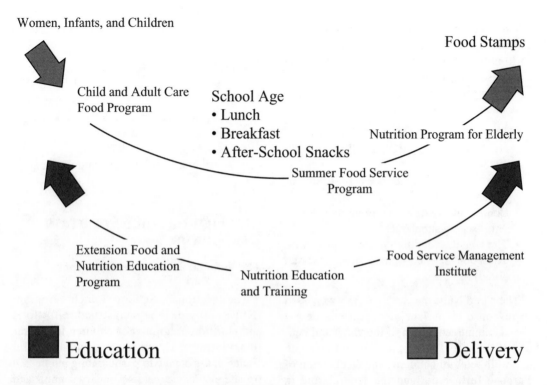

Figure 3–2 Child Nutrition Programs: A Continuum of Services

grams, and various commodity donation programs for needy families on Indian reservations, low-income mothers and children, children in summer camps, persons in charitable hospitals and institutions, the homeless, and those suffering from disasters.

THE NATIONAL SCHOOL LUNCH ACT OF 1946 AND THE CHILD NUTRITION ACT OF 1966

The NSLA of 1946 provided a foundation for the development of a strong national child nutrition policy and established the NSLP on a permanent basis. Note the words in the Declaration of Policy, which eloquently states the congressional commitment.

> Declaration of Policy
> *It is hereby declared to be the policy of Congress, as a measure of national security, to safeguard the health and well-being of the Nation's children and to encourage the domestic consumption of nutritious agricultural commodities . . . by assisting the states . . . in providing nonprofit school lunch programs.*
> —NSLA, June 4, 1946.
> *Source:* Reprinted from *The National School Lunch Act of 1946*, Public Law 79-396, Declaration of Policy, Stat. 281, Section 2, 1946.

Although Congress has amended the NSLA many times since 1946, expanding, revising, and modifying food and nutrition services for children, the policy has not changed. The school lunch program provided the framework and conceptual foundation for the structure of child nutrition programs to be authorized by Congress over the next half-century and beyond. Amendments to the NSLA since 1946 have authorized establishment of

- The CACFP, initiated in 1966 and permanently authorized in 1978 and renamed in 1988
- The Summer Food Service Program for children (1966)
- Commodity distribution program (1946)
- After-school supplements
- The homeless children nutrition programs
- The Food Service Management Institute (1989)

The Child Nutrition Act of 1966 was passed in response to the social conditions of the 1960s and in recognition of the value and benefit of the school lunch program to the health and well-being of children. The Declaration of Purpose further defined the federal role in building a strong child nutrition policy linking food and nutrition education.

Declaration of Purpose

In recognition of the demonstrated relationship between food and good nutrition and the capacity of children to learn and develop, based on the years of cumulative successful experience under the national school lunch program with its significant contributions in the field of applied nutrition research, it is hereby declared to be the policy of Congress that these efforts shall be expanded, extended, and strengthened as a measure to safeguard the health and well-being of the nation's children, and to encourage the domestic consumption of agricultural and other foods . . . to meet more effectively the nutritional needs of our children.

Source: Reprinted from the *Child Nutrition Act of 1966,* Public Law 89-642, Declaration of Purpose, Section 2, p. 2, 1966.

The CNA has also been amended many times to strengthen and expand programs. It authorized establishment of

- The special milk program (1966)
- State administrative expense (1966)
- The School Breakfast Program (initiated as a pilot program in 1966 and permanently authorized in 1976)
- The WIC program (1973)
- Nutrition Education and Training Program (1977)

OVERVIEW OF CHILD NUTRITION PROGRAMS

The National School Lunch Program

The National School Lunch Program (NSLP) provides the infrastructure for food and nutrition programs for children in institutional settings. The program provides federal financial assistance to participating public and private elementary and secondary schools and residential child-care institutions to help support the program infrastructure and provide meals for all children. Cash reimbursement and commodities are provided for each lunch served. There are three provisions for financial assistance: (1) Section 4, the General Cash for Food Assistance, provides a basic cash reimbursement for all lunches served; Section 4 provides funds to support program infrastructure; (2) Section 6 provides commodities for all lunches served; (3) Section 11 provides additional cash reimbursement for lunches served needy children. Reimbursement rates are established by Congress and adjusted annually for inflation. A national average payment for each category of meal (paid, free and reduced-price) and a maximum payment for each is set annually. This provision allows states and school districts some discretion in setting rates of reimbursement for local school districts. The NSLA requires states to match federal dollars derived from Section 4 on a three-to-one basis using all sources of non–federal funds to do so.

The NSLA prescribes five major requirements for schools to participate in the program[5]:

1. Lunches are to be based on nutritional standards.
2. Children unable to pay the full price of the lunch are to be served at a reduced price or free, and there shall be no discrimination between paying and nonpaying children.
3. The program will be operated on a nonprofit basis.
4. The program must be accountable.
5. Schools must make use of the commodity program.

Although modifications have been made to clarify or expand these requirements since 1946, the basic intent has not changed.

The Nutrition Component

Section 9 of the 1946 NSLA stated, *"Lunches served by schools participating in the school lunch program under this Act shall meet minimum nutritional requirements prescribed by the Secretary on the basis of tested nutritional research."* The congressional commitment to high nutrition standards for meals was strengthened in 1994 with the Healthy Meals for Americans Act. This amendment to the NSLA states that *"schools participating in the school lunch or school breakfast program shall serve lunches and breakfasts under the program that are consistent with the goals of the most recent Dietary Guidelines for Americans . . . and provide, on the average over each week, at least ⅓ of the daily RDA [Recommended Daily Allowance] with respect to lunches and ¼ of the RDA with respect to breakfast as established by the Food and Nutrition Board of the National Research Council of the National Academy of Sciences."*

Congressional concern over the number of young men who could not qualify for the World War II draft for reasons related to malnutrition and hunger created an awareness of the relationship of food to national security. The nation's primary nutrition concern in 1946

was the elimination of deficiency diseases and malnutrition. A five-component lunch pattern established by USDA subsequent to the NSLA was designed to provide one-third to one-half of the RDA of a school-age child. The nutrition focus for the program began to change in the 1970s as research related diet to chronic disease and health care costs escalated. Alarming statistics presented to the Senate Select Committee on Nutrition and Human Needs related food habits to chronic disease and created a major congressional concern. This awakening to a greater need for food than just to prevent malnutrition focused congressional attention on the need for dietary guidance to promote positive health practices and prevent disease. The first Dietary Guidelines for Americans were developed in 1980 and contained the nutrition principles of lowering fat with special attention to reducing calories from unsaturated fat; increasing the consumption of fruits, vegetables, and grains; and proposing moderate use of sugar and salt in the diet.

The nutrition principles of the Dietary Guidelines for Americans were incorporated into menu-planning procedures by many school food and nutrition professionals in the 1980s. The USDA eliminated the butter requirement from the meal pattern and schools were given an option to offer skim and low-fat milk, in addition to whole milk with the meal. Guidance material from USDA encouraged the regular and frequent offering of vitamin A- and vitamin C-rich fruits and vegetables with special attention to iron-rich foods.

The 1970s were filled with triumphs and trials. The programs grew in every direction, and student school lunch participation increased to 26 million meals per day. However, the nation was faced with an energy crisis that had an impact on public perception. The issues of conservation and waste were debated by Congress and publicized by the media. A major city newspaper ran a series of articles entitled "The War on Waste," based on a private research study of extensive waste in school lunch programs in one very large school district. Congress responded to this issue by enacting the offer versus serve (OVS) provision in 1976, which authorized schools to allow high school students to select as few as three of five meal components. The legislation provided an option for middle and elementary schools to implement the OVS. Prior to OVS schools were expected to serve all five components: milk, meat or meat substitute, two vegetables and/or fruits, and butter and bread.

OVS marked the beginning of school food and nutrition managers' focusing attention on matching customer needs with their wants in meal planning. On the surface, the OVS provision is logical; however, it has been used in some places as a springboard to increase profit. If a student takes only three of the meal items, costs are reduced and profits generated as the school receives the same reimbursement rate for the meal regardless of the number of items taken. If the meal selected contains only three of the four items, the child's nutrition needs may not be met even though the meal was planned to provide one-third of the RDA and meet recommendations of the Dietary Guidelines for Americans. Although the student may select three items and have a reimbursable meal, the items selected may well be the items with the greatest amount of fat.

In the majority of schools, OVS has created an awareness of the need for more customer involvement in menu planning, greater marketing efforts, and increased attention to offering quality foods and more effective management of service. The OVS provision should serve as a challenge to the school food and nutrition leader to provide nutritious, customer-focused meals that students cannot resist.

In the early years of the school lunch program, the majority of schools offered only one menu choice each day. In response to a variety of social and economic factors, including the rapid growth of the fast-food industry and its encroachment into schools, it is the prevailing practice for schools to include a variety of meal combinations or choices within the framework of the menu option. The School Nutrition Dietary Assessment (SNDA) study in

1993 indicated that the average elementary school lunch menu met or exceeded one-third of the RDA for most all nutrients for 7- to 10-year-old children; also that 44 percent of the schools in the survey offered lower-fat choices within the meal components, such that if selected by the student, the meal would have less than 30 percent of the calories from fat.[6]

Since the Dietary Guidelines for Americans were first published in 1980, school lunch leaders have promoted the use of the guidelines for planning meals. In the early 1980s, as in the 1970s, an economic crunch resulted in a major program shift. With the national deficit escalating, Congress drastically reduced Section 4 reimbursement rates by one-fourth, commodity entitlement was reduced, and the non–food assistance program was eliminated. At the same time federal education funds were reduced and school districts expected school nutrition programs to assume more of the indirect cost burden. This economic crisis resulted in many schools opting to meet student wants without regard to their nutritional needs. The focus for some became the bottom line. Several hundred schools dropped out of the NSLP, and others, while remaining on the program, expanded à la carte food offerings to increase revenues. Program participation dropped from 26 million student meals daily to 24 million. The program assumed a greater overtone of a welfare program. However, with intensive marketing, student involvement, and training and retraining of personnel to promote participation, the March 1998 reports indicate that national participation once again reached 26.7 million. The loss of participation in the 1980s occurred rapidly with the cut in federal money, and the recovery of the lost participation required at least 15 to 17 years. School nutrition leaders believe now that maintaining student customers should be a priority for all programs.

The Dietary Guidelines for Americans jointly published by USDA and the Department of Health and Human Services (DHHS) provided an impetus for Congress and USDA to reaffirm support for school meals that reflect the nutrition principles of these guidelines. The Healthy Meals for Americans Act (1994) required schools to implement the Dietary Guidelines for Americans in school meals by 1996; however, a waiver provision extended the implementation to 1998. Subsequently, the USDA Food and Nutrition Service published regulations describing menu-planning options, including both food-based and nutrient standard menu planning. The latest option is referred to as "any reasonable approach" and was authorized by Congress (1996) in response to requests from school food and nutrition professionals. While "any reasonable approach" offers some flexibility, it requires that meals meet the recommendations of the Dietary Guidelines. The regulation for implementing this last option is scheduled to be finalized in 1999. (For a complete discussion of meal pattern options, see Chapter 9.) Regardless of the menu option chosen, meals are required to meet the Dietary Guidelines for Americans when analyzed over a week's time.

With the implementation of the Healthy Meals for Americans Act (1994), the nutrition standards for school meals have been expanded to ensure that school meals are not only geared toward meeting basic nutrition needs for growth, development, and maintenance, but also that the menus offered promote positive healthy eating practices and disease prevention.

Access to All Children

The second major requirement of the 1946 NSLA states: *"Such meals shall be served without cost or at a reduced cost to children who are determined by local school authorities to be unable to pay the full cost of the lunch. No physical segregation of or other discrimination against any child shall be made by the school because of his inability to pay."* Access is more than having the program available in the school. Access has four dimensions[4]:

1. The *setting*: The schools must have meals available during the school day to all children, including those who are disabled, and must provide an environment that ensures that no child will experience discrimination of any sort.
2. The student must have *resources* to purchase the meal or be eligible for and approved for a free or reduced-price meal.
3. The school must *offer quality food that meets nutrition standards*.
4. The child must have *time* to be served and to eat.

The first and second dimensions of access include the setting and resources: Wherever the program is offered, it is available to all children. There are three categories of students: paid, free, and reduced price. All three categories are affected by these dimensions. The congressional intent was clear. It was to be a program to serve all children nutritious meals. The school receives a federal reimbursement for each meal served, which meets meal requirements. Amount per meal is related to category of students.

Lunches served to children eligible for free or reduced-price meals are reimbursed with funds provided under Section 4 and an additional amount from Section 11. For almost 20 years after passage of the NSLA, the only reimbursement for lunches came from Section 4 The General Cash for Food Assistance provided. In 1962, Congress authorized the first financial support for schools with high levels of needy children. Up to that time, local school administrators were expected to find ways to serve meals to needy children. And they did their best. Even so, only about 10 percent of all meals were served to needy children. The 1962 amendments established Section 11 which provided for a pilot program of limited assistance for a few needy schools.[7] This assistance, provided in the form of special foods, was called the Special Commodity Assistance Program (SCAP). The Child Nutrition Act of 1966 revised Section 11 to provide supplemental funding (to Section 4 funds) for all schools with high levels of economic need. The 1970 NSLA amendments (PL 91-248) authorized Section 11 funds to be used to supplement Section 4 funds for meals served at a free or reduced price in all schools.[8] Section 11 was extensively amended in 1973 to include the provision that payments would be based on numbers of meals served by category (performance funding) rather than an annual appropriation to states.[9] Performance funding replaced fixed funding in 1973. Up to 1973, the amount of funding available to states was based on an annual appropriation.

As a means of ensuring that all children from low-income families have access to free or reduced meals at schools, the NSLA was amended in 1972 to provide consistency in procedures for providing meals to low-income children. These include the following:

- Eligibility criteria for free or reduced-price meals: Children who come from homes with income no higher than 130 percent of the poverty level qualify for free meals, and those whose family incomes range between 131 percent and 185 percent of the poverty level qualify for reduced-price meals.
- Congress required USDA to establish income guidelines annually for schools to use in determining eligibility for free and reduced-price meals.
- NSLA required states to prepare guidelines or a prototype free and reduced-price meal policy and required schools to have a state-approved free and reduced-price meal policy consistent with state guidelines. The policy must outline
  1. procedures to be used in notifying caregivers of the availability of meals and eligibility requirements
  2. procedures for making application
  3. the school's responsibility for reviewing and approving applications and maintaining a current roster of eligible participants

4. the school's plan to protect the anonymity of children receiving free or reduced-price meals and to avoid overt discrimination.[10]

The Act provides for children whose families qualify for food stamps or Aid for Dependent Children or those enrolled in Head Start to be automatically eligible for free meals with appropriate documentation. A 1996 amendment eliminated the required annual filing of applications by school districts and requires the filing only when there are substantive changes to the policy. Schools have tried many ways to protect the anonymity of the child receiving a free or reduced-price meal. Computer programs with point-of-service software and scan cards have contributed to success in protecting the child's anonymity and to simplifying the process. Congress has continued to legislate provisions to simplify the application process. PL 105-336 contained a provision that allows an option whereby under certain conditions schools participating in provisions 2 and 3 may take applications every 4 years. Attempts have been made to provide meals at no cost to all children. Since the early 1970s, the NSLA has contained provisions for schools to serve all children without cost provided sufficient funds are available from non–federal sources to offset the additional costs accrued by serving free meals to noneligible children. A pilot universal program was approved in 1994, and several cities, including Philadelphia, were approved to participate in the pilot program. Hardly a year goes by without legislative changes to the procedure for managing the free and reduced-price provisions. Based on past history, more changes can be expected from Congress. For specific information about current requirements, contact the state agency or the Federal Register or the Internet.

Lunches served to children from families whose income is above 185 percent of the federal poverty guidelines are reimbursed at the basic rate from Section 4 funds. These children are referred to as paying students, and the meals are referred to as paid meals. Schools receive Section 4 funds for all meals served, including those served to paying students. This basic reimbursement helps to support the infrastructure of the program. There is national concern that the number of paying children continues to decline. Research conducted by Emmons et al.[11] in New York concluded that nutritionally needy and economically needy were not synonymous. All children need to have their school-day nutritional needs met and to develop healthy food practices. Being well nourished is a prerequisite to being ready to learn.

Many factors affect participation, and two of these are meal price and the perception of the program as a welfare program. Some studies have shown a direct relationship between meal price and participation. In order to maximize access to the school food and nutrition program, the price of meals should be within reach of the majority of paying children so they can afford to buy their meals. Changes in meal prices generally result in a participation decline. Another factor thought to affect adversely participation of both the paying children and those eligible for free or reduced-price meals is the welfare stigma. USDA reports that more than four million children eligible for free or reduced-price meals do not eat. Another closely related factor, which accounts for decline in paid meal participation, is the competition from à la carte food service. Providing a setting conducive for all children to eat with focus on choosing nutritious meals is an essential aspect to making the program accessible to all students.

The 1946 NSLA did not mention children with disabilities or special nutritional needs; however, the intent of the program was to reach all children. This concern for providing access to school meals for children with disabilities was clarified with the passage of the Rehabilitation Act of 1973 and later with passage of the Americans with Disabilities Act in 1991 (ADA). The ADA requires that children with disabilities have access to the same pro-

grams as all other children. Congress directed USDA to work with the department of education and the attorney general to develop guidance for accommodating the medical and special dietary needs of children with disabilities as prescribed in Section 504 of the Rehabilitation Act of 1973. In 1995, USDA and DHHS reissued an instruction that clearly delineates responsibility of the child nutrition programs to meet special needs of children with disabilities.[12] (See Chapter 12 for an in-depth discussion of meeting the special food and nutrition needs of children with disabilities.)

The school lunch program is available in 95,326 schools, including 5,885 residential child-care institutions (RCCI). A record 51.7 million children entered the nation's classrooms for the 1996–1997 school year.[13] Almost 59 percent of enrolled students eat lunch at school.[14] Of the 26.7 million children eating lunch at school in March 1998, approximately 57 percent were eligible for either free or reduced-price meals (See Exhibit 3–1). A review of this participation data indicates that schools have a great challenge to increase participation if the goal of reaching all children is to be achieved. Slightly more than 70,000 schools participated in the breakfast program in March 1998, with more than 7 million children participating each day. These participation figures provide an indication that many children enrolled in participating schools may or may not have access due to lack of time, money, or personal reasons.

The third dimension of access is related to the quality of food offered. Implementing the recommendations of the Dietary Guidelines for Americans is a major step in promoting quality meals. About the same time Congress enacted legislation requiring that meals meet the Dietary Guidelines for Americans, they also provided funding to develop materials and provide training. Materials made available to schools in support of improving meal quality include *A Tool Kit for Healthy School Meals: Recipes and Training Materials, Serving It Safe* (an independent learning module also is

Exhibit 3–1

Student Participation in National School Lunch Program and Meals Served by Category

March 1998

Number children enrolled 1996–1997 school year	Total Number Participating	Paid Meals	Reduced Price Meals	Free Meals
51.7 million	26.7 million	11.36 million	2.2 million	13.16 million

Source: Reprinted from U.S. Department of Agriculture, Food and Nutrition Service, *Program Information Report: U.S. Summary*, March 1998, Financial Management, Food and Nutrition Service, U.S. Department of Agriculture, and Code of Federal Regulations, Agriculture 7CFR 210.2, Definitions: Nonprofit School Food Service, Child Nutrition Programs, Office of the Federal Register, p. 9, 1966, U.S. Government Printing Office.

---

available on compact disc). Team Nutrition Materials distributed to schools include *Choice Plus* (a purchasing manual), posters, marketing, and nutrition education material. The National Food Service Management Institute (NFSMI) has been in the forefront in providing satellite teleconferences around the theme of *Managing Child Nutrition Programs To Teach Healthy Food Practices*, in collaborating with states to develop materials such as *Culinary Techniques for Healthy School Meals* and in providing the *Healthy Cuisine for Kids Workshops* in collaboration with the Culinary Institute of America. NFSMI also provides *Hands-on-Training*, a technical assistance initiative, upon request to assist schools in improving program quality. The American School Food Service Association's *Healthy Edge* is a basic course supporting quality meals. Focus on quality is an ongoing process and the responsibility of the school food and nutrition leader. For more information regarding quality of meals, refer to Chapters 9 and 10.

The fourth dimension of access is time to be served and to eat. School participation in the program is only a step in providing access. Equally important to meeting the issue of access is scheduling adequate time for children to be served and to eat and space for them to be seated. Meal schedules should provide students with time to wash their hands and time to eat. Traditionally the lunch schedule took into con-

sideration the number of children that could be served within a reasonable amount of time and the amount of seating available. More recently the block schedule is used in secondary schools, which often releases hundreds of students at one time for lunch. To ensure that all children have time to eat, the school food and nutrition director must be extremely creative in providing a sufficient number of serving outlets to accommodate students without their having to stand in line an excessive length of time. However, in some respects, providing access to students at breakfast presents an even greater challenge than lunch. In most schools, the breakfast period precedes the opening of the school day. Many students are bused or have private transportation to school. Unlike lunch, when, in most elementary and middle schools and some secondary schools, students are scheduled into the cafeteria on a staggered basis or multiple meal periods are provided, most students arrive at school each morning at the same time. Having space and arrangements to accommodate all students within a short period of time creates both an administrative and management challenge to ensure that all children have access to the breakfast program. Chapter 17 contains useful information in determining space needed for seating children and factors affecting scheduling.

Congress has been reluctant to address the issue of time to eat, as it is perceived to be a local issue. However, in the 1990s with pressures for more time on classroom tasks, mealtimes were severely compressed, particularly at the middle and secondary school level. Many children complained about not having enough time to eat, and Congress heard. A proposal was included in the 1998 Reauthorization Bill for Congress to include statutory language related to adequate meal service periods. Although this proposal was not included in the final bill approved by Congress and signed by the president (PL 105-336), the Conference Committee included the following statement in the Conference Report

> The conference committee believes that the benefits derived from meals provided in schools depend to a considerable extent on the environment in which they are provided and consumed, and that school administrators and the entire school community play an essential role in assuring that children receive the full benefit of such meals. Accordingly, the conferees call on the Secretary to encourage schools to make every effort to establish meal service periods that provide children adequate time to fully consume their meals and to provide an environment conducive to eating those meals.

Source: Reprinted from Analysis of William F. Goodling/Child Nutrition and WIC Reauthorization Amendments of 1998: http://connection.asfsa.org/legislation.

Operating a Nonprofit Program[15]

As noted in the Declaration of Policy of the NSLA, the basic philosophy of Congress reflects that federal support will be provided to carry out nonprofit programs. CFR 210.2 defines *nonprofit school food service as meaning* [that] *all food service operations conducted by the school food authority are principally for the benefit of school children; all of the revenue from which is used solely for the opera-*

tion or improvement of such food services. A non-profit private school is defined as one exempt from income tax under section 501c-(3) of the Internal Revenue Code.

Schools are generally allowed to have no more than three and one-half months' operating balance on hand without being charged as having an excessive balance or making too much profit. Not-for-profit organizations such as schools are designed to provide services or goods to meet a social need and do not operate for personal financial gain. In schools, as in other tax-supported institutions, the public is viewed as the owner; its interest is in the efficiency of the organization and, for school food service, in seeing that the nutritional needs of children are met in the most cost-effective way. Any revenues over costs should be used to improve the program for children. This may mean increasing the amount of budget allowed for food, decreasing the meal price, purchasing needed equipment, ensuring that the compensation scale is adequate, or supporting a work environment conducive to a high-production workplace.

The Program Must Be Accountable

Section 12 of the NSLA requires participating schools and state education agencies to maintain accounts and records to verify the use of funds and to verify that provisions of the act are met. These records must be available for review upon request. Reporting and accounting requirements include accountability for funds received by category of meal served (paid, free, or reduced price) and used. Much more than financial accountability is required. Accountability includes assurance that appropriate reimbursement is claimed by meal category, that applications for free and reduced-price meals are correctly approved and rosters maintained on a current basis, that children who qualify for free or reduced-price meals are being served with no discrimination, and, finally, that meals meet the nutrition standards (menu option) for the age group. Accountability embraces being nutritionally accountable for the meals served; financially accountable for the way resources are claimed and used; and customer accountable for the way meals are approved, counted, claimed, and served. Shirley Watkins[16] uses the word *integrity* to describe her passion for seeing that the programs are accountable in every way. She points out that integrity "is a necessity to maintain the trust of the American people who invest in the program, and to the Americans these programs serve." The total federal cost for fiscal year 1997 for the NSLP was $5,525,039,585, a staggering amount of public money that demands guardians to ensure that each dollar is used effectively toward the program's mission.

School Breakfast Program

The School Breakfast Program was authorized as a pilot program by the Child Nutrition Act of 1966 and permanently authorized in 1975. In the process of making the program permanent, Congress stated: *As a national nutrition and health policy, it is the purpose and intent of the Congress that the school breakfast program be made available in all schools where it is needed to provide adequate nutrition for children in attendance.* The School Breakfast Program, like the school lunch program, is a voluntary federal program; however, a large number of state legislatures have mandated these programs either in all schools or in schools serving a relatively high percentage of needy children. The framework for the School Breakfast Program is similar to that for the school lunch program. The requirements of access, resources, quality, and accountability are applicable to breakfast as to lunch.

Federal cash assistance is available to states for distribution to public and nonprofit elementary and secondary schools and to residential child care institutions that serve breakfasts that meet nutrition standards. One major difference between federal assistance for lunch and breakfast is that there is no commodity entitlement for the breakfast program. Bonus

commodities may be made available for use in the breakfast program. Nutrition standards reflected in the meal pattern for school breakfasts are designed to provide one-fourth of the child's RDA and meet the recommendations of the Dietary Guidelines for Americans. The caloric goals for both breakfast and lunch are based on the age or grade group of the child. The menus are required to meet the Dietary Guidelines for Americans when analyzed over a week's time. Schools may choose to use the traditional food-based meal pattern or the nutrient standard option.[17]

As in school lunch, schools receive federal cash assistance on the basis of the number and category (free, reduced price, and paid) of breakfasts served. All breakfasts served to children are eligible for reimbursement. Under certain conditions, schools may qualify for severe-need funding, an amount in excess of the regularly assigned reimbursement rate.[18] Reimbursement rates are set by Congress and adjusted annually for inflation, usually each July 1. The breakfast program funding is based on performance, or the number of meals served by category. The level of family income and number of family members determine whether a child is approved to receive a free or reduced-price breakfast or pays the regular sale price. The family application for free or reduced-price meals is used for determining eligibility for both lunch and breakfast. The maximum charge that schools can make for a reduced-price breakfast is 30 cents.[19] The breakfast meal price is set by the school district. The program is operated on a nonprofit basis, and any funds accruing in excess of costs are to be used for program improvements. There are no matching requirements for breakfast funds.

The breakfast program has expanded rapidly in the past few years. Factors influencing this expansion include the following:

- The Food Research Action Committee (FRAC), a Washington, DC–based advocacy group, has actively worked to promote school participation and has been a strong voice in getting state-legislated mandates.

- State legislatures have mandated breakfast programs.
- Some research findings have related higher test scores to breakfast participation. A Harvard study[20] concluded that students who increased their school breakfast participation were significantly more likely to show decreased child-reported depression and anxiety, decreased parent-reported overall psychosocial symptoms, decreased teacher-rated hyperactivity in the classroom, improved grades, and decreased absences and tardy rates on school records. As early as 1962, the Iowa Breakfast Studies reported the positive impact of breakfast on academic success.[21] Other studies relate classroom performance to transient hunger.[22]
- Congress provided start-up money for schools to get breakfast programs under way. State agencies and USDA have worked collaboratively to market the program, conduct outreach efforts, and improve public education to enhance the image of the program.[22]

Promoting the importance of an adequate breakfast to academic success is not new, but maybe, just maybe it is a concept whose time has come. There appears to be a moment of truth appearing with school administrators that a hungry child will not do as well on tests as a well-nourished one. Anecdotal information from many school districts indicates that principals encourage parents and teachers to emphasize the need for students to eat breakfast during test week. In some schools, breakfast has been provided to all students during test week. As stated in the section on school lunch, hunger is not a socioeconomic issue. Any student who skips or does not have access to breakfast can suffer learning and health deficits.[23] The School Breakfast Program is a natural ally for school leaders in helping to address the education goal to have children ready to learn when they enter the classroom. An adequate breakfast and a daily adequate diet are closely associated.

More than seven million children were eating a school breakfast in the 1997–1998 school year, an increase of three million since 1994. Approximately 86 percent of the seven million served are needy children. The 1997–1998 statistics indicate a slight increase in the number of paying children participating in the program over previous years. Federal assistance for the School Breakfast Program in fiscal year 97 was $1.2 billion.[24] Research relating the breakfast program and a child's success in school provided impetus for the American School Food Service Association to advocate for a universal school breakfast program in the elementary schools. In 1998, Congress authorized a pilot program to test the concept of a universal breakfast program in elementary schools.

Child and Adult Care Food Program

The Child and Adult Care Food Program (CACFP) is permanently authorized under Section 17 of the National School Lunch Act of 1946.[25] It provides financial assistance for breakfasts, lunches, suppers, and snacks for lunches served to children in licensed child-care centers, family or group day-care homes, and disabled elderly persons in adult day-care facilities. Commodity assistance or a cash-equivalent is available to support lunches and, may also be used for breakfasts. The legislation provides for meal supplements for children in after-school care. The program serves children not over 12 years of age, migrant children under age 15, and handicapped children (no age limit). The majority of the children served are between three and five years of age.[26] Unlike school nutrition programs, which are generally administered at the state level by the state education agency, CACFP administration at the state level varies. It may be administered by the state education agency, the health and human services agency, or another agency designated by the governor. In those states that have not agreed to administer the program, it is administered by the USDA/FNS regional office. Legislation enacted in 1998 related to seamless programs would simplify record-keeping requirements if all child nutrition programs were administered by the same state agency.

The CACFP sponsorship is generally restricted to public and private nonprofit sponsors. Several legislative and societal changes forebode the continued growth of the CACFP, including more after-school care programs; the back-to-work program, which creates a need for child care; and emphasis on the importance of early childhood education. The term sponsor in the CACFP is analogous to the school board in school nutrition programs. The school board often sponsors a CACFP. The term provider describes the site-based operator where the service is actually delivered to recipients.

The CACFP has five components: child day care, family and group home care, adult day care, after-school meal supplements, and homeless children under age six in emergency shelters. All children enrolled in participating day-care centers, like those in school lunch and school breakfast programs, are eligible to receive subsidized meals or snacks regardless of their family income. However, the amount of reimbursement for each meal or snack varies according to need as determined by the free and reduced-price meal application or in some instances those children who qualify under a categorical designation such as participation in Head Start, approval for aid for families with dependent children (AFDC), a Title XX Program, or similar prior approvals. Child care centers are reimbursed for up to two meals and a snack for each child in care more than eight hours per day. The reimbursement rates for meals served in centers are the same as those provided for school lunches and breakfasts; there are also rates set for the snack served. All rates are established legislatively and are adjusted annually for inflation. As in schools, meal patterns based on reliable nutrition research are set by USDA/FNS.

The after-school supplement component may be provided by the school or another organization. In most instances, the school must have a separate agreement with the CACFP administering organization in order to participate in the after-school snack program. With national emphasis on the need for schools to offer after-school programs, the school nutrition leader has opportunity to collaborate with the instructional program in planning a nutritionally sound snack program. The after-school snack program can also be a source of revenue for the school nutrition program. For a complete discussion of CACFP program requirements, refer to Chapter 10. PL 105-336 expanded the after-school snack program to reach children up to the age of 18 in certain after-school programs. Specifically,

- the after-school program must be located in a geographical area served by a school in which 50 percent or more of the children enrolled are certified as eligible for free or reduced-price meals;
- the programs must be organized primarily to provide after school hours, on weekends and holidays during the regular school year and have an educational or enrichment purpose;
- only one meal supplement per child per day will be reimbursed; and
- supplements must be served to children at no cost.

Another provision in the 1998 amendments provides flexibility to state agencies and local school districts by allowing a single claim to be submitted for both the school meals program and the provisions of the CACFP. USDA issued policy memoranda early in December outlining implementation procedures for all the provisions contained in the 1998 amendments.

Several significant changes were made to the CACFP in 1996,[27] including the provision for food service to children under the age of six who reside in homeless shelters, and modification of the funding mechanism for family day-care homes. The family and group home care component of the CACFP operates differently from the child care center program. A sponsoring organization may oversee a few or hundreds of homes. Administrative payments are provided for sponsors of family and group day-care homes at a set rate per month. The provider of the day care or group home is responsible to the sponsor for meeting program requirements. The sponsor monitors the operation in the day-care homes and provides training to providers.

Prior to 1996, there was no income test for children served in family day-care homes. The Personal Responsibility and Work Opportunity Reconciliation Act of 1996 established a two-tiered reimbursement system for child-care homes participating in the CACFP. The goal of that provision was to better target benefits to low-income children. Tier I homes are those located in low-income areas or those in which the provider's household income is at or below 185 percent of the federal income poverty guidelines. All meals served to children enrolled in tier I homes are reimbursed at essentially the same rates received before tiered reimbursement, except the rates are adjusted for inflation. Tier II homes, in contrast, do not meet the criteria for location or provider income, and meals served in these homes are reimbursed at lower rates. The day-care home provider may elect to have the program sponsor collect free and reduced-price meal applications from the households of enrolled children. If applications are taken, the reimbursement pattern is similar to the school meals program, with meals being categorized and reimbursed as paid, free or reduced price.

The CACFP is the fastest growing federal food assistance program. The federal cost to the program for meals and supplements in the CACFP in fiscal year 1997 was $1,568,473,203. School food and nutrition leaders can be valuable resources for the CACFP. Leaders can serve as advocates for high standards, assist with in-service training, and share nutrition education and training materials. Helping young children establish positive food practices will truly give them a head start in academic tasks as well as in social responsibility when they get to kindergarten or first grade.

Summer Food Service Program[28]

Initially authorized as the special food service program in 1968, it was renamed the Summer Food Service Program (SFSP) in 1975 under Section 13 of the National School Lunch Act of 1946.[29] The program has been reauthorized every four years since its initial establishment. Since neither the SFSP nor the WIC program is permanently authorized, each must be considered for reauthorization every four years unless Congress gives them permanent status.

The primary purpose of the SFSP is to provide food service to children from needy areas during the time schools are closed for vacation. Programs may be operated by school or local municipal or government agencies, public and private nonprofit summer camps, and colleges and universities participating in the national youth sports program (NYSP). The law also allows private nonprofit sponsors to operate programs in areas where there is no public sponsor or where no public sponsor has operated a program for at least a year. The program is available to daytime summer programs and to children in residential camps whose family income is below 185 percent of the federal poverty guideline. Meals served in the SFSP must meet meal quality standards established by USDA and must demonstrate that food safety and sanitation practices are in place. Periodic inspections by local health authorities are required.

Federal financial assistance is provided for breakfast, lunches, suppers, or snacks served to children in areas where 50 percent or more of the children have family incomes below 185 percent of the poverty guidelines. Rates for meals in the SFSP are generally higher than in school programs, since it is fully federally supported and no local or state matching money is required. The program receives commodities based on meals served. The number of meals reimbursed is limited to two per day (lunch and breakfast or one meal and a snack), except in camps and summer programs serving primarily migrants, where up to four meals per day may be subsidized. All meals and snacks are provided free to participants in daytime summer programs regardless of the family income. Children in residential summer camps whose family income is below 185 percent of the poverty guidelines receive free meals, and others pay as in school programs. Program sponsors receive administrative reimbursement for each meal served under a two-tiered system providing higher administrative payments to programs operating in rural areas and have on-site preparation of meals.

The program generally operates in the summer. Colleges and universities that participate in the SFSP as NYSP sponsors are permitted to receive reimbursements for a limited number of meals and snacks served to NYSP participants during the academic year. Reimbursement for the meals served during the academic year is paid at the rate received by schools. A special allowance is made for snacks served to NYSP participants.

There is a recognized need to expand the SFSP and the CACFP, as both these programs are intended for vulnerable groups. In fiscal year 1997, 2.2 million children participated in the SFSP at 28,880 sites. The need for expansion is obvious when SFSP participation of 2.2 million children is compared with the free and reduced-price meal participation of about 15 million per day during the school year. Children deprived of nutritious meals in the summer will lose physically and cognitively. The SFSP program cost for fiscal year 1997 was $242,582,410.[30]

Many school districts recognize three distinct benefits accruing from sponsoring of the SFSP. It provides a continuing food service for needy children; provides summer employment for food service personnel desiring summer work; and generates revenue for the school food and nutrition program. School food and nutrition leaders seeking to provide consistent service and nutrition messages will seize the opportunity to be an SFSP partner, if not a sponsor.

Special Milk Program

The special milk program (SMP), initially begun in 1954, was permanently authorized in 1970 by the Child Nutrition Act of 1966.[30] Through the years the program has been modified a number of times. Participation in the SMP is currently limited to schools and institutions that are not participating in the school lunch program, school breakfast program, or the CACFP. Schools that operate half-day kindergartens where the children do not have access to a meal service may be reimbursed for milk served to enrolled children.

The federal assistance is based on a half-pint of milk, and under no circumstances will a school be paid more than the cost of milk. The milk may be provided at a partially subsidized price per half-pint (known as the paid rate), with the difference made up by charges to the recipient, or it may be provided free to children with family income below 130 percent of the income poverty guideline. There is no reduced price rate for special milk.[30]

Commodity Assistance for Child Nutrition Programs[31]

The National School Lunch Act (NSLA) of 1946 permanently authorized commodity assistance for lunches, and this authority has been extended to the School Breakfast Program, the Child and Adult Care Food Program, and the Summer Food Service Program. As noted in the NSLA Declaration of Policy, one of its purposes is to expand the consumption of nutritious agricultural commodities. Two types of commodity support are offered to programs: entitlement commodities authorized under Section 6 of the NSLA to meet a legislatively specified level for each lunch served, and bonus commodities. The bonus commodities are offered when the USDA needs to reduce commodity holdings or move an unexpected agricultural surplus. The NSLA provides for a commodity entitlement per meal. The entitlement rate is set by Congress and adjusted annually for inflation. USDA notifies states of their commodity entitlement, which is based on the number of lunches served the preceding school year.

USDA seeks information from states and school food authorities regarding commodity preferences. States request the type of commodities they want based on school district preferences. USDA works with a commodity advisory committee consisting of school food and nutrition leaders to evaluate the commodity program and suggest preferences. Since 1992, USDA has revised specifications to procure foods that are more consistent with the nutrition principles of the Dietary Guidelines for Americans.[31]

USDA purchases some commodities specifically for child nutrition programs. For the most part, commodities are acquired for farm price support and surplus removal reasons. It is estimated that commodities comprise approximately 20 percent of the food used, while 80 percent is bought on the open market by local school districts or through purchasing cooperatives. There is a prevailing practice for states or local school districts to contract with processors to convert commodities into products easily usable in meal programs. In some cases, USDA will ship commodities directly to the food processor. States are not required to match the value of the USDA commodity food items.

Entitlement commodities (those mandated under Section 6 of the NSLA) generally are bought by USDA for farm support or surplus removal reasons. In the event that these purchases do not meet the mandated monetary value set for lunches served, the USDA must either purchase items for these programs on the open market or provide cash in lieu of the value of the commodities. States may choose to receive cash in lieu of commodities for the CACFP. A pilot program has been in existence for several years that allows certain school districts to receive equivalent cash value for the commodities or a commodity letter of credit (CLOC).

Bonus commodities are foods that USDA needs to move off the market to relieve a surplus or prevent spoilage. These include dairy and grain products held in USDA inventory or more perishable foods (meats, poultry, fruits, or vegetables) that must be purchased on a short-term notice to relieve a surplus. Schools commonly receive butter, cheese, nonfat dry milk, flour, and cornmeal as bonus items. These price-supported commodities are less perishable and usually come from USDA inventories.

Special Supplemental Food Program for Women, Infants, and Children

The purpose of the WIC program is to provide supplemental foods and nutrition education for pregnant, postpartum, and breast-feeding women, infants, and young children (through the age of four) from families with inadequate income. It is designed to serve as an adjunct to good health care during critical times of growth and development, to prevent the occurrence of health problems, and to improve the health status of these persons.[32] To be approved for assistance through the WIC program, a person must be at nutritional risk and economically needy. Recipients receive monthly food packages designed to meet their nutritional needs.

The WIC program is administered by state health agencies. Benefits to recipients are provided through a health-related local agency. Benefits are provided on a monthly basis and consist of actual food items or vouchers authorizing the purchase of specific food items in retail stores. Authorized supplemental food that may be included in WIC food packages include iron-fortified infant formula, infant cereal, milk, cheese, eggs, iron-fortified breakfast cereals, fruit or vegetable juices, dry beans and peas, and peanut butter.

The state agency is allowed to set its income criteria no higher than 185 percent of the poverty level and no lower than 100 percent of the poverty level. WIC operates in all states and the territories. (Chapter 10 has more information about the WIC program.) School food and nutrition leaders would find it helpful to work with the agency administering WIC, and with WIC recipients who have children in school, for the purpose of coordinating nutrition education messages.

Another federal assistance program aimed at this same population is the commodity supplemental food program (CSFP). The food benefits offered under the CSFP are government-acquired commodities purchased under various farm support programs. Recipients are not required to meet the criteria for nutritional risk to receive this support. However, the agency is required to provide nutrition education to recipients. These benefits may be provided for children up to the age of six. The WIC and CSFP may operate in the same area. Recipients are allowed to receive benefits from one program only.

Evaluation of the WIC program has demonstrated its value in reducing infant mortality and birth defects. Because of the built-in evaluation requirement for the program, it is recognized as a valuable program that has shown positive results. It is currently funded by an annual appropriation.[33] Efforts have been made for it to be given entitlement status as a means of ensuring that all needs will be met.

Nutrition Education and Training Program

The purpose of the Nutrition Education and Training (NET) Program is to provide funds to states to formulate and carry out a nutrition information, training, and education program. The NET program was authorized in 1977 under Section 19 of the Child Nutrition Act of 1966. Funding was authorized for an amount equal to 50 cents per child enrolled in a state. Congress only provided the 50 cents per child for fiscal years 1978 and 1979. Since 1980 NET funding has been fragile and erratic. NET funding, along with other child nutrition program funding, was drastically reduced by the Budget Reconciliation Act of 1981. However, in 1994 Congress permanently authorized NET with an annual appropriation of $10 million. It appeared that the program was back on a stable basis, but this was not the case. When the Personal Responsibility Act and Work Opportunity Reconciliation Act became law in August 1996,[34] NET funding was once more made discretionary and not funded. The Secretary of Agriculture transferred $3.75 million from other sources for NET in fiscal year 1997 and this amount was appropriated for 1998. An effort was made during the 1998 reauthorization process to have the permanent status restored was not successful and no funds were appropriated for NET for fiscal year 1999. In looking back over almost 60 years of the National School Lunch Program, congressional history reveals an advocacy for nutrition education and training. Therefore, it is difficult to comprehend congressional resistance to providing funding for nutrition education and training. As the link between diet and chronic disease is tightened, the link between wellness and productivity more pronounced, and the data available to reflect the cost of health care attributed to diet-related causes, surely Congress will come to recognize that nutrition education is an investment in the future.

NET has provided the only federal money for state use to meet specific state needs based on an assessment. Funds were used to

- provide nutritional training of educational and food service personnel
- train school food service personnel in the principles of food service management, in cooperation with materials developed by NFSMI

• conduct nutrition education activities in schools, child care institutions, and institutions participating in the SFSP

As noted in Chapter 2, the preamble to Section 19 of the Child Nutrition Act of 1966 succinctly describes the conceptual framework and rationale for managing a child nutrition and nutrition education program.[35] NET funds have not been adequate to meet state needs. Extra sources of funds have helped to fill the gap left when NET funding was reduced. The three sources of funds for developing training and education materials and conducting training are as follows:

1. Team Nutrition: Discretionary funds appropriated annually for use by the USDA, FNS. Materials developed are generic and can be used or adapted for use by all states. A portion of the Team Nutrition Funds has been granted to states on a competitive basis for meeting state identified needs.
2. *NET:* Discretionary authorization since 1996 and not funded for fiscal year 1999. The purpose of NET is to provide grants to states for meeting state identified nutrition education and training needs. States need these funds for developing a delivery system to use effectively the materials developed by USDA, FNS and the NFSMI.
3. *NFSMI:* These funds are used to develop materials and training programs and to conduct training that will help states develop training networks for getting training to the local school level.

Each of the fund sources has a specific role to fulfill in the nutrition education and training system. While there is some overlap, there is no unnecessary duplication of effort. Each organization receiving funds for developing material and providing training has a specific role to fulfill in achieving program goals.

The task of training school food service personnel in 95,000 schools and thousands of child-care programs, as well as providing training for parents and teachers, is awesome. Full-funding for each of the three entities would barely begin to meet the need. Some congressional decision makers see these three sources of education and training as duplication of effort. Consequently, the NET program has not been adequately funded.

The National Food Service Management Institute

The NFSMI was authorized in 1989 by Section 21 of the NSLA of 1946. Initial funding was appropriated in fiscal year 1991 to establish the institute at the University of Mississippi. The act provides for the NFSMI to be operated in cooperation with the University of Southern Mississippi. The NFSMI was permanently authorized in 1994 with a base level of funding.

The purpose of the NFSMI is to conduct activities to improve the quality of operation in the federally funded child nutrition programs and other federal food and nutrition programs. The congressional charge to NFSMI is fourfold: (1) to conduct applied research leading to improved nutrition and cost effectiveness of operations; (2) to develop training materials, conduct workshops, and provide technical assistance to school food service personnel; (3) to develop a network of trainers; and (4) to operate a clearinghouse for the dissemination of research, studies, findings, and reports, including those developed by the NET program.

The applied research division is located at the University of Southern Mississippi, with the education division and the clearinghouse responsibility located at the University of Mississippi. The Healthy Meals for Americans Act included NFSMI as a collaborator with USDA/FNS in developing and providing technical assistance to help schools and districts implement the nutrition requirements related to the Dietary Guidelines for Americans. The 1994 legislation also authorized USDA/FNS to enter into noncompetitive cooperative agreements with NFSMI to carry out responsibilities related to implementing the provisions of the act.[35] Congress appropriated $3,000,000 in 1995 to be matched by state funds for a permanent headquarters building on the University of Mississippi campus. Groundbreaking for the NFSMI building was held in March 1998.

State Administrative Expenses

State administrative expense funds are authorized under Section 7 of the Child Nutrition Act of 1966. These funds are provided to assist states with the cost of operating federally assisted child nutrition programs. The amount available each year is about 1.5 percent of federal cash payments for the institutional meals programs and totaled almost $100 million in 1996.[36] As a condition for receiving SAE funds, states must maintain a level of funding for administrative costs out of state revenues. The level of state administrative funds to be maintained must be not less than the amount the state expended in 1977.

SUMMARY

The child nutrition programs described in this section are authorized by two basic laws: the National School Lunch Act of 1946 and the Child Nutrition Act of 1966. Congressional commitment to the child nutrition programs reflects a bipartisan effort. The development of the nation's comprehensive child nutrition program has been advocated and supported by school food and nutrition professionals working as partners with education, professional, and public interest groups, and working collaboratively with Congress and USDA.

This overview is by no means comprehensive. The dynamic nature of federal legislation makes it imperative that school food and nutrition leaders maintain a process for keeping abreast of changes in legislation and regulations. The most timely source of information is the Internet. Since state agencies are responsible for administering programs, school food and

nutrition professionals are advised to maintain regular and frequent contact with the state agency for specific program requirements and interpretations. Becoming a regular user of the USDA Web page, American School Food Service Association (ASFSA) home page, and the FNIC connection will provide the reader with current information on programs. All action taken by the House of Representatives and the Senate is reported daily in the *Congressional Record*.

This chapter has reviewed federal programs. Many states have state legislation to support programs. ASFSA tracks state legislation for child nutrition programs and this can be accessed through the ASFSA Connection. An attempt has been made over the years to draft a state prototype bill that would be help state leaders in seeking reinforcement of federal policy or legislative provisions for issues not covered under federal law, such as staffing, personnel qualifications, standards for foods and beverages, nutrition education, dining room supervision, and extent of programs.

The chapter has not discussed USDA rules and regulations disseminated for implementing laws passed by Congress. Based on the reports from congressional committees, the discussions in the House and Senate and the laws, the USDA has an extensive process for writing and publishing rules. Most rules are first published in proposed form, and a considerable amount of time is allowed for public comment. After consideration of the comments received and considered, the rule is published in final form. Rules and regulations are published in the Federal Register and carry a Code of Federal Regulations (CFR) designation. Directors and other leaders help to make rules workable by carefully studying proposed rules and sending responses to USDA on a timely basis.[37] Proposed rules, policy memoranda, and copies of public laws are available on the Internet.[38]

Public policy is the force that shapes child nutrition programs. Professionals in all areas of food and nutrition programs have opportunities to become architects for the best possible programs for children. The Congress, the USDA, and the state legislature respond to public comment. Public policy occurs when issues of broad concern need to be addressed. Participation in legislative conferences sponsored by professional associations provides basic as well as advanced training in the public policy area.

The future begins now. Students, practitioners, and the public have a vested interest in seeing that carefully crafted child nutrition programs are designed for the future. The future belongs to the children in school, today, tomorrow, and in the new millennium.

CASE STUDY
SHARING THE UNIVERSAL VISION:
HOW ONE STATE ASSOCIATION INFLUENCED PUBLIC POLICY

Mary Begalle

With the change in the administration in Washington in the early 1990s, school food and nutrition professionals for the first time in over a decade seized the opportunity to rekindle the vision of serving all children nutritious school meals with a universal school meals program. In Minnesota, this idea appeared to be a natural, since the concept was championed by one of Minnesota's favorite sons, the late U.S. Senator Hubert Humphrey. But this was not an easy task. School food and nutrition professionals had spent the decade of the 1980s staving off cuts to child nutrition programs at the federal level. At the center of the battle was preserving Section 4 funding, the basic rate paid for the full-price meal. The challenge now was to convince policy makers that not only should funding for all meals be preserved, but expanded to include meals at no cost to all children.

The Minnesota School Food Service Association (MSFSA) had worked for several years to become actively involved in Minnesota's public policy and legislative process. Association leaders knew that this formidable task needed to be approached in small steps at the grass-roots level. Association leaders had become regulars at the Minnesota legislature, providing expert testimony before a variety of legislative committees in both the House and Senate on many issues related to child nutrition. MSFSA members, as well, had developed relationships with legislators. Each year MSFSA held a legislative conference at the state capitol that included visits by members to legislative offices. Contacts were maintained with legislators throughout the school year with invitations to visit school cafeterias and letter writing campaigns.

It was this ongoing relationship and the efforts to educate legislators about child nutrition programs that allowed association members to introduce the concept of universal school meals in Minnesota. The legislative committee of MSFSA wrote an issue paper on universal school meals. The committee also collected a variety of research studies showing the link between nutrition and learning. Key legislative contacts were cultivated in both the Minnesota House and Senate education committees. School breakfast was specifically the issue that resonated well with legislators. School breakfast had received much attention nationally, thanks to the efforts of the Food Research and Action Council, a Washington-based hunger advocacy group. The Minnesota legislature had in fact already passed a legislative mandate in 1989 for school breakfast programs in schools where up to 40 percent of the students were from low-income families. MSFSA also forged coalitions with allied education and health groups to support the concept of a universal school breakfast program in Minnesota.

These efforts to educate and collaborate with policy makers and children's advocates resulted in legislation being introduced during the 1994 session to establish a universal school breakfast pilot program. This initial one-year pilot program included a $167,000 appropriation that was adequate to fund four elementary schools. Through intense lobbying efforts by association members and the relatively small price tag (compared with the state's multibillion dollar education budget) the legislation was passed into law. Two additional elementary school sites were later added through corporate donations.

The legislation that resulted in the new law was carefully crafted with the help of association leaders and a professional lobbyist to include two significant elements. First, the law directed the commissioner of the department of education to submit a report on school meals in Minnesota. To accomplish this task, the department of education formed a school meals advisory group, which included representatives from a wide variety of education, health, and business organizations in the state. Even though there were child nutrition professionals on the advisory group, it was a calculated risk to have such a diverse group evaluate the effectiveness of school meals programs and make formal recommendations to the legislature. The result of months of meetings culminated in a comprehensive report to the legislature that recommended a universal school breakfast program statewide. Even though the cost of the proposal was prohibitive ($62 million) it established a recognition by a collaboration of education, health, and business professionals for the value of feeding all children a nutritious school breakfast at no charge.

The second important element of the law was that the legislature also directed the department to evaluate the four pilot sites. The evaluation was to determine the impact of school breakfast on children's school performance, including discipline, test scores, attendance, and other measures of educational achievement. The independent evaluation, conducted by the Center for Applied Research and Educational Improvement at the University of Minnesota, reported that when all students are involved in school breakfast they are more attentive, have improved attendance, and there is a general increase in learning and achievement. The study finally proved what teachers and school food and nutrition professionals knew all along—hungry children can't learn.

It was these two tangible documents, a legislative report with recommendations from a representative group of respected professional organizations and the research study produced by a major university, that provided the vehicle for school nutrition professionals to share the message about the importance of feeding children's minds and bodies. Not only was the information shared with school administrators, teachers, and allied groups, but it was also re-

ported back to the legislature during the 1995 session. MSFSA again lobbied the legislature in 1995, this time to continue the pilot program and the University of Minnesota study to assess the long-term effect of universal breakfast over a three-year period on student achievement. Convinced by the compelling evidence of the two reports and the continued lobbying efforts of the association members, the legislature extended the original one-year pilot for two additional years.

By the end of the second year of the pilot program, it was clear that the research data pointed to very high levels of participation, increased student attendance, improved student behavior, reduced visits to the nurse's office, a general increase in composite math and reading scores, and positive social benefits for children. This set the stage for the association to attempt to establish a permanent universal breakfast program in Minnesota. But the strategy had to change. By 1997, welfare reform had taken hold and the concept of a universal program needed to take on a new look. Policy makers were looking for strategies to target tax dollars to the neediest citizens. So the proposed program took on a new name and a new focus. The targeted school breakfast program legislation introduced during the 1997 legislative session would expand the pilot program sites to include grant awards to schools with at least 33 percent of the school lunch participants qualifying for free or reduced-price meals. This provision targeted the money to school sites serving low-income children.

The grant program also required a local commitment from the grant recipients. The schools receiving grants were required to identify and implement strategies to integrate school breakfast into the educational day of students. Grant recipients were also required to match one dollar for every three dollars of grant money received from the state. This match could be in the form of in-kind contributions such as staff time or volunteer time or donations from outside organizations. This type of local commitment and the fact that the grants were targeted to lower-income schools helped to convince even the more conservative policy makers that the legislation had merit.

At the end of the 1997 legislative session, Governor Arne Carlson signed into law legislation that appropriated $1,037,000 to establish the targeted school breakfast program. Thirty-one elementary school sites statewide received grants for the 1997–1998 school year. Nearly 9,000 children will benefit physically, socially, and educationally by eating a nutritious breakfast every school day in a supportive environment. School administrators, teachers, and parents in these schools recognize and support the critical role school breakfast plays in educating their children. Many more schools that have applied for the grant are on the waiting list. The grant amount, while significant, is not nearly enough to meet the need.

The MSFSA is working to collect additional information and gather additional research data to illustrate the need to expand the program in the future. This information is also being shared with other state and national advocates for child nutrition issues. Twenty groups supported the MSFSA in its quest for universal breakfasts, including the Children's Defense Fund, Congregations Concerned for Children, Food First Coalition, MN Association of Alternative Programs, Minnesota Association of School Administrators, Minnesota Association of School Business Officials, Minnesota Association of Secondary School Principals, Minnesota Business Partnership, Minnesota Chapter of the American Academy of Pediatrics, Minnesota Children's Initiative, Minnesota Community Action Association, Minnesota Department of Health, Minnesota Dietetic Association, Minnesota Early Childhood Care and Education Council, Minnesota Education Association, Minnesota Elementary School Principals' Association, Minnesota Federation of Teachers, Minnesota FoodShare, Minnesota School Boards Association, and the School Nurse Association of Minnesota.

The vision of healthy children, ready to learn, lives on.

REFERENCES

1. Congressional Research Service, *CRS Report for Congress. Child Nutrition: Program Information, Data, and Analysis.* [Summary] (1993).

2. Congressional Research Service.

3. S. Watkins, *Historical Perspective on the School Meals Program: The Case for Strong Federal Programs.* Presented at the Ceres Forum on School Meals Policy, Georgetown University, Washington, DC, November 1997.

4. J. Martin, "Food Summit Reaffirms Basic Values in Child Nutrition," *CNI Nutrition Week* 26, no. 47 (1996): 4–6.

5. J. Martin, "Child Nutrition Program Legislation." *Topics in Clinical Nutrition,* 9, no. 4 (1994): 9–19.

6. J. Burghardt and B. Devaney, *The School Nutrition Dietary Assessment Study: Summary of Findings* (Princeton, NJ: Mathematica Policy Research, Inc., 1993), 8–10.

7. Public Law 87-823, 76 Stat. 946, 1962.

8. Public Law 91-248, 84 Stat 211, 1970.

9. Public Law 93-150, 87 Stat 561, 1973.

10. Public Law 92-433, 86 Stat. 726, 1972.

11. L. Emmons et al., "A Study of School Feeding Programs," *Journal of the American Dietetic Association* 61 (1972): 262–265

12. US Department of Agriculture, Food and Nutrition Service. *Accommodating Children with Special Dietary Needs in School Nutrition Programs: Guidance for School Food Service Staff* (Alexandria, VA: 1995).

13. "Echo Boom Hits U.S. Schools," *The Futurist,* March–April, 1997.

14. USDA, Food and Nutrition Service, *Program Information Report: U.S. Summary, March 1998,* Financial Management, 1998.

15. Code of Federal Regulations, Agriculture 7CFR 210.2. Definitions: Nonprofit School Food Service. Child Nutrition Programs, Office of the Federal Register, U.S. Government Printing Office (1996), 9.

16. Watkins, *Historical Perspective on the School Meals Program.*

17. USDA, *Nutrient Analysis Protocols for the School Nutrition Program* (Alexandria, VA: Food and Nutrition Service, 1998), 1.

18. 7 CFR. Reimbursement payments. 220.9 (Alexandria, VA: Food and Consumer Service, USDA).

19. Public Law 97-35. Stat 95 1981. Omnibus Reconciliation Act of 1981.

20. Harvard 1997.

21. Cereal Institute, Inc., *A Complete Summary of the Iowa Breakfast Studies.* (Chicago, Ill: Cereal Institute, Inc., 1976). (Originally published in 1962).

22. Congressional Research Service.

23. D. Derelian, *Breakfast and Learning: Better Breakfast–Better Learning.* (Sacramento, CA: California Department of Education, 1994).

24. USDA, *Program Information Report.*

25. Martin, "Child Nutrition Program Legislation," 17.

26. Congressional Research Service.

27. Public Law 104-193, 110 Stat. 2294, Sect 17, 1996.

28. Congressional Research Service.

29. Public Law 94-105. 89 Stat. 515: Sect 13:1975.

30. Congressional Research Service.

31. Congressional Research Service, 7.

32. Congressional Research Service.

33. Congressional Research Service, 6.

34. J. Richardson, *CRS Report for Congress: Child Nutrition Legislation in the 104th Congress.* Congressional Research Service, the Library of Congress, January 1997.

35. Martin, "Child Nutrition Program Legislation."

36. Congressional Research Service.

37. USDA: http://www.usda.gov/

38. Library of Congress: http://thomas.loc.gov/

PART II

Administration

CHAPTER 4

Nutrition Integrity

Dorothy Caldwell

A guaranteed level of performance that assures that all foods available in schools for children are consistent with recommended dietary allowances and dietary guidelines and, when consumed, contribute to the development of lifelong, healthy eating habits.

—American School Food Service Association,
Five-Year Planning Conference, 1990 [1]

School nutrition services: Integration of nutritious, affordable, and appealing meals; nutrition education; and an environment that promotes healthy eating behaviors for all children. Designed to maximize each child's education and health potential for a lifetime.

—Health is Academic: A Guide to Coordinated
School Health Programs, 1998 [2]

OUTLINE

- Introduction
- Historical Perspective
- Factors Influencing Nutrition Integrity
- Support for Nutrition Integrity
- Application
- Summary
- Case Study: State
- Case Study: Local

INTRODUCTION

For more than a century, school meals have helped students avoid hunger during the school day as well as improve their nutrition, health, and learning readiness. They have been enormously successful. As the twenty-first century approaches, it is important to examine the role of school meals, determine the degree to which their integrity of purpose is being maintained, and implement changes if needed.

There is consensus today that school food and nutrition programs are important to learning readiness, health promotion, and disease prevention.[3–6] Numerous governmental entities and nongovernmental organizations include the National School Lunch Program (NSLP), School Breakfast Program (SBP), and Nutrition Education and Training (NET) Program in strategies to meet short- and long-term health and education goals. Increasingly, the Summer Food Service Program (SFSP) and the Child and Adult Care Food Program (CACFP) are being added to the menu of services schools provide to contribute to children's health and learning after school and when the school has a long vacation. Yet, despite the clear connection of nutrition to health and education, there is great diversity in how states, communities, and schools view the programs and provide policies and resources to maximize their effectiveness.[7]

The epidemic in childhood obesity in the 1990s provided a rallying point to move children's nutrition and physical activity higher on the public agenda. Obesity became the third most prevalent nutritional disease of children and adolescents in the United States, affecting one in five.[8] And indications are that the current generation of children will grow into the most obese generation of adults in U.S. history.[9] Obese children tend to become obese adults, facing increased risk for diabetes, cardiovascular disease, and many other chronic diseases.[10] Childhood obesity is not only a predictor of adult disease, but also has widespread psychosocial consequences for children and adolescents.[11] An increased prevalence of behavioral and learning difficulties has been observed among children who are gaining weight rapidly.[12] As the severity of childhood obesity and its consequences become better understood by policy makers, health professionals, community leaders, and parents, the relationship of school meals, physical education, nutrition education, and a total school environment that is supportive of healthy eating and physical activity may also receive greater attention.

Many schools and communities view school meals as an integral part of the total education program. Adequate resources are allocated to ensure quality and maintain affordability. Support is provided for integrating the school cafeteria into the total school program as a laboratory for learning. Policy decisions are made with the goal of providing all students the skills, social support, and environmental reinforcement they need to adopt short- and long-term, healthy eating behaviors. Schools with these policies and practices in place have high participation in school food and nutrition programs, with increasing numbers of students learning to select and consume meals that contribute to learning readiness and to a healthy lifestyle now and in the future.

This is not the case in all schools, however. Often there is no clear identity established for school food and nutrition programs. Expectations are not defined. Policies are often unwritten and generally have been developed in reaction to problems as they arise. There is general acceptance of a role for the program in children's health and education, but there is no champion or group of supporters who promote that role. Resource allocation reflects a low priority for the program. Frequently this leads to mediocrity and unfulfilled potential.

In many other schools the food and nutrition program is viewed strictly as an auxiliary service. There may be a substantial set of policies and standards, but they are limited to fiscal affairs and do not address issues of nutrition, affordability, and equal access to services by all students. The success of a program is measured almost totally by its bottom line. There is often inadequate local support to fund cafeteria construction with adequate space for the production of a variety of tasty, appealing meal choices and for timely meal service to all students. Financial support for program operations is often minimal or nonexistent, indirect costs are assessed at the highest legal level, and some programs are required to make a profit that is paid to the general fund.

The problem is exacerbated by the operation of snack bars and vending machines by other entities within the school in competition with the school food and nutrition program. No nutrition standards are required for food and beverages sold in snack bars and vending machines, and profits from such sales are popular sources of funding for many projects and activities not included in the regular school budget. Such practices are being adopted by an increasing number of school districts.

It is easy to understand the differences of opinion on how school food and nutrition programs should be viewed and supported. Tight school budgets make it convenient for administrators to look at the programs as primarily federal programs. However, federal support for school meals declined dramatically in 1980 and 1981. Support was further eroded by reductions in bonus commodities and, in the 1990s, by the rounding down of reimbursement rates for paid, free, and reduced priced meals. The decline in both federal and local support has challenged the social, economic, and nutritional viability of school food and nutrition programs. As a result, the nutrition integrity of school food and nutrition programs is in jeopardy. To ensure that nutrition integrity is maintained, it is important that the opportunity for all students to develop and practice healthy eating behaviors become an established goal of each school. The degree to which there is a school and community commitment to that goal will influence greatly the degree to which food and nutrition programs will be managed for excellence in the twenty-first century.

This chapter will assist in the development of a basic understanding of nutrition integrity.

Specific objectives are to discuss the complex issues related to nutrition integrity, outline areas for policy development, provide the framework for a local nutrition integrity assessment, and suggest strategies to promote nutrition integrity.

HISTORICAL PERSPECTIVE

The concept of providing nutritious food for students has a long history and is deeply rooted in our society. Long before the National School Lunch Act (NSLA) was passed in 1946, school administrators, parents, and other community leaders were coordinating efforts to provide nourishing, affordable "hot lunches" as part of the school day. In many schools, volunteers prepared food donated by parents and other members of the community, teachers served the meal, and students helped with the dishes. Civic groups and philanthropic organizations often joined forces to raise funds for organized school meal programs. (For more historical information, see Chapter 2.)

Such grass-roots efforts had varying levels of local and state support with widely disparate results. In 1946, a growing awareness of the relationship of nutrition to good health and learning was a major factor in the passage of the NSLA that provided national requirements and federal support for local programs. Across the country, boards of education committed local resources to build cafeterias, purchase equipment, and otherwise subsidize school lunches to make them affordable to as many students as possible. The program grew and was implemented successfully in thousands of schools. By the early 1960s, however, it had become apparent that schools with large numbers of low-income students were unlikely to have sufficient resources to operate programs with access for all students. Although schools participating in the NSLP agreed to serve meals to students who could not pay for them, no additional federal subsidies were available for these meals, and local funds were often inadequate to provide all the free meals that were needed. The vast majority of school meals were served to students who could pay most of the cost of the meal.

In 1962, Congress responded to concerns about this gap by approving a new special assistance program that provided meals free or at a reduced price to students who could not afford to pay for them. The concepts that would be defined more than 25 years later as nutrition integrity were becoming institutionalized in many schools. They were strengthened in 1977, when Congress authorized the NET program. This program established a system of grants to state agencies for the development of comprehensive nutrition information and education programs that fully use school food and nutrition programs as a learning laboratory.

Budget cuts of the early 1980s altered school food and nutrition programs and diminished their role to provide broad-based nutrition and education support for all children. Although the NSLA of 1946 provided infrastructure support for local programs in the form of a small reimbursement for meals served to all students, critics ignored the foundation on which school meals were built and questioned the need to subsidize meals for the "paying child." The resulting legislation slashed reimbursement rates for paying students, reduced income eligibility criteria for free and reduced-price lunches, and cut NET funding and commodity spending. Adjusted for inflation, federal funding for school lunch in 1990 was only 58 percent of its initial 1946 level.[13]

Among the arguments made to the Congress in opposition to the elimination or drastic reduction of funds was the question of whether child nutrition programs would turn into welfare programs, lose their broad support, and become more vulnerable to cutbacks in state and federal funding. There was a concern that reduced federal funding would result in higher meal prices and lower participation, which, in turn, would lead to increased unit costs for producing meals. Another concern was the difficulty of protecting the anonymity of low-income children if fewer paying students eat

school meals. Many of these fears proved valid. In 1982, almost four million fewer students ate the school lunch than the average number eating in 1979, prior to the budget cuts.

FACTORS INFLUENCING NUTRITION INTEGRITY

Many schools responded to the new environment by strengthening efforts to make a nutritious school lunch the meal of choice for students. They expanded reimbursable meal choices to include more popular fast-food items as well as more salad bars and ethnic options. They developed more efficient food service systems to reduce costs while maintaining quality. They increased revenues by expanding services such as breakfast programs, contract meals for child care and elderly feeding programs, and catered functions to meet school and community needs. They invested in upgrades for serving and dining areas to meet changing student expectations, and they adopted marketing plans that promoted school meals in the school and community.[14] They were proactive in the development of local policies that ensured resources and administrative support for healthful and appealing meals, adequate time to eat, classroom nutrition education that integrated the cafeteria as a laboratory, and total school environments that supported the goal of healthy eating. Where this was successful, participation increased and the effectiveness of the program was maintained.

Many other schools compensated for the loss of federal funds by raising prices for reimbursable meals and increasing the sale of à la carte foods. This had far-reaching consequences. Almost four million fewer students ate the school lunch in 1981 than in 1979. This resulted in more students making food selections for which there were no nutrition goals and decreased the number of paying students eating the school lunch, thus contributing to divisions among the student body based on socioeconomic status. Students with ample money often selected meals from à la carte foods, and many students who could not afford a complete lunch of à la carte foods either skipped lunch or selected snacks from the à la carte program, vending machines, or snack bar. In some schools the growth of these profit-driven options resulted in the reimbursable meal's identity changing to a program primarily for low-income students. Many declined to eat to avoid peer-perceived stigma. A United States Department of Agriculture (USDA) study found that more than four million low-income students did not apply for free or reduced-price meals, but would have been eligible had they done so.[15] A later study found that 26 percent of eligible students did not become certified, and their concern about the stigma associated with receiving free meals was one of the causes cited.[16] As this image grew, more paying students chose not to participate, perpetuating elitist attitudes and social distinctions that are counterproductive to education goals.

Increasing enrollment, the high cost of school construction, and shrinking local budgets often resulted in facilities inadequate to prepare and serve school meals in ways that make them appealing to students. In some schools, the lunch period began as early as 10:30 AM and ended as late as 1:00 PM due to inadequate seating capacity. School improvement plans began to call for longer class periods, but did not make recommendations to maintain lunch schedules adequate for the development of healthy eating. The profitability of selling food to students led to the growth of local decision making based primarily on the bottom line. Vending machines and snack bars required less investment than cafeterias, provided quick service to students, and produced profits for schools. In the absence of policies that precluded the practice, foods and beverages with no nutrition standards became widely available to students, with profits earmarked for band uniforms, field trips, or other activities approved by the school. This egregious competition for students' dollars and appetites put additional pressures on food service programs to provide à la carte foods that would

bring students into the cafeteria, even if their contribution to the development of healthy eating was questionable.[17]

While federal regulations address competitive foods, political pressures over the years have diminished their effectiveness. Current regulations require that the local school food authority maintain a nonprofit school food service, observe limitations on the use of nonprofit school food service revenues, and control competitive food service.[18] They further define competitive foods as "any foods sold in competition with the program to children in food service areas during the lunch period."[19] The responsibility and authority to control the sale of foods in competition with lunches served under the program are granted to state agencies and local school food authorities, with one exception. The sale of foods described in federal regulations as "foods of minimal nutritional value" is limited to areas outside the food service area during the lunch period.

The flexibility of these regulations has resulted in local and state policies that vary greatly throughout the country. At one end of the spectrum is a state limitation of à la carte sales to those items that are a component of the school lunch menu.[20] At the other end of the spectrum are states that exercise almost no control. In most states, schools have wide latitude to serve foods without nutrition standards as à la carte and in some states schools serve foods of minimal nutritional value, primarily carbonated beverages, as a free bonus with a school lunch. The latter practice requires that the food or beverage not be marketed as an option for a required meal component (i.e., soda for milk) and that a paper trail exist to show that a source other than school meal revenues is used to purchase the foods of minimal nutritional value. School or school district revenues from lucrative sole-source contracts for soft drinks often are provided to food service programs to fund this practice.

At the same time difficulties such as these were escalating, students' food preferences were changing. Highly advertised fast foods and other snack foods with low nutrient density were becoming student favorites. More than 84 percent of young people exceed national recommendations for total fat intake.[21] More than 90 percent exceed recommendations for saturated fat, less than 21 percent eat the recommended five or more daily servings of fruits and vegetables, and 29 percent eat less than one serving a day of vegetables that are not fried.[22] The competing priorities of promoting healthy eating and providing what students want to eat presents a significant challenge for schools. Schools are making great progress in planning reimbursable school meal menus that meet the new nutrition standards. However, this will not ensure that student intake will be consistent with the Dietary Guidelines if fruits and vegetables are declined and french fries, nachos, or other high-fat à la carte items are selected in lieu of or in addition to the reimbursable meal. Because the foods students favor tend to be higher in fat than the vegetables and fruit they shun, it is safe to assume that children are getting a less balanced diet than they would by eating the whole school meal.[23] Research is needed to determine the extent to which this is a problem.

SUPPORT FOR NUTRITION INTEGRITY

There is growing recognition that schools alone cannot be held accountable for improving students' eating behaviors.[24] Other powerful influences include the family, socio-cultural and economic factors, the food industry, and the mass media.[25] However, schools are a critical part of the social environment that shapes young peoples' behaviors. To maximize its effect, schools must create a school environment that provides opportunities and reinforcement for healthy eating and physical activity, have the support of students' families and the larger community, integrate nutrition services into the coordinated school health program, and gain the cooperation of all school staff.[26]

The American School Food Service Association (ASFSA) framed the debate around these issues in the early 1990s when it defined nutrition integrity and established core concepts for use by state and local boards of education.[27] The definition and core concepts established healthy eating for all students as the desired outcome and nutrition integrity as the umbrella term for a comprehensive approach to school nutrition services that goes far beyond school menus.[28] These core concepts include the following:

- Nutrition standards will be based on the Dietary Guidelines for Americans and the Food Guide Pyramid.
- Student preferences will be considered in menu planning. Since foods must be eaten to provide nutrients, menu changes will be gradual to ensure acceptance.
- Meals will contain adequate calories and variety of foods to support growth, development, and healthy weight.
- The nutritional value of school meals will be evaluated over a period of days, rather than a single meal or food item.
- Purchasing practices will ensure the use of high-quality ingredients and prepared products to maximize flavor and acceptance. School food service and nutrition professionals will work with industry to develop appetizing, affordable products that meet nutrition standards.
- Foods will be prepared in ways that ensure a balance between optimal nutrition and student acceptance.
- Foods offered in addition to meals will be limited and will be selected to ensure optimal nutrition quality to foster healthful eating habits.
- Pleasant eating environments will be provided. This includes adequate time and space to eat school meals, positive supervision, and role modeling at mealtimes.
- Nutrition education will be an integral part of the curriculum from preschool to twelfth grade. The school cafeteria will serve as a laboratory for applying knowledge and skills taught in the classroom.

- Professional development will be provided for school food service and nutrition personnel and other school community members to build teams of competent, caring individuals with common goals.
- Promoting nutrition integrity in child nutrition programs will be a cooperative effort between nutrition professionals and other school community members working with legislative and other government agencies.

The core concepts were endorsed by education and nutrition groups, who agreed to work toward their implementation in all schools. Among these groups were the American Academy of Pediatrics, American College of Nutrition, American Dietetic Association, National Education Association, National Parent-Teacher Association, National School Boards Association, and Society for Nutrition Education. The Association of School Business Officials gave a partial endorsement, declining to support the recommendation to limit foods served in addition to the school meal. Some members of ASFSA also expressed the view that it is unrealistic to expect school food and nutrition programs to operate in the current fiscal environment without substantial menu offerings beyond the reimbursable meal. In October 1994, ASFSA's executive board deleted the limitation language from the core concepts.

Research-based nutrition integrity standards were developed for the core concepts by the National Food Service Management Institute.[29,30] These standards were later used as the basis for *Keys to Excellence: Standards of Practice for Nutrition Integrity.*[31] Schools and school districts will find *Keys to Excellence* useful as a self-assessment tool and guide for continuous improvement of their school food and nutrition programs.

The Centers for Disease Control and Prevention (CDC) developed "Guidelines for School Health Programs to Promote Healthy Eating," which are useful to schools interested in improving or maintaining the nutrition in-

tegrity of school food and nutrition programs.[32] The guidelines make recommendations in seven areas to assist schools in improving the eating behaviors of students and their potential for learning and good health:

1. School nutrition policy
2. Sequential, coordinated nutrition education curriculum
3. Developmentally appropriate and fun instruction
4. Integration of food service and nutrition education
5. Staff development
6. Family and community involvement
7. Program evaluation

The CDC recently completed another project that provides support for nutrition integrity in schools. More than 70 national organizations and 300 individuals were involved in writing and reviewing a guide to coordinated school health programs, which includes nutrition services as one of its eight components.[33] The guide cites poor eating habits as the second of six preventable behaviors established in childhood that account for most of the serious illnesses and premature deaths in the United States. The risky behaviors occur in all socioeconomic and ethnic groups, and many of the skills necessary to prevent or reduce risky behaviors are common to more than one risk. The guide's definition of health as more than the absence of disease—as complete physical, mental, and social well-being—effectively addresses the preventive and social aspects of learning to eat healthy for a lifetime.[34] The definition of school nutrition services and its recommendations are consistent with the ASFSA nutrition integrity definition and core concepts. The collaborative process that led to the guide's publication, as well as its content, strengthens the role of nutrition in the broader context of school health programs and makes recommendations for integrating it fully with comprehensive school health education and other components of coordinated school health programs. The guide's target audience is school administrators and other key decision makers, whose support is key to local implementation.

USDA's School Meals Initiative for Healthy Children and Team Nutrition are also supportive of nutrition integrity. Statutory and regulatory requirements of the School Meals Initiative are limited primarily to nutrition standards of reimbursable meals.[35] However, policy guidance and training and technical assistance materials recognize that planning and serving school meals that meet the new standards is only one part of the solution.[36–39] If there is no demand for the nutritious meals, school food and nutrition programs will be unable to continue to provide them, and children's health and education will not be improved. Team Nutrition was developed as a tool to help implement the School Meals Initiative in ways that will get students to avail themselves of the healthier meals. When implemented fully, Team Nutrition results in modest, but significant changes in knowledge, motivation, and behavior.[40]

Team Nutrition recommends a school nutrition team in each school, as well as public-private partnerships that promote healthy eating. This combination of school and community leaders contributes to success with a multichannel approach that includes the following: 1) classroom activities, 2) food service initiatives, 3) school-wide events, 4) home activities, 5) community events, and 6) media events and coverage. Almost 28,000 schools have enrolled as Team Nutrition schools. Beginning in school year 1997–1998, schools that had not enrolled were given the opportunity to order Team Nutrition materials as an incentive to become Team Nutrition schools and implement recommendations fully.

Team Nutrition objectives are: (1) to provide training and technical assistance to school food and nutrition personnel to help them serve meals that look good, taste good, and meet nutrition standards; (2) to provide multifaceted, integrated nutrition education for children and parents so that children will have the skills, motivation, and support for making healthy food choices as part of a healthy lifestyle; and (3) to provide support for healthy eating by involving school administrators and other school and community partners. The third objective was added in 1998 to formalize federal support for food and nutrition program directors and other staff in raising the priority of school meals and nutrition education within the education community.

The report of the Institute of Medicine's Committee on Comprehensive School Health Programs in grades kindergarten through 12 included school food and nutrition programs as a key contributor to children's health and optimization of the education process.[41] The report described nutrition's role in health education and health services and its relevance in the coordinated approach to school health in ways that were consistent with nutrition integrity concepts. Appendix B, adapted from the American School Health Association, provides recommendations for policy and administrative support that reflect a commitment to meeting the nutritional needs of all students in an environment fostering positive attitudes and social skills. Specific recommendations include the following:

- Establishment of goals and objectives
- Professionally trained directors and managers
- Staff development for all staff
- Menus that meet established nutrition standards as well as ethnic and cultural food preferences
- Standards for foods available in addition to federally reimbursable meals
- Pleasant eating environments, including time to eat, positive supervision, and role modeling
- Confidentiality of free and reduced-priced status to protect the dignity of students
- Involvement of students and families in planning and evaluation
- Cafeteria nutrition education that complements the classroom curriculum
- Ongoing evaluation that ensures continuous improvement

Additional support for nutrition integrity was provided by the inclusion of a developmental objective in *Healthy People 2010 Objectives: Draft for Public Comment.*[42] One of the Healthy People 2000 objectives had focused only on the fat and saturated fat content of school meals. The 2010 draft objective has a broader nutrient focus and includes both meals and snacks eaten at school. The proposed objective calls for an increase in the "proportion of children and adolescents 6 to 19 years of age whose intake of meals and snacks from all sources contributes proportionally to good overall dietary quality."

Rationale for the new draft objective stated that students' food choices are influenced by the total eating environment created by schools. This includes the types of foods available throughout the school as well as nutrition education provided in the classroom, point-of-choice nutrition information in the cafeteria as well as the rest of the school, and nutrition promotions that reach families and affect the choice of foods brought to school. This objective is expected to encourage school administrators, other policy makers, and community groups to develop strategies that promote healthy eating by all students during the school day.

APPLICATION

School food and nutrition programs, like all other components that make up a local education system, are a reflection of the community. They vary greatly from school district to school district, and often from school to school within a district, depending on the perceived needs, resources, and priorities of the school and community.[43] If the community wants a school food and nutrition program that reflects the principles of nutrition integrity, such a program can become a reality. Creating or maintaining a demand for nutrition integrity in schools has a strong role for the food and nutrition program director and manager. It also has strong leadership roles for

school and community leaders and for state and national partners.

There are four primary areas in which local, state, and national efforts must be coordinated in order to ensure nutrition integrity:

1. Healthy meal choices in child nutrition programs
2. Comprehensive, sequential nutrition education in pre-kindergarten through grade 12
3. School nutrition policies and practices that include adequate resources and reflect nutrition integrity as a priority
4. Partnerships that promote nutrition as an integral component of health and education in the school and community

Figure 4–1 shows how these four points are interdependent and interrelated. Nutritious meals and nutrition education are overlapped to illustrate the importance of the school cafeteria as a learning laboratory for nutrition education. These services are provided within a school environment that is supported by comprehensive nutrition integrity policies, and the school is surrounded by school-community partnerships that extend to the state and national level.

Action steps for developing nutrition integrity policies include the following:

1. Establish a coordinating group to assess school nutrition needs, develop a strategic plan to address those needs, and develop and implement policies that reflect healthy eating as a high priority for the school. Ensure that participation in the group includes key members of the school administration, board of education, teachers, and parents.[44] Provide good information and ensure time in the planning process for the group to come to a consensus on the role it sees for school food and nutrition programs to advance children's health and education. The use of the strategic planning process as a tool to develop a shared vision,

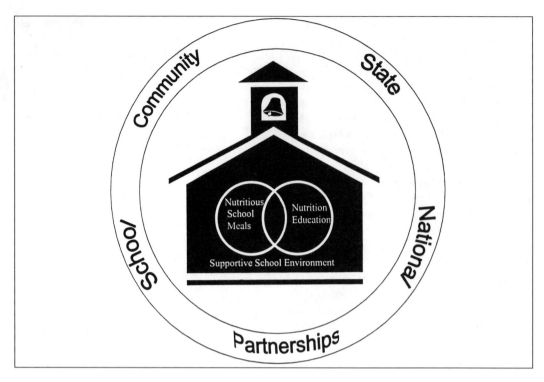

Figure 4–1 Ensuring Nutrition Integrity through Community, State, and National Partnerships

a clear identity, and a commitment to achieving success as defined by the team will provide a sound foundation for later decisions when competing priorities are brought to the table.

2. Ensure that policies are comprehensive. Effects of nutrition intervention on children's cognitive performance and health status provide a compelling argument for universal nutrition programs and services in schools.[45–49] When administrators and community leaders understand these connections, they are more likely to support sound policies. CDC's "Guidelines for School Health Programs to Promote Lifelong Healthy Eating,"[50] ASFSA's *Creating Policy for Nutrition Integrity in Schools,*[51] and *Keys to Excellence,*[52] and the National School Board Association's *Policy Update: School Nutrition Programs*[53] are useful references for policy

development. It is important that policies not be limited to "competitive food" issues, but rather are addressed in a comprehensive fashion in relation to school and community value and goals.[54]

3. Get "buy-in" from other school staff. Participate in staff meetings and promote staff wellness activities. Seek opportunities to collaborate with others involved in coordinated school health, and train cafeteria managers to collaborate with classroom teachers in ways that support the classroom/cafeteria connection. Collaboration between food and nutrition personnel and other school staff is more the exception than the rule.[55] A 1994 survey found that health education, physical education, and health service staffs reported organizing fewer joint activities or projects with food service staffs than with any other

school health component. When a large number of school staff is invested in the goal of healthy eating, competing priorities are more likely to be resolved in support of the goal. Working in tandem with other school staff who care about children's health and well-being can help expand school and community support for policies and practices that promote healthy eating.

4. Support nutrition education that is behavior focused, fun, and multichanneled. Build a strong team of school and community leaders to effect change in students' nutrition knowledge, motivation, and behavior through consistent messages in curricula, cafeteria and other school-based activities, community events, and mass media.[56] Promote the understanding that nutrition knowledge is not enough to produce behavior change, and seek support for making the cafeteria and any other food options available in school effective extensions of classroom nutrition lessons. School environments that are supportive of healthy eating will ensure that all students, regardless of income, view the cafeteria as a relaxing place to enjoy food and friends, and normative lifestyle behaviors will be improved.

SUMMARY

Nutrition is widely recognized as important to health and quality of life. Yet for many Americans, it does not become a priority until they have a nutrition-related health problem. Schools have the opportunity to help change that for the next generation. Helping children learn to eat as part of a healthy lifestyle that will improve learning readiness and reduce the prevalence of childhood obesity and the future risk of chronic disease is an important role for schools in partnership with families and the community.

It is a role that is embraced rhetorically by many decision makers. However, just as many individuals do not make nutrition a strong personal priority, many educators and boards of education do not make nutrition a school priority. School personnel view nutrition as a priority only to the extent that it facilitates their primary mission—education.[57] Educators show they believe that school meals facilitate education by going to great lengths to ensure that students eat a healthy breakfast on the day standardized tests are scheduled. Strong teams of parents and other school and community leaders can provide encouragement and support to school decision makers that will make nutrition integrity a local priority every day.

School administrators are under enormous pressures and have limited resources to meet community expectations. If school food and nutrition programs are to reach their potential, they must become an important part of community expectations. Increasingly, schools are looking at entrepreneurial ways to supplement limited resources. Not everyone is comfortable with schools getting into the profit arena.[58] Particularly disturbing to some is the practice of granting companies exclusive vending contracts in return for large sums of money, and selling advertising on buses, in classrooms, and at sports facilities.[59] Parents and other school and community leaders can help ensure that school food service and nutrition program goals and resources are important parts of this discussion and of the decision-making process.

USDA's Team Nutrition articulates the following principles that, when shared by supporters at the local, state, and national levels, will create success[60]:

- We believe that children should be empowered to make food choices that reflect the Dietary Guidelines for Americans.
- We believe that good nutrition and physical activity are essential to children's health and educational success.
- We believe that school meals that meet the Dietary Guidelines for Americans should appeal to children and taste good.

- We believe our programs must build upon the best science, education, communication, and technical resources available.
- We believe that public/private partnerships are essential to reaching children to promote food choices for a healthful diet.
- We believe that messages to children should be age appropriate and delivered in a language they speak, through media they use, in ways that are entertaining and actively involve them in learning.
- We believe in focusing on positive messages regarding food choices children can make.
- We believe it is critical to stimulate and support action and education at the national, state, and local levels to change children's eating behaviors successfully.

Local teams should examine these principles, assess the degree to which the values of their school and community are aligned with the principles, and use that assessment as the basis for planning strategically.

In *The One Place,* the Young and Rubicam Foundation gives the following advice to educators, parents, and community leaders who want to work together to change local schools: "The answer does not lie in any prescribed structure or schedule, but in the adoption of a different concept. . . . The only valid guide to what a particular school in a particular community should be and do is the determination of what children need to develop, learn and become the masters of their own destinies."[61] When there is true agreement on what the community wants its school food and nutrition program to be, decisions will be made to ensure success.

Stephen Covey reminds us to begin with the end in mind, to consider the law of the farm, and plan for a harvest of what we have planted and nurtured.[62] There is often a great chasm between rhetoric and reality. Local supporters of nutrition integrity can begin to close that gap. It is time to move beyond words . . . to walk the talk. Every school and community can design a school food and nutrition program that meets its identified needs and priorities and they can implement that design with integrity.

CASE STUDY
STATE

State agencies can work closely with public and private partners at both the national and local levels to facilitate school food and nutrition programs that promote healthy eating and learning readiness. The state agency role is far more than regulatory. Effective leadership at this level can provide strong support to advance the availability, quality, and acceptance of school food and nutrition programs that are an important part of the school day.

Beliefs

The following planning foundation laid by the Arkansas Department of Education Child Nutrition Unit is an example of the way many state agencies are beginning their planning process today:

- Nutritious, tasty, affordable school lunches and school breakfasts should be available for all students in Arkansas schools.
- School environments that make available only healthful food choices, provide adequate time for their selection and enjoyment, and promote their consumption through pleasant surroundings and positive adult role modeling should be the norm for Arkansas schools.

- Nutrition education in the classroom and the cafeteria to promote critical thinking that will result in the development of healthful eating behaviors, improved learning readiness, health promotion, disease prevention, and pleasure in eating should be a priority for all schools.
- Local, state, and federal commitments to child nutrition programs as integral components of education, evidenced by adequate financial resources effectively managed to provide quality services, are necessary for a healthy school.

Vision

Every Arkansas student and staff member will exhibit an understanding of nutrition concepts by selecting healthful meals at school and away from school.

Mission

To foster the service of nutritious meals and the development of school environments supportive of healthful eating behaviors of all students and staff.

CASE STUDY
LOCAL

In 1992, the food service department of the South Side Area School District in Hookstown, Pennsylvania, was losing student and faculty participation and also losing money. The department was considered an independent support function, primarily concerned with profit and loss. The new food service director, Andrew Adams, was charged with turning things around. He chose to look beyond the financial bottom line.

His school district had completed district-level strategic planning and implementation as well as site-based planning to produce a plan for the elementary programs. Adams had been part of the district-level planning team, but school food service was only peripherally addressed. He became convinced that the concept of strategic planning offered his department the opportunity to stretch for the ideal, stimulate proactive leadership, reverse the operating deficit, and improve customer satisfaction. His superintendent of schools, George Szymanski, Ph.D., was a strong proponent of strategic planning and together they concluded that the food service department's organizational structure would be a good fit for the site-based planning process.

Team Selected

The planning team included the food service director and representation from school food service managers, food service assistants, students, teachers, parents, administrators, board members, and food purveyors, along with a food service director from another school district and a staff member from the Pennsylvania Department of Education.

Data collected for the team included detailed participation records, potential growth, payroll and staffing, current literature related to universal school lunch, school breakfast and learning, nutrition trends, and planning processes. The district's belief statements and strategic plan were thoroughly examined as the first order of business. The group decided to lay aside their preconceived notions of the food service department as an independent support function and think outside the box in ways they had never before thought about student nutrition.

Strengths and Weaknesses

Strengths

Departmental strengths identified by the team included the following:

- High-quality food
- Cooperative, competent, friendly, and efficient staff
- Student and parent involvement
- Computerized meal purchases
- Incentives for increased participation
- Special services for other school programs
- In-house staff rather than management company
- Visible willingness to make changes

Weaknesses

Departmental weaknesses to be addressed in developing the improvement plan included the following:

- Constraints on time to eat
- Low staff participation
- Repetitive menus
- Sterile appearance of dining areas
- Old equipment and delayed repairs
- Lack of cleaning between meal periods
- Breakfast participation below potential
- Staff and substitutes inadequately trained
- Confidentiality of application information sometimes violated
- Inadequate parent information on computer accounts
- Inadequate nutrition education for students

External Analysis

As the team members looked at local data and needs, they also discussed social, economic, demographic, and political factors as well as assumptions that would affect the future of the food service program.

- Latchkey children
- Single-parent families
- Growing number of dysfunctional families
- Unemployment
- Collective bargaining agreements
- Elections
- Commodities
- Expansion of the greater Pittsburgh International Airport
- Fast foods and fast-food trends
- Advertising

Vision and Mission

The group process for examining critical issues was slow and difficult. As the process progressed, however, it was clear that the time was a good investment. Adams said that this is not an area that can be rushed—or the outcomes will be diminished. The clear, concise vision became a consensus objective for the team. While it was futuristic, given the current state of the department, the planning team made it clear that time was not to be wasted in making the vision a reality. The mission was written to be a road map for effective change.

Vision

The South Side School food service and nutrition program will ensure that each student's readiness to learn will not be impaired by nutritional inadequacies.

Mission

The mission of the South Side School food service and nutrition program is to remove the nutritional barriers to learning and ensure that students are capable of making healthy food choices by providing appetizing and nutritious meals to all students, in a courteous, respectful, and stress-free environment while supporting a district-wide nutrition education program and remaining fiscally responsible.

Strategies

Areas requiring the greatest effort and allocation of resources were identified. Adams said the level of excitement and intensity rose as concrete strategies were developed and priorities established. Heading the list were the following:

- Student nutrient intakes
- Nutrition education
- Communication
- Cafeteria environment
- Equipment and facilities
- Staff development
- Finances
- Reorganization

Action plans were developed for each strategy. Strategic policies had been developed previously for the district and the team chose to accept them, but made the following additions they believed were critical to successful operation of the food service and nutrition program:

- We will ensure that there is opportunity for students to adhere to the 1990 Dietary Guidelines for Americans.
- We will not allow any breach of confidentiality.
- All decisions will be made in the best interest of our students.
- We will not tolerate any behavior that demeans the human worth or dignity of anyone.
- We will implement practices that are environmentally responsible.
- No child will be denied a meal because of the inability to pay.

Implementation

The team was pleased with its plan and determined that it not remain on the shelf. Within six weeks, teams were further studying facilities, equipment, and the home/school community. Working cooperatively within the five-year curriculum cycle, a nutrition education strategy in health education was developed and an NET grant proposal was submitted to the state department of education. Catering opportunities were explored and consideration was given to providing meals for Head Start. Short- and long-term reorganization plans were developed.

Results

The NET grant proposal was successful, and a proposal was also funded the following year. Increased emphasis on nutrition education and nutrient analysis of expanded menu cycles resulted. High school participation doubled within two years and significant gains were made in elementary schools. Innovation became the norm, as all employees began looking at possibilities differently. One popular result was "summer lunch on the bus." The summer food service program at the high school met the needs of children who could get there for meals; however, there were others in the rural district who were not being served. Adams had the four back seats in a school bus removed to make space for insulated food carriers, serving tables, and wastebaskets. When the bus pulls into a serving site, students climb aboard the bus to be served and to eat their lunch, then the bus moves on to another site. "By taking good tasting, nutritious lunches to some of our most at-risk students during the summer, we are not only providing for their physical needs, but we are sending the message that we care about them and that their needs are important to us," Adams said. "We believe this is making a difference in the way these students develop, grow, and learn." At the same time the program was better meeting the needs of students, the financial picture was improving. The program had had deficits of $24,853 over the previous two years. At the end of the first year after the new planning process was implemented, revenues exceeded expenditures by $17,083. The second year the program was able to replenish reserves with $24,000 to build a comfortable operating balance that would support further program improvements.

Adams said less tangible results were equally important. "Team members felt energized and excited. Our department connected with the rest of the education program and gained much-needed support." Szymanski said the experience infused optimism and excitement into the district's strategic plan. "It connected the loop and made a strong statement about support services and their impact on student learning," he said.

Continuous Planning and Improvement

Adams was quick to say that the planning process was not a one-time thing. "We looked at it as an ongoing process, with adjustments made along the way as situations changed. The key was having a clear identity that was defined not by us, but by representatives of the total school and community," he said. This clear identity provided direction for planning and implementation, and was also useful in assessing the effectiveness of continuous improvement.

In 1997, a new planning team was convened. The same process was used and some of the players were the same. However, new people were added to bring new perspectives and keep the process dynamic. Adams said some changes were made, but the team elected to keep the original vision and mission. One result of the process is that Adams's services have been sold to a neighboring school district to manage their school food service and nutrition program. Adams said that the South Side program is operating so well that he can focus some of his energies on the new venture without fear of failure at home. "We have great staff and a great school and community that values our contribution to the education of our students. It is clear now that there is no way the community would consider anything but an education-focused school food service and nutrition program," Adams said.

REFERENCES

1. G. White, "Nutrition Integrity Defined," *School Food Service Journal* 48, no. 1 (1994): 21–22.

2. E. Marx et al., Preface, *Health Is Academic: A Guide to Coordinated School Health Programs* (New York: Teachers College Press, 1998).

3. Committee on Diet and Health, National Research Council, *Diet and Health: Implications for Reducing Chronic Disease Risk* (Washington, DC: National Academy Press, 1989).

4. U.S. Department of Health and Human Services, *The Surgeon General's Report on Nutrition and Health* (Washington, DC: U.S. Government Printing Office, 1988).

5. U.S. Department of Health and Human Services, *Healthy People 2000: National Health Promotion and Disease Prevention Objectives.* DHHS Publication No. (PHS) 91–50213, Public Health Service (Washington, DC: U.S. Government Printing Office, 1991).

6. U.S. Department of Agriculture, *Healthy Kids: Nutrition Objectives for School Meals.* (Washington, DC: 1994).

7. Institute of Medicine, *Schools and Health: Our Nation's Investment*, eds. D. Allensworth et al. (Washington, DC: National Academy Press, 1997).

8. W. Dietz, "Health Consequences of Obesity in Youth: Childhood Predictors of Adult Disease," *Pediatrics* 101, no. 3 (1998): 518–525.

9. J. Hill and G. Trowbridge, Childhood Obesity: Future Directions and Research Priorities, *Pediatrics* 101, no. 3 (1998): 570–574.

10. F. Braddon, "Onset of Obesity in a 30 Year Birth Cohort Study," *British Medical Journal* 193 (1986): 299–303.

11. Dietz, "Health Consequences of Obesity in Youth."

12. T. Melbin and J. Vuille, "Further Evidence of an Association between Psychosocial Problems and Increase in Relative Weight between 7 and 10 Years of Age," *Acta Paediatrica Scandinavica*, 78 (1989): 576–580.

13. Citizen's Commission on School Nutrition, *White Paper on School Lunch Nutrition.* (Washington, DC: Center for Science in the Public Interest, 1990).

14. V. Pilant, "Current Issues in Child Nutrition." *Topics in Clinical Nutrition* 9, no. 4 (1994): 1–8.

15. Abt. Associates, *Final Report: Study of Income Verification in the National School Lunch Program* (Arlington, VA: 1990).

16. P. Gleason, "Participation in the National School Lunch Program and the School Breakfast Program," *American Journal of Clinical Nutrition* 61(S) (1995): 213–220.

17. American Dietetic Association (ADA), "Position: Competitive Foods in Schools," *Journal of the American Dietetic Association* 91 (1991): 1123–1125.

18. Child Nutrition Programs Rule, 7 C.F.R. 210.9(a)(1).

19. Child Nutrition Programs Rule, 7 C.F.R. 210.11(a)(1).

20. Mississippi State Board of Education, "Policy on Competition and Extra Food Sales" (1985).

21. C. Lewis et al., "Healthy People 2000: Report on the 1994 Nutrition Progress Review," *Nutrition Today* 29, no. 6 (1994): 6–14.

22. S. Krebs-Smith et al., "Fruit and Vegetable Intakes of Children and Adolescents in the United States," *Archives of Pediatric and Adolescent Medicine* 150 (1996): 81–86.

23. *Consumer Reports,* "Is Your Kid Failing Lunch?, September 1998, 49–52.

24. Institute of Medicine, *Schools and Health.*

25. S. Crockett and L. Sims, "Environmental Influences on Children's Eating," *Journal of Nutrition Education* 27(suppl.) (1995): 235–249.

26. D. Caldwell et al., "School Nutrition Services," in *Health Is Academic: A Guide to Coordinated School Health Programs,* E. Marx et al., eds. (New York: Teachers College Press, 1998).

27. White, "Nutrition Integrity Defined."

28. American School Food Service Association (ASFSA), *Creating Policy for Nutrition Integrity in Schools* (Alexandria, VA: 1994).

29. J. Sneed and M. Gregoire, "Setting the Standard," *School Food Service Journal* 48, no. 1 (1994): 27–30.

30. M. Gregoire and J. Sneed, "Standards for Nutrition Integrity," *School Food Service Research Review* 18, no. 2 (1994): 106-111

31. ASFSA, *Keys to Excellence: Standards of Practice for Nutrition Integrity* (Alexandria, VA: 1995).

32. Centers for Disease Control and Prevention (CDC), "Guidelines for School Health Programs To Promote Lifelong Healthy Eating," *Morbidity and Mortality Weekly Report* 45, RR-9 (1996).

33. E. Marx et al., Preface, *Health is Academic.*

34. F. McKenzie and J. Richmond, "Linking Health and Learning: An Overview of Coordinated School Health Programs," *Health Is Academic: A Guide to Coordinated School Health Programs,* E. Marx et al., eds. (New York: Teachers College Press, 1998).

35. Child Nutrition Programs, School Meals Initiative for Healthy Children Rule, 7 C.F.R. Parts 210 and 220 (1995).

36. USDA, *USDA Team Nutrition Strategic Plan for Training and Technical Assistance to Achieve Healthy School Meals: Executive Summary* (Washington, DC: 1994).

37. USDA, *A Menu Planner for Healthy School Meals: To Help You Plan, Prepare, Serve, and Market Appealing Meals* (Washington, DC: 1998).

38. USDA, "Healthy School Meals" in *Healthy Kids: A Leadership Guide for School Decision-Makers* (Washington, DC: 1997).

39. USDA, *A Tool Kit for Healthy School Meals: Recipes and Training Materials* (Washington, DC: 1995).

40. USDA, *Evaluation of Team Nutrition Pilot Communities* (Washington, DC: 1999).

41. Institute of Medicine, *Schools and Health.*

42. U.S. Department of Health and Human Services, Office of Public Health and Science. *Healthy People 2010 Objectives: Draft for Public Comment* (Washington, DC: 1998).

43. Institute of Medicine, *Schools and Health.*

44. D. Caldwell, "Clear Vision Leads to Success: Foodservice Strategic Planning," *School Business Affairs,* November 1994, 19–22.

45. White, "Nutrition Integrity Defined."

46. ASFSA, *Legislative Issue Paper: Universal Vision: American's Children Ready to Learn* (Alexandria, VA: 1992).

47. ASFSA, *Consensus Conference: Building Healthy Children Ready to Learn: Executive Summary* (Alexandria, VA: 1993).

48. American Dietetic Association (ADA), Society for Nutrition Education, and ASFSA, "School-Based

Nutrition Programs and Services," *Journal of the American Dietetic Association* 95, no. 3 (1995): 367–369.

49. M. Nestle, "Societal Barriers to Improved School Lunch Programs: Rationale for Recent Policy Recommendations," *School Food Service Research Review* 16, no. 1 (1992): 5–10.

50. CDC, "Guidelines for School Health Programs."

51. ASFSA, *Creating Policy for Nutrition Integrity.*

52. ASFSA, *Keys to Excellence.*

53. National Association of State Boards of Education, *Policy Update: School Nutrition Programs* (Alexandria, VA: 1997).

54. Institute of Medicine, *Schools and Health.*

55. B. Pateman et al., "School Health Policies and Programs Study: School Food Service," *Journal of School Health* 65 (1995): 327–332.

56. USDA, *Evaluation of Team Nutrition.*

57. ADA et al., "School-Based Nutrition Programs."

58. K. Vail, "11 Ways To Make Money: When Traditional Funding Isn't Enough," *American School Board Journal,* May 1998, 30–33.

59. K. Vail, "Insert Coins in Slot: School Vending Machines Generate Funds and Controversy," *American School Board Journal* (February 1999):28–31.

60. USDA, *Community Nutrition Action Kit: For People Where They Live, Learn and Play* (Washington, DC: 1996).

61. Young and Rubicam Foundation, *The One Place: A New Role for American Schools* (New York: St. Martin's Press, 1991).

62. S. Covey, *Principled Centered Leadership* (New York: Simon & Schuster, 1992).

CHAPTER 5

Human Resources

Martha T. Conklin

OUTLINE

- Introduction
- Leaders in Child Nutrition Programs
  - The Ideal CNP Leader
  - Qualifications of District Directors and Single-Unit Managers
- Development of CNP Leaders
  - Education and Lifelong Learning
  - Certification
  - Role of NFSMI
  - Recruitment of CNP Leaders
- Management of Human Resources
  - Staffing and Diversity
  - Labor Productivity
  - Training
- Summary
- Case Study: The Successful Turnaround of a Child Nutrition Program, 1992–1998
  Gail M. Johnson

INTRODUCTION

A ship without a rudder goes nowhere or anywhere, totally dependent on the current for direction. Child nutrition programs (CNPs) without competent leaders and employees are similarly set adrift, constantly buffeted by forces competing for the finite resources necessary to provide education to children. Effective leadership makes the difference between the perception that food and nutrition services are simply a "necessity" to feed children and the knowledge that providing nourishing meals to children is just as important to the educational process as textbooks and transportation to school.

The American School Food Service Association (ASFSA) recognizes the importance of competent leadership and human resource management to the profession. ASFSA's *Keys to Excellence* identifies human resources as a major area leading to program excellence. Key Achievement Five of the *Keys* states that "The school foodservice and nutrition staff is qualified to implement the goals of the school foodservice and nutrition program."[1(p5)] The importance of effective human resource management also is addressed by research on the knowledge and skills required of competent CNP district directors.[2]

The objectives of this chapter are to discuss who will be the leaders in CNPs in the next century and how these leaders will be developed. Specific objectives are to (1) define leadership in CNPs, (2) describe the qualifications of CNP district directors/supervisors and single-unit managers, (3) identify the process for developing competent leaders, and (4) discuss issues in effective human resource management in CNPs.

LEADERS IN CHILD NUTRITION PROGRAMS

The Ideal CNP Leader

Administrators are charged with the control of tasks and the direction of people to carry out tasks. Within this responsibility, administrators always have discretionary power or a range of actions they may take, but do not have to take. It is in the realm of discretionary power that leaders are created. Leaders are people within an organization who have the power of position and use their discretionary power to carry out a vision that moves the organization to meet its goals.[3] Leaders can be found at various levels in CNPs but for purposes of this chapter, the discussion focuses on characterizing the district food and nutrition program director as leader. The district director is the person designated by the school food authority to administer the CNP. District directors lead by doing the following:

- Articulating to all stakeholders the role CNPs play in educating children from pre-kindergarten to high school graduation
- Engendering support for the CNP from school administration, teachers, parents, and the community
- Participating as a full partner in delivering nutrition education within a comprehensive school health curriculum
- Designing and directing CNP operations to meet the needs and desires of customers while maintaining the nutrition and fiscal integrity of the program
- Managing a CNP that is accountable to taxpayers and the congressional intent of child nutrition legislation
- Embracing change as the only constant in the program milieu
- Committing to continuous quality improvement by benchmarking program performance with best practices in CNPs throughout the nation
- Advocating for a variety of CNPs and services within the community
- Collaborating with education, public health, and other professional groups to deliver seamless services to children

District directors as leaders are self-assured and confident when relating to others because they have knowledge backed by sound research that proper nourishment is a vital component of the educational process. When district directors act as leaders, they will be recognized as such and sought out by their community as the person who can provide information on food and nutrition services for children.

Qualifications of District Directors and Single-Unit Managers

Just as the image of Betty Crocker has changed from the comforting mother figure to the busy working mom, the image of the "nice lady or man in the lunchroom" is no longer current. District directors may be pleasant people, but they are foremost professionals with a specific body of knowledge and skills directed to providing a vital service to the community while managing a million-dollar budget.

Federal SCANS Report

What does it take to be successful in administering food and nutrition programs for children? The federal government has a partial answer for all employees regardless of their position. The Secretary's Commission on Achieving Necessary Skills (SCANS) was established in 1990 to define skills needed for employment in today's workplace. This commission identified two types of skills: competencies necessary for success in the workplace (Exhibit 5–1) and foundation skills and qualities that underlie the competencies (Exhibit 5–2). The relative importance of the SCANS competencies/foundations is dependent on the needs of a specific job. For example, the competence required of a food service manager in *allocating money* is much greater than similar skills required of a secretary.[4] Key points to be

Exhibit 5–1 SCANS Competencies

COMPETENCY	EXPLANATION
Resources	Allocates time Allocates money Allocates material and facility resources Allocates human resources
Information	Acquires and evaluates information Organizes and maintains information Interprets and communicates information Uses computers to process information
Interpersonal	Participates as a member of a team Teaches others Serves clients and customers Exercises leadership Negotiates to arrive at a decision Works with cultural diversity
Systems	Understands systems Monitors and corrects performance Improves and designs systems
Technology	Selects technology Applies technology to task Maintains and troubleshoots technology

Source: Reprinted from U.S. Department of Labor, The Secretary's Commission on Achieving Necessary Skills. *Skills and Tasks for JOBS: A SCANS Report for America 2000*, pp. 1–4, 1992, Washington, DC: U.S. Government Printing Office.

derived from the SCANS document are that basic competencies are required of any type of work, and the foundation skills and beginning levels of these competencies should be attained by high school graduation. Figure 5–1 illustrates how these competencies and foundation skills support job performance in the school food and nutrition program.

National Food Service Management Institute Competency Research

Researchers at the National Food Service Management Institute (NFSMI) conducted two national surveys to determine the functions and tasks associated with management positions in school food and nutrition programs.[5,6] Differences exist in the roles of district director and site-based manager. The role of district director is more complex. The district director's job has 16 functions versus 12 for the manager, and they are performed with less consistency. The most important function rated by district directors responding to the Gregoire and Sneed survey[6] was customer service, followed by functions associated with managing a safe and sanitary food service, financial management and record keeping, food production, procurement, and program accountability (Exhibit 5–3).[6,7] Single-unit managers meet with the customer every day, but their perceptions of their management role placed customer service third in importance to their job. Issues of program accountability were rated as primary, followed by sanitation and safety, customer service, equipment use and care, and food production as the top five roles of this position (Exhibit 5–4).[8,9]

Figure 5–2 compares similar job functions of the district director with those of the single-unit manager. This comparison is made only on the 10 broad functions each position had in common, and the exact tasks under each job function differed depending on the level of management involved. Single-unit managers

Exhibit 5–2 SCANS Foundation Skills

FOUNDATION SKILLS	EXPLANATION
Basic Skills	Reading Writing Arithmetic Mathematics Listening Speaking
Thinking Skills	Creative thinking Decision making Problem solving Seeing things in the mind's eye Knowing how to learn Reasoning
Personal Qualities	Responsibility Self-esteem Social Self-management Integrity and honesty

Source: Reprinted from U.S. Department of Labor, The Secretary's Commission on Achieving Necessary Skills. *Skills and Tasks for JOBS: A SCANS Report for America 2000,* pp. 1–5, 1992, Washington, DC: U.S. Government Printing Office.

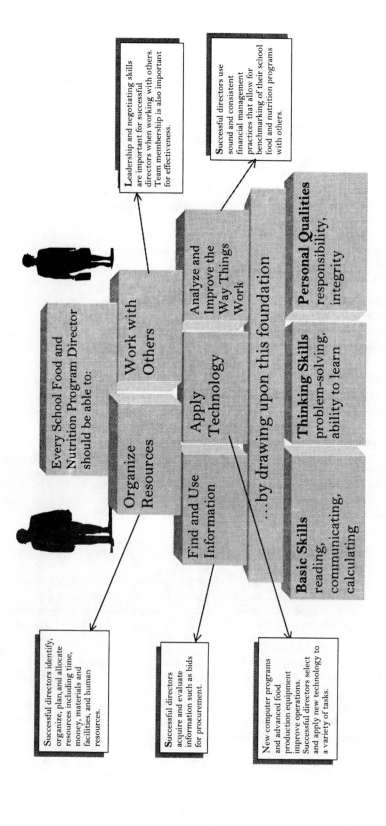

Figure 5-1 SCANS Competencies Applied to School Food and Nutrition Program Directors. *Source:* Adapted with permission from Chrysler Learning Connection, How To Help Your Child Love to Learn, *Learning Together*, No. 3, © 1996, The Chrysler Corporation.

Exhibit 5–3 Job Tasks Rated as "Very Important" by District Directors for the Six Most Important Functions of Their Job

CUSTOMER SERVICE
- Develops standards for prompt, courteous, and efficient service.
- Evaluates efficiency of serving area.
- Establishes quality standards in the presentation, merchandising, taste, and service of food.
- Evaluates serving methods to ensure students are served quickly.
- Recommends solutions to problems with the service of food.

SANITATION AND SAFETY
- Facilitates development of sanitation procedures and cleaning schedules.
- Ensures proper storage and handling of chemicals and cleaning supplies.
- Maintains an effective insect and rodent control system.
- Establishes safety standards and rules.
- Monitors food service unit compliance with health and safety rules established by federal (OSHA), state, and local agencies.
- Considers safety requirements when ordering equipment.

FINANCIAL MANAGEMENT AND RECORD KEEPING
- Operates program within budget.
- Implements control in all cost categories (e.g., labor, food, supply, operating).
- Establishes financial objectives for the food service operation.
- Supervises free and reduced-price meal applications and verification process.
- Establishes a system to ensure food service fiscal accountability.

FOOD PRODUCTION
- Evaluates food quality.
- Established procedures to ensure appropriate temperatures of foods during preparation, transportation, and service.
- Establishes procedures for portion control. Delegates authority and responsibility for food production and service to unit managers and assistants.
- Establishes procedures to provide and preserve maximum nutritional value of food.
- Works with unit managers to evaluate the food production system and food quality, and revises the system as needed to improve operations.

PROCUREMENT
- Determines the type and quality of food and supplies to be purchased based on student needs and resources available.
- Maintains a system for proper storage and distribution of food and supplies throughout the district.
- Ensures that food, supplies, and equipment are purchased to meet specifications.
- Maintains a purchasing system consistent with USDA and state purchasing guidelines.
- Establishes a purchasing system to secure food and supplies used by district food service units.

PROGRAM ACCOUNTABILITY
- Assesses program compliance with federal, state, and local regulations.
- Revises school food service program operations based on changes in federal, state, and/or local regulations.
- Informs administrative staff and school food service program personnel of federal, state, and local government regulations that affect program operations.
- Communicates changes to school food service personnel.

continues

Exhibit 5–3 continued

• Cooperates with federal agencies and personnel responsible for the administration and review of district food service programs.

Source: Reprinted with permission from M.B. Gregoire and J. Sneed, Competencies for District School Nutrition Directors/Supervisors, *School Food Service Research Review*, Vol. 18, pp. 89–99, © 1994, American School Food Service Association.

---

have greater daily operational responsibilities than directors. Managers are supervising, overseeing, and coordinating school-level CNP activities, and they collect information for decision making at the district level. District directors' responsibilities involve planning, coordination, and administration for the entire school food authority.

Overall, single-unit managers rated the functions of their job (Figure 5–2, *solid line*) as *more important* than district directors rated similar job functions (Figure 5–2, *dotted line*). An exception is found with the functions of financial management and record keeping and nutrition and menu planning. Directors viewed these two functions as more important to their job than single-unit managers rated these same functions in their jobs. This is understandable because the prime objective of school food authorities should be to administer a food and nutrition program that has both nutrition and fiscal integrity, and the district director is assigned this responsibility.

District directors performed the functions of their jobs on an episodic basis. No job functions were performed daily, and most were performed on a monthly or periodic basis. The highest frequency of performance was found with the functions of customer service and food production. These findings suggest that the effective role of district director be that of a generalist with excellent time management skills. Directors need to be able to do many tasks and must be flexible enough to deal with the potential of performing different tasks each day. Educational preparation and continuing professional development should be in a broad range of areas related to food, nutrition, and business management.[10]

Change Leadership

Leaders in CNPs know strategies for managing change.[11] Effective district directors must respond to changes in this federally sponsored program, but they also must initiate change in their operations to survive in today's educational and business climate. They do not need to know all the answers, but they do need to ask the right questions. Leaders must engage people in confronting challenges, adjusting values, changing perspectives, and learning new habits.[12] The crucial attribute is the ability to initiate and deal with change as an overriding prerequisite to success.

A study of change leaders in Fortune 500 companies found that they were technically skilled people who were very capable in personal relationships. Change leaders were tough decision makers who were results oriented. Few of these managers went to business school, but they came from a technical specialty such as engineering or accounting.

They honed their skills on the job by encountering problems and finding solutions. Their most distinctive competence was their ability to operate with more than one leadership style. They did whatever works, depending on the situation. When speed was essential, they would tell their people what to do. When a change in behavior was needed, they would change gears and become coaches. Change leaders were totally focused on results, not methods, so they tried anything that helped them achieve their goals.[13]

Exhibit 5–4 Job Tasks Rated as "Very Important" by Single-Unit Managers for the Five Most Important Functions of Their Job

PROGRAM ACCOUNTABILITY
- Follows federal, state, and local regulations.
- Prevents discriminations by protecting the identity of students receiving free and reduced-price meals.

SANITATION AND SAFETY
- Practices and enforces personal hygiene.
- Maintains sanitations standards for equipment, personnel, food, and facility.
- Controls insects and rodents.
- Follows safety standards for equipment, personnel, food, and facility.
- Follows procedures to maintain safe and sanitary conditions in the storage, preparation, and service of food.

CUSTOMER SERVICE
- Serves food at correct temperatures.
- Operates serving line with prompt, courteous, and efficient service.
- Maintains a serving line with proper conditions (for example, time and temperature) to keep nutitive value of foods.
- Encourages employees to be pleasant and helpful when serving meals, exchanging monies, and maintaining facilities.
- Improves food service by making sure the dining and kitchen areas are clean and attractive.

EQUIPMENT USE AND CARE
- Maintains safety standards.
- Trains employees to use safety precaustions when operating and cleaning equipment.
- Reports faulty operation of equipment.
- Monitors cleaning and maintenance of large equipment.
- Supervises employees in the proper use and care of equipment.

FOOD PRODUCTION
- Directs the preparation of foods that taste good and are nutritious.
- Maintains daily menu and food production records.
- Monitors effectiveness of food production, distribution, and service procedures.
- Sets up and maintains standards for control of quality and quantity food production and distribution.
- Monitors and improves productivity.

Source: Data from J. Sneed and K.T. White, Development and Validation of Competency Statements for Managers in School Food Service, *School Food Service Research Review*, Vol. 17, pp. 50–61, © 1993, and M.T. Conklin, Job Functions and Tasks of School Nutrition Managers and District Directors/Supervisors, *NFSMI Insight,* No. 2, © 1995, National Food Service Management Institute.

Change leaders speak and write well, and they especially know how to listen. They have the ability truly to hear what others are saying, and, when necessary, to be led by those who lack formal authority over them.[14] They know the value of teamwork and the multidisciplinary approach to program planning, especially in a community setting. Change leadership reduces to two essential capabilities: (1) the ability to identify the right solution at the right time to meet objectives, and (2) the ability to understand and orchestrate the human variables necessary to gain support and commitment from those affected by change deci-

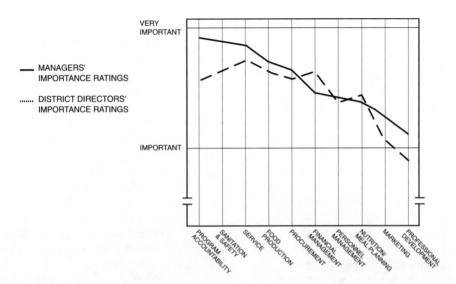

VERY
IMPORTANT

—— MANAGERS'
IMPORTANCE RATINGS

······ DISTRICT DIRECTORS'
IMPORTANCE RATINGS

IMPORTANT

PROGRAM ACCOUNTABILITY
SANITATION & SAFETY
SERVICE
FOOD PRODUCTION
PROCUREMENT
FINANCIAL MANAGEMENT
PERSONNEL MANAGEMENT
NUTRITION/ MEAL PLANNING
MARKETING
PROFESSIONAL DEVELOPMENT

Figure 5–2 Comparison of District Directors'/Supervisors' to School Nutrition Managers' Job Function Importance Ratings. *Source:* Reprinted with permission from M.T. Conklin, Job Functions and Tasks of School Nutrition Managers and District Directors/Supervisors, *NFSMI Insight*, No. 2, © 1995, National Food Service Management Institute.

sions.[15] Both abilities encompass the use of technological advancements to improve and simplify processes to support decision making at the lowest level possible in the organization.

Although the overall goal of CNPs has remained unchanged for more than 50 years, the precise emphasis of the program changes with political administrations. CNP leaders characterized at the beginning of this chapter will not be blindsided by these political forces because they keep abreast of the needs of all their constituents. Others, however, may need to call upon their change leadership skills to respond to new government initiatives. For the past several years, CNPs have been instructed to alter menus to meet minimum nutrient goals for calories and vitamins within maximum guidelines for total fat and saturated fat content. This has created the greatest change in CNPs since offer versus serve regulations in the 1970s. In this instance, the primary objective for the change was dictated by government regulation. Effective change leaders would have identified the right solutions to meet the

School Meals Initiative for Healthy Children in their districts by the date required. They also would have provided resources and training while coaching their employees to gain support and commitment for these changes.

Recently, the emphasis on running CNPs as a sound business has reemerged. The impact on the successful district director is to foster the ability to deal with and promote change to survive in a business climate. Effective directors welcome and promote change as a necessity in running a successful program. They seek to benchmark their program with best in practice and work with employees to "build better mousetraps" in their own operation. Continuous quality improvement is required to operate a successful CNP with nutrition and fiscal integrity.

DEVELOPMENT OF CNP LEADERS

Qualified CNP leaders are in demand now, and evidence exists that this demand will increase in the next few years. In a survey of state directors, nearly half (41 percent) of the 43 respondents answered yes to the question, "Do you believe there will be a shortage of qualified food service directors in the year 2000?"[16(p4)] This belief was held the strongest by state directors in the Midwest and Northeast regions of the country.[16]

Researchers at the National Food Service Management Institute conducted nationwide, random surveys that collected information in the early 1990s on the demographics of district food and nutrition program directors.[17–19] Analysis of demographics from these research samples shows that 43 percent of single-unit managers and district directors had between 11 and 20 years of food service experience, and approximately 30 percent had more than 20 years experience. If the average working life of an individual is 40 years, about one-third of the professionals involved in the management of CNPs had fulfilled more than half their years of employment. One could conclude from these data that in the early years of the twenty-first century, there will be a substantial turnover of these professionals. The demographics are alarming while challenging, because this degree of turnover in the profession provides an opportunity to increase professional standards for individuals filling vacated positions.[20] An opportunity exists to swell the ranks of district directors as CNP leaders.

Education and Lifelong Learning

School food and nutrition programs function within an educational setting in a knowledge-based world economy. Knowledge, preceded by information, is the primary resource for individuals and for the economy.[20] School systems and school administrators have traditionally valued the acquisition of knowledge through formal education culminating in advanced degrees. The reward systems in schools are based on education attained, continuing professional education, and certification in professional disciplines. If district directors

want to be recognized as full partners in providing services to children in the school environment, they need to be evaluated and found equal to teachers and administrators using similar criteria. Therefore, district directors should attain at least a baccalaureate degree and seek certification as a food and nutrition professional.

This is not a new idea, but one whose time has come. In Chapter 2 the author recalled that as early as the 1920s, Emma Smedley wrote that the school lunch program provided professional opportunities for trained cafeteria managers or dietitians who should have the same rank as teachers of home economics.[21] In the 1930s, Mary de Garmo Bryan stated that the cafeteria manager should be as well trained as the classroom teacher. She believed that technical qualifications were not enough because managers must be able to work with people, have a scientific attitude toward problem solving, and have an appreciation for the social significance of their work.[22] These characteristics remain vital today if not more so due to the complexity of government and societal systems in the millennium. John F. Kennedy wrote that leadership and learning are indispensable to each other.[23]

Data show that of the district directors with more than 20 years of school food service experience, approximately 30 percent had attained a baccalaureate degree and beyond, and 40 percent had earned a high school diploma as their highest level of education. On the contrary, 66 percent of district directors with less than five years experience in school food service held at least a baccalaureate degree, and 9 percent had only graduated from high school. Increasing educational level with decreasing experience in school food service held true at other levels of experience.[24] Data indicate that younger professionals were more likely to assume the role of district directors equipped with degrees comparable to those of teachers and administrators. This trend must continue for the entire profession to earn respect as a full partner in the educational process, to handle the multimillion-dollar budgets associated with this program, and for individuals to have the self-confidence in the school setting to advocate for the CNP and for children's nutritional needs.

A baccalaureate education has unique advantages over a high school or even a technical degree in light of future needs of the profession. A B.S./B.A. degree, constructed with a firm foundation in liberal education, will enable individuals to adapt more easily to a shifting environment. Liberal education encourages critical thinking skills, communication, foreign language, and knowledge of other cultures. The importance of integrating and synthesizing learning from a variety of disciplines is emphasized.[25] By the time a child born today finishes college, knowledge may have quadrupled; by the time that child is 50, knowledge will have grown 32-fold.[26] Much of what is learned in technical courses is obsolete a few years after graduation. Education should prepare twenty-first century professionals to be critical thinkers and change leaders when processes and opportunities are created, not recalled. A bachelor's degree also will allow individuals to earn over a lifetime twice the income they would earn with a 10th grade education.[27]

With the explosion of information in our society, even a four-year degree will not be sufficient to allow individuals to remain in the forefront of their profession. Professionals should be prepared, as a vital part of their education, actively to engage in learning throughout their life span. Continuing education should be viewed as a necessary extension of professional preparation. Students should be encouraged to pursue advanced degrees and to apply for scholarships made available through professional associations such as the American Dietetic Association, the American Association of Family and Consumer Sciences, and the American School Food Service Association. They should be taught the use of the Internet for asynchronous education and training. Students also should learn to value professional

meetings and networking as a source of information to upgrade knowledge and skills.

Certification

Certification seeks to ensure minimum competence of professionals, thereby protecting consumers, be they patients, clients, or employers. Certification is usually attained by entry-level education requirements, professional experience, and successful completion of a national examination. These programs also recognize the importance of lifelong learning by requiring continuing professional education to maintain certification status.

Several certification programs are designed for food and nutrition professionals, but not all school food and nutrition professionals have valued attaining this designation. Research has shown that approximately 35 percent of district directors were not certified in the early 1990s. Of directors who were certified, approximately 11 percent were registered dietitians, 40 percent maintained ASFSA certification, and 20 percent were certified through their state departments of education.[28]

Many states require state certification for the individual administering the school food and nutrition program. The Georgia Department of Education established in the 1960s an entry-level certificate for school food and nutrition program directors, which was mandated a requirement in 1980 except in very small districts. Educational requirements for entry-level certification include a bachelor's degree with at least six semester hours in food and nutrition at the upper division level. In addition, they must meet American Dietetic Association (ADA) membership requirements or complete 15 quarter hours or 10 semester hours in the areas of psychology or sociology of the school-age child or adult, personnel management, and methods and principles of education, with no more than 10 hours in any one area. School food and nutrition program directors with a master's degree are issued a professional certificate. Entry-level directors with a bachelor's degree receive a provisional certificate and have a maximum of five years to complete a master's.[29]

The department of education in the state of Louisiana requires that a CNP director/supervisor have a master's degree in home economics, institutional management, nutrition, dietetics, business administration, food technology, or public health nutrition from an accredited institution of higher education. In addition, there are work experience and specific course work requirements, including a requirement to audit a portion of the prescribed training course for school food service manager certification, during the first year of employment. Regulation further stipulates that payment from school food service funds shall be made only for CNP director/supervisors and acting supervisors who meet all the certification requirements.[30]

State certification programs are required, but there also are voluntary, national certification programs structured to enhance professional development. The most directly applicable national certification program is the one offered by the ASFSA. Research showed that district directors with fewer years of experience were significantly less likely to hold ASFSA certification. Twenty-three percent of directors with less than five years of school food service experience were ASFSA–certified versus 48 percent of directors with more than 20 of years experience. Perhaps new professionals were not informed of this type of certification, or employers had not seen the value of hiring someone with this type of preparation.[31] ASFSA has taken strides recently to develop higher standards for the certification process by developing a national examination based on competencies of district directors,[32] which, when passed, will yield credentials as a school foodservice and nutrition specialist (SFNS). The rigors involved in developing and validating a national examination will lend credibility to this certification. In turn, acquiring the SFNS credential will result in increased recognition and self-esteem for in-

dividuals who choose this route to ensuring and maintaining professional competence.[33]

There are other national certification programs that may meet the needs of specific people better, depending on their educational background and professional goals. Table 5–1 shows various food and nutrition certification programs with education, professional experience, and continuing education requirements. The important aspect of any certification program is that individuals make a commitment to attaining competence by successfully challenging a national exam, and then seek to maintain their proficiencies by continuing professional development. No matter the particular route taken, the certification process is a necessary step in maintaining the knowledge and skills for performance in the information age.

Role of NFSMI

The National Food Service Management Institute was created by Congress in 1989 to enhance the quality and cost effectiveness of CNPs by conducting applied research and educational activities using appropriate technology. The institute was formed through a grant with the U.S. Department of Agriculture (USDA) and a partnership between two universities in Mississippi: The University of Mississippi (UM) and The University of Southern Mississippi (USM). Administrative offices and the education division of the institute are housed in a new building on the UM campus in Oxford. The applied research division is at USM in Hattiesburg, 250 miles south. The NFSMI has a national mandate to deliver services to persons involved in food and nutrition programs for children that are administered by the USDA. This includes the National School Lunch and School Breakfast Programs, Summer Feeding Program, and the Child and Adult Care Food Program. Lifelong learning and continuous quality improvement are underlying tenets of the institute. Primary target audiences are state and district directors of CNPs. Continuing professional education activities

Table 5–1 Certification Programs for Food and Nutrition Professionals

Credential	Title	Education	Professional Experience	National Examination	Continuing Education
CDM[a]	Certified dietary manager	Five pathways—combination of formal education and experience	Varies with formal education	Yes	45 Clock hours over three years-required
DTR[b]	Dietetic technician, registered	Associate degree plus completion of a dietetic technician program approved by the American Dietetic Association	450 Hours of supervised practice	Yes	50 Clock hours over five years-required
FMP[c]	Food service management professional	Five options—combination of education and experience	Five options—varies with management experience and education	Yes	50 Continuing education points over five years-voluntary
RD[b]	Registered dietitian	Baccalaureate degree plus completion of didactic program in dietetics approved by the American Dietetic Association	900 Hours of supervised practice	Yes	75 Clock hours over five years-required Professional development portfolios effective in 2001
SFNS[d]	School foodservice and nutrition specialist	Associate degree or culinary arts certificate	One year experience in school food service and nutrition	Yes	45 Clock hours over three years-required

[a] Certified by the Certifying Board for Dietary Managers, Dietary Managers Association.
[b] Certified by the Commission on Dietetic Registration, The American Dietetic Association.
[c] Certified by the Educational Foundation, National Restaurant Association.
[d] Certified by Certification Governing Board, American School Food Service Association.

are specifically targeted to these audiences. A national advisory council composed of university and industry leaders gives direction to the NFSMI, and each year the program of work is approved by USDA.

Programming for the institute begins with research. The applied research division is unique in that it is the only USDA-funded unit to conduct research on operational issues in food service management. The current focus of this unit is research on customer satisfaction and financial management. Research findings are then used as the basis for educational activities targeted to specific audiences. A clearinghouse for information on CNPs also is administered by NFSMI. The clearinghouse can be reached by calling the main number of NFSMI, 1-800-321-3054. Other NFSMI programs of note are a short course for new and aspiring directors of school food and nutrition programs offered each summer and satellite seminars for single-unit personnel broadcast nationwide at least twice a year.

Recruitment of CNP Leaders

To encourage more baccalaureate-trained professionals to chart a career in CNPs, college and university faculty in dietetics, food service management, and hospitality need to participate fully in recruitment. DeMicco et al.[34] suggested several ways students can be introduced to school food service:

- Expose college students in dietetics and hospitality programs to information about career opportunities in school food service management. Packets of information could be prepared by ASFSA and sent to educators for distribution.
- Send representatives from school food service management to college campuses to recruit, serve as guest speakers, and participate in career fairs.
- Sponsor structured and organized internships for students similar to the ones developed by the National Association of

College and University Food Service/Association of College University Housing Officials.
- Develop a mentoring/internship program for current university students.
- Invite students to attend regional, state, and national conferences sponsored by school food service associations.

By introducing young professionals to child nutrition programs, they will become aware of a career setting that combines food service administration and nutrition education proficiencies in a work environment that favors children and family life.[35]

MANAGEMENT OF HUMAN RESOURCES

Staffing and Diversity

Staffing the child nutrition program with competent, able-bodied food service employees is a constant challenge. The equation is really quite simple. District directors and single-site managers want to hire workers who are willing and able to do the jobs required of them. Employees, on the other hand, want to work in a setting where they can get the most fulfillment and compensation for their labor. Compensation primarily used to be wages, but non–wage benefits have become increasingly important.[36] Today's workers would like full benefits, including health insurance, sick leave, and ample personal leave. All this has to be at a location in which they want to live with work schedules that dovetail with other priorities in life. "Soft" benefits such as compressed workweeks, meals, paid vacation leave, and job sharing also are in demand.[37]

Workers sell their labor to the highest bidder, and employers hire workers who can do the job at the least cost to the organization. The economic concepts of supply and demand apply. When the supply of labor is short, as happens when the unemployment rate is low, the demands of workers for increased wages and better benefits will be met by employers who are competing for qualified staff. When labor is in abundance, the opposite may be true.

School food service work has negative and positive attributes that affect the employment equation. On the positive side, schools function only on weekdays, hours of work correspond to the school day, and holidays are matched to the school calendar. The customers are children and the program exists for a noble cause, nourishing children so they can learn. School food service is a business that will hire employees with low skills and train them. It is an ideal setting for persons with limited skills who wish to work in an environment that is conducive to family life, especially families with children in the primary or secondary grades.

On the other hand, most work in this setting requires high physical demands in a hot, damp environment as with all food service jobs, but the pay and benefits may not match those in other food service segments. Work is not available all year in school systems with the traditional summer vacation, few employees are scheduled for eight-hour days, wages may not compete successfully with other employment settings, and ample benefits may not be available. This all adds up to less annual compensation, placing school food service at a disadvantage in competing for skilled employees unless these workers want part-time jobs matched to the school calendar. Back in the days of Ozzie and Harriet, this was the case. Most school food service employees were women who wanted to earn or supplement an income in a setting coordinated to their children's schedules. They could use skills developed as a homemaker to deliver services to students.

Currently, Harriet needs to work full time because two incomes are needed to raise a family, schools have become a threatening place for some students and adults, and few homemakers come into the work force with basic food preparation skills. So the workers available for school food and nutrition employ-

ers to hire may be individuals who cannot obtain work elsewhere: people who lack special skills, people with age or language barriers to other employment, and people with disabilities. If school districts move to year-round, full-day schooling with child nutrition programs serving three meals per day plus snacks, the total number of full-time employees will undoubtedly increase but the people available for this type of work still will come mostly from the same labor pool.

Immigrants

Immigrants are a source of labor for school food service. According to a labor market survey, the unemployment rate for immigrants was higher than the rate for native-born workers, and the weekly earnings of immigrants who worked full time were lower than those of natives. The proportion of immigrants who had completed less than 12 years of schooling was nearly twice the proportion of U.S. natives. Approximately one-third of the immigrants spoke English "not well" or "not at all." This pattern varied little by gender, but there were large differences across racial and ethnic groups. Fifty-three percent of Hispanics spoke little or no English compared with 29 percent Asian, 13 percent white, and 10 percent black immigrants.[38]

Immigrants who moved to the United States during the 1980s were much more likely than natives to work in occupations that are generally lower paying. Nineteen percent of recent immigrants versus 9 percent of U.S. natives worked in service occupations such as food service, child care, and janitorial services. The median weekly earnings for immigrant men who worked full time was 78 percent of the median for U.S. natives.[38] By the year 2005, more than four million new jobs will be created in all segments of the food service industry. School food service needs to look to immigrants for this labor pool. Hispanics are the fastest growing food service minority, more than doubling in past years.[39]

Returning Welfare Workers

Recent changes in the welfare system will create individuals returning to the work force. Many of these workers have few skills for the demands of the current marketplace, except for service jobs such as those available in the food service industry. Several communities have formed training programs in hospitality to help welfare recipients find jobs.[40] An example is D.C. Central Kitchen in Washington, D.C. The director stated that their success as a food service training and placement program depends on a first-rate screening process. Before trainees are accepted in the program, they must be drug and alcohol free, able to read and comprehend basic instructions and food safety information, willing to attend class consistently and on time, interested in the restaurant industry, and motivated to work.[41] These same workers would be very suited for employment in school food service providing they have a commitment to children and working in an educational environment.

Workers with Disabilities

Persons with disabilities will find opportunities to work in school food service, depending on the nature of the disability. One survey found that the food service industry had the largest number of employees with disabilities.[42] Another study found that food service managers thought that employees with disabilities were punctual and loyal, and showed a positive attitude toward job responsibilities. Overall, they felt workers with disabilities were an asset to their organizations.[43]

Older Workers

The American work force also is being transformed in age categories. Since the early 1980s, workers aged 18 to 34 have become a decreasing segment of the work force. One response to this trend is to employ older workers.[44] Older workers possess good work habits, and many are looking for part-time work with flexible hours and job sharing. Part-time work

by older people has increased dramatically. For example, from 1960 to 1986, the female and male workers aged 65 and older increased from 43 percent to 61 percent.[44] As opposed to employees younger, older workers will more likely display traditional work ethics and concentration on the job. Younger workers may like the hours and the work schedules offered in school food service, but they also will want to learn skills for advancement and earn many "soft" benefits to allow time for their various lifestyle pursuits.[45]

Managing Diversity

With the types of employees seeking work in school food service, many district directors and single-site managers deal with issues of diversity daily. They may, however, just accept the situation as part of the job and not think of it as "diversity issues." A recent survey of district directors sponsored by ASFSA found that 22 percent of their employees were non–Caucasian, and an average of 44 percent of workers was non–Caucasian in districts with 25,000 or more students. Age and racial diversity were the issues that the directors felt presented the most challenge to overall management of school food and nutrition programs. In general, when asked to rate how they felt different types of diversity (racial, ethnic, gender, religious, age, and domestic partner) affected operations on a scale of 1 (no challenges) to 5 (significant challenges), the highest score was only a 2 for racial diversity.[46]

Managing diversity is a process of acknowledging difference through action. In school food and nutrition programs this involves welcoming heterogeneity. Valuing diversity means being responsive to a wide range of people. This range covers race, gender, class, native language, national origin, physical ability, age, sexual orientation, religion, professional experience, personal preferences, and work styles. Valuing diversity means using the "platinum rule" of treating others as *they* wish to be treated.[47] A recent survey found that most directors are female (86 percent) and Caucasian/European American/white (92 percent).[48] Current directors will be challenged to respond to the needs of a work force that is very different from themselves. Bilingual recipes, policies, and procedures may need to be developed for use by food service staff. Benefits such as after-hours instruction in English might be offered. Special attention may need to be paid to lighting, flooring, and work surface heights to accommodate workers who are older or have disabilities. Managers and directors may need to be sensitized to idiomatic expressions and body language that translate differently to various national and ethnic groups.

Demographics show that the faces of American workers are changing. The work force of tomorrow will be nonwhite and will speak another language more fluently than English. Administrators of school food and nutrition programs will need to meet the challenges of managing a diverse work force even more in the years to come.

Labor Productivity

If labor is in scarce supply or too expensive, management strategies may be to increase the productivity of current workers on the payroll and/or replace workers with technologically advanced machines or systems. Many CNPs use a combination of these strategies in addition to buying production labor incorporated in ready-prepared food products.

Measuring Productivity

The first step in deciding how to increase the productivity of current workers is to measure it. Productivity is the ratio of output divided by input. The major unit of productivity in CNPs is meals, and a traditional method for analyzing productivity is to compare meals served in a given period with the labor hours used to generate those meals in the same period. The productivity index of *meals per labor hour* is obtained when meals are divided by labor hours. Industry leaders quote anywhere from 16 to 20 meals per labor hour as a reason-

able level of productivity given the large variation in food delivery systems and form of food purchased in CNPs.

When calculating this index, determination of labor hours is straightforwardly obtained from time cards or work schedules showing actual hours worked. The measurement of meals can be more problematic if CNPs have sources of revenue other than the traditional breakfast and lunch programs. A count can be obtained for all adult meals and student-paid, free, and reduced-price meals, but catered, contract, and à la carte meals produced by the same work force are more difficult to determine. A standard method of calculating these meals is to establish meal equivalents from different revenue sources.[49] All calculations equate other types of meals to a standard: the lunch meal served to students. Formulas for meal equivalents are detailed in Exhibit 5–5.

If the answers calculated in Exhibit 5–5 were added to a lunch meal count for the period of 862, the total meals and meal equivalents served would be 1528 (862 + 200 + 147 + 319). Total meals can then be divided by the total labor hours for this period, and the *meals per labor hour* index results (e.g., 1528 meals ÷ 85 labor hours = 18 meals per labor hour).

The key factor associated with the reliability of this productivity index is to calculate it correctly and consistently from one period to the next. Factors of validity are harder to surmount when using meals per labor hour. For example, pricing structures may confound the calculation of meal equivalents by being understated. À la carte, catered, and contract meals may be priced lower than break-even because a school food and nutrition program director may incorrectly consider these "added" sales and only variable costs are used for establishing prices.[50] Counting student meals is made even more difficult by offer versus serve regulations. A meal under this regulation can consist of three to five traditional meal components. In addition, variation in menus and food production systems makes the use of this type of index very suspect when comparing one CNP

Exhibit 5–5 Formulas for Calculating Meal Equivalents in CNPs

Breakfast
Meal Equivalents = $$\frac{\text{\# Breakfast meals}}{2}$$

e.g., 400 ÷ 2 = 200 meal equivalents*

À la Carte
Meal Equivalents = $$\frac{\text{À la carte \$ales}}{\text{Free lunch reimbursement}}$$
                                                       +
                                                       Commodity value/ meal

e.g., \$300 ÷ \$2.04 (1.89 + .15) = 147 meal equivalents

Catered/Contract
Meal Equivalents = $$\frac{\text{Catered \$ales}}{\text{Free lunch reimbursement}}$$
                                                       +
                                                       Commodity value/ meal

e.g., \$650 ÷ \$2.04 = 319 meal equivalents

*Some school food service experts use a figure of 3 to convert breakfast to lunch meal equivalents. If this were used, the resulting answer would be 134 meal equivalents.

Source: Adapted with permission from *Financial Management Information System*, © 1998, National Food Service Management Institute.

with another. It would be better to use meals per labor hour as an internal benchmark to track a site-based manager's performance in increasing labor productivity or possibly use for a similar comparison among schools in a homogeneous school district. It is not a good parameter for benchmarking among CNPs.

In the 1980s, Mayo and colleagues suggested that the ratio of servings produced per labor hour would be a better statistic for productivity in school food service because it helps to negate the problem of defining a meal. This figure includes servings of all food items that have to be processed divided by the total number of labor hours. The number of servings produced is taken from the daily production sheets. Milk is not included if the deliveryman places the milk directly into service dispensers.[51,52] The justification for using servings produced per labor hour has merit, but the index has not been widely adopted by the school food service industry. Perhaps the attainment of reliable figures for servings produced has been problematic. Other researchers have since argued that a *total-factor productivity model* that relates organizational output to all input resources should be applied to food service settings so that all factors under a food service administrator's control such as capital, energy, materials, and labor would be considered in the equation.[53] Recently, Reynolds detailed his preferred measure of productivity for school food service. It is a partial-factor statistic with the following formula:

Productivity = Revenue for period ÷ productive labor cost for period + cost of goods used for period

Revenue is all government reimbursements and all sales from operations, including off-premise sales and satellite operations. *Productive labor cost* includes productive hourly wages and salaried positions (gross salary divided by the appropriate number of periods; e.g., gross salary divided by 9 if the period is a month and salary is paid for a 9-month school year). If food is prepared off site, labor costs associated with food preparation is factored into the cost of goods. *Cost of goods* includes purchased food and commodities, chemicals, paper, and all other variable costs. By including labor, food, and other costs in the productivity index, the form of food purchased and factors associated with the food production and meal delivery systems are considered.[54] A year-to-date figure calculated annually would be most meaningful because it would take into account the variances in cost of goods used that naturally occur from one period to the next. This index, which is a ratio of revenue to variable costs, could be easily calculated from data already required of CNPs, and it could be used for benchmarking across CNPs in all regions of the country.

Increasing Productivity

Regardless of the parameter used to measure it, if labor productivity is determined to be too low, there are two main ways to approach the issue. Both methods assume that the quality of output or meals will remain constant. Quality entails the nutritional, sensory, and microbiological attributes of food as well as courteous, timely service to customers in clean and pleasant surroundings. The first method to increase productivity is to increase meals with the same amount of labor. If a school district has not implemented a breakfast program, this might now be considered as a means to increase the productivity of current staff by increasing meals produced and thus revenue. Efforts can be made to increase CNP participation in the lunch program as well. Customer surveys can be conducted with follow-up focus groups to find out students' opinions of the CNP. Continuous quality improvement initiatives can be implemented to better the program in the eyes

of its clientele. Research has determined that high student satisfaction and participation are directly related.[55] Marketing and promotions can be used to interest students and teachers in eating school breakfast and lunch. Other approaches might be to seek add-on business-producing meals or meal components for child-care centers, adult-care centers, nutrition program for the elderly sites, vending, and catering.

The second method to increase productivity is to reduce labor while keeping the number of meals constant. The master schedule controls the number of labor hours used. Many CNPs have severely limited the number of full-time employees hired. Rather, they have staffed their facilities with part-time workers who can be scheduled for peak hours of service. School district policies such as minimum shift lengths, maximum shift lengths associated with paying benefits, lack of labor available for short shifts, and other constraints further complicate this scheduling process.[56] Other methods to decrease the labor force are to trim staff by natural attrition, hiring freezes, and interdepartmental transfers. All reduce labor costs while creating less employee unrest than layoffs.[57] The case at the end of this chapter details one district's experience in reducing labor costs and, therefore, increasing productivity.

Any discussion about increasing productivity in food service facilities would be remiss if the impact of food delivery systems and the use of labor-saving equipment were not mentioned. Commissary operations enable school districts to centralize food production staff, maximizing the skills of highly trained and paid employees as well as minimizing the production equipment necessary in individual schools. If a cook-chill system is incorporated into the commissary concept, employees can work on a factory schedule and cook food products to inventory. Chapter 14 discusses aspects of these types of systems. Robots also could be used to reduce labor costs while maintaining or enhancing productivity of commissaries and other large-volume food production operations. Robots are in use in hospitals to deliver late trays,[58] but the practical use of robots for use in school food service has yet to be determined except with warehousing functions. Researchers state, however, that the potential for automated processes exists with 64 different food-related job functions.[59] Directors who wish to increase their labor productivity will need to watch for development of technologically advanced equipment in the future.

Training

Training and human resource management are synonymous in the food service industry, and school food service is certainly no exception. An unskilled work force necessitates training on the job, and this type of training is prevalent in food service operations. Training is related to decreased labor turnover and greater job satisfaction. When specific aspects of a restaurant's culture were studied in relation to profitability, researchers from the National Restaurant Association found that providing formal training for employees, especially hourly employees, was related to higher profitability and, conversely, not offering formal training to employees was related to lower profitability.[60] A recent Gallup survey found that younger employees particularly view training and education on the job as a major attraction. They believe on-the-job training is a way to improve their chances of getting ahead.[61] School food and nutrition program directors know the relationship of training to success. They regularly train in vital areas such as food production skills, food safety and sanitary food handling, USDA regulations, work simplification, customer relations, and others. School food service operations exist in a legislative environment that also creates the necessity to train callow and seasoned workers on new systems prompted by changes in regulations such as the School Meals Initiative for Healthy Children.

Most of the training that occurs in school food service happens on the job except for staff development days at the beginning of the school year, which may be used for formal training. In general, formal or classroom training is basically ineffective. It's expensive, and learning retention is low because this type of training is passive. Since approximately 80 percent of critical job skills learning occurs on the job anyway, situations in the work unit should be used to promote effective training.[62] Process-activated training (PAT) is an on-the-job training system that involves all employees in a food service facility. A process is all the little things done in a work site, such as hand washing. This system uses hands-on practical training on the spot and just in time in the work unit. PAT uses a network of subject matter experts (SMEs) identified by their fellow workers and managers as being proficient in at least one job process. These SMEs become the teachers of coworkers. The training is done in 15 minutes in the work unit. The curriculum for this training is written by SMEs and stored in a computer for immediate retrieval when there are productivity lulls during the day, and there is time for training instead of an unscheduled break. After the training is completed, the SME submits a learning voucher to the office containing the learner's name and signature, and any comments by the SME. All employees must accumulate a specific number of vouchers to demonstrate learning throughout the year.[63]

The PAT system uses high-touch techniques. Coworkers who are experts in a given process deliver the training in a familiar and nonthreatening atmosphere. Teaching time is short and the emphasis is on learning skills directly related the job. The SMEs who develop training expertise in several processes are considered potential candidates for advancement, which provides an incentive to learn and teach more.

The high-tech approach also will work to deliver on-the-spot, just-in-time training, and new technology will advance this trend into the new millennium. Various tools such as computer software, compact disc, read-only memory (CD-ROM), compact disc-interactive

(CD-I), interactive video, video conferencing, computer networks through the Internet, and virtual reality are used now and will be used even more in the future as vehicles for learning.[64] Some methodologies such as satellite transmissions and video conferencing deliver training simultaneously to large audiences while other technologies such as CD-ROM and Internet courses provide asynchronous learning opportunities.[65] The average school food service worker may be coming late to the world of computers and other technologies, but training in computer usage and, therefore, potential for being comfortable with multimedia technologies, can be effective particularly with younger workers.[66]

The emphasis for any training activity should be on student learning. The delivery method should then be matched to the learning process. A written workbook with graphics might be a very effective method of training food service workers at their own pace, and the technology has been around for centuries. On-the-job coaching and teaching by example may be the best method for training employees in the "soft" skills so important to student satisfaction. Working with people and developing a caring attitude with children are among the interpersonal areas that need to be stressed. Interactive multimedia presentations are appropriate for subject matter that needs to be repeated and reinforced frequently, such as USDA regulations, food safety and personal hygiene, basic food production techniques, and storage and receiving techniques. Researchers have evaluated the traditional classroom method with interactive computerized programs and found there was little difference in student learning,[67] so the decision framework for school food and nutrition program directors is cost and availability of the newer training methods versus the cost and availability of trainer/supervisory time necessary to implement more traditional methods of training. The outcome in student learning appears to be the same.

SUMMARY

This discussion has not attempted to be all inclusive, but rather to highlight human resources issues of critical importance to CNPs in the next century. Human resource management at all levels of CNPs is and will undoubtedly continue to be a top priority in the future. Leaders in the child nutrition profession should be working now on strategies to develop their replacements in the next century and beyond. Potential school food and nutrition program directors and site-based managers will need to be identified and nurtured to meet the needs for qualified personnel in school districts. Issues of educational requirements and certification are fundamental to these strategies. Labor costs and productivity will be a foremost consideration of school food and nutrition program directors as they balance finite resources to manage effectively the CNP as a business within the school setting. CNPs need to be staffed with personnel willing to be trained to care for children by serving them wholesome and appealing food. Chapters 15 and 16 also speak to the importance of training in food production and customer relations skills. This is a current need, and it will not cease in upcoming years. The future of CNPs is bright only if issues in human resource management are emphasized and effectively addressed.

CASE STUDY
THE SUCCESSFUL TURNAROUND OF A CHILD NUTRITION PROGRAM, 1992–1998

Gail M. Johnson

EBRP Child Nutrition Program Facts and Figures

The East Baton Rouge school system consists of 100 schools and is the 50th in the nation in enrollment of students. The child nutrition program has a budget of $22,000,000 and has 106 feeding sites.

In 1992 the child nutrition program employed 675 full-time employees, 659 of whom were assigned to the school cafeterias. Sixteen employees worked in the administrative office of the child nutrition program. During the 1992 school year, the child nutrition program was in financial trouble, with a deficit of $2,500,000.

The child nutrition program serves 16,500 breakfast meals and 42,500 lunch meals on a daily basis. The principal expenditure of serving these meals is labor. To reduce this, a three-year plan of action was put into place. The major component of this plan was to eliminate 84 full-time job equivalents. As director, it was my job to accomplish this downsizing without terminating any employees. I was compelled to take an aggressive position by ensuring the following:

• That each employee understood that the child nutrition program would continue to operate as a business
• That each employee would strive for efficiency

The Key Components of Downsizing and Cost Control

1. All employees were informed of the financial problems of the child nutrition program.
2. Several meetings were held with the child nutrition staff to explain why job equivalents had to be cut.
3. All permanent employees were assured that they would not lose their jobs, and they would not experience a decrease in salary. A two-tiered salary schedule was established to accommodate current salaries with a lower level for newly hired employees.
4. In 1992 a hiring freeze was put into place.
5. In 1993 the glass ceiling was removed and promotional opportunities were provided for all child nutrition employees. Formerly all managers in the East Baton Rouge child nutrition program were required to have a degree in food and nutrition or home economics. At present only a high school diploma is required. When the new non-degreed position was put into place 26 managers were trained through in-house training.
6. Convenience foods were purchased to facilitate downsizing. At the time of the downsizing, 120 convenience foods had been introduced. For every 10 convenience items used, 15 minutes of labor time was reduced at each school. Originally the average meals per labor hour were 8.5. The meals per labor hour continue to increase with the addition of other convenience items. The introduction of convenience items at breakfast and the addition of provision 2 have eliminated even more labor hours. The present meals per labor hour are now 14. Some of the convenience items, which the child nutrition program is presently serving, are listed on the following page.
7. Outsourcing of several food items was instituted (e.g., USDA commodity ground beef was sent to a processing plant to be made into hamburger patties).

8. Installation of computers in all school cafeterias, which allowed for reduction in serving time and more accurate, accessible, and time-relevant records.
9. Monitoring food cost at the school level was instituted by following a 14-step plan as follows:

14-Step Food Cost-Control Plan

1. Issue a food cost allowance (director). This is a monthly average (determined by precosting central breakfast and lunch menus).

Portion-control	Jellies, jam, mayonnaise, mustard, catsup, and fruit juice
Breakfast items:	Breakfast burrito, Danish pastry, muffins, pancakes, pancake and sausage on a stick, super buns, waffles, French toast, funnel cakes
Lunch items: packs:	Hash brown potato patties, chicken nuggets, chicken patties, seafood patties, stuffed pizza, barquito (Mexican pizza), taquito, shrimp poppers (precooked)
Precut items:	Broccoli florets, broccoli-slaw mix, chopped cabbage, cabbage slaw, carrot sticks, shredded carrots, celery sticks, diced celery, chopped lettuce, lettuce salad mix, diced onions, diced pepper, sliced radishes

2. Translate being "over budget" into dollar values (director).
3. Determine the cost of the breakfast and lunch each day. Use the daily issue/withdrawal form (manager). (Manager can monitor food costs throughout the month.)
4. Determine "average cost of lunch" and "average cost of breakfast" for purchased food (manager). (Sent to the Child Nutrition Program office for preparation of a district summary.)
5 Monitor (area supervisors.) monthly food costs at each school and observe and report the following:
   - Overordering or overproduction
   - Theft and waste
   - Portion control
   - Failure to use standardized recipes
6. Meet in a group with managers who still have problems maintaining their food budgets. Implement a food budget assistance plan for individual managers who are having problems (director).
7. Plan a managers' meeting on food cost control. Use a panel discussion format with managers who exhibit good food cost control as presenters and panelists (director).
8. Send out food cost reminders during the year (director).
9. Submit to the child nutrition program office monthly inventory totals (managers).
10. Prepare a summary of purchased and commodity food. Set parameters for year-end inventory. Monitor year-end inventories (director).
11. Send letters to managers who leave food in their freezers over the summer (director).
12. Send letters to managers documenting noncompliance of inventory control (director).
13. Monitor schools with high–purchased food or commodity inventories (director).

DOWNSIZING RESULTS	EMPLOYEES 1992–1993	EMPLOYEES 1997–1998
Administrative	15	14
Cafeteria	633 (7-hour)	539*
Maintenance	15	10
Warehouse	12	10

*Sixty-nine employees work six hours per day. The six-hour employee was created after an evaluation of labor hours was completed. It was discovered that employees completed tasks within five and a half to six hours. Therefore, in the beginning of the 1996–1997 school year the child nutrition program hired all new employees other than a technician III (head cook) to work six hours rather than seven hours. Since the labor at present is approximately $18.50 per hour, this saves a considerable amount of money. Because of the new six-hour position that was created, we had vacancies in approximately 40 seven-hour positions. Using those figures it will take about seven years to complete the transition. In addition, any substitute employee who works for a permanent seven-hour employee works only six hours. Formerly, substitute wages totaled $1,110,000.00; presently, substitute wages total $736,000.00. This is an overall saving in substitute wages of $374,000.00.

14. Evaluate the process of monitoring inventory and set new parameters each school year (director).

Outcome of the Child Nutrition Program Three-Year Plan

As of May 1998, the number of job equivalents that were reduced has exceeded the 84 anticipated. Staff in the East Baton Rouge Parish child nutrition program has been reduced by 102 job equivalents. We now have 573 employees. This is a reduction of 15 percent, which is greater than the estimated reduction of 12 percent. All newly hired employees below a technician III grade are hired as six-hour employees. This is being continued to eliminate the number of hours worked daily.

Conclusion

The East Baton Rouge Parish child nutrition program has successfully reduced and continues to reduce labor and overall food costs. This was accomplished by implementing the three-year plan, which includes doing the following:

- Downsize by reducing labor hours without reducing a large number of employees or reducing their salaries. In those schools where labor was reduced, the employees were often transferred to another location and not laid off. All newly hired employees were hired to work six hours instead of seven.
- Allow for employees to rise to their own potential by training and promoting within the department.
- Control the cost of food purchased and used by implementing such procedures as reprocessing commodities and the 14-step food cost-control plan.
- Pay attention to all areas of budgetary costs with special attention to labor, productivity, cost of purchased food, and cost of food used.
- Install computers and computer training for employees. This allows for reduced time spent during lunch periods, and more accurate and accessible records.

REFERENCES

1. American School Food Service Association, *Keys to Excellence: Standards of Practice for Nutrition Integrity* (Alexandria, VA: 1995).

2. D.H. Carr et al., eds., *Competencies, Knowledge and Skills of Effective District School Nutrition Directors/Supervisors* (University, MS: National Food Service Management Institute, 1996).

3. A.P. Carnevale and S.C. Stone, "Managers and Leaders: What's the Difference?" *Training and Development* 48 (1994): 22–39.

4. U.S. Department of Labor, the Secretary's Commission on Achieving Necessary Skills, *Skills and Tasks for Jobs: a SCANS Report for America 2000* (Washington, DC: U.S. Government Printing Office; 1992).

5. J. Sneed and K.T. White, "Development and Validation of Competency Statements for Managers in School Food Service," *School Food Service Research Review* 17 (1993): 50–61.

6. M.B. Gregoire and J. Sneed, "Competencies for District School Nutrition Directors/Supervisors," *School Food Service Research Review* 18 (1994): 89–99.

7. M.T. Conklin, *Job Functions and Tasks of School Nutrition Managers and District Directors/Supervisors. NFSMI Insight*, No. 2 (University, MS: National Food Service Management Institute, 1995).

8. Sneed and White, "Development and Validation of Competency Statements."

9. Gregoire and Sneed, "Competencies for District School Nutrition Directors/Supervisors."

10. Conklin, "Job Functions and Tasks of School Nutrition Managers."

11. Carr et al., *Competencies, Knowledge and Skills.*

12. R.A. Heifetz and D.L. Laurie, "The Work of Leadership," *Harvard Business Review*, 1997; January–February 1997: 124–134.

13. S. Sherman, "Wanted: Company Change Agents," *Fortune*, 132, no. 12 (December 11, 1995): 197–198.

14. E.K. Warren and M. Goldstein, "Dealing with Change," *CPA Journal* 76, no. 8 (1997): 68–69.

15. M.J. O'Connell, "Marketing-Driven Change Management," *Journal of Health Care Marketing* 16, no. 1 (1996): 11–13.

16. F.J. DiMicco et al., "In Search of School Food Service Leaders: The Next Millennium," *School Food Services Research Review* 21, no. 1 (1997): 2–4.

17. Sneed and White, "Development and Validation of Competency Statements."

18. Gregoire and Sneed, "Competencies for District Directors/Supervisors."

19. Gregoire and Sneed, "Continuing Education Needs of District School Nutrition Directors/Supervisors," *School Food Service Research Review* 18 (1993): 16–22.

20. M.T. Conklin et al., "Preparing Child Nutrition Professionals for the 21st Century," *School Food Service Research Review* 19, no. 1 (1995): 6–13.

21. E. Smedley, *The School Lunch: Its Organization and Management in Philadelphia* (Philadelphia: Innes & Sons, 1920).

22. M.G. Bryan, *The School Cafeteria* (Bridgeport, CT: F.S. Crofts & Co., Inc., 1936).

23. J.F. Kennedy, Remarks prepared for delivery at the Trade Mart in Dallas, Nov. 22, 1963, in *Barlett's Familiar Quotations*, 16th ed. J. Kaplan (Boston: Little, Brown and Company, 1992): 742–747.

24. Conklin et al., "Preparing Child Nutrition Professionals."

25. R.A. Armour and B.S. Fuhrmann, "Confirming the Centrality of Liberal Learning," in *Educating Professionals: Responding to New Expectations for Competence and Accountability*, eds. L. Curry et al. (San Francisco: Jossey-Bass, Publishers, 1993): 126–147.

26. G.T.T. Molitor, "Trends and Forecasts for the New Millennium," *Futurist* 32, no. 6 (1998): 53–59.

27. "College Degree Better Investment Than T-Bills," *USA Today* 123, no. 2599 (1995): 14.

28. Conklin et al., "Preparing Child Nutrition Professionals."

29. Georgia Professional Standards Commission, *Teacher Certification Rules-505–118: School Nutrition Director:* 1997.

30. *Louisiana Food and Nutrition Programs Policies of Operation*, Bulletin no. 1196 revised. State of Louisiana, Department of Education, 1995.

31. Conklin et al., "Preparing Child Nutrition Professionals."

32. Carr et al., *Competencies, Knowledge and Skills.*

33. Conklin et al., "Preparing Child Nutrition Professionals."

34. DiMicco et al., "In Search of School Food Service Leaders."

35. M.T. Conklin, "Opportunities for Registered Dietitians in Child Nutrition Programs," *Topics in Clinical Nutrition* 9, no. 4 (1994): 54–60.

36. M.H. Kosters, "New Employment Relationships and the Labor Market," *Journal of Labor Research*, 18 (1997): 551–559.

37. National Restaurant Association Research Department, *Business Culture's Impact on Restaurant Perfor-*

mance (Washington, DC: National Restaurant Association, 1995).

38. J.R. Meisenheimer II, "How Do Immigrants Fare in the U.S. Labor Market?" *Monthly Labor Review*, 115, no. 12 (1992): 3–19.

39. M. Delucca, "Is Diversity the Answer to Labor Woes?" *Restaurant Hospitality* 81, no. 4 (1997): 16.

40. M. Sheridan, "Difficult Labor," *Restaurants and Institutions* 108, no. 17 (1998): 79–88.

41. D. Detzel, "Pulling Themselves Up by Their Apron Strings," *National Restaurant News*, 18, no. 9 (1998): 13–17.

42. D.E. Craig and W.E. Boyd, "Characteristics of Employers of Handicapped Individuals," *American Journal of Mental Retardation* 95 (1990): 40–43.

43. J. Barrios and J. Boudreaux, "Foodservice Managers' Perceptions of Issues Related to the Employment of Individuals with Disabilities," *Journal of Child Nutrition & Management* 22, no. 1 (1998): 3–5.

44. B. Crawley, "The Transformation of the American Labor Force: Elder African Americans and Occupational Social Work," *Social Work* 37, no. 1 (1992): 41–46.

45. M. Cetron, *American Renaissance*, 2nd ed. (New York: St. Martin's Press, 1994).

46. "Diversity Today," *School Foodservice & Nutrition* 52, no. 6 (1998): 64–72.

47. A.P. Carnevale and S.C. Stone, "Diversity Beyond the Golden Rule," *Training & Development* 48, no. 10 (1994): 22–39.

48. "Diversity Today."

49. Financial Management Information System (University, MS: National Food Service Management Institute, 1999).

50. D. Reynolds, "Productivity Analysis," *Cornell Hotel and Restaurant Administration Quarterly* 39, no. 3 (1998): 22–31.

51. C.R. Mayo et al., "Variables That Affect Productivity in School Foodservices," *Journal of the American Dietetic Association* 84, no. 2 (1984): 187–193.

52. C.R. Mayo, and M.D. Olsen, "Food Servings per Labor Hour: An Alternative Productivity Measure," *School Food Services Research Review* 11, no. 1 (1987): 48–51.

53. D.M. Brown and L.W. Hoover, "Productivity Measurement in Foodservice: Past Accomplishments—A Future Alternative," *Journal of the American Dietetic Association* 90, no. 7 (1990): 973–978.

54. Reynolds, "Productivity Analysis."

55. M.K. Meyer and M.T. Conklin, "Variables Affecting High School Students' Perceptions of School Foodservice," *Journal of the American Dietetic Association*, 98, no. 12 (1998): 1424–1428.

56. R.C. Tart and R.G. Taylor, "Optimizing School Food Service Employee Scheduling," *School Food Service Research Review* 21, no. 1 (1997): 24–27.

57. J.C. Hutchinson et al., "The Impact of Downsizing on School Food Service Personnel," *School Food Service Research Review* 21, no. 1 (1997): 11–17.

58. C. Snow, "Technology Keeps Food Costs on Diet," *Modern Healthcare* 25, no. 41 (1995): 92–93.

59. E.A. Adams and A.M. Messersmith, "Robots in Food Systems: A Review and Assessment of Potential Uses," *Journal of the American Dietetic Association* 86, no. 4 (1986): 476–480.

60. National Restaurant Association, *Business Culture's Impact*.

61. "Training Key to Attracting, Retaining Talented Gen Xers," *Hattiesburg American*, September 7, 1998, 1A.

62. S. Caudron, "Your Learning Technology Primer," *Personnel Journal* 75, no. 6 (1996): 120–136.

63. D.C. Fisher, "Give Employees a PAT: Process Activated Training: The Self-Trained Work Team Concept," in *Preparing Child Nutrition Program Professionals for the 21st Century*, eds. J. Sneed and M. Conklin (University, MS: National Food Service Management Institute, 1993), 97–116.

64. K.J. Harris and J.J. West, "Using Multimedia in Hospitality Training," *Cornell Hotel and Restaurant Administration Quarterly* 34, no. 4 (1993): 75–82.

65. Caudron, "Your Learning Technology Primer."

66. R. Gould and B. Barrett, "Post-Then-Pre Evaluation of Computer Classes for School Foodservice Personnel," *Journal of Child Nutrition & Management* 22, no. 1 (1998): 40–45.

67. Harris and West, "Using Multimedia."

CHAPTER 6

Evaluation and Procurement of Computer Technology

Penny E. McConnell and Jean B. Shaw

OUTLINE

INTRODUCTION

Child nutrition programs are experiencing a time of rapid, fundamental, and philosophical change. To remain a competitive provider of nutritious food to those in the school and community, food and nutrition service professionals must use time wisely, have accurate data on which to make decisions, and employ tools for analyzing current trends and projecting future outcomes.

Computerization in child nutrition programs is crucial. Financial restraints experienced by virtually all school systems are dictating that we contain costs, manage people, and design programs to be self-supporting. To survive, we must be entrepreneurs.

From this chapter, the reader should be able to make educated judgment decisions regarding computer applications that are currently available. Primary to these decisions, child nutrition professionals must know where to go or what to look for in computerization. With this knowledge the pros and cons of various aspects of computer programs or systems available such as features, costs, and training requirements can be evaluated to determine program needs. Specific chapter objectives are to provide an overview of the role of technology in managing child nutrition programs; assist school food and nutrition directors in making decisions related to selecting, purchasing, and using computers; and identify the application of computers and telecommunication technologies in managing child nutrition programs.

West et al. wrote in 1988, "Computers are being used to some degree almost universally today, although foodservice organizations have been slower than other industries to convert to their use, especially for decision-making support. While many food service functions have become computerized, the industry remains behind others in the business world."[1(p622)] Since that statement was written, the food service industry has seen a remarkable increase in the use of computers. Because of the demand for in-creased accountability and the political influence on child nutrition programs, we have become leaders in food service computerization.

Effective use of computer technology in program management and operations allows time for the school food and nutrition director to address program needs in relation to nutrition education, marketing, partnerships, and customer services.

WHAT IS A COMPUTER? WHAT IS A COMPUTER SYSTEM?

A computer is a programmable electronic device that can store, retrieve, and process data.[2] Child nutrition professionals do not need programming skills, but they do need to be computer literate.[3-4]

A computer system may be defined in several ways. A simple computer system includes hardware, software, and peripherals. Think of the computer system as having three layers; the *hardware, software,* and *peripherals.* The *hardware* consists of all the physical parts of the system, such as keyboard, central processing unit, and monitor. The *software* consists of two major parts: an operating system such as Windows or MS-DOS and the programs or applications. The operating system runs the *programs/applications* which perform the functions that you want done such as word processing or free and reduced-price meal application processing. The *peripherals* include such things as printers and scanners. A more complex computer system may employ many computers or terminals into which data is entered and transmitted to a specific location from which it is used to generate useful information. When several complex systems are employed, the entire package is known as a Management Information System (MIS). Keiser and DeMicco[5] caution, however, "Today computer systems are available that can greatly extend the skills of experienced managers. They do not necessarily replace people, but rather provide management tools that maximize the manager's skill, experience, and management time."[5]

The Computer System		
Hardware	Software	Peripherals
All physical components, such as monitor, keyboard, central processing unit	Two parts: Operating system, which runs Programs/ Applications	Printers, scanners, etc.

THE DECISION-MAKING PROCESS

Depending on the organization's size and policies, certain questions should be answered prior to beginning the decision-making process.

- Who will be involved in the actual decision-making process? Who will be involved in the approval process once decisions are made?
- Is the food service department centralized or decentralized?
- What is the size of the operation?
- How advanced are the computer skills in the department?

To reach a workable solution regarding computer needs, school food and nutrition professionals should examine where they are today and where they want to be in the future. In finding a solution, the method to be used in transmitting data may need to be addressed. A local area network (LAN) is used to exchange information within a single organization.[6] As a rule, a LAN can connect computers in sites a maximum of 300 feet apart.[7] As an example, a computer in the school office could notify computers on each serving line when students are absent, thus possibly preventing an unauthorized free or reduced-price meal. A wide-area network (WAN) is used when schools communicate with district offices and subse-

quently with the state level. WANs may be wireless, but most use telephone high-speed data circuits. Once these decisions are made, whether the school system is large or small, centralized or decentralized, not computerized, partially computerized, or fully computerized, long-range plans should be written.

To determine computer needs, a feasibility study should be conducted by a committee of key personnel who will use and be affected by future computerization. In this way, an accurate, realistic description of needs is developed. Recommendations can thus be made on the basis of initial costs, projected actual costs, resources, sophistication, and ease of implementation.

From the initial feasibility study, decisions can be made regarding what must be accomplished and when it must be done. Computerization is a long-term project that is generally accomplished in phases. Priorities must be established:

- What must be done now
- What must be done in the future
- What needs to be done in the interim period[8]

Once a short-term and long-range plan is developed, budgets can be established to ensure implementation of a total program.

During the decision-making process, consideration must be given to the organizational structure. A school system may have a mainframe computer through which food service data is processed. Other foodservice computer systems may be self-contained within the department.

Hardware and Software

As a rule, software should be considered before hardware. School food and nutrition directors managing food service operations that are not computerized should define first what they want the system to do

- approve free and reduced-meal applications

- process point-of-service transactions
- facilitate school kitchen production and purchasing
- set financial controls, and so forth.

Once the purposes are defined, the software should be chosen that best meets established needs. Care must be taken to ensure that all software selected can be used in the same computer hardware. For computerized school food service departments, the decision must be made to adapt software to existing hardware or to find compatible software.

During this phase of the decision-making process, district size, skills, and budget are relevant. The needs of small school districts may be relatively simple and easily satisfied through other departments. Medium-sized school districts require a longer time frame and greater resources for adaptation. Large school districts may need a more sophisticated system and have specialized personnel on staff to implement the computerization process.

Purchase Software or Customize

Most software can be classified as customized, full-featured, or generic.

- Customized software is written specifically for an operation. The user is actively involved in determining the functions to be performed. Many times the written, manual system is used as the basis for the design of computer-generated reports. Considerable resources are required to customize software.
- Full-feature software is generally less expensive than customized software, and it has usually been widely tested and sold. Examples of full-featured software are inventory and purchasing control and nutrient analysis of menus.
- Generic software programs include word processing, electronic spreadsheets, database management, and graphics.[9]

Kavulla[10] reports greater control and flexibility with customized programs. If a full-feature software program is adapted to a specific food and nutrition operation by the vendor, the cost may be equal to that of a customized program. In addition, the full-feature software company controls the rate of price increases for technical and maintenance support. With custom software the school district owns the source code and the program in which it was written. Finally, school food and nutrition professionals are cautioned to inquire about proprietary programs or equipment that may not be adaptable to other software. Customized programs, while initially more expensive, are fully adaptable, are owned by the school district, and there are no fees for use of the program. However, data may become outdated due to the rapidly changing food industry, and program upgrades would not be readily available.[10]

Search and Test

Once decisions are made to implement an integrated system, upgrade an existing system, or implement a newer version of an existing component, it is crucial that the market be thoroughly searched. With the exploding computer market, software or hardware deemed desirable a few weeks ago may be antiquated today.

Hardware must be powerful enough to handle efficiently the projected task, with excess capacity to accommodate future expansion. Speed is time. An adequate computer working with a slow printer causes frustration. If your goal is to print multipart forms, a dot matrix printer should be specified. For professional-quality printing a laser printer should be considered; if you are using color, an ink jet printer may be adequate.[11]

From the feasibility study, needs have been established. Next a list must be made of hardware, software, and peripherals available to meet each need. There are many sources of this information. After first checking with computer-knowledgeable experts in your organization, answers may be found through:

- Annual state and national school food service association conferences
- Professional trade associations
- Trade shows
- Local vendors
- Reputable nationwide vendors
- Other school food and nutrition directors[12]

Request for Proposal

From each vendor request the same information in writing to ensure that features are truly comparable:

- Hardware and software documentation
- List of current customers
- Sample report forms and training materials
- Annual financial statements
- Cost, including purchase/lease options
- User support and maintenance programs, as well as availability and cost of upgrade
- A copy of the users' manual and demonstration disk[12]

In addition, questions should be asked regarding adaptability. Some believe that the most important feature of any software application package is that it is open ended. This means that it allows users to build upon it and customize it to fit their unique needs. Software that allows this kind of flexibility has what is commonly called "open architecture."[13] If the system is nonproprietary it can be added to or modified to include open architecture or networked processor-based devices that enable the user to design a system flexible enough to meet the needs of each operation.[14]

As data are gathered they are sorted according to previously established criteria to facilitate the evaluation process. An example of a simple evaluation tool is shown in Exhibit 6–1. Products that appear to be acceptable should be demonstrated. Manufacturers' representatives may be involved in this phase. After this demonstration several of the most promising programs may be pilot tested. For pilot testing, actual school food and nutrition program sites

should be used. Depending on local purchasing practices, a purchase request may need to be developed for this phase of the selection process.

Bid Evaluation and Award

Obtaining Hardware or Software

During pilot testing, detailed records should be kept of problems encountered, such as bottlenecks and overtime incurred. These results are, in turn, used to develop a bid. Prior to preparing a bid for hardware or software, the child nutrition professional should investigate local options including sources within the school system. Frequently, software programs are purchased by other departments through which the child nutrition department can obtain a copy. For most specialized hardware or software, the school food and nutrition department must prepare an invitation for bid (IFB) or a request for proposal (RFP). In an IFB, the exact items required are specified. Care must be taken to specify exactly what you want. With an RFP, the purchaser outlines what the product(s) are expected to do and the bidders respond by telling the purchaser how these needs can be met. Because of the complexity of most computer systems, an RFP is frequently used. Exhibit 6–2 may serve as a checklist in preparing an RFP. The RFP may be written to include a pilot program using several vendors, after which the successful or best vendor is chosen to complete the project. This is frequently the method used when several schools are involved and a universal system is desired for the school district.

APPLICATION

Operating systems are generally included with the computer hardware when purchased. Software application programs are loaded into operating systems. Computer operating systems and application programs allow school food and nutrition departments to handle effi-

Exhibit 6–1 Software Evaluation

Name of Program: _____

Manufacturer's Information:

• Hardware Requirements	
• Software Requirements	
• Current Customers	
• Sample Report Forms	
• Sample Training Materials	
• Annual Financial Statement	
• Purchase/Lease Options	
• User Support	
• Maintenance Programs	
• Availability of Upgrades	
• Cost of Upgrades	
• Approximate Total Cost	
• Users' Manual	
• Demonstration Disk	

Information from current users of this software in systems of similar size:

• What problems have their systems had? _____

• How long did it take to get the system fully functioning? _____

• Is the vendor providing adequate support and service? _____

• What would they have done differently? _____

• Is the software meeting the department's needs? _____

• What effect has the software had on personnel? _____

Exhibit 6–2 Essential Components of a Request for Proposal

Components	Comments
Scope of Contract ☐ What the Child Nutrition Department is looking for	
☐ How many sites will be affected?	
☐ Brief discussion of project requirements	
Background ☐ What led up to this RFP being prepared?	
Tasks to be performed ☐ In outline form, tasks should be defined to meet the department's objectives.	
Technical Proposal ☐ What is the vendor's organization like? Where is it? What is its size? How is the business structured?	
☐ What are the qualifications of key people in the vendor's company and of the people who will be assigned to your project?	
☐ Data are required on the vendor's financial stability.	
☐ If subcontractors are to be used by the bidder, what are their credentials and financial stability? Also, what is the scope of their responsibility?	
☐ What is the experience of the vendor and the subcontractor?	
☐ The bidder supplies a brief synopsis that demonstrates a clear understanding of the project. It should contain a brief statement of the salient features of the proposal.	
☐ Ask the vendor to provide a technical plan. It should include detailed descriptions of hardware, software, and peripherals that will be used.	
☐ If the components are to communicate, the vendor should describe in detail how this is to be accomplished.	
☐ Training of food service personnel is a must. Vendors should submit a timeline and description of the training plan.	
☐ Vendors should describe their plan and business location.	

continues

Exhibit 6–2 continued

Business Proposal	
☐ All items should be priced separately.	
☐ Vendor supplies complete breakdown of all costs associated with the proposal. Included are one-time costs (for hardware, for example).	
☐ If licensed software is to be used, all costs should be listed.	
☐ Financial arrangements: vendor should describe how the purchaser will acquire items in the proposal—lease, lease/purchase, or direct purchase.	
☐ Maintenance service costs	
☐ Supply costs	
Contract Completion	
☐ When (date/time) does the food service department require the work to be completed?	
Pricing	
☐ How the vendor is to supply the pricing: if a fixed price for the total installation is required, it should be stated.	
Period the Proposal Remains Valid	
☐ The length of time the vendor must maintain the price quoted	
Basis for Award	
☐ A selection committee should review and evaluate all RFPs submitted. Technical responses are evaluated first.	
☐ The selection committee conducts a preliminary evaluation of the ability of each vendor to perform, past performance, ability to meet time requirements, personnel assigned to the project, and an understanding of the work to be performed.	
☐ Next, business proposals are reviewed from those vendors whose technical proposals rated highest on the established criteria by the selection committee.	
☐ Additional meetings with these vendor(s) may be required and may include oral presentations.	

continues

Exhibit 6–2 continued

Contract Is Negotiated	
Bid Is Awarded	
☐ Purchase orders are prepared.	

ciently inventory, labor scheduling, cost accounting, and electronic mail, and piggyback onto existing school computer programs for enrollment. The goal is to type in the data only once.[15] Currently, a typical computerized food service operation uses several proprietary software systems. This means that a user cannot alter a software program, but has to use it "as is." In addition, traditional proprietary software offers little means for connecting information systems.

Child nutrition professionals must be able to work on more than one task at a time. Using an "operating platform," a variety of functions can be integrated.[16] Current technology favors the use of a relational database. In a relational database, information is stored in such a way that data can be related to each other. Using and retrieving information is three-dimensional, in that "stacks" of tables of data can share data cross-sectionally. The principal advantages of a relational database system are powerful data management, query, and reporting capabilities. Desirable features are speed, multitasking performance, and seamless exchange of data in "real time," where data move from one program to another as they are entered. In other words, data that are updated in one location are automatically updated everywhere.[16]

For classification purposes, software vendors or companies can be grouped according to the application their software encompasses. Applications may include free and reduced-price meal application processing, point-of-service accountability, nutritional analysis, inventory control, food production and distribution, personnel management, financial management, training, and implementation support.

- Comprehensive systems perform functions within a minimum of four application areas.
- Point-of-service or point-of-sale (POS) systems primarily perform point-of-service functions, but also may offer additional features.
- Specialized modules perform functions within one to three application areas.[17]

While some companies specialize in POS applications, most vendors deal in comprehensive systems or specialized modules.

FOOD SERVICE MANAGEMENT FUNCTIONS

Food service management functions include purchasing, delivery systems, inventory, warehousing, menu planning and nutrient analysis, recipes, food production and record keeping, equipment, and vending.

Purchasing

Regardless of the size of the school entity, purchasing is one area where an effectively managed program can truly save money.[18] Most child nutrition programs follow established procedures of bidding competitively for food and supplies. Depending on state and local regulations, the person responsible for purchasing prepares bid specifications and instructions to which potential vendors respond. Specialized programs have been written for purchasing management. Some are broad and include specification writing, bid distribution (including mailing labels), bid evaluation, tabulation, and a final report showing the selected vendor.

In the absence of specific purchasing software, certain purchasing aids should be computerized. A database of suppliers, brokers, or manufacturers' representatives should be a priority. In addition to their name, address, telephone, and fax numbers, types of products supplied and quality of products supplied should be listed. Other useful information in the database includes suppliers, brokers, or representatives' responsiveness; delivery and service performance; adherence to product specifications; cost competitiveness; integrity; knowledge of their product(s) line; and their understanding of the product application to child nutrition programs and their overall operating environment.[18]

Computers can be used to generate a purchase order automatically if a reorder point and a maximum level has been established.[19] With the unpredictable nature of child nutrition programs and fluctuating availability of United States Department of Agriculture (USDA) commodities, most child nutrition professionals prefer to use the reorder point system only for standardized, routinely served items such as fluid milk.

Instead, most child nutrition purchases are menu driven. The computer program prints out the ingredients needed for a meal or order period. This way the correct amount of food is ordered at the right time to meet food production demands. The purchasing module may forecast amounts needed in portions, convert the amount to purchase units, calculate the amount of food on hand and the amount committed to interim meals, and the vendor's delivery schedule.[20]

This process can be expedited further through either direct ordering or electronic ordering. With direct ordering, the food service manager or operation supervisor communicates directly with the supplier, using his or her own computer and a modem. With electronic ordering, the communication is through the computer and a modem via electronic mail (E-mail). Both computerized ordering options can

be specified in the bid process. The greatest advantages are in time saved, accuracy, and closer inventory control.

Controls and security must be considered when ordering electronically. To maintain menu and program integrity or standards, all involved in the purchasing process should have a password. For example, a purchasing clerk can review a file, but cannot build on it, change established prices, or change a selected vendor. To ensure continuity and quality, only the child nutrition professional can make product substitutions. To accomplish this, ramifications of each level of authority should be considered before assigning system rights to users. Some rights may be assigned in groups, such as ingredient menu functions; others are assigned item by item through data field flags designated "yes" or "no" for each user. In turn, each employee's customized menu of computer choices is used as a training guide.[21]

These same controls apply to multiple vendors or a prime vendor. No vendor should be allowed to substitute any food item automatically. When the order is transmitted to the vendor either directly or by E-mail, an electronic confirmation should be returned to the food service operator. If not enough product is available or if the vendor is out of a selection, school food and nutrition professionals should select the acceptable substitution and notify the vendor. They should not allow the vendor, who may have a database of substitutions, to select for them. Only the school food and nutrition professionals are aware of their child nutrition program standards.[21]

Once the order is placed, a receiving list is automatically produced or printed for use by the individual checking in the order. Receiving personnel, in turn, check the goods received against the order shown, possibly on the computer terminal. The receipt can be acknowledged through the terminal, allowing the computer to include the received goods in its inventory, in daily or meal food costs, and nutrient analysis at the same time accounting personnel are notified of the receipt of goods.[22]

Delivery Systems

Food service delivery systems are major management decisions that are already in place or must be chosen early in the computerization process. The most commonly used system is the conventional system, in which all delivery subsystems are located on the same premises. The services on this premises may be centralized, where food is portioned in one place as it is served, or decentralized, where bulk quantities of food are sent by heated or refrigerated carts or modules to serving facilities on the same premises.[23]

In a commissary or satellite system, procurement and possibly food production are centralized. Prepared food is distributed to several service locations. Food is transported in specialized equipment such as trucks outfitted with equipment to keep food hot or cold. Other variations of commissary systems are the ready-prepared or cook-chill or cook-freeze systems and the assembly serve system, where completely prepared foods are purchased and only minor heating and preparation are done on the premises.[23]

In establishing a computerized delivery system, each ingredient or premade product must have a recipe or item number, either previously assigned by the software manufacturer or assigned by the computer operator as new ingredients and recipes are added to the file. In addition, large operations may also assign storage location numbers to various foods used. When food and supplies are stored in assigned locations, care must be taken by receiving personnel to ensure that food and supplies are always stored in the correct slot or location. Exhibit 6–3 shows item numbers and storage locations.

Operators of child nutrition programs are aware of the need to maintain accurate food and supply costs for each location. To fully understand the operation in all serving locations, detailed computerized reports must be generated daily. In a conventional or commissary system, the process begins when food and sup-

plies enter the door and are included in the inventory. Exhibit 6–4, Purchase Requisition, may be used for this purpose. As they are ordered and dispensed to the various preparation or serving locations, a record is kept as shown in Exhibit 6–5, Issue Requisition, and Exhibit 6–6, Dispatch Invoice. As they are sold to a customer, another record is produced indicating the amount sold and the amount left over. Exhibit 6–7, Service Summary, report may be used to accurately show what was used.

The scenario described above is merely an example of how a delivery system can be computerized. As a rule, software programs are extensive and offer the user various options for the delivery system. In applying the information gathered, the child nutrition professional should search for a computer system or program that uses double entry to produce a profit-and-loss statement by school site, by preparation site, and for the district.

In arguing for delivery systems computerization, one must remember that it is hard to produce the information manually in time for the rapid decision making required in food service. Computers, with appropriate software, are ideal for performing these functions rapidly and accurately, freeing managers to manage with assurance of tight financial control and of availability of information in time to be fully utilized.[24]

Inventory

Inventories are lists of items available in various areas of an operation. Two types of inventories are commonly maintained by food service operations: physical and perpetual. A physical inventory deals with the physical count of all items on hand at the end of a specified period of time, usually a month. A perpetual inventory is a continuous record of purchases and issues. At the time of interpretation, all inventories are converted to dollar values.[25]

Traditionally, inventory has been physically counted, manually recorded, and extended. This system is extremely time consuming and

Exhibit 6–3 Item Numbers and Storage Locations

REPORT #: 289 * * * CBORD FOODSERVICE MANAGEMENT SYSTEMS * * * PAGE: 1
OPTION : 7.5.3.6.5 MENU MANAGEMENT SYSTEM - 6.2 DEC 09 96
USERS : 4 FAIRFAX COUNTY PUBLIC SCHOOLS 0954 HOURS
DETAILED ISSUE ANALYSIS

UNDEFINED INVENTORY UNIT

Unit : 3   FINISHING KITCHEN

Item Number	Item Name	Req Membr	Storage Location	Issue Date	Quantity Issued	Issue Unit	Price	Extension	Item Subtotals
236	BISCUITS, FROZEN 140/CS	3	11-FREEZER	112096	0.500	CASE	8.5900	4.295	4.295
4	CHICKEN NUGGETS	3	11-FREEZER	112096	3	CASE	15.5000	46.500	46.500
1053	EGG ROLL, PORK, 60/CS TONYS	3	11-FREEZER	112096	2	CASE	28.5300	57.060	57.060
990	JUICE, FZN GRAPE K-PAC96/C	3	11-FREEZER	112096	0.500	CASE	11.0200	5.510	5.510
808	MUFFIN, BLUBERY 1 oz 4X60/C	3	11-FREEZER	112096	3	TRAY	6.3275	18.983	18.983
646	PANCAKEnSAUSAGE STIK 48/C	3	11-FREEZER	112096	1	CASE	12.5600	12.560	12.560
925	ORANGES, FRESH 138/CS	3	20-REFRIGERATOR, PRODUCE	112096	1.500	CASE	12.6000	18.900	18.900
761	CEREAL, CHEERIOS 96/CS	3	21-CONDIMENTS - STAPLES	112096	1	CASE	13.5400	13.540	13.540
759	CEREAL, CIN. TOAST CRUNCH	3	21-CONDIMENTS - STAPLES	112096	1	CASE	13.5400	13.540	13.540
176	JELLIES, ASSORTED 200/CS	3	21-CONDIMENTS - STAPLES	112096	0.500	CASE	6.6900	3.345	3.345
318	RICE, WHITE, 25LB	3	21-CONDIMENTS - STAPLES	112096	7	LB	0.4236	2.965	2.965
704	SWEET/SOUR SAUCE PACKETS	3	21-CONDIMENTS - STAPLES	112096	2	CASE	5.7100	11.420	11.420
183	SYRUP, IND. PKTS. 100/CS	3	21-CONDIMENTS - STAPLES	112096	2	CASE	5.1800	10.360	10.360
92	PEARS, HALVES 6/CS	3	23-DRY STORAGE - CANNED	112096	4	CAN	3.2411	12.965	12.965
146	POTATOES, DEHYD. 6/CS	3	23-DRY STORAGE - CANNED	112096	2	CAN	3.7884	7.577	7.577
1015	FORK & NAPKIN KIT, 1000/CS	3	32-PAPER AND SUPPLIES	112096	1	CASE	27.8700	27.870	27.870
382	TEASPOONS, BLACK, 1000/CS	3	32-PAPER AND SUPPLIES	112096	0.500	CASE	5.8100	2.905	2.905
904	TRAY, TAN STYRO SEN.250/C	3	32-PAPER AND SUPPLIES	112096	1.670	CASE	13.3400	22.278	22.278
91	BUTTER PATS, USDA 30LB/CS	3	99-NOT IN USE - FOOD	112096	1	5 LB BOX	5.3074	5.307	5.307
TOTAL(S)								297.880	

SUBTOTAL NUMBER OF RECORDS PRINTED   19

Courtesy of The CBORD Group, Inc., 1997, Ithaca, New York.

Exhibit 6–4 Purchase Requisition

```
REPORTS#:  175    * * * CBORD FOODSERVICE MANAGEMENT SYSTEMS * * *     PAGE: 1
OPTION    : 7.5.2.6.2.      MENU MANAGEMENT SYSTEM - V6.2              DEC 09 96
USER#     : 4               FAIRFAX COUNTY PUBLIC SCHOOLS             0957 HOURS
                                   PURCHASE REQUISITION
PR Number  : 2                         Unit  : S 100
PO Number  : 456                       Status :
Order Date : WEDNESDAY   11/20/96      Vender: FOOD SERVICE CENTER FROZ.
Deliver Date : THURSDAY  11/21/96
Vendor Invc#: 456
Terms     :
Contract # :
Ship to   :
Reference :
Req Type              :           Signature: _____
```

| — Item — | | Vendor | | | Purchase | |
Number	Name	Order #	Quantity	Unit	Price	Extension
4	CHICKEN NUGGETS	_____	5	CASE	15.500	77.500
TOTAL(S)			5.000			77.500

Courtesy of The CBORD Group, Inc., 1997, Ithaca, New York.

fraught with potential for human errors. Many computer systems are designed for a periodic physical inventory, which provides data only on completion of the physical count. On the other hand, a computerized perpetual inventory system provides the current status of inventory as well as what has been received and used during the month.[26] In addition to data entry required to create the inventory master file, goods received and storeroom issues must be entered. The advantage here is the ability to provide a food usage cost shortly after the meal is served.[27] When questions arise regarding possible food loss or theft, this becomes a valuable aid.

Computer inventory programs provide the operator with many useful tools. If items are manually counted according to established inventory-taking procedures, the software should provide a tally sheet onto which the amounts in inventory are recorded. An example of a tally sheet is found in Exhibit 6–8. From this, the computer operator enters the physical inventory counts into the computer and generates an inventory extension, which may be by category or storage location. Physical Inventory Transactions, Exhibit 6–9, and Inventory Valuation Summary, Exhibit 6–10, illustrate this.

A good computer application would also provide other inventory options to the user, such as the ability to inquire about an inventory item's status. Food in process is considered by some as inventory until it is served. For accuracy, foods that are not on the shelf but have been pulled, prepared for tomorrow, or left over are counted as part of the inventory. Finally, be sure the inventory software has the ability to convert purchase units, issue units, and weights automatically to allow for easy tracking of items from inventory through production.

An additional inventory area of great concern to child nutrition professionals is large and small equipment inventory. Programs for this purpose are available into which the computer operator records when the equipment was purchased; lists the serial numbers, warranty information, and model numbers;

Exhibit 6–5 Issue Requisition

```
REPORT #: 264        * * * CBORD FOODSERVICE MANAGEMENT SYSTEMS * * *        PAGE: 1
OPTION    : 7.5.3.6.2.          MENU MANAGEMENT SYSTEM - V6.2                 DEC 09 96
USER#     : 4                 FAIRFAX COUNTY PUBLIC SCHOOLS                  0959 HOURS
                                    ISSUE REQUISITION
```

Req Nmbr : 3
Unit   : S3 FINISHING KITCHEN   Prep Area:
Commit Dt : WEDNESDAY 11/20/96   Reference:
Issue DT : WEDNESDAY 11/20/96   Invoice # :
Status   : I   Req Type :
Ship To   :

Bin Nmbr	Item Nmbr	Name		Quan	Issue Unit	Price	Extension
11-FREEZER							
_____	(236)	BISCUITS, FROZEN 140/CS	—	0.50	CASE	8.5900	4.295
_____	(4)	CHICKEN NUGGETS	—	3	CASE	15.5000	46.500
_____	(1053)	EGG ROLL, PORK, 60/CS TONYS	—	2	CASE	28.5300	57.060
_____	(990)	JUICE, FZN GRAPE K-PAC96/C	—	0.50	CASE	11.0200	5.510
_____	(808)	MUFFIN, BLUBERY 1oz 4x60/C	—	3	TRAY	6.3275	18.983
_____	(646)	PANCAKEnSAUSAGE STIK 48/C	—	1	CASE	12.5600	12.560
20-REFRIGERATOR, PRODUCE							
_____	(925)	ORANGES, FRESH 138/CS	—	1.50	CASE	12.6000	18.900
21-CONDIMENTS - STAPLES							
_____	(761)	CEREAL, CHEERIOS 96/CS	—	1	CASE	13.5400	13.540
_____	(759)	CEREAL. CIN. TOAST CRUNCH	—	1	CASE	13.5400	13.540
_____	(176)	JELLIES, ASSORTED 200/CS	—	0.50	CASE	6.6900	3.345
_____	(318)	RICE, WHITE, 25LB	—	7	LB	0.4236	2.965
_____	(704)	SWEET/SOUR SAUCE PACKETS	—	2	CASE	5.7100	11.420
_____	(183)	SYRUP, IND. PKTS. 100/CS	—	2	CASE	5.1800	10.360
23-DRY STORAGE - CANNED							
_____	(92)	PEARS, HALVES 6/CS	—	4	CAN	3.2411	12.965
_____	(146)	POTATOES, DEHYD. 6/CS	—	2	CAN	3.7884	7.577
32-PAPER AND SUPPLIES							
_____	(1015)	FORK & NAPKIN KIT, 1000/CS	—	1	CASE	27.8700	27.870
_____	(382)	TEASPOONS, BLACK, 1000/CS	—	0.50	CASE	5.8100	2.905
_____	(904)	TRAY, TAN STYRO SEN. 250/C	—	1.67	CASE	13.3400	22.278
99-NOT IN USE - FOOD							
_____	(91)	BUTTER PATS, USDA 30LB/CS	—	1	5 LB BOX	5.3074	5.307
TOTAL(S)			—	35.17			297.880

NOTES: 1. _____ _____ _____ _____
        2. _____ _____ _____ _____
        3. _____ _____ _____ _____
        4. _____ _____ _____ _____

Courtesy of The CBORD Group, Inc., 1997, Ithaca, New York.

Exhibit 6–6 Dispatch Invoice

REPORT#:   266   * * * CBORD FOODSERVICE MANAGEMENT SYSTEMS * * *   PAGE 1
OPTION :   7.5.3.7.3.   MENU MANAGEMENT SYSTEM - V 6.2   DEC 09 96
USER#   :   4   FAIRFAX COUNTY PUBLIC SCHOOLS   1000 HOURS
                                         DISPATCH INVOICE
                                    UNDEFINED INVENTORY UNIT

Req Number : 3   Unit   :S3   FINISHING KITCHEN
Commit Date: WEDNESDAY 11/20/96   Reference   :
Issue Date : WEDNESDAY 11/20/96   Invoice Nmbr:
Ship To   :

Bin Nmbr	Item Nmbr	Name	Quantity	Issue Unit	Price	Extension
11-FREEZER						
_____	(236)	BISCUITS, FROZEN 140/CS	— 0.50	CASE	8.590	4.295
_____	(4)	CHICKEN NUGGETS	— 3	CASE	15.500	46.500
_____	(1053)	EGG ROLL, PORK, 60/CS TONYS	— 2	CASE	28.530	57.060
_____	(990)	JUICE, FZN GRAPE K-PAC96/C	— 0.50	CASE	11.020	5.510
_____	(808)	MUFFIN, BLUBERY 1oz 4x60/C	— 3	TRAY	6.328	18.983
_____	(646)	PANCAKEnSAUSAGE STIK 48/C	— 1	CASE	12.560	12.560
20-REFRIGERATOR, PRODUCE						
_____	(925)	ORANGES, FRESH 138/CS	— 1.50	CASE	12.600	18.900
21-CONDIMENTS - STAPLES						
_____	(761)	CEREAL, CHEERIOS 96/CS	— 1	CASE	13.540	13.540
_____	(759)	CEREAL, CIN. TOAST CRUNCH	— 1	CASE	13.540	13.540
_____	(176)	JELLIES, ASSORTED 200/CS	— 0.50	CASE	6.690	3.345
_____	(318)	RICE, WHITE, 25LB	— 7	LB	0.424	2.965
_____	(704)	SWEET/SOUR SAUCE PACKETS	— 2	CASE	5.710	11.420
_____	(183)	SYRUP, IND. PKTS. 100/CS	— 2	CASE	5.180	10.360
23-DRY STORAGE - CANNED						
_____	(92)	PEARS, HALVES 6/CS	— 4	CAN	3.241	12.965
_____	(146)	POTATOES, DEHYD. 6/CS	— 2	CAN	3.788	7.577
32-PAPER AND SUPPLIES						
_____	(1015)	FORK & NAPKIN KIT, 1000/CS	— 1	CASE	27.870	27.870
_____	(382)	TEASPOONS, BLACK, 1000/CS	— 0.50	CASE	5.810	2.905
_____	(904)	TRAY, TAN STYRO SEN.250/C	— 1.67	CASE	13.340	22.278
99-NOT IN USE - FOOD						
_____	(91)	BUTTER PATS, USDA 30LB/CS	— 1	5 LB BOX	5.307	5.307
TOTAL(S)						297.880

NOTES: 1. _____ _____ ____ _____
              2. _____ _____ ____ _____
              3. _____ _____ ____ _____
              4. Received by: _____

Courtesy of The CBORD Group, Inc., 1997, Ithaca, New York.

Exhibit 6–7 Service Summary Report

REPORT#: 28	OPTION: 7.1.5.1.6.	USER#: 4	*** CBORD FOODSERVICE MANAGEMENT SYSTEMS ***

MENU MANAGEMENT SYSTEM - V6.2
FAIRFAX COUNTY PUBLIC SCHOOLS
SERVICE SUMMARY REPORT

PAGE: 1
DEC 09 96
1002 HOURS

UNIT : 3 Area :   FINISHING KITCHEN

Day : THURSDAY 11/21/96
Meal: 2 LUNCH

Cy-Mo-Wk:
Cust Cnt : 100
Act Cust :

— Recipe — Mmbr Name	Serving Utensil / Serving Pan	Fcst	DA#	Portions Prepared - Leftover Served	Time Ran Out	Ptn Size / Ptn Desc	Sell Price
5 CHICKEN NUGGETS (4-12)	TONGS 9" / 12" × 20" × 2" STEAMTABLE	125<	DA#11	>< >=<	<	3.25 / 5 NUGGETS	1.250
645 EGG ROLL, PORK (1)		100<	DA#15	>< >=<	<	3.00 / 1 EGG ROLL	1.000
573 PANCAKE n SAUSAGE STIK 48/CS		25<	DA#21	>< >=<	<	2.85 / EACH	1.250
342 CEREAL, CHEERIOS 96/CS/		10<	DA#22	>< >=<	<	0.63 / 1 BOWL	0.400
738 CEREAL, CINNAMON TOAST CRUNCH		10<	DA#23	>< >=<	<	0.75 / 1 BOWL	0.400
681 POTATOES, WHIPPED (3/8 CUP) PURCH#10 DISHER = 3/8 CUP	12" × 20" × 4" STEAMTABLE	225<	DA#17	>< >=<	<	2.70 / 3/8 Cup	0.750
587 ORANGE, FRESH		150<	DA#18	>< >=<	<	3.64 / 1 ORANGE	0.500
88 PEAR HALVES, CANNED	#8 DISHER = 1/2 CUP / 18" × 25" × 1" DISPLAY	75<	DA#19	>< >=<	<	4.44 / 1/2 CUP	0.500
265 JUICE, FROZEN GRAPE K-PAC	18" × 25" × 1" DISPLAY	40<	DA#20	>< >=<	<	4.00 / 1/2 CUP	0.400
367 MUFFIN, BLUEBERRY 1 OZ. 60/TRAY	18" × 25" × 1" DISPLAY	125<	DA#10	>< >=<	<	1.00 / 4 OZ CUP	0.300
132 RICE, STEAMED	TONGS 9" / 12" × 20" × 2" STEAMTABLE	150<	DA#16	>< >=<	<	3.75 / 1 PIECE	0.500
151 BISCUITS, FROZEN	#8 DISHER = 1/2 CUP / 12" × 20" × 2" STEAMTABLE	20<	DA#24	>< >=<	<	1.00 / 1 BISCUIT	0.300
402 MILK, WHOLE		180<	DA#32	>< >=<	<	8.00 / 1/2 PINT	0.350
128 MILK, 1%		180<		>< >=<	<	8.00	0.350

continues

Exhibit 6–7 continued

Item #	Description		DA#	Qty		Unit	Value 1	Value 2
694	SWEET/SOUR SAUCE PACKETS		DA#33	200<	>< >=<	1/2 PINT	1.00	0.000
200	JELLY, ASSORTED PACKETS		DA#27	100<	>< >=<	1 PKT	0.50	0.050
252	SYRUP, IND. PACKETS		DA#29	200<	>< >=<	1 PKT	1.50	0.150
325	FORK & NAPKIN KIT, 1000/CS		DA#30	1000<	>< >=<	1 PACKET	0.26	0.80
600	TRAY, ROSE STYRO 250/CS		DA#25	400<	>< >=<	EACH	0.01	0.100
603	TEASPOONS, PLASTIC		DA#26	500<	>< >=<	EACH	0.01	0.050
102	BUTTER, PATS, USDA 30LB/CS		DA#31	100<	>< >=<	1 EACH	0.18	0.050
			DA#28			ONE PAT		

Courtesy of The CBORD Group, Inc., 1997, Ithaca, New York.

Exhibit 6–8 Inventory Tally Sheet

```
REPORT#  :  40   * * * CBORD FOODSERVICE MANAGEMENT SYSTEMS * * *    PAGE: 1
OPTION   :  8.1.1.        MENU MANAGEMENT SYSTEM - V6.2              DEC 09 96
USER#    :  4            FAIRFAX COUNTY PUBLIC SCHOOLS              1005 HOURS
                         INVENTORY TALLY SHEET
```

Unit Name: Taken By: _____
Nmbr: 100   Date: ____/____/____ Time: _____

Storage Location: 11 FREEZER

Item Name	FIDF Nmbr	Units on Hand	Stock Unit	Price per Stk Unit	User FIDF Number
BISCUITS, FROZEN 140/CS	236	<_____-___>	CASE	8.590	_____
CHICKEN NUGGETS	4	<_____-___>	CASE	15.500	_____
EGG ROLL, PORK, 60/CS TONYS	1053	<_____-___>	CASE	28.530	_____
JUICE, FZN GRAPE K-PAC96/C	990	<_____-___>	CASE	11.020	_____
MUFFIN, BLUBERY 1oz 240/CS	897	<_____-___>	CASE	25.310	_____
PANCAKEnSAUSAGE STIK 48/C	646	<_____-___>	CASE	12.560	_____

SUBTOTAL NUMBER OF RECORDS PRINTED 6

Courtesy of The CBORD Group, Inc., 1997, Ithaca, New York.

Exhibit 6–9 Physical Inventory Transactions

```
REPORT#:  39   * * * CBORD FOODSERVICE MANAGEMENT SYSTEMS * * *    PAGE: 1
OPTION :  8.3.         MENU MANAGEMENT SYSTEM - V6.2               DEC 09 96
USER#  :  4           FAIRFAX COUNTY PUBLIC SCHOOLS               1010 HOURS
                      PHYSICAL INVENTORY TRANSACTIONS
```

Unit   : S 101
Inventory Date : 11/18/96
Storage Location: 11 FREEZER

Item Name	Item Nmbr	Units On Hand	Stock Unit	Price/ Stk U	Inventory Value
BISCUITS, FROZEN 140/CS	236	.5	CASE	8.5900	4.295
CHICKEN NUGGETS	4	2	CASE	15.5000	31.000
EGG ROLL, PORK, 60/CS TONYS	1053	1	CASE	28.5300	28.530
JUICE, FZN GRAPE K-PAC96/C	990	.5	CASE	11.0200	5.510
MUFFIN, BLUBERY 1oz 240/CS	897	.5	CASE	25.3100	12.655
PANCAKEnSAUSAGE STIK 48/C	646	.33	CASE	12.5600	4.145

STORAGE LOCATION SUBTOTAL   86.135

Courtesy of The CBORD Group, Inc., 1997, Ithaca, New York.

Exhibit 6–10 Inventory Valuation Summary

```
REPORTS: 37              * * * CBORD FOODSERVICE MANAGEMENT SYSTEMS * * *                    PAGE: 1
OPTION  : 8.1.2.                   MENU MANAGEMENT SYSTEM - V6.2                             DEC 11 96
USERS   : 4                      FAIRFAX COUNTY PUBLIC SCHOOLS                             0847 HOURS
                                   INVENTORY VALUATION SUMMARY
        Unit     :  S 100
Inventory Date   :  11/19/96
```

Product Group	Inventory Value		Storage Location	Inventory Value	
			11 FREEZER	86.135	24.542%
11 FREEZER	86.133	24.542%	19 REFRIGERATOR	73.300	20.885%
19 REFRIGERATOR	73.300	20.885%	21 CONDIMENTS - STAPLES	15.164	4.321%
20 REFRIGERATOR, PRODUCE	8.475	2.415%	23 DRY STORAGE - CANNED	19.727	5.621%
21 CONDIMENTS - STAPLES	15.164	4.321%	32 PAPER AND SUPPLIES	141.105	40.204%
23 DRY STORAGE - CANNED	19.727	5.621%	97 NOT IN USE - PAPER	1.867	0.532%
			99 NOT IN USE - FOOD	13.678	3.897%
TOTAL FOODS	202.801	57.782%	UNSPECIFIED ROLLUP GROUP	330.976	100.000%
31 COMMODITIES	5.203	1.482%			
TOTAL COMMOITIES	5.203	1.482%			
39 PAPER SUPPLIES	142.972	40.736%			
TOTAL PAPER/CLEANING	142.972	40.736%			
TOTALS	350.976	100.000%		350.976	100.000%

Courtesy of The CBORD Group, Inc., 1997, Ithaca, New York.

records original costs and calculates its depreciated value; and shows where it is located, when it was moved, and its maintenance record.

For inventory accuracy and time saving, a relational database is a must to ensure that data updated in one location are automatically updated everywhere. At the same time, the hardware should have adequate power to accommodate future technology.[28]

Warehousing

Many school food and nutrition programs have central warehousing, although some warehousing is limited to USDA commodities. Some school food service programs share warehouse space with other departments or the entire school district. The warehousing objective should be to provide positive item identification while conserving time, labor, and equipment.

Warehousing as we know it today is relatively new. Forty years ago, a warehouse was thought of as a place to store goods and not as a part of a distribution network. Little or no attention was placed on materials handling equipment. This is easy to understand when one recognizes that the forklift is a modern invention and was used for the first time in 1939. It became important to commerce only after World War II.[29]

Just as we are concerned about labor costs and efficiency in food service production, we should be equally as aware of costs and inefficiency in warehousing. Smaller child nutrition programs may find the computerized inventory and distribution tools previously discussed to be adequate. However, those districts that have a large warehouse or share a warehouse can realize significant savings through computerized automation. When selecting a computerized warehouse receiving and distribution system, the child nutrition professional should look for the features found in Exhibit 6–11.

USDA–donated commodities receipt, allocation, and delivery are major considerations of child nutrition professionals. The receipt of USDA commodities may be handled the same as purchased goods; however, the computer programs should be designed to substitute USDA commodities for purchased products. Conversely, when the USDA commodity is expended, the computer should automatically designate an acceptable substitution. For those who must allocate USDA commodities to various sites, software is available that automatically allocates the amount received by participation. In turn, a report can be generated for USDA accounting purposes by the individual school or the entire district.

With a computerized warehousing system, a perpetual inventory is established. However, periodic physical inventories should be taken to balance the computer-generated inventory against the physical, on-hand balance. With a printed variance report, inconsistencies between the actual amounts on hand and the computer-projected inventory are spotted immediately. Thus data entry errors, damaged goods, and theft are controlled. Because of the vastness of most warehouses and the volume of goods stored, electronic applications are advised. With a computer-compatible universal marking or bar code system, a simple bar code wand or a hand-held bar code scanner may be used. A hand-held bar code scanner computer,

equipped with item numbers and memory that are subsequently downloaded into the computer, is ideal. Recent innovations such as waterproof labels securely attached to frozen and refrigerated products have advanced this form of inventory taking in the food service industry. If bar code readers are being considered, care must be taken to ensure that manufacturers and processors place universal codes on each unit and case. This may require a bid modification.

Additional peripheral applications in a warehouse are robots and receiving scales with output that connects to a printer or computer for data collection. Robots can be programmed to select and move food and supplies in a warehouse, thus decreasing labor costs associated with picking and assembling food and supplies ordered.

For child nutrition professionals, operating a warehouse in heavily populated or expansive areas, computerized routing systems for deliveries should be considered. Recently these delivery systems have become sophisticated to the point of enabling the driver to watch a display screen inside the vehicle that indicates its location and where turns are to be made.

Exhibit 6–11 Steps to Warehouse Computerization

---

1. Warehouse receiving personnel physically check each arriving shipment against the appropriate document.
2. The computer selects a storage location according to the type of goods and space available. Good software should be able to handle multiple warehouse/freezer/refrigerated locations.
3. Goods received are entered into a computerized daily receiving report.
4. Orders from production site(s) are electronically transmitted to the warehouse, where the computer automatically checks all of the schools' orders against current inventory quantities on hand and prints an exception list of all items that are out of stock.
5. Substitutions can be made automatically for out-of-stock items.
6. Areas or screens can be set up for supervisors to check their schools' orders.
7. Pick tickets with designated storage locations are generated along with delivery tickets and printed shipping labels.
8. Orders are assembled according to a computerized delivery schedule, thus ensuring energy-saving, efficient deliveries.
9. For billing purposes, shipping reports are generated to indicate which items were shipped to each school.

Menu Planning and Nutrient Analysis

The food service manager used computer systems in the 1960s to replace time and personnel. By the 1980s, managers were using computer systems to assist in decision making to use resources in an optimal way.[30]

Textbooks tell us that menus are the basis of the entire food service operation. The menu determines the inventory to be purchased, the food items needed to produce and serve, the precost and postcost of meals, and their nutritional adequacy. Menu planning with the aid of a computer allows food service managers to pinpoint costs prior to service and to evaluate all the implications of presenting a menu—from purchasing and inventory to production and service.[31]

In 1969, Helen McGee, president of the American School Food Service Association (ASFSA), indicated computers should be used by school food and nutrition service programs. She went on to say, ". . . we need to look at the expanded school lunch program—perhaps not only a free, nutritionally balanced lunch, . . . but also a free breakfast where needed, total food service for the elderly, evening meals for the children of working mothers, and family meals for the increasing members participating in adult education."[32(pp233–234)] Most menus written by child nutrition professionals are based on the recommended dietary allowances (RDAs) and the Dietary Guidelines for Americans. Whether menus are being planned for school-aged children in child nutrition programs, infants, children in day care, or senior citizens, RDAs have been established.[33] Using the RDAs, USDA devised food-based meal patterns for the National School Lunch Program (NSLP)[34] School Breakfast Program (SBP),[34] Child and Adult Care Food Program (CACFP),[34] Summer Food Service Program (SFSP),[34] and the Meal Pattern for Adults.[35] Many child nutrition providers offer a combination of these programs. In addition to serving breakfast and lunch to enrolled students, their food service operation may serve as a contractor for meals or snacks to day-care centers, to summer programs, and to adults in senior nutrition and day care programs. While USDA has provided options for designing NSLP and SBP menus, a food-based menu plan is required for the CACFP, SFSP, and the Meal Pattern for Adults.

In the early 1970s, five school districts tested the Computer-Assisted Nutrient Standard (CANS) menu planning method. While CANS was used for costing menus and establishing purchasing needs, most food service professionals found it too complex and difficult to use. During the 1983–1984 school year, 18 food service authorities participated in a nutrient standard menu planning pilot. By the next year, 39 percent of the participants no longer used the system because of an inadequate nutrient database for processed foods, difficulty in using the computer software, and the costs and skills required to run the program.[36]

Child nutrition programs are faced with tremendous challenges and opportunities for improving the health of America's children, as outlined in the Surgeon General's *Healthy People 2000*.[37] The School Meals for Healthy Children Act reflects the mandate of *Healthy People 2000*. In 1994, USDA amended the traditional food-based meal patterns to reflect the most current *Dietary Guidelines for Americans* and the *Food Guide Pyramid*.[38,39]

To improve the nutritional quality of children's meals, different methods of meal planning have been established

- Nutrient Standard Menu Planning (NSMP)
- Assisted Nutrient Standard Menus (Assisted NSMP)
- Food-Based Menus that meet the Dietary Guidelines for Americans (Traditional and Enhanced)
- Menus planned by "reasonable approach" to meet the Dietary Guidelines for Americans, including the traditional NSLP and SBP patterns.

NSMP and Assisted NSMP are planned using computer software programs approved by USDA. With this new focus, child nutrition professionals must provide one-third of the RDA for protein, calcium, iron, Vitamin A, Vitamin C, and calories for lunch, and one-fourth of the RDA for the same nutrients for breakfast. In addition, fat is limited to 30 percent of total calories, and saturated fat to less than 10 percent of total calories. Nutrients for these meals are averaged over a week's cycle of menus. Both NSMP and food-based menus are structured to require higher levels of nutrients for older children or adolescents.

To facilitate uniform computerization of menu planning and nutrient analysis for the NSLP and SBP, USDA developed a database of nutritional values for over 7,000 ingredients or prepared products. In addition, USDA established criteria for software to be used in constructing NSMP and Assisted NSMP. Software systems approved to implement NSMP, Assisted NSMP, and for state monitoring of food-based menus all use menu planning programs of their own design or designed by another approved software company and sold under authorization of the owner. When considering menu planning software systems child nutrition professionals should carefully evaluate all features as shown in Table 6–1. Nutrient standard menu planning should not be confused with nutrient analysis of menus planned using traditional food-based meal patterns. For years, some child nutrition professionals have analyzed their school lunch menus planned with meal pattern components.[40]

The database of nutrient analysis programs must be accurate, well documented, and large enough to perform all intended tasks. Nutrient databases vary among programs depending on the number of food items and nutrients included, whether the most recent USDA data have been incorporated, and the degree to which non–USDA sources (such as food industry and scientific literature) or estimated calculations are used to replace missing nutrient values.

Other important operating features include the ease and speed with which food items can be entered into a program; quality of the user's manual and help screens; ability to preview single food nutrients while entering foods; ability to assign different volume or weight measures to food items; ease of editing the food list; limit in number of food entries; ease of averaging multiple days of dietary input; and ability to compare results with a variety of dietary standards. Users should also consider the program's costs and ability to print a variety of reports and export data. The inability of a program to export data is a distinct disadvantage for those wishing to analyze data statistically.[41]

Software for nutrient analysis, as a rule, provides an extensive review of many nutrients. Nutrient information required for NSMP and Assisted NSMP is not as detailed as that supplied by good nutrient analysis software. All users are cautioned to choose a nutrient analysis program carefully that will meet their specific needs. As the general public has become more aware of the relationship between nutrition and health, their demand for nutrition information has been heard, and child nutrition professionals have responded. Many school food service operations provide detailed, printed nutrient analyses of all menus or menu offerings. Often students request an analysis of a specific menu prior to purchasing a meal. This can be accommodated by posters or pamphlets like those used in fast food operations. Innovative managers provide this information as a Nutrition Facts label for every choice in the cafeteria. Others have placed interactive computers with touch screens in the dining room. Students browse the menu and design their meal before buying or selecting.[43] In other operations, cash registers can be programmed to provide an analysis of the items selected when customers pay for their meal.

As child nutrition professionals continue to meet their customers' needs, there is a growing demand for ingredient lists and a database of food additives. With an increasing awareness of food and ingredient sensitivities and ethnic

Table 6–1 Menu Planning Software Systems

Desirable Features	*Features To Avoid*
Can be used with any of the approved menu-planning methods.	Cannot be used with all approved menu-planning methods.
Has user-friendly, on-screen help for every menu-planning step.	Lack of user-friendly, on-screen help for every menu-planning step.
Demonstration workbook and disks are user-friendly.	Lacks demonstration workbook or disks.
Computer experience is not necessary.	Extensive computer experience and training required.
Walks the user through adding to menu item master list and recipes.	No provisions are made for the addition of regional menu items or ingredients.
Uses terms common to school food service such as #10 cans, pounds, cups, quarts, tablespoons, etc.	Uses very technical terms and portions that must be manually converted.
Adjusts recipes to portion sizes.	User is required to adjust portion sizes.
Can add, modify, or deactivate ingredients.	Must use only the ingredients included in the software.
Uses USDA *Food Buying Guide.*[42]	Does not use the USDA *Food Buying Guide.*[42]
Uses USDA database.	Does not use the USDA database.
Has a branded product database.	Has no branded product database.
Provides menu and recipe costing.	Lacks menu and recipe costing ability.
Nutritional analysis is available on screen and in printed form.	Nutritional analysis is not readily available in usable form.
Guards against common data entry errors through nutrient checkup.	No mechanism is available to signify data entry errors.
Automatically generates production records and shopping lists.	No additional features are available—plans and analyzes menus only.
Has a toll-free customer support line.	All customer support must be paid by the user.
Is child nutrition user-friendly—analogies are to situations familiar to food service professionals.	Does not use food service terminology. Uses computer or technical terminology, which requires detailed translations.
Has an ingredient search feature enabling the use of USDA commodities or excess inventory.	Has no ingredient search feature.
Is the track record good? How many use it and how long has the company been in business?	Poor track record and weak promotional material.
Company is within the geographic area. Response to needs is immediate.	Company is far away and uses a network of dealers, sometimes in protected territories. Response time is poor.
Able to interface with other systems.	Discourages use of other systems.
Additional software can be installed by a specialized staff person.	Must rely on the vendor to install software.
Can use existing hardware providing it has enough power and memory.	Wants you to buy their hardware and software.
Printed menus and portions are easy to read in everyday language.	Printed menus and portions require a key to decipher.
Field-level access or system rights can be assigned; only designated people can change menus, ingredients, or amounts.	Field-level access or system rights cannot be assigned; anyone can change a menu, ingredient, or amount.

diversities, we must provide ingredient and additive information to concerned adults, parents, and students as well as those in the medical community.

The term *nutrition integrity* belongs to school food and nutrition programs. As early as 1990, ASFSA defined it as a guaranteed level of performance that ensures that all foods available in schools for children are consistent with recommended dietary allowances and dietary guidelines and, when consumed, contribute to the development of lifelong, healthy eating habits.[44]

Recipes

A standardized recipe is one that has been tested to provide an established yield and quality through the use of ingredients that remain constant in both measurement and preparation methods.[45] Unless the food service department uses standardized recipes for every item produced, there is little point in planning menus that accurately fulfill nutrient requirements and meet cost limitations. The ingredients used in each recipe must be issued through a controlled procedure, and production workers must follow recipes exactly.[46] Robertson goes on to say, "It can be costly to have each cook add a personal touch to foods. In fact, many people swear by the 'ingredient room' concept, where the ingredients for a recipe are premeasured and delivered to the cook for preparation."[47(p27)]

According to Keiser and DeMicco, "Standardized recipes are paramount to effective and efficient food production and cost controls. . . . Recipes must be developed precisely and adhered to in the kitchen. Failure to enforce this policy in a computerized operation will result in overproduction, waste, inconsistent product, inventory shortages, and meaningless costing projections. Enforcing standard recipe use will yield the payoffs of greatly reduced food costs, minimum waste, accurate accounting, and streamlined, efficient inventory control."[48(p43)]

The availability of accurate recipes adjusted to the required yield is especially valuable to

food service production personnel. Yield of recipe ingredients is usually coded into the food item database. The yield of the food varies depending on the exact prepreparation and preparation instructions in the recipe. A recipe database that allows adjustment of the ingredient yield factors at the recipe level more accurately projects food to purchase and product yields.[49] Consequently, with accurate yields, reliable precosts and postcosts can be obtained.

USDA approved software for menus contain USDA recipes, ingredients, and yields. In addition, the approved software allows for adding new recipes and nutritional analysis or to modify existing recipes and nutritional analysis. As a word of caution, operators have to know what the computer doesn't know and how to make the right adjustments.

- Somewhere in the software a "yield factor" should be entered to adjust for food growing or shrinking as it is prepared. Pasta grows during preparation and meat shrinks.
- Nutritional information in a recipe must be consistent. Raw pasta and cooked pasta have the same kinds of nutrients, but in different proportions. For example, some vitamins flow out of foods during cooking more than others. When cooked pasta is used, the computer needs to be told to use nutrition information for cooked pasta by "coding" for cooked, not dry, pasta.
- When raw or frozen vegetables are cooked, the recipe should list raw or frozen vegetables—the actual ingredients cooks are to use—and the nutritional information code should be for cooked vegetables.
- When food is cooked in salted water, the amount of sodium remaining should be included.

When making recipe adjustments, the computer operator must keep a list of coding decisions made to ensure consistency from recipe to recipe.[50] More and more food service professionals are calling for a computer software industry standard database. Until there is a nutrient database that is adapted as the standard and made available to all vendors, the databases (of nutrients and ingredients) will continue to vary, leaving child nutrition professionals with the responsibility of carefully choosing or altering a program to meet their specific needs and tasks.[51–53] All USDA–approved software has the ability to generate a recipe with different portion sizes. The wise operator will select software that prints a recipe in portions and terms familiar to school food and nutrition program personnel.

With accurate recipes and inventory, menus can be precosted. When menus are precosted on the basis of a forecasted demand, pertinent data for management decision making can be made before the menu is finally approved or food purchased. With an up-to-date inventory file, actual, not theoretical, precosts are derived. To avoid bottlenecks caused by the time required to input new costs as ingredient prices fluctuate, the child nutrition program operator should use software that will accept electronic updates from vendors and that will update prices globally on receipt.[54]

In postcost analysis, actual customer counts and quantity of menu items prepared and sold are entered into the computer. The computer then provides detailed consolidations and summaries of daily production results, including food usage. Unused prepared food is returned to inventory, and a postcost is derived. Postcosting is an advanced feature of a sophisticated menu-planning system and provides important financial information such as comparison of portions prepared to portions sold, costs and margins for each item, and for the item on a per-customer averaged basis. In addition, data are stored and can be reported over long periods of time, thus defining trends in costs and usage of various menu items over time.[55]

Food Production and Record Keeping

The menu is the driving force for all program activity, from planning to purchasing, production, service, cleanup, and the ultimate satisfaction of our customers' appetites.[56] In the previous section, computerized menus were discussed, including the need for child nutrition professionals to extend or decrease a recipe. In a food production system, computer applications have shifted from haphazard forecasting, intuitive marketing research, seat-of-the-pants decision making, and indiscriminate data collection for strategic planning to automated information systems.[57]

Crucial to a sound production system is the need for accurate participation figures. An integrated food service management system collects and computes actual historical service quantities as the basis of the forecast rather than past production quantities. Some authorities recommend gathering these statistical data five times before implementing them as a reliable forecast figure.[58] A computerized POS system permits every food item selected by a student to be itemized. In this way, a historical file of menu items sold is developed. Such accurate sales reports are used to forecast the amount of food to purchase and produce in the future. At the same time, production sheets can be generated comparing the amount of food prepared to the amount served.[59]

In programs where the ability is not available to accurately count individual portions sold, other forecasting methods must be used. Using participation and revenue (PAR) (sometimes referred to as participation and deposit, or PAD) reports generated by a POS system and computer-generated service summary reports (Exhibit 6–7), relatively accurate forecasting data can be derived.

School food and nutrition professionals are aware of the need for detailed record keeping. In addition to POS systems, a good computerized production and record-keeping system will consist of various modules. Depending on the size of the program and the food delivery system chosen, the food service operator may use several modules or many of them. Examples of readily available computerized production modules are found in Exhibit 6–12.

Equipment

In addition to computer software for the production process and record keeping, computers are utilized extensively in production equipment. As appliances for the home have become "smart," with computer controls and other modular features, the food service equipment industry has responded to requests for similar features in commercial applications. Cooks and managers realize the convenience of setting controls and allowing equipment to do the work intelligently. Food service operators realize the cost benefits associated with shorter, controlled cooking time, reduced labor needs, and a uniform, standardized, perfectly cooked product. In large central production facilities, elaborate computer systems may be tied into the cook-chill equipment to record pertinent production data such as cooking times and food temperatures.[60] In light of food safety issues and Hazard Analysis Critical Control Points (HACCP) requirements, computerized printouts of temperatures throughout the cook-chill process provide the needed audit trail. In single-unit kitchens, "smart" ovens are found with controls that are programmed by the cook for the perfect temperature in the right amount of time. In addition, these ovens have load timer pads that determine the cooking time for each shelf in the oven. If the operator causes a temperature change by opening the oven door or adding extra cold foods, the computer automatically compensates by adjusting itself for a longer cooking time. Actual temperature readings and cooking times remaining are available on a lighted, digital readout. With modular "plug-in" control units and self-diagnostic systems, service calls are limited and repair times are reduced. Combination steamers and ovens (combi-ovens) are remarkable in that they save valuable equipment dollars by combining two pieces of equipment into one and they have such features as microprocessor-based oven controls, programmable memory, self-diagnostic control panels, and digital time and temperature displays. Deep-fat fryers may have process controllers that allow like foods to be

Exhibit 6-12 Available Food Service Production Module

- Point-of-Service (POS) systems
- Modules that interface with POS registers to report flow of sales, menu items, and trigger need for additional food to be prepared
- Production schedules that produce forecast-adjusted recipes. One worksheet is generated for each menu item.
- Employee daily production schedule modules through which the manager can schedule employees by task, preparation procedures, time of service, equipment availability, and the employee's time schedule
- Production reports indicating employee labor used and costs as well as purchased and USDA foods used and costs
- Storeroom-issue request modules that produce a printout of items to be issued from the storeroom; also a computer-analyzed menu plan that indicates whether or not there is adequate stock on hand and deletes inventory used
- Advanced freezer withdrawal modules that produce a printout of frozen foods called for in recipes to be used in days ahead
- Advanced or preparation module-generated lists that alert cooks to schedule items (such as gelatin) far enough in advance to have them ready when needed.
- Modules that update recipe costs as new purchases are made and calculate automatic leftover costs that are added to inventory with a "use by" date[61]

fried at the same time and temperature by selecting a particular setting. The fryer automatically cools to 275°F when it is not immediately reused, thus prolonging the life of the oil.[62]

Vending

Many child nutrition programs have inventively adopted alternative styles of food service because of a diverse customer pool and alternative serving facilities. Vending machines were considered an additional serving area when school food service managers first used them for à la carte sales in the early 1980s. Those machines were equipped with a standard coin mechanism. By the mid 1980s, the demand for bill validators increased as inflation caused prices to rise and customers requested more variety. When these demands continued into the 1990s, vending machines had to become more in tune with the times. Coinless vending and smart machines are now available.

With the advent of POS systems in school food and child nutrition programs came the magnetic strip or debit card. With today's technology, debit card readers can be included in all vending machines. Two options for transmitting data from the card reader to a computer in a LAN are available by wired or wireless technology. The latter transmitting options have increased satellite vending locations in a single location by enabling a customer to draw down on his or her food service account.

The next wave of vending payment options is the "smart card" or stored value card. Smart cards in child nutrition programs in the foreseeable future will entail placing cash, a check, or an electronic transfer from an existing account to the individual customer's account. In turn, the smart card with its computer chip can be used for vending machine purchases. In the more distant future vending machines will be equipped to accept credit cards.

Without electronics, vending machine restocking decisions take place at the machine when it is being serviced by the route person. When a central system electronically gathers the machine's stock level information via wireless technology, those responsible for replenishing know before they leave the central vending supply facility exactly what each machine will require. Time-of-day and day-of-week information can also allow stocking in anticipation of use rather than in response to it. Time-of-day information tells the central facility how long a choice has been unavailable. It also eliminates stocking bias on the part of the person filling the machine.

Benefits of electronic data in vending machines are that choices can be stocked appropriately and walkaways from one machine can mean a lost sale in another machine. For example, if you are out of cookies, you could also lose a sale for milk. At the same time, determining a machine's customer usage pattern allows for more attractive choices, while hard sales information helps managers deal with small, vocal groups of customers and project performance of additional machines and prices acceptable to the customer. Finally, condition alarms mean faster maintenance and less downtime while age of stock information helps reduce spoilage, lost sales and unhappy customers.[63]

In specifying vending machines with advanced computer capabilities, the contract should include a multidrop bus (MDB) interface standard and a vending industry Data Transfer Standard (DTS). The MDB governs vending machine add-ons or peripherals such as coin mechanisms, bill validators, and card readers. With MDB, it is easier to add peripherals because it ensures they will all work together in a standard compliant vending machine. The term *bus* means a system into which components can be fitted. A building's electric wires are a bus into which electric devices can be plugged. You know they'll work because the plugs and outlets conform to standards. An MDB will accept as many as 36 peripherals, which means it has space for future expansion.[64]

The DTS has been adopted by the vending industry and works hand in hand with MDB.

Data transfer standards specifically govern how data are transmitted or received. Many hand-held computers, such as those used in inventory taking, currently utilize the DTS. Data are transmitted through a hand-held computer, where they are stored until being downloaded instantaneously into a computer, or they can be transmitted to the computer through wireless technology. While MDB and data transfer standard are two different protocols, their role in enhancing data retrieved is interrelated.[65]

With MDB, the following advantages can be realized:

- Future computerized upgrades in vending machines are easily accomplished without removing the machine for retrofitting.
- Data retrieval can be added as a peripheral that collects data from one machine or from an entire bank of MDB equipped machines.
- Troubleshooting and repair are easier, thus reducing lost sales, repair time, and costs.

In the future with MDB-equipped machines, operators will be able to know what is selling as it is being purchased. An internal bar code scanner can record this information or it can, through wireless transmission, alert the vending supply operation when the machine needs to be stocked with what product(s). In turn, the receiving computer tells the delivery person when to fill the machine with what product.[65]

Depending on the food service operator's needs, budget, and clientele, decisions can be made for a vending operation. Regardless of the peripheral potentials in vending, all specifications for lease or purchase of machines should require MDB and data transfer standard on all machines. Smart cards are used predominantly in colleges and universities and several school systems. Their initial cost is currently seven and one-half times that of a magnetic strip card. On the other hand, it is often easier for the user to put money on the card through cash to card machines or automated teller machines (ATMs).[66] The operator accepts the smart card at the POS for the amount of the transaction. Funds for the transaction are electronically transferred from the cardholder's account to the operator's account.

BUSINESS FUNCTIONS

In some school food and child nutrition programs, business functions may be assigned to another department of the school district; others may have total responsibility for all business functions; and still others handle selected functions such as budget development and personnel. Regardless of where the business functions are performed, all school food and child nutrition directors must have a working knowledge of computer applications and program requirements in this vital area.

Free and Reduced-Price Meal Application Approval

Perhaps the earliest use of computers by school food and nutrition professionals was for processing free and reduced-price meal applications. In selecting application-processing software, the food service operator may want to establish a committee to determine what is needed. Once the criteria are developed, a search can begin for appropriate software, or a customized program can be written.

Free and reduced-price meal application processing software uses a specialized database. With this software, users are able to select from multiple tasks found in Exhibit 6–13. Regardless of the software used, free and reduced-price meal application processing remains a labor-intense task for child nutrition programs. Many school districts are forced to use temporary data entry personnel during this busy time to meet the required schedules for completion. With the advent of scanners, particularly ones now available that can process handwritten information, the day may be near when the approval process is not as labor intense. While these scanners were relatively expensive initially, the cost has dropped and they should

Exhibit 6–13 Features of Free and Reduced-Price Meal Application Software

Standard Features
- Process both direct-certified and nondirect-certified meal and milk-only application.
- Process an unlimited number of applications for any number of schools.
- Flags incomplete applications and prints letters requesting needed information.
- Calculates total income based on weekly, biweekly, monthly, or yearly figures.
- Calculates multisource, multifrequency income totals.
- Assigns eligibility status.
- Retrieves family information when entering applications for additional family members, thus ensuring that all family members have the same eligibility status.
- Assigns temporary eligibility when no income or case number is provided.
- Prints a "temporary status expiring" letter for temporarily approved, nonresponsive applicants.
- Compiles a dated history of activity for each application. Included are the original eligibility assignment, letters generated, verification activity, reasons for change to the application, and movement of the student(s) from school to school.
- Generates lists, reports eligibility counts, and multilingual parent letters.
- Selects random or focus verification sampling with letters printed notifying applicants of their selection.
- Tracks verification progress with warning letters printed for those who fail to respond.
- Prints status change letters for those whose status changed as a result of the verification process.

Additional Useful Features
- Automatically updates federal eligibility guidelines.
- Exchanges data with the school board information database.
- Searches for a student or family by name or identification number.
- Processes applications on site or at a central location.
- Enters a foster care child as a family of one.
- Generates student lists by school, track, grade, homeroom, etc.
- Generates a free and reduced-eligibility report.
- Generates mailing labels for letters.
- Completes daily and monthly edit checks.
- Produces year-end grade promotion and school transfer for graduating students.

soon be affordable by even small school districts, particularly when the cost of additional labor is considered.

Point-of-Service Systems

More and more school districts are investing in state-of-the-art electronic POS systems to replace existing cash boxes, cash registers, and manual meal count systems. These electronic systems use computers to track meal eligibility (free, reduced price, and full price) and meal receipt by individual students. Electronic systems also make it easier to comply with reviews required by USDA regulations. Since these reviews (essentially audits) impose punitive monetary fines where adequate, child-specific documentation is not demonstrated, the POS investment dollar amount could very possibly, instead, be spent in countless manual hours or monetary fines. A final bonus of the latest POS systems is the opportunity to cease using student meal cards. Instead a personal identification number (PIN) number similar to that of an ATM system is proving to be workable, fast, and efficient. Student meal cards consume food service time and school administration time.[67]

At the school level, many believe the POS systems have produced faster service through the cafeteria line in addition to the documented meal service tracking accuracy. POS registers are probably the single greatest application of computers in food service. They are really minicomputers that can store data received through transactional keys and manipulate these data to provide a wide variety of reports. A POS register has been defined as "a computer that thinks it's a cash register."[68(p49)] Today, wireless POS registers are as affordable as plug-in units. Wireless units are mobile, making possible the use of carts in out-of-the way locations and outdoor service.[69]

Free and reduced-price meal applications can be processed on site and the information retained in the individual school's computer. In systems where meal applications are processed at a central location, modems may be used. By using existing telephone lines, the central office computer communicates each night with schools that have a POS system. The overnight communication function through the WAN allows the central office computer to send student eligibility, transfer changes, meal payments, and menu changes to the computer located in each school. During this communication, the central office computer also receives information such as the day's breakfast and lunch participation counts, à la carte sales, student account balances, etc. The software in the central office performs the federal edit checks and consolidates meal counts and à la carte sales districtwide. In addition, if a school has changed a student's eligibility without central office authorization, the next day the central office prints an error report listing the school, the student, and the issue in question.[70]

Of major concern to students, school food and nutrition professionals, and school administrators is the ability to process customer transactions rapidly. Before a POS system is implemented, decisions must be made regarding functions to be performed by the system. Customers move rapidly when the cashier vi-sually scans the selected meal components and à la carte items to make visual decisions regarding reimbursable meals. The result is sales information only. When each food item on the customer's tray is itemized by the cashier, the computer software analyzes the meal for needed components and alerts the cashier if the meal is not reimbursable. If the customer chooses not to take a reimbursable meal, the system will charge the student for each item at an à la carte price level and will not count the meal for reimbursement. The second function of itemization is menu forecasting. A good POS system can create a history file of menu items sold daily, which can be used to forecast the amount of food needed to purchase and produce in the future. A good system can also generate a production sheet that compares the amount of food prepared and served.[71] With this system, the speed of the customer through the serving area is directly related to the ability of the cashier to key in the selected items. On the other hand, the information generated is valuable and a potential, reliable source of management information while reducing redundant paper work.

Various peripherals transmitting to POS registers are currently in use. In place of the time-consuming student meal cards, many food service operators use student identification, debit cards equipped with a magnetic strip, or a bar code. A magnetic strip card is swiped through an input device that reads the customer identification number. A bar code card is waved past a laser, which reads the bar code and translates it into the customer's identification number assigned to his or her account, from which payment is deducted. Both types of identification systems at the POS enable customers to receive a free or reduced-price meal or to debit a prepaid account. An acceptable computer POS program generates the reports necessary for meal accountability and also can print a notice for parents when the student's prepaid balance is at a certain level. In some school districts, the child nutrition program student identification card meets other student identification needs such as access to athletic events, borrow from the library, and shop in the school store. For additional positive identification, the card may also contain the customer's name, the school's name, and possibly the customer's picture.[72] Generally, picture identification cards are more expensive and time consuming to produce. Current input devices include the following:

- A box with a magnetic strip reader through which the customer or cashier swipes the card
- A numeric key pad into which customers enter their identification number at the POS, or the cashier enters the identification number through the computer's keyboard. (Some systems automatically respond with a video image of the customer, and a computerized voice announces a complete or incomplete transaction. A system such as this may free the cashier for other tasks during serving time.)
- Thumbprint pads, hand scanners, or retina scanners that automatically display the customer's image on the screen
- Laser bar code readers and bar code wands that automatically display the customer's picture or name on the screen.

In the future, a POS terminal that can accept debit cards or smart cards will also be able to authorize credit card purchases. The advantage of both is immediate payment and the absence of fraudulent checks.

Reports

Food service must be understood and addressed as a business. In general, individual units or sites maintain operational data, and central offices need strategic data such as payroll, revenue, product cost, and statistical information. Using a unit-level database, information can be organized in various ways and transmitted to a central location for further processing and storage. Many child nutrition programs use electronic store-and-forward techniques or on-line data transmission. Telecommunication, involving telephone circuits and modems, is currently the best way to move data within a multiunit operation.[73]

Information links with the central office allow communication between schools and the central office in an on-line, real-time environment or in a dial-up file transfer environment. In many schools, reimbursement information is electronically transmitted to the state child nutrition office. Financial reporting data are also electronically passed to some states' child nutrition computer systems for analysis and consolidation[74] (see Figure 6–1).

As daily reports are received from individual sites, those responsible for accounting are able to take immediate action with the use of financially specific software. This software should be able to integrate data received fully to produce desired results and avoid duplication. Eventually a reimbursement claim form and other required monthly reports can be generated. Desirable features include, but may not be limited to, instant notification of overshorts with systemwide consolidation, processing of multiple POS terminals in one site and transmission to a central location, ability to review and modify POS information, instant notification of actual participants versus qualified participants, edit check reports, and automatic reimbursement claims.

Accounting

In food service operations, computers can complete such general accounting functions as accounts payable, general ledger accounts, accounts receivable, payroll (including deductions for payroll and benefits and generation of such forms as year-end W-2s), and sales and cash controls.

School food and nutrition programs with purchasing responsibility generate purchase orders and receiving reports. Years ago, com-

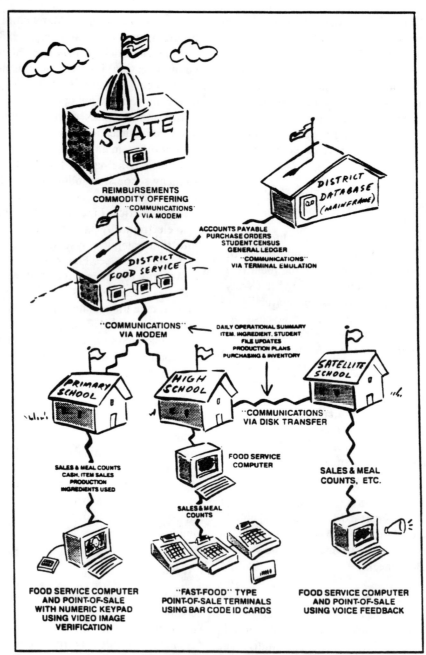

In a computerized school food service network, open architecture software can offer multiple options of what, where and how information flows. The network in this illustration, reaching from the point of sale to the state office, is one of an unlimited number of possible configurations.

Figure 6–1 A Computerized School Food Service Network. *Source:* Reprinted with permission from C. van Almelo, Getting the System You Want, *School Foodservice Journal,* Vol. 45, No. 1, p. 38, © 1991, American School Food Service Association.

puters had the ability to generate purchase orders when goods were received and the arrival entered into the inventory list. In turn, the computer generated a request for payment that was forwarded to the accounting department for payment. Finally, the computer regularly compared prices and inventory figures to prevent errors or fraud.[75]

Today's more sophisticated systems go even further as they audit received inventory versus ordered inventory, track purchase orders, determine cash requirements for payables, produce a payable detail including vendor due dates, select and audit invoices for payment, post payables to the general ledger, and automatically write checks through an interface with the general ledger. Conversely, the same systems are designed to gather data for goods or services sold; bill and follow through to the contractor, and post amounts received to the general ledger. For those not responding in a timely manner, follow-up letters or action may be initiated through the computer.

While billing and payments within an institution are frequently submitted and paid by an electronic transfer of funds, this is not always possible with outside vendors. To be able to pay bills electronically, both the vendor and the purchaser have to have identical configurations in their computer systems that enable them to communicate. Recently, entrepreneurs have established services through which orders can be placed electronically to the vendor. The invoice requesting payment is returned electronically through the service and the purchase is paid for by electronic transfer, again through the service. Usually, there is a one-time cost to users for the software and a monthly service fee to the distributor or vendor. The monthly service fee may be passed on to the purchaser. Careful evaluation of all costs involved for manual and electronic transfers should be performed before accepting this method of payment. Until electronic transfers are universally available, child nutrition professionals may want to negotiate the transfer of orders and payments for goods received as part of the original contract.

In addition to accounts payable and accounts receivable, good software has general ledger capabilities. Such a system is designed to receive data from other modules and generate reports such as income and expense statements and property management items. Such modules can be programmed to detail sales by category or perform statistical analysis on individual sites or profit centers. Reports can be prepared for any time period such as sales expenses per meal, per day, per week, per year, or any other period desired.[76] The child nutrition professional should select only software that ensures complete integration with all related modules; thus information is entered once and not touched again.

Good general-ledger software has many characteristics such as the ability to update multiple accounts based on predefined parameters; automatic sales tax calculations; journal entry screens for posting to the general ledger; out-of-balance condition detection; ledger audit trails; ability to print selected account codes; and balance sheets reflecting debits and credits for assets, liability reserve, and fund balance reports.

Even if responsibility for all other food service business functions belongs to other departments, as a rule budget development is confined to the school food and nutrition program. Budget forecasting can be risky if not based on sound data. To obtain sound data, computerized tools such as spreadsheets and database preparation are frequently used.

If you need your software to generate reports in various forms, your software will be database oriented. For example, a membership data bank list can be produced by alphabetical order, last name then first name and vice versa, by state, by title, by zip code—the list could go on and on. Database management allows you to manipulate and process raw facts and figures and create customized reports from that information.[77] An example of a specialized database is a software program that processes free and reduced-price meal applications or one that contains recipes or food nutrients.

Spreadsheets are modeled after traditional ledger sheets used by accountants; a computer spreadsheet uses a few simple commands to add, subtract, multiply, and divide rows and columns of figures to provide requested information almost instantly. On the computer screen, a spreadsheet is a block of empty boxes or "cells." For cells that require certain calculations, formulas must be inserted using cell identification codes and the mathematical functions that will result in the desired computation.[78] Unlike databases with the ability to generate the same data in various forms, spreadsheets generate selected, specific data in a comparison format.

When budgets are developed, managers require the most current information. In turn, it is used by budget preparers to project costs and forecast income. This is frequently designed by using the "what if" system. What would happen if prices or participation were increased by incremental amounts? Would labor have to be decreased by corresponding amounts? If these things happen, what innovations are proposed that could financially offset the anticipated changes? With computerized information, answers to questions such as these are rapidly available. Productivity, facilities, and equipment are inextricably linked. What is not budgeted for and spent up front, for up-to-date equipment, is lost through overworked personnel, a declining customer base due to problems in quality or speed of service, and wages paid for time-consuming tasks that could be automated.[79] In preparing the budget factors such as these should be examined.

Personnel

Functions typically found in computerized labor-management systems include time and attendance recording, control of overtime and lost time, labor-requirement forecasting, employee scheduling, labor cost analysis, and data preparation for payroll generation.[80] Depending on the size and structure of the operation, child nutrition professionals may use one or all possible computerized functions avail-able for handling personnel. Employee scheduling provides a plan by work area, skill position, and work time. A model for food service scheduling may include the various lengths of time in a workday for which any part-time or full-time worker could possibly be scheduled, all possible starting times, number of employees needed at each location for each period of the day, the ability to handle multiple classes of employees (such as staff members and supervisors), average cost per hour for each class of employee, limits on the number of employees who might be available within a certain class of employee for particular times of the day or at particular sites, and the need to preschedule certain individuals such as skilled, tenured employees.[81] Child nutrition providers with large production facilities or those engaged in summer meal programs where many variables are found may benefit most from computerized employee scheduling.

There is software available for scheduling substitute employees by using an interactive voice response system. Substitute employees are screened and registered in the system. When a permanent employee is unable to work, the manager calls the number of the interactive voice response system, notifying it of the employee's absence and requesting substitute help with specific skills (cook, cashier, etc.) for a specific length of time. In turn, the system automatically begins calling previously registered substitutes and stops calling once the assignment has been accepted. The substitute receives specific information about the position and work location and has the ability to accept or decline the assignment. Managers can specify acceptable substitutes, and substitutes can selectively eliminate certain work sites.

Paramount to employee scheduling is an employee master file and a skills inventory file. In these files is a running history of employees: positions, full- or part-time status, times they can work, how many hours they accrue as the week progresses, and special requests. Akin to scheduling files is technology that allows absenteeism, employee accidents, and workers' compensation claims to be tracked individually as well as by unit or system. In one system where employee absenteeism was tracked and posted, substantial reductions in Monday and Friday absences were noticed. This same technology enables management to track employee turnover by reason.[82]

In analyzing labor costs, time sheets, time cards, or printouts of times worked from a computerized key pad are valuable tools. Overtime and lost time directly influence labor costs. Currently computerized time clocks are available that automatically transmit employees' hours worked to a central location and instruct the computer to print paychecks. Such a system requires flags, which prevent abuse and unauthorized use of overtime.

Tracking Trends and Theft Control

The wise school food and child nutrition program manager will have someone on staff who knows the food service business and understands the entire computer system. This "trend analyst" should be assigned to audit various aspects of the operation, track trends within various units, and control theft.

For systems where various cost centers have been established, the accountant can produce an individualized, computerized profit-and-loss statement. The trend analyst periodically analyzes all cost centers, establishes acceptable norms, tracks variations, and makes recommendations to resolve problems. Computer programs are available that forecast production, control purchasing, compute the cost to produce a meal, and compare the theoretical to the actual preparation and service costs.[83]

When income and expenses are tracked in the monthly periods in which they occur, patterns will emerge that point to areas that need adjustment or change. In tracking such information, it is useful to list monthly income and expenses by dollars, then by applicable percentage. A second set of columns of the same information computed for the fiscal year to date is useful as well.[84]

A trend analyst, familiar with the computer system(s), should be able to trace uncovered problems to their source. For example, food usage comparisons showing percentage of food used versus percentage of participation can reveal problems such as possible theft, over- or underproduction, standardized recipes or portions not being followed, etc. Further records of computerized analyses should indicate which areas to track next.

OFFICE FUNCTIONS

Databases, as previously discussed, were accounting, nutrient analysis, and inventory applications were largely constructed from other computerized sources within the department. Databases may also be purchased and adapted for use with specific-application software such as that used for free and reduced-price meal application processing and POS systems. Regardless of the database used, time is required to gather information and insert it in the appropriate location. Hastily constructed or edited databases result in poor, incomplete, or even useless information. Baltzer et al. state, "Although there is no time algorithm to project how many labor-hours will be required for database development, the experience of personnel in other food service organizations can be used as a guide. For example, food item database development took 1,000 labor-hours to complete in a large food service organization (750 meals per mealtime) that had complete and effective manual records to use in development. This development project utilized an additional 1,000 hours of labor from the computer support department to develop the database file structure and to key in the data."[85(p240)]

Other types of assistance needed for database development require food service expertise. Gathering information and cross-referencing databases requires sufficient experience in a food service to make the various decisions needed to code the fields of the database. More time is required to structure and develop a database than to use a purchased one. Other time required to input data reflective of the specified food service organization may be similar for either option, however. The time needed to customize a purchased system may be less than, equal to, or greater than the time needed to gather and enter data into a system developed on-site.[85(p241)] Nevertheless, databases are absolutely essential to a well-managed program. Wise operators are willing to invest the time and skills necessary to ensure a useful final product.

Word Processing

Since the turn of the century typewriters have made the handwritten word obsolete. The latter half of this century saw high-quality computerized copy machines, which not only copied the printed word, but graphics as well. Today, manual and electric typewriters have given way to word-processing equipment, and copying machines are used to reproduce documents created with a word processor.

The keyboard used for word processing is similar to a typewriter with additional function keys. Many schools now teach keyboarding instead of typing. Once a text or document is prepared it is given a file name for easy retrieval and saved on a diskette for future reference. When a document has been input, many things can be done with it prior to final preparation. It can be printed in large type and double spaced for ease in editing. The font or typeface and type size can be changed by the click of a button or "mouse." Both operating systems and printers have fonts. If neither of these has the preferred font, additional font packages can be installed in the system.

Akin to word processing is the ability to reproduce graphics. Software is available with many graphics, which can be copied and imported into the word processing program. The ability to draw is also available as an advanced word-processing function enabling such refinements as customized maps and floor plans.

As a rule, software that reproduces graphics or draws requires a great deal of memory.

Along with word processing and drawing is computer simulation, which has been used in food service management since the 1960s but until recently was not applied to the school food and nutrition program arena. Simulation is a process that uses a computer to design a model of a real system. The purpose of simulation modeling is to help the decision maker solve a problem. Recent research was conducted using computer simulation to find solutions to operational problems in school food service. Research scientists at the National Foodservice Management Institute (NFSMI) used simulation to show that altering staffing patterns and arrival times of classes into the cafeteria can greatly affect the time it takes students to go through the serving line. By using computer simulation, various strategies for evaluating meal schedules without physically moving students and disrupting the academic day can be explored.[86]

Desktop Publishing

Desktop publishing can be defined as using a microcomputer to write, design, and produce publications. Desktop publishing can reduce or eliminate many of the expenses historically associated with producing printed pieces. It can save time and money, provide flexibility, and help management control important operational factors.[87]

Perhaps the greatest uses of desktop publishing in child nutrition programs are to prepare menus and design forms, brochures, and promotional flyers. Each year food service operations spend many dollars to print multiple forms designed in the central facility. Recently, school districts have been sending diskettes to computer-equipped schools, with all forms available for printing on site. Thus, the problem of too many, too few, or obsolete forms is eliminated. Brochures and promotional flyers are forms of marketing. The catchier and more colorful they are the more successful the promotion will be. One director summed it up by saying, "selling is just selling what you have, but marketing is selling what the customer wants."[88(p16)] With innovative brochures and promotional flyers we are attracting customers and giving them what they want.

Perhaps the menu sent home to parents is the programs' greatest marketing tool and most powerful sales communication device. In a computer-designed menu parents can learn about what is going on in the child nutrition program and access nutrition information and students can take advantage of eye-catching promotions and nutrition-focused puzzle activities. With a computer-designed menu, it is easy to print different name banners on menus for different schools.[89]

E-Mail, Voice Mail (V-Mail), and Fax

The Internet is a global collection of computers interconnected by networks and able to share information using common communication protocols. In the United States, computer networks are grouped into seven categories called domains:

— .com commercial sites in the United States

— .edu educational sites in the United States

— .gov United States government sites

— .mil United States military sites

— .net network administrative organizations

— .org United States non-profit organizations

— .int international

Each site or address on the Internet has a unique, four part address. Cheryl Harris, author of *An Internet Education*,[90] uses her address to explain as shown on the next page.

Some computers on the Internet provide information and are called servers. With appropriate software called the client on your computer you can communicate with these servers and obtain information from them. One type of client-server system is gopher, which locates information through a series of menus. Another is the World Wide Web (WWW), which presents information through a succession of linked hypertext pages.[91] Hypertext transfer protocol (HTTP) is the uniform standard used to send documents across the WWW. The client software that displays the documents to the user is called a browser. Browsers perform basic functions: they send requests to remote Internet servers, receive data, and display files on the computer screen.[92]

In addition to servers and browsers, file transfer protocol (FTP), USENET news, and mailing lists must be understood. FTP is a standard tool used for transferring files from one computer on the Internet to another. USENET news is a collection of discussion or news groups, and mailing lists are electronic mail services that allow people on the list to communicate. Unlike USENET, in which messages are sent to a news group, mail list messages are delivered to a user's mailbox.[92]

Child nutrition professionals and their operations benefit immensely from the Internet and the ability to receive mail electronically, download files to a computer, participate in discussion groups, and retrieve information on many topics. For example, the Internet provides the school food and nutrition director with immediate access to federal regulations, proposed and status of legislation, and an abundance of resources. Keep in mind that although increasing numbers of recognized health organizations are providing publicly accessible information, much of the nutrition information on the Internet is not peer reviewed in the manner traditionally used by scientific journals. Inaccurate nutrition information, nutrition-related misbeliefs, health fraud, and quackery flourish.[92]

Once you have appropriate hardware the possibility of your organization's already hav-

charris	@	ccvax.fullerton	.edu
↑	↑	↑ ↑	↑
User name	at	Server names	Signifies an educational institution

ing access to the Internet should be investigated. If your organization does not have Internet access you can access it directly or you can access it indirectly by joining a commercial on-line service. The commercial Internet service providers are businesses that provide Internet access. They typically supply a variety of Internet services, including E-mail, telnet (a program that allows you to log on to a remote computer and run programs on it), USENET (a system of public discussion groups), and file downloading. Fees may range from $10 per month plus an hourly charge to $250 per month with no hourly charge.[93]

Regardless of the means by which the Internet is accessed, the modem is an absolute requirement. Modems can be internal in your computer or external. Modem speed is definitely important. Although the initial cost of a high-speed modem is greater, it helps save time and money in direct costs to on-line users.[93]

In the food service industry E-mail has alleviated the paperwork shuffle. Recipients of E-mail messages can read them and respond while the sender is still at the sending terminal. Or the message can be saved to disk, printed for filing, or left for later reply. The speed with which documents can move from point to point is unmatched by traditional mail ("snail mail") (Figure 6–2). Multiunit food service managers can have rapid written communication with customers, vendors, and coworkers—sending, for example, catering contracts, emergency orders, and menu revisions.[94] Voice mail and fax machines are mentioned here because of their almost universal use and their high degree of computerization.

A high volume of incoming telephone calls may lead to a search for an alternative to live-attendant services. V-mail is composed of three features: voice messaging, voice response, and automated call routing. Voice messages are more accurate and direct than E-mail, for instance, because they are a recording of the caller's voice with its original tone and emphasis. V-mail messages are not recorded on magnetic tape; they are digitized and stored in electronic mailboxes. A V-mail system's greatest advantage over tape recording is its flexibility in storing, routing, and delivering messages. Users can edit their messages before sending them and, with password controls, V-mail can ensure confidentiality. Voice responses can be randomly accessed by the caller. Using their push-button phones, callers choose which messages they want to hear. Voice responses are made available through the installation of a plug-in voice board in a computer. The voice board digitizes speech and provides the interface between the phone system and the computer. Automated call routing deals with incoming calls without an operator. It answers calls, screens them, and forwards them to in-house extensions, remote phones, or an operator.[94(p78)]

As a word of caution, personal experience suggests that many of today's V-mail systems tend to be consumer unfriendly to the point of discouraging and irritating callers. To prevent this, systems should be selected carefully and, once implemented, evaluated periodically. A good test is to dial into your system and see how unsuspecting callers are treated.

Fax machines with fax modem software exploded onto the office scene in the 1990s. They use telephone lines for communication. In addition to printers that use plain paper as opposed to thermal fax paper, today's fax machines are able to interface with a computer, which enables the computer terminal operator to input the document directly to the fax machine. The same interfaced machine receives a

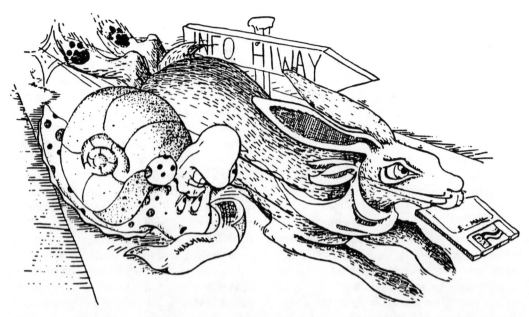

Figure 6-2 Snail Mail versus E-Mail. *Source:* Reprinted with permission from Elsevier Science, Inc., from Computers in Multiunit Foodservice Operations, by M. L. Kasavana, *Cornell Hotel and Restaurant Administration Quarterly,* Vol. 35, No. 3, pp 73–75 and 77–78. Copyright by Cornell University.

fax directly into the computer where it is stored in memory or printed on command from the terminal operator. The fax machine printer may be designed to receive faxed messages, print faxed messages, and print word-processed documents, independent of the fax feature.

TRAINING

Computer training has been discussed throughout this chapter for those who will be installing and using hardware and software in child nutrition programs. Traditional training techniques are frequently used when introducing a computerized process. Initial training should take place in a low-stress, simulated environment; then in simulated, pressured on-the-job training; and finally in on-line transactions or applications with the trainer standing by.[95] For very large applications such as the installation of a POS system, out-of-town trainers can be expensive, even if their services are included as part of the contract. It is wise for

the food service operation to have a staff member trained. In turn, that person will oversee future training.

For child nutrition professionals introducing computerization for the first time, phobias may need to be overcome. One restaurateur explained, "It took me three or four months to make the decision to invest in the equipment and then it was, 'I've put this big beast in here, nobody touch it or it'll crash.'" Gradually, fears were overcome as the operator gained experience with the machine.[96]

Besides a natural aversion to change, some think computerization will eliminate their jobs. In reality it has been documented that personnel become proficient with computerized applications in 6.3 days.[97] Variations in training for your system may include peer training where cashiers from one school move to the next school to train their cashiers. One director favors a gradual approach to computerization by introducing one new program at a time and allowing personnel to become comfortable with one operation before implementing another.[98] Nevertheless, training is the key to success. Ample time should be allowed for training, for even knowledgeable people need time to really learn a system.

Some food service operators have tried different approaches for training such as increasing training opportunities, limiting the length of workshops, and offering workshops closer to the employees' work site. Others have turned to computerized applications for training, continuing education, and advanced academic preparation.

Distance learning by way of satellite courses and computer network learning is becoming more common. Changing student demographics and the cost of higher education will force more education programs to consider new options to resident instruction. Computerized technology will allow educators to provide flexible and individually tailored learning situations with the ability to integrate cost-effective real-world expertise into the educational process.[99]

The Internet and E-mail are currently being used by universities for distance learning. Students enrolled in one independent learning program receive their books and materials from the institution through the mail. Assignments and problems are addressed by E-mail.[100] Another institution has a home page on the WWW. It is used to improve communication, allow greater student access to materials, and make better use of student and instructor time. Weekly quizzes are via the computer terminal. Students are quizzed on previously studied information and they hone their information-seeking skills by searching the WWW for answers to other quiz questions. To keep grading confidential, students send completed quizzes to the instructor's mailbox. Quizzes are graded on-line and then returned to the student's private mailbox.[101] Recently, another university tested an eight-week Internet-based course on nutrition for K–12 teachers.[102]

Most child nutrition professionals agree that increasing demands of technology are going to change professional development requirements dramatically. USDA has pushed this requirement to the forefront with the NSMP concept. Training materials furnished by USDA are accompanied by a variety of CD-Rom and computer-based training (CBT) diskettes, thus enabling the materials to be used with various available hardware. Food service operators should be cautioned, however, regarding this method of training. Implementing the NSMP program in California early test programs pointed to a need for a considerable amount of time and training. It took an average of six months before the program could produce a menu for one school level. It took at least two years for a district to implement the program for all schools and grade levels.[103]

The current focus on making education fun and entertaining will continue to expand. Although few of us got into the business to be actors, it is clear that we will have to be more creative in the delivery of educational programs and experiences. Technology will provide an avenue to add images, animation, and interaction to educational experiences. We are faced with a generation of students (and employees) who grew up with educational technology and entertainment.[104] Child nutrition professionals should become familiar with and use presentation software. Presentation software enables the user to create a professional-looking presentation that delivers your message in any situation. Your presentation can gain life with extended animated builds, sounds, and action. For many the additional feature of conferencing, when a remote audience reviews your presentation over the network as you present, is an added advantage.

SUMMARY

Any process that can be defined and taught to another human for manual performance can be computerized. In the future, fast-track food service managers will be as comfortable with computers as they once were with calculators. Computer literacy—understanding what computers are capable of and being comfortable in their use—is essential for food service person-nel. Computer proficiency is becoming an-other credential for upwardly mobile food ser-vice managers. To maximize excellence in managing CNPs in the twenty-first century, the knowledge and skills of the school food and nutrition directors must include implementing and updating computer applications in child nutrition programs and training staff to apply computer technology in program operations in the central office and at the school site.[105]

Successful school food and nutrition admin-istrators will delegate the responsibility for computerization to an individual to search for hardware and software to meet the programs' specific needs. Both the administrator and the computerization expert must have a food ser-vice background and be knowledgable of child nutrition programs. In addition, there must be a continual awareness of the manual processes employed for each computerized function. Computers are machines that can malfunction.

A back-up system should always be available. While computers can sort out a logical solution to a problem, they are not a substitute for con-ceptual work that a designer brings to a job.

Child nutrition professionals must continu-ally evaluate their computer needs and look to the future. The future is inevitable. Today, the newest buzzwords in the computer technology vocabulary include open systems, open archi-tecture, seamless, and integration which means one company's software interfaces with soft-ware developed by other companies. Tomor-row there will be a new set of buzzwords which must become a part of the school food and nutrition director's technology vocabulary. Change is now the norm. It is thrilling to see child nutrition programs enter a new century as a food service industry leader in the use of computer technology. And if we use it wisely, the new technology will help us all do a better job in providing healthful foods to the nation's children in a cost effective manner.

CASE STUDY
SELECTION AND INSTALLATION OF A POINT-OF-SERVICE SYSTEM

Fairfax County, Virginia, is the 12th largest school system in the United States, with 153,000 students in 234 schools and centers. Geographically, Fairfax County covers 400 square miles in metropolitan Washington, DC. The current food and nutrition services budget is $43.8 million. This narrative describes how a computerized system was chosen and implemented in a large school system.

The Office of Food and Nutrition Services began searching for information about point-of-service (POS), computerized systems that utilized bar-coded or magnetic strip cards. Elementary schools used rosters, and middle and high schools used monthly tickets. The rosters and tickets were difficult to use, prone to errors, and time consuming, and account balances had to be transferred manually at the end of each month.

Representatives from various POS companies were contacted to learn what equipment and systems were available in the market. One POS system, tested in an elementary school for two months, demonstrated that the printed reports were inadequate and the software was inflexible. Four school systems in the geographic area of comparable size were visited to observe student acceptance, serving line speed, and the manager's comfort with the system.

It was decided to develop a request for proposal (RFP) as opposed to an invitation for bid (IFB), since various POS systems had different features and options available. We knew we wanted the system to interface with our student record system and daily transfer of data between the central food service office and the managers' computers. We had input from our department of information technology (DIT) regarding what type of hardware to buy, the compatibility with transferring student data, and necessary communication.

An advisory committee was established to write the RFP and evaluate the responses. The committee was composed of the director of food services, the food services management analyst, five representatives from the DIT, four food service managers and three school principals. The proposal was issued and 11 vendors responded. The committee narrowed the responses to the top three that came closest to our specifications. Each of the three was invited to provide a demonstration for the advisory committee emphasizing how the various systems worked and the pros and cons of each. The committee members were encouraged to ask questions of the vendors for a better understanding of the various systems.

The committee recommended the company that met all of our specifications and had some extra features we liked. In addition, the committee wanted the system tested for 60 days in an actual school food service environment. Two elementary and two high schools with varying free and reduced-price meal participation were chosen to test the system.

The successful vendor and food services planned a training program with installation scheduled for all schools. Each week the computers were set in place and the software installed in six schools. Current managers were invited to apply for positions to install computers and train school personnel. The vendor trained our trainer-managers. An installation and training calendar was established and published for the school system.

Because of the necessary link between POS and the free and reduced-price meal system, an application processing module was also purchased from the same vendor. This permitted overnight communication of free/reduced status to POS systems in the schools. This was a big improvement over the old method of mailing free/reduced lists to managers weekly. The new meal application processing module instantly calculates the status of an application, enters it into the central database, generates a parent notification letter, and transfers students to individual schools. Free and reduced-price meal lists can be printed both centrally and at the school.

During the summer, a file server was installed in the central food service office with five stations. Five were selected to allow simultaneous entry of free and reduced-price meal applications at five computers during the anticipated September rush. Also during the summer, the school systems's electronic systems services office (ESSO) was instructed by the vendor as to the communication wiring needs in each school, and a schedule was established for installation of a communication cable from each serving line to the computer in the manager's office.

Classroom training for managers was conducted three days before the new POS system was to start in their schools. This included becoming familiar with the parts of the computer system, the computer menus, various reports or printouts, and how to enter money on a student's account. On the third afternoon, the cashiers joined their managers and all were instructed in cashiering. A trainer-manager was assigned to each school for the first three to five days the school was on the system to answer questions, help reinforce what was covered in the classroom, and general trouble-shooting.

Before a school began, the food service supervisor visited the school principals to remind them that the system was coming, to ask that it be advertised to the parents and students, and to answer any questions. While the trainer-managers set up the computers and installed the software at each school about a week before the start date, the management analyst worked with ESSO to ensure that the installation of cabling was on schedule, that the computers had been delivered, and that all new equipment from the POS vendor had arrived.

Installation and training went as planned with only minor problems such as incorrectly installed cabling. Since most of our managers were not computer literate, some of them required more "hand holding" than others. Having one trainer-manager on hand per school for the first three to five days was an asset to the successful POS installation. Trainer-managers were able to calm nerves, to reassure cashiers and managers, and to relate to the school administrators how well installations had gone in other schools.

The POS system greatly improved our prepayment balance, made serving lines move faster, and reduced paperwork for both the manager and the cashier. All cards look the same, and only the computer has the correct meal eligibility code. Approximately 85 percent to 95 percent of elementary students use the bar-coded cards, and the number of secondary school users increases every year. This is due to the high school students having "grown up" with the use of cards in elementary and middle schools and their familiarity with them.

REFERENCES

1. B.B. West et al., *Foodservice in Institutions*, 6th ed. (New York: Macmillan Publishing, 1988).

2. C.S. George, Jr., *Supervision in Action the Art of Managing Others*, 4th ed. (Englewood Cliffs, NJ: Prentice Hall; 1985), 54.

3. West et al., *Foodservice in Institutions*, 622.

4. C. Getz, "Computer Literacy, Part 1." *School Foodservice and Nutrition* 48, no. 6 (1994): 26–27.

5. J. Keiser and F.J. DeMicco, *Controlling and Analyzing Costs in Foodservice Operations*, 3rd ed. (New York: Macmillan Publishing, 1993).

6. T. Watts, "Computer Trends for the Future," *School Food Service Journal* 46, no. 1 (1992): 24–29.

7. S. Grossbauer, Linking up with Off-Site Units: Wide-Area Networks," *Food Service Director* 9, no. 9 (1996): 178.

8. P.N. Pugh, "Computer System Feasibility Study for Public School Food Service," *Effective Computer Management in Food and Nutrition Services*, ed. F.A. Kaud (Gaithersburg, MD: Aspen Publishers, Inc., 1989), 159–177.

9. B.A. Byers et al., *Foodservice Manual for Health Care Institutions* (Chicago: American Hospital Association Publishing, Inc. 1994), 231, 232.

10. T.A. Kavulla, "Purchase or Develop?" *School Food Service and Nutrition* 49, no. 2 (1995): 20, 62.

11. S.L. Geiger, *Buying and Using Personal Computers* (Monologue developed by SL Geiger, Ph.D., for use in her business as a microcomputer trainer and consultant; Address available on request), 40, 41.

12. K.P. Brewerand F.J. DeMicco, "Being Wise When You Computerize," *School Food Service Journal*, 47, no. 1 (1993): 23–28.

13. C. van Almelo, "Getting the System You Want," *School Food Service Journal* 45, no. 1 (1991): 38–40.

14. M.L. Kasavana, "Computers and Multiunit Food-Service Operations," *Cornell Hotel and Restaurant Administration Quarterly* 35, no. 3 (1994): 72–80.

15. P. McLaren, "The Year in Review: The Industry," *School Foodservice and Nutrition* 48, no. 11 (1994): 34–39.

16. *Foodservice Software Dynamics (FSD) 1996 White Paper: Foodservice and Computer Technology*. Downloaded from the Internet from http://www.fsdinc.com.

17. American School Food Service Association, "Child Nutrition Software Buying Guide," *School Food Service Journal* 46, no. 1 (1992): 30–33.

18. D.L. Learn, "Beyond Filling Orders: The Purchasing Professional's Expanding Role," *School Business Affairs* 60, no. 11 (1994): 23–27.

19. L.N. Robertson, "Cost Containment 101," *School Foodservice and Nutrition* 49, no. 9 (1995): 25–27.

20. Keiser and DeMicco, *Controlling and Analyzing Costs*, 40, 41.

21. S. Grossbauer, "Controlling Security and Substitutions Are Essential: Checkpoints That Safeguard Your Purchase Orders," *Food Service Director* 9, no. 7 (1996): 134.

22. J. Keiser, *Controlling and Analyzing Costs in Foodservice Operations*, 2nd ed. (New York: Macmillan Publishing, 1989), 190.

23. M.A. Khan, *Concepts of Foodservice Operations and Management*, 2nd ed. (New York: Van Nostrand Reinhold, 1991).

24. Keiser and DeMicco, *Controlling and Analyzing Costs,* 34.

25. Khan, *Concepts of Foodservice Operations and Management,* 202, 203.

26. B. Connell, "Applications: Food and Labor Production Services in Health Care Services," in *Effective Computer Management in Food and Nutrition Services*, ed. F.A. Kaud (Gaithersburg, MD: Aspen Publishers, Inc., 1989), 2–34.

27. Keiser, *Controlling and Analyzing Costs,* 212.

28. Foodservice Software Dynamics, 3, 5.

29. S.L. Frey, *Management's Guide to Efficient, Money-Saving Warehousing* (Chicago: Dartnell Press, 1982), 29.

30. J.R. Bender and M.E. Matthews, "Computer Systems in Food Services: A Review of Applications and Potential Benefits," *School Food Service Research Review* 13 (1989): 150–156.

31. K.S. Christensen, "Computerizing? Start with Menu Planning," *School Food Service Journal* 45, no. 1 (1991): 46–50.

32. J. Caton, *The History of the American School Food Service Association: A Pinch of Love* (Alexandria, VA: American School Food Service Association, 1990).

33. Food and Nutrition Board, *Recommended Dietary Allowances*, 10th ed. (Washington, DC: National Academy Press, 1989).

34. *Food Buying Guide for Child Nutrition Programs* (Washington, DC: United States Department of Agriculture, 1984). USDA (Food and Nutrition Services) Program Aid 1331.

35. *Child and Adult Care Food Program Adult Day Care Handbook* (Washington, DC: United States Department of Agriculture, 1993). USDA (Food and Nutrition Services).

36. A.G. Tufts et al., "School Meals under Construction," *School Food Service Journal* 48, no. 3 (1994): 25–28.

37. *Healthy People 2000* (Washington, DC: United States Department of Health and Human Services, 1991).

38. *Dietary Guidelines for Americans*, 4th ed. (Washington, DC: United States Department of Agriculture and United States Department of Health and Human Services, 1995). Home and Garden Bulletin No. 232.

39. *The Food Guide Pyramid* (Washington, DC: United States Department of Agriculture, 1992). USDA (HNIS) Home and Garden Bulletin No. 252.

40. M. Briggs et al., "Nutrient Standard Menu Planning in Child Nutrition Programs," *Topics in Clinical Nutrition* 9, no. 4 (1994): 37–46.

41. R.D. Lee et al., "Comparison of Eight Microcomputer Dietary Analysis Programs with the USDA Nutrient Data Base for Standard Reference," *Journal of the American Dietetic Association* 95 (1995): 858–867.

42. *Food Buying Guide for Child Nutrition Programs*.

43. S. Grossbauer, "How Computers Can Help: Nutrition Talk," *Food Service Director* 9, no. 4 (1996): 124.

44. P. Birkenshaw, "Nutrition Integrity in School Menu Planning," *School Business Affairs* 60, no. 11 (1994): 4–8.

45. National Food Service Management Institute, *Creating Healthy Meals for the Mainline*. Part II. Satellite broadcast, 1995.

46. Byers et al., *Foodservice Manual*, 385.

47. Robertson, "Cost Containment 101," 27.

48. Keiser and DeMicco, *Controlling and Analyzing Costs*, 43.

49. L.E. Baltzer et al., "Food Service Database Management," in *Effective Computer Management in Food and Nutrition Services*, ed. F.A. Kaud (Gaithersburg, MD: Aspen Publishers Inc., 1989), 233–265.

50. S. Grossbauer, "Yields, Coding, Cooking Impact Data: Recipe Analysis," *Food Service Director* 9, no. 10 (1996): 156.

51. Lee et al., "Comparison of Eight Microcomputer Dietary Analysis Programs," 867.

52. K. Schuster, "Can School Programs Cut the Fat and Keep Their Customers?" *Food Management* 31, no. 8 (1996): 26–34.

53. P. McLaren, "Industry: Doing Flips for School Foodservice," *School Foodservice and Nutrition* 49, no. 11 (1995): 23–28, 70.

54. Foodservice Software Dynamics, 6.

55. B.R. Lane, "Point of Sale and Menu Management Systems," in *Effective Computer Management in Food and Nutrition Services*, ed. F.A. Kaud (Gaithersburg, MD: Aspen Publishers, Inc., 1989), 58–77.

56. Briggs et al., "Nutrient Standard Menu Planning," 43.

57. Kasavana, "Computers and Multiunit Food-Service Operations," 73.

58. S.K. Leinen, "A Menu-Focused Computer System for Health Care," in *Effective Computer Management in Food and Nutrition Services*, ed. F.A. Kaud (Gaithersburg, MD: Aspen Publishers, Inc., 1989): 35–57.

59. M. Begalle, "Planning Student-Driven Menus," *School Food Service Journal* 48, no. 3 (1994): 36–41.

60. P. King, "Central Production Scores in America's Heartland," *Food Management* 27, no. 9 (1992): 58–63.

61. West et al., *Foodservice in Institutions*, 642.

62. T. Lydecker, "How To Extend Its Life and Hold Food Quality: Deep-Frying Oil," *Food Service Director* 9, no. 9 (1996): 148.

63. G.E. Lackey, "By Using Electronic Data Banks: Incoming Vend Sales/Turns," *Food Service Director* 9, no. 9 (1996): 176.

64. G.E. Lackey, "What They Mean to Operators: The New Vending Standards," *Food Service Director* 7, no. 4 (1994): 162.

65. R. Gitlin, "MDB Technology To Give Equipment More Versatility," *Automatic Merchandiser* 38, no. 10 (1996): 16–24.

66. L. Lenzner, "Smart Cards: Can Vending Use the Technology?" *Vending & OCS* 4, no. 2 (1996): 44–48.

67. J.M. Boehrer, "Managing To Meet the Bottom Line," *School Business Affairs* 59, no. 11 (1993): 3–8.

68. Keiser and DeMicco, *Controlling and Analyzing Costs*, 49.

69. McLaren, "The Year in Review," 38.

70. T. Pellegrino, "Point of Sale Perfection," *School Food Service Journal* 48, no. 4 (1994): 31–35.

71. Begalle, "Planning Student-Driven Menus," 38, 39.

72. R.E. Conn et al., "Keep the Line Moving," *School Food Service Journal* 48, no. 4 (1994): 37–38.

73. Kasavana, "Computers and Multiunit Food-Service Operations," 74.

74. P. Montague, "Weights and Measures," *School Foodservice and Nutrition* 49, no. 9 (1995): 36–46.

75. National School Boards Association, "Quick! Tell Me How To Buy . . . Computerized Cash Registers," *American School Board Journal* 175, no. 5 (1988): 14.

76. Keiser and DeMicco, *Controlling and Analyzing Costs*, 47, 49.

77. C. Getz, "Computer Literacy, Part 3," *School Foodservice and Nutrition* 48, no. 10 (1994): 27, 92.

78. C. Getz, "Spreadsheet Basics," *School Food Service Journal* 48, no. 4 (1994): 39–41.

79. Boehrer, "Managing To Meet the Bottom Line," 6.

80. Kasavana, "Computers and Multiunit Food-Service Operations," 78.

81. R.G. Taylor and S.P. Mayeux, "Building an Optimal and Flexible Schedule for School Food Service Employees," *School Food Service Research Review* 18 (1994): 101–105.

82. K. Cogdell and G. Richardson, "Outstanding Employees = Success," *School Business Affairs* 60, no. 11 (1994): 44–45.

83. D. Roycroft, "Technology Rules," *Food Management* 31, no. 7 (1996): 94–98.

84. Boehrer, "Managing To Meet the Bottom Line," 4.

85. Baltzer et al., "Food Service Database Management," 241.

86. M.F. Nettles and M.T. Conklin, "Using Computer Simulation To Solve School Foodservice Problems," *National Food Service Management Institute Insight* 5 (1996).

87. Kasavana, "Computers and Multiunit Food-Service Operations," 74, 75.

88. M. Ward, Sr., "Jane Boehrer," *School Foodservice and Nutrition* 49, no. 2 (1995): 14–16.

89. J. Bennett, "Menus with Punch," *School Food Service Journal* 48, no. 3 (1994): 43–48.

90. C. Harris, *An Internet Education: A Guide to Doing Research on the Internet* (Belmont, CA: Wadsworth Publishing Company, 1996).

91. S.E. Feldman and L. Krumenaker, *The Internet at a Glance* (Medford, NJ: Information Today, Inc., 1995), 2.

92. K. Davidson, "Finding Nutrition Information on the Net," *Journal of the American Dietetic Association* 96 (1996): 749–750.

93. D.H. Morris, "Locating the Information Superhighway On-Ramp: You <u>Can</u> Get There from Where You Are," *Journal of the American Dietetic Association* 96 (1996): 14–15.

94. Kasavana, "Computers and Multiunit Food-Service Operations," 77.

95. P. Rhodes, "Piloting Pays Off!" *School Food Service Journal* 45, no. 1 (1991): 52–55.

96. M. Kass, "Computerize Your Menu," in *Winning Food-Service Ideas*, ed. M. Bartlett (New York: John Wiley & Sons, 1994), 102–104.

97. Keiser and DeMicco, *Controlling and Analyzing Costs*, 31.

98. Christensen, "Computerizing?" 47.

99. S.C. Parks, "Challenging the Future: Impact of Information Technology on Dietetics Practice, Education, and Research," *Journal of the American Dietetic Association* 94 (1994): 202–204.

100. B.E. Egan, "Correspondence School Nineties-Style," *School Foodservice and Nutrition* 96, no. 10 (1996): 42–48.

101. Davidson, "Finding Nutrition Information on the Net," 750.

102. P.A. Beffa-Negrini et al., "Evaluation of an Internet-Based Nutrition Education Course for K–12 Teachers," *Journal of the American Dietetic Association* 96 (suppl) (1996): A-10 [abstract].

103. Tufts, "School Meals under Construction," 28.

104. Parks, "Challenging the Future," 204.

105. D.H. Carr et al., "Competencies," in *Knowledge and Skills of Effective District School Nutrition Directors/Supervisors* (University, MS: National Food Service Management Institute, 1996), 157–161.

CHAPTER 7

Financial Management

Dorothy Pannell-Martin and Gertrude B. Applebaum

OUTLINE

INTRODUCTION TO FINANCIAL MANAGEMENT

Today financial management is essential to effective management of school food and nutrition programs because more and more school district administrations expect these programs to operate like a business and to be self-supporting. The emphasis on the school food and nutrition programs' being self-supporting is due to school districts' budgets being tighter and thus the necessity for administrations to look for ways to reduce costs and increase revenues in their budgets. School food and nutrition directors face the challenge of maintaining focus on operating a nutritionally sound program that is cost effective.

It is difficult to be self-supporting today because revenue generally has not kept pace with expenditures. At the same time, the student customers in schools and changes in the United States Department of Agriculture (USDA) requirements are more demanding. Many of the favorite foods are higher in costs, and foods necessary to meet Dietary Guidelines for Americans may be more costly.

For effective financial management, detailed timely information regarding finances must be available and accessible to the school food and nutrition director/manager. If school food and nutrition program directors are to be held responsible for operating a self-supporting program, it is essential that they know the goals set by the school board, the administration, and the customer, and to manage financial aspects of the program according to high standards of business and accounting practice. Competencies needed by directors to meet this goal include establishing financial goals and objectives, directing the operation of the schools' food and nutrition program within established guidelines for a financial management system that provides a cost-effective program of high integrity, and implementing efficient management techniques to ensure that all records and supporting documentation are maintained in accordance with federal, state, and local requirements.[1]

If directors are to meet the goal of managing a self-supporting program, coupled with the goals of meeting nutrition needs of students, increasing the number of customers served, meeting the customers' demands, and at the same time doing all for less, new strategies and skills are needed. It is the objective of this chapter to provide some guidelines to financial management, including (1) a better understanding of cost control management, (2) ways to determine revenue and expenses, (3) ways to analyze costs, (4) ways to use financial data when making management decisions, (5) suggested corrective action, and (6) a case study on how the Brownsville, Texas, independent school district director reduced labor costs.

REQUIREMENTS FOR FINANCIAL MANAGEMENT

Requirements for financial management begin with an understanding of the school districts' goals for the Child Nutrition Program and access to a good accounting system. Responsibility for the financial management of school food and nutrition programs may be different from that for other departments in a school district. School food service, unlike other parts of the school, must generate revenue to cover costs. The accounting system for school food and nutrition must be consistent with requirements of the local school district, state, and the federal government. The accounting system used for the school food and nutrition program should parallel that used for a business, because both a product and a service are being sold to students and adults. The accounting system used by school districts may be one of three types: accrual, modified accrual, or cash. School food service may use modified accrual or an accrual system. Accrual and modified accrual accounting, unlike cash accounting, recognizes revenues when they are earned, expenses when incurred, and inventory value as an asset.

Good Accounting System

A good accounting system is one that provides accurate, meaningful reports on a timely basis. These should be capsule-type reports that are readable and easy to understand. They should provide a school food service director/manager the information needed in a straightforward way and should compare the current data with a local standard that has been set in previous months or years. *Timely* can be defined as within 15 days of the close of an accounting period or sooner.

A uniform system of accounts for schools has been established by the Association of School Business Officials and should be used, and it certainly should be a computerized system. Unfortunately, there is no one software package at this time that is widely used for the school food and nutrition programs. Many school food and nutrition program directors are taking lengthy records that fill reams of paper produced by the districts' many computer packages; they then put the needed data into capsule reports, using popular spreadsheet software programs (e.g., Lotus 1-2-3) to produce profit-and-loss (P&L) statements—adding accruals (accounts receivable and accounts payable and value of inventory). These P&L statements should cover revenues and expenditures for the same period of time (generally for a calendar month).Timely information about successful financial management programs is available from the state child nutrition agency.

With computerization, a weekly P&L statement is possible and desirable; however, a monthly P&L is more common. The director and/or manager needs to know when a change occurs, such as when expenditures increase or revenue increases/decreases. Today management should be managing by numbers; for instance, if breakfast sales decrease, management should find out why and take immediate action to increase those sales.

The financial documents that a school food service director needs are as follows:

Balance sheet: A balance sheet is a snapshot view of the fund. It tells management what the fund balance is at any given time and summarizes the assets and liabilities.

Budget: The budget is an annual plan for what the fund expects to accomplish (it will be discussed later).

Income or P&L statement: The P&L shows management how the fund has performed for a given period of time (see Tables 7–1 and 7–2). This statement is generally management's favorite report. It will be meaningless, however, if not compared, analyzed, and acted upon. Regardless of the size of the school district, comparisons of how revenue has been spent should be made with as many of the following as are available:

- Industry standards
- Prior period of time
- Other schools in the district (e.g., high schools compared with other high schools)
- Other school districts
- Goals set by the budget

Comparisons should be made using percentages of costs to total revenue. Schools or school districts of any size can be compared when percentages are used because variances in percentages are easy to spot, as illustrated in Tables 7–1 and 7–2. To arrive at the percentage of costs to revenue or the percentage of revenue from different sources, use the formulas shown below:

These percentages would be compared with budgeted figures, with previous month, with industry standards, and, if available, with other school districts. Table 7–1 shows a comparison of three months. How much a school district charges and how much is paid for labor and food will differ from district to district. As a

Table 7–1 Sample Monthly Profit-and-Loss Statement for a Small School District

Category	September	%	October	%	November	%	Year-to-Date	%
REVENUE								
Breakfast—elementary								
Paying—full-price students	$1,648	0.006	$1,932	0.006	$1,569	.006	$5,149	0.006
Breakfast—secondary								
Paying—full-price students	1,440	0.005	1,656	0.005	1,296	.005	4,392	0.005
Paying—reduced-price students	390	0.001	483	0.002	405	.002	1,278	0.002
Federal reimbursement								
Full-price students	774	0.003	885	0.003	700	.003	2,359	0.003
Reduced-price students	932	0.003	1,155	0.004	968	.004	3,055	0.004
Free students	16,280	0.060	18,487	0.059	14,633	.059	49,400	0.060
Adults	1,000	0.004	1,150	0.004	900	.003	3,050	0.004
Lunch—Elementary								
Paying—full-price students	71,250	0.263	82,110	0.263	64,395	0.262	217,755	0.262
Lunch—secondary								
Paying—full-price students	52,920	0.195	61,180	0.195	48,195	0.195	162,295	0.196
Paying—reduced-price students	1,200	0.004	1,426	0.005	1,108	0.005	3,734	0.005
Federal reimbursement								
Full-price students	13,798	0.051	15,921	0.051	12,508	0\.051	42,227	0.051
Reduced-price students	4,312	0.016	5,124	0.016	3,984	0.016	13,420	0.016
Free students	55,125	0.203	63,774	0.204	50,042	0.203	168,941	0.204
Adults	7,200	0.027	8,280	0.027	7,290	0.030	22,770	0.027
Other revenue								
À la carte sales								
Elementary schools	4,450	0.017	5,119	0.016	4,005	0.016	13,574	0.016
Secondary schools	14,650	0.054	16,847	0.054	13,185	0.054	44,682	0.052
Catering	3,730	0.014	4,600	0.015	3,690	0.015	12,020	0.015
Interest	550	0.002	632	0.002	369	0.002	1,551	0.002
USDA commodities	16,805	0.062	18,555	0.059	14,569	0.059	49,929	0.060
State matching	2,638	0.010	3,044	0.010	2,395	0.010	8,077	0.010
TOTAL REVENUE	$271,092	100%	$312,360	100%	$246,206	100%	$829,658	100%

Category	$	%	$	%	$	%	$	%
EXPENDITURES								
Food purchased	$94,158		$112,639		$88,521		$295,318	
+ Starting inventory	3,260		3,653		3,843		10,756	
− Ending inventory	3,653		3,843		3,730		11,226	
Cost of food used	93,765	0.346	112,449	0.360	88,634	0.360	294,848	35.5
USDA Commodities	17 344		18,128		14,798		50,270	
+ Starting inventory	4,600		7,544		6,930		19,074	
− Ending inventory	7,544		6,930		6,956		21,430	
Value of commodities used	14,400	0.053	18,742	0.060	14,772	0.060	47,914	0.058
Supplies, detergents purchased	14,074		15,256		12,292		41,622	
+ Starting inventory	4,020		4,691		4,640		13,351	
− Ending inventory	4,691		4,640		4,622		13,953	
Cost of supplies and detergents used	13,403	0.050	15,307	0.049	12,310	0.050	41,020	0.050
TOTAL FOOD AND SUPPLIES AND DETERGENTS COST	$121,568	0.449	$146,498	0.469	$115,716	0.470	$383,782	0.463

continues

Table 7–1 continued

Category	September	%	October	%	November	%	Year-to-Date	%
Labor Cost								
School-based salaries/wages	$75,582		$91,834		$72,384		$239,800	
Substitutes	1,111		1,311		1,034		3,456	
Fringe benefits	34,455		38,046		29,988		136,944	
Total school-based labor	111,148	0.410	131,191	0.420	103,406	0.42	380,200	0.458
Central office salaries/wages	11,223		13,119		10,450		34,792	
Fringe benefits	5,042		5,623		4,322		14,987	
Total central office labor	16,265	0.060	18,742	0.060	14,772	0.06	49,779	0.060
TOTAL LABOR COST	$127,413	0.470	$149,933	.480	$118,178	0.48	$429,979	0.518
Equipment/supplies								
Small equipment/office supplies	$2,711	0.010	$1,562	0.005	$2,462	0.012	$6,735	0.008
Computerization	3,253	0.012	3,748	0.012	2,954	0.012	9,955	0.012
Large equipment	5,421	0.020	3,124	0.010	3,693	0.015	12,238	0.015
Other operating expenses								
Telephone	63	0.003	62	0.0002	49	0.0002	174	0.0002
Maintenance	1,870	0.007	1,874	0.006	1,477	0.006	5,221	0.006
Utilities	4,302	0.015	3,124	0.010	2,462	0.010	9,888	0.012
TOTAL OTHER EXPENSES	$17,620	.067	$13,494	.043	$13,097	.055	$44,211	.053
TOTAL EXPENDITURES	$266,601	0.983	$309,925	0.992	$246,991	(1.003)	$823,517	.992
PROFIT (OR LOSS)	$4,491	0.017	$2,435	0.008	($785)	(0.003)	$6,141	.008

result, each district needs to set its own standards based on what is possible—and this may not be easy for a director.

The P&L for the school district is essential, but it needs to be broken down for each cost center (all schools with food services, warehouse, etc.). These reports become very meaningful to school food service managers, as well as to the school food service director/supervisor. They point out where problems exist. They help the school food service director to see data for similar types of schools compared (an elementary school compared with an elementary school [see Table 7–2], middle school with another middle school) in a spreadsheet arrangement. A school food service director can more easily spot problems, such as high food costs, when using percentages of revenue comparisons, as shown in Table 7–2 with John Doe Elementary School.

Knowledgeable Food and Nutrition Program Supervisors/Directors/Managers

All the accurate, timely reports are meaningless unless the person in charge knows how to read them. It is essential that those responsible have a good working knowledge of accounting, be able to read and understand reports, be able to analyze data, know what to do when costs are up and/or revenue is down, and be willing to do something about costs that are too high.

School food and nutrition management staff may not come to their jobs with this knowledge, mainly because accounting and financial management may not have been in their college curriculum. Independent study courses or community college courses in accounting can be most helpful, because a director (or the department accountant) will need to provide training to others in management roles if the data are to be used as they should be.

Table 7–2 Example of Profit-and-Loss Statement Comparison for Three Schools

Category	Jones Elementary	%	John Doe Elementary	%	Marion Elementary	%
REVENUE						
Breakfast—elementary						
Paying—full-price students	$420	0.012	$840	0.026	$672	0.021
Paying—reduced-price students	95	0.003	95	0.003	76	0.002
Federal reimbursement						
Full-price students	104	0.003	208	0.006	166	0.005
Reduced-price students	226	0.006	226	0.007	181	0.006
Free students	4,808	0.140	2,137	0.065	2,030	0.064
Adults	525	0.015	656	0.020	525	0.017
Lunch—elementary						
Paying-full-price students	2,363	0.069	12,600	0.381	10,012	0.315
Paying-reduced-price students	168	0.005	126	0.004	121	0.004
Federal reimbursement						
Full-price students	280	0.008	1,491	0.045	1,211	0.038
Reduced-price students	604	0.017	452	0.014	452	0.014
Free students	20,066	0.590	7,332	0.222	10,612	0.334
Adults	1,418	0.04	1,418	0.043	1,418	0.044
Other Revenue						
À la carte sales						
Elementary schools	2,100	0.061	4,200	0.127	3,179	0.100
Catering	300	0.008	450	0.014	375	0.012
Interest	200	0.006	250	0.007	225	0.007
USDA commodities	200	0.006	250	0.007	225	0.007
State matching	369	0.011	323	0.009	321	0.010
TOTAL REVENUE	$34,246	100%	$33,054	100%	$31,801	100%

Category	$	%	$	%	$	%
EXPENDITURES						
Food purchased	$12,461		$12,934		$11,759	
+ Starting inventory	3,200		4,106		3,505	
− Ending inventory	3,915		4,246		3,816	
Cost of food used	11,746	0.343	12,794	0.387	11,448	0.360
USDA commodities	1,908		1,974		1,913	
+ Starting inventory	340		190		185	
− Ending inventory	205		196		190	
Value of commodities used	2,043	0.059	1,968	0.060	1,908	0.060
Supplies, detergents purchased	1,746		1,644		1,597	
+ Starting inventory	475		160		480	
− Ending inventory	553		164		519	
Cost of supplies and detergents used	1,668	0.049	1,640	0.049	1,558	0.049
TOTAL FOOD AND SUPPLIES AND DETERGENTS COST	$15, 457	0.451	$16,402	0.496	$14,914	0.469

continues

Table 7–2 continued

Category	Jones Elementary	%	John Doe Elementary	%	Marion Elementary	%
Labor cost						
School-based						
salaries/wages	$12,702		$ 12,241		$11,865	
Substitutes	140		134		130	
Fringe benefits	1,116		1,075		1,043	
Total school-based labor	13,958	0.407	13,450	0.410	13,038	0.410
Central office salaries/wages	1,847		1,660		1,609	
Fringe benefits	161		144		140	
Total central office labor	2,008	0.059	1,804	0.055	1,749	0.054
TOTAL LABOR COST	$15,966	.466	$15,254	.465	$14,787	.464
Equipment/supplies						
Small equipment/office	$340	0.010	$328	0.010	$318	0.010
supplies	409	0.012	394	0.012	381	0.012
Computerization	647	0.019	328	0.010	318	0.010
Large equipment						
Other operating expenses						
Telephone	7		7		6	
Maintenance	204	0.006	197	0.006	190	0.006
Utilities	511	0.015	459	0.014	381	0.012
TOTAL OTHER EXPENSES	$2,118	0.062	$1,713	0.052	$1,594	0.050
TOTAL EXPENDITURES	$33,541	0.979	$33,369	100.9	$31,295	0.984
PROFIT (OR LOSS)	$705	0.021	($315)	0.009	$506	0.016

$$\frac{\text{Costs in dollars}}{\text{Total revenue in dollars}} = \text{Percentage of revenue spent for a specific category}$$

Example: $$\frac{\$55,500 \text{ in Labor}}{\$150,000 \text{ total revenue}} = 0.37 \text{ or } 37\% \text{ of revenue spent for labor}$$

$$\frac{\text{Revenue by source}}{\text{Total revenue in dollars}} = \text{Percentage of revenue from a specific source}$$

Example: $$\frac{\$20,500 \text{ breakfast revenue}}{\$150,000 \text{ total revenue}} = 0.136 \text{ or } 13.6\% \text{ of revenue from breakfast program}$$

Staff Training in Financial Management

When financial reports are provided to school food service managers and supervisory staff, it is imperative to give them training in basic accounting, what the financial reports mean, how to evaluate them, and how to analyze the data. Otherwise, reports may be put in a desk drawer and not used. Also, the standards or goals established by the school food and nutrition director should be provided to managers and discussed. For example, how much of the revenue should be spent for food? One shouldn't take for granted that any of the management staff understand accounting reports, because they may not. Those coming from other food service industries will need to be trained in how a self-supporting, USDA school food and nutrition program differs from other food service operations (e.g., hospital food services, commercial restaurants, and university/college food services).

KNOWING SOURCES AND AMOUNT OF REVENUE

School food service management today needs to manage by numbers, and some of the most important numbers have to do with how much revenue is received for different services provided, particularly breakfast and lunch. School food service programs that are operated under federally subsidized school food and nutrition programs are unique, and are unlike any other segment of the food service industry because of the various funding sources. However, knowing about the different sources is basic to determining how much revenue can be spent on food, labor, and other items. Before describing how to arrive at the average revenue for a breakfast and a lunch, it is important to know the sources of revenue that most school food and nutrition programs will have, which are

- Student and adult cash payments
- Federal reimbursement on student meals
- Commodities (lunch only)

- State matching funds (if available)
- Local funds (if available)

The amount of revenue from the federal government changes from year to year on the basis of legislation, the type of meal, or the funding categories. The amount of federal revenue is based on the number and category of meals served. The per meal amount is adjusted and published annually by USDA to reflect changes in the food away from home series of the Consumer Price Index. The income scale published by USDA includes the national average payment per meal based on income level and size of household. How to determine the revenue is illustrated in Tables 7–3 through 7–6, which provide examples of funding for a breakfast and a lunch in the 1996–1997 school year.

Breakfast Revenue

The revenue for a subsidized breakfast comes from what students pay, federal funds, and state/local funds, as shown in Tables 7–3 and 7–4. The federal funding varies on the basis of the poverty levels of the children's families. The schools that qualify for "severe need" funding under the breakfast program

---

Table 7–3 Example of the Revenue Available to a School District for Breakfast Using 1997–1998 Federal Rates

Source	Elementary Paying Student	Secondary Paying Student	Free Regular	Free Severe Need	Reduced-Price Regular	Reduced-Price Severe Need	Adult
Cash payments[a]	$0.80	$0.80	N/A	N/A	$0.300	$0.300	$1.30
Federal reimbursement	0.20	0.20	$1.045	$1.245	$0.745	$0.945	N/A
Local funds[b]	N/A	N/A	N/A	N/A	N/A	N/A	N/A
State matching funds[c]	0.02	0.02	0.020	0.020	0.020	0.020	N/A
TOTAL	$1.02	$1.02	$1.065	$1.265	$1.065	$1.265	$1.30

[a]Prices are set by local school district.
[b]Local funds may be from profits made on à la carte sales or catering.
[c]States may or may not provide revenue toward breakfast. Check with state department to determine what funding is available.

Table 7–4 Example of the Average Revenue for a Breakfast Based on Data from Table 7–3 and Average Participation

Category	Average Number Served per Day	(X) Revenue by Category	(=) Revenue by Category
Full-price students	20	$1.020	$20.40
Free students	100	$1.065	$106.50
Reduced-price students	10	$1.065	$10.65
Adults	10	$1.300	$13.00
TOTALS	140		$150.55
AVERAGE REVENUE FOR A LUNCH	$ 150.55 ÷ 140 = $1.075 or $1.07[a] for breakfast		

[a]Round down to avoid overstating the revenue.
Note: Revenues from sales of adult meals, à la carte items, and catering activities often offset the difference in revenues received for the paying and the nonpaying child.

School Meal Categories

The three funding categories for meals are based on the income level and size of households in each school. The three funding categories are:

Paid: The rate paid for meals served to students whose household income is above 185% of the Federal Income Poverty Level.

Reduced: The rate paid for meals served to students whose household income is between 130% and 185% of the Federal Income Poverty Level.

Free: The rate paid for meals served to students whose household income is at or below 130% of the Federal Income Poverty Level.

and the school districts that qualify for "Supplemental Funding (Safety Net)" under the national school lunch program receive additional subsidies; however, this funding changes annually and can be discontinued at any time. The qualifying criteria are different for breakfast

and lunch, and many schools/school districts have not realized that this extra funding has been available.

"Severe need" breakfast funding is available to schools that served 40 percent or more of the lunches free or at reduced prices two years ago and have breakfasts costs higher than the regular breakfast reimbursement rates. Table 7–3 shows the additional funding available in 1997–1998. Unless a state agency collects school data, it is generally necessary for a school district to initiate a request for severe need rates for eligible schools and to submit cost information demonstrating their eligibility. The cost data to demonstrate eligibility for the severe need rate is obtained through a costing out of the breakfast by the school/school district and submitted to the state agency. Some states do the costing using a "prorated" figure from the financial report, however, this is not as accurate as actual costing of the meal. It should be noted that qualifying for severe need breakfast funding is school by school; a school district may have to apply for the additional funding (if the state does not collect data on each school in the district), and the cost of the breakfasts must equal or exceed the rate of reimbursement for the school. The cost data may be obtained by the state departments of education from financial data provided to the state, or through a costing-out of the breakfast done by the school/school district and submitted to the state. It is important to be aware of the use of these data and to make sure that all costs for producing and serving a breakfast are included. For example, the administrative costs, equipment and computerization costs, and all overhead should be prorated over all programs, whereby the full cost of the breakfast program is calculated. For specific information regarding applying for severe need rates, contact the state agency responsible for administering child nutrition programs.

The price charged the "full-price" student for breakfast is set by the local school district within state criteria, but the price should have some relationship to the cost of the meal. Even the full-price student's breakfast is federally subsidized, and the difference in that subsidy and the cost is a logical price to set. Unfortunately, most school districts do not price meals in this way; as a result, breakfast and lunch prices are often set too low.

The price charged a student who qualifies to receive a reduced-price breakfast is limited by federal regulations (at 30 cents in the 1997–1998 school year). The breakfast can be set at a lower price but not higher.

The price an adult is charged is a local decision as long as it is in accordance with state and/or federal regulations. Again, the cost of the meal should have a direct relationship to the price charged an adult. However, the minimum adult payment should reflect the price charged to students paying the school's designated full price, plus the current value of Federal cash and donated food assistance (entitlement and bonus) for full price meals. (FNS Instruction 782-5:NSLP/SBP Pricing of Adult Meals. Rev 1: 6/6/88) Some school districts use à la carte prices (not set meal prices) for determining how much an adult will pay; this practice allows for flexibility.

Lunch Revenue

The price of lunch the full-price students are charged is a local school district decision, and, as in the case of breakfast, that price should make up the difference between federal subsidy (cash and commodity) state and local sources and the cost of producing and serving that lunch. Many school districts have kept the

Table 7–5 Example of the Revenue Available to a School District for Lunch Using 1997–1998 Federal Rates

Source	Elementary Paying Student	Secondary Paying Student	Free	Reduced Price	Adult
Cash payments[a]	$1.50	$1.75	N/A	N/A	$2.25
Federal reimbursement	0.18	0.18	$1.89	$1.49	N/A
Entitled commodity value[b]	0.15	0.15	0.15	0.15	N/A
Local funds	N/A	N/A	N/A	N/A	N/A
State matching funds[c]	0.02	0.02	0.02	0.02	N/A
TOTAL	$1.85	$2.10	$2.06	$2.06	$2.25

[a]Prices are set by local school district.
[b]In 1997–1998 the entitlement commodity was set at $0.15; however, school districts may refuse commodities, and the value is usually less than the entitlement.
[c]States may or may not provide matching funds in the form of cash for a lunch meal.

Table 7–6 Example of the Average Revenue for a Lunch Based on Data from Table 7–5 and Participation

Category	Example of Average Number Served per Day	(X) Revenue per Lunch by Category	(=) Total Revenue by Category
Full-price students	215	$1.85	$397.75
Free students	190	2.06	391.14
Reduced-price students	18	2.06	37.08
Adults	15	2.25	33.75
TOTAL	438		$859.72
AVERAGE REVENUE FOR A LUNCH			$846.39 ÷ 438 = $ 1.9628 or $1.96[a]

[a]Round down to avoid overstating the revenue.

prices charged students extremely low in order to maintain the highest level of student participation. The free and reduced-price student lunches are subsidizing the full-price students' lunches (see Tables 7–5 and 7–6).

The price charged a student who qualifies to receive a reduced-price meal is limited by federal regulations (at 40 cents in the 1997–1998 school year). The price charged may be lower but not higher. The price adults are charged is a local decision, but state and/or federal regulations will affect the price charged. Check with the state department of education for those regulations.

Supplemental Lunch Funding

In order for a school district to qualify for supplemental need lunch funding, it has to have served 60 percent or more of the lunches free and at reduced prices two years ago. This qualifies the district for a higher federal reimbursement (in 1997–1998 this meant two cents more for all student lunches served).

Value of Donated Foods

The school district receives USDA donated commodities based on the number of lunches served (known as entitlement commodities). The per lunch value of donated food assis-

tance (entitlement commodities) is adjusted annually to reflect changes in the Price Index for Foods Used In Schools and Institutions. For the 1997–1998 school year, entitlement commodity value has been set at 15 cents per student lunch. It is important that school districts check the value of entitlement commodities received each year with the amount set as entitlement. Some districts receive and use far less than entitlement (e.g., seven to eight cents), mainly because they refuse some of the commodities offered. The value of commodities actually used is needed when determining the revenue for lunch; otherwise, the revenue may be overstated. (Note in Table 7–5 the value of USDA entitlement commodities.)

Bonus commodities are often made available to school districts, but the dollar value of these commodities fluctuates from year to year, based on market conditions.

À la Carte Sales and Other Sources of Revenue

À la Carte Sales

In some states, state regulations control/ prohibit or limit the sale of extra food items; in other states, only federal regulations control the sales. Local school districts' philosophy may determine what, if anything, will be sold à la carte. The prices established for à la carte items should be high enough not to compete with breakfast and lunch prices. The prices should be determined on the basis of cost of food, cost of labor, amount of profit desired, how much the competition charges for that same item, and how much the customer is willing to pay.

Catering

Catering is another means for schools' food service departments to increase revenue and make a profit, if services are priced to yield a profit. This profit can be used to help offset the costs of producing and serving the meals under the school food and nutrition programs. It is important to determine the total cost of catering and set the prices accordingly. Good financial data are essential, and if not available, catering may be costing the school food and nutrition programs instead of helping them.

Providing Food Services to Senior Citizens, Day-Care Centers, and Other Programs

Profits can be made and a good service can be provided by the local school district's food service department by providing services to groups other than those within the school food and nutrition program. However, none of these services should be provided at the expense of the federally subsidized programs. Before considering taking on any additional responsibility, the food service department should be well organized, have well-trained employees with high productivity, employ good purchasing practices, have a good accounting system, and have a contract(s) approved by the administration and school board.

ANALYZING COSTS AND KNOWING WHAT THEY SHOULD BE

How much should a school breakfast and a school lunch cost? What do they usually cost? Abt Associates found in a 1993 USDA study that the cost of producing and serving a lunch averaged $1.88. The average cost of producing and serving noted by the authors of this chapter while teaching cost-control seminars are shown in Table 7–7. A school food service director needs preset standards or norms against which to compare costs. These standards or norms become a benchmark, and a variance should cause management to search for answers and find out why. However, each district will need to set its own standards, and these may resemble those shown in Table 7–7. The average costs of producing and serving lunch may differ from those provided as a suggested norm because the prices paid for food and supplies differ, as do the costs of a labor hour.

Often the labor costs of school food and nutrition programs exceed 40 percent, and this results in less for food or other costs—or the results will be a deficit. The labor costs are usually the most difficult area in which to reduce costs. This is mainly because it involves people.

Table 7–7 Sample Percentages of Revenue Spent—An Industry Standard

Expenditure	Percentage of Revenue
Labor cost for school-based employees (including all fringe benefits)	40%
Food cost (including the value of USDA commodities)	40%
All other costs	<u>20%</u>
	100%

Source: Reprinted with permission from D. Pannell-Martin, *School Food Service Management*, 5th ed., © 1998, in TEAM Associates, Inc.

Exhibit 7–1 Example of Fringe Benefits Included in Labor Costs

- Federal Insurance Contribution Act (FICA) taxes
- Worker's compensation
- Health and life insurance
- Retirement plans
- Unemployment taxes
- Employee uniforms and laundry
- Employee meals
- Vacations, holidays, sick leave
- Employee training

Labor Costs

Labor costs include salaries, wages, and fringe benefits for school-based and central office employees, and all labor-related expenses as shown in Exhibit 7–1.

The labor costs for central office employees are often listed under "administrative costs," particularly in commercial companies, and are something for self-operated school districts to consider. The main approach to determining how many labor hours a school can have is based on productivity rates, which are measured by number of meals prepared and served. Some school districts determine the number of labor hours based on the revenue.

The productivity rate of the employees (e.g., meals served per labor hour [MPLH]) is most frequently used by school food and nutrition program directors for determining the number of labor hours to assign schools. The number of hours of labor assigned is determined by dividing the average number of meal equivalents the school serves a day by the productivity rate established. A frequently used guide is shown in Table 7–8.

Some labor costs may be considered fixed (minimum labor essential to operation and/or the labor hours of people under an annual contract), whereas other labor costs are considered variable costs (part-time and substitute employees). School food service management determines how much labor with which to staff each school. Few managers in school food service, if any, determine how much labor will be placed at a school based on dollar amounts set aside for labor. Instead, the school food and nutrition director determines how much labor the school manager (or principal) "thinks" is needed. This has often resulted in low productivity rates and high labor costs (more than 50 percent of the revenue being spent on labor).

Probably the best approach to staffing a school is based on productivity and use of a guide, as shown in Table 7–8. It is based on a reasonable productivity rate as related to size operations. This entails determining how much work an employee can do—or the productivity of each employee. Productivity may be measured in many different ways, but basically it is based on "output." Output can be number of meals, number of customers, or number of dollars taken in. Since lunch is the major meal service, often school food and nutrition programs are staffed based on equivalent lunch meals. The number of breakfasts served and the amount (in dollars) sold à la carte need to be converted to meal equivalents as well as other services (e.g., snacks, Head Start meals). These equivalents should reflect comparable work. Several formulas are being used to arrive at equivalent meals. For example, preparing and serving two or three breakfasts is equivalent in time required to preparing and serving one lunch, and selling $2 or $3 in à la carte sales is a meal equivalent. A state department of education may set the meal equivalent standards. Timing work is by far the most reli-

Table 7–8 Staffing Guideline for On-Site Production

Number of Meal Equivalents[1] (1)	Meals per Labor Hour (MPLH)/Total Hours	
	Conventional System[2] MPLH (2)	Convenience System[3] MPLH (3)
Up to 100	8	9
101–150	9	10
151–200	10–11	12
201–250	12	14
251–300	13	15
301–400	14	16
401–500	14	18
501–600	15	18
601–700	16	19
701–800	17	20
801–900	18	21
900+	19+	22+

Source: Reprinted with permission from D. Pannell-Martin, *School Food Service Management,* 4th ed., © 1990, in TEAM Associates, Inc.

[1] Meal equivalent is a common measurement of output (breadfast, à la carte sales, and snacks) based on the lunch.
[2] Conventional system is preparation of food from raw ingredients on premises (using some bakery breads and prepared pizza and washing dishes).
[3] Convenience system is using many processed foods (for example, using mostly bakery breads, prefried chicken, and preportioned condiment) and using disposable dinnerware.

able, but very little work has been done in this area. Frequently used meal equivalents are as follows.

3 Breakfast Meals	=	1 Equivalent Meal
1 Lunch Meal	=	1 Equivalent Meal
$3 in à la Carte Sales	=	1 Equivalent Meal

Source: Reprinted with permission from D. Pannell-Martin, *School Food Service Management,* 5th ed., © 1998, in TEAM Associates, Inc.

School food service management must forecast the number of meals and the volume of sales in order to determine meal equivalents. Once the meal equivalents have been established, the guidelines in Table 7–8 may be used for on-site production schools. For example, if a school serves 450 lunches and 210 breakfasts and sells $60 in à la carte sales, the meal equivalents are

Breakfast—	210 ÷ 3	=	70 Meal Equivalents
À la Carte—	$60 ÷ 3	=	20 Meal Equivalents
Lunch —	450	=	450 Meal Equivalents
			540 Meal Equivalents

If the school still prepares some food from raw ingredients and washes dishes, it would be considered a conventional school and be staffed at 15 MPLH; 540 meal equivalents should be divided by 15 to determine the number of labor hours (36).

Food Costs

Food costs, including the value of USDA commodities, are the other prime costs in school food and nutrition programs, using approximately 40 percent of the revenue. Food waste probably accounts for 5 to 10 percent of the food costs. Once revenue has been forecasted and management determines what percentage will be used for food, foods that can be served within those criteria can be determined. The cost of food includes the value of food received from USDA, as well as purchased foods used, and it is determined as shown in Exhibit 7–2.

A standardized food system of operation makes it easier to control costs, which means using a cycle menu and standardized recipes, with each school in the district purchasing food products at the same bid prices. Many school districts do not use standardized recipes, and the excuses are many. Example of excuses and responses follow:

- The cook doesn't need a recipe. He or she has been cooking for many years.
  Response: How many years one has cooked has nothing to do with the need to use a standardized recipe. The cook may have standardized recipes committed to memory.
- The cook has secrets that he or she does not want to share.

Response: School food and nutrition programs can't afford to have cooks that keep secrets. What is to happen when the person is absent ?
- It would take so long to develop standardized recipes.
  Response: There are many already standardized recipes available to school food service personnel. It isn't necessary for the food service manager to develop standardized recipes.

The cost of food is affected by many factors, starting with the prices paid for the food items. After that, how the inventory is handled, the production procedures, and the portion-control methods used will affect the final cost of producing and serving the food. Finally, the service of the food will affect the food cost. Steps for controlling food costs include these:

- Step 1: Purchase food at the best price possible.
  — Use competitive bids.
  — Consider cooperative purchasing.
  — Investigate prime vendors' potential (grouping purchases and reducing number of vendors).
  — Investigate central warehousing; determine whether there would be any savings.
  — Determine the most advantageous delivery frequency.

Exhibit 7–2 Determining Food Cost—Purchased and Commodity

+ Beginning Inventory of Purchased Foods
+ Food Purchases during the Period of Time
<u>− Ending Inventory of Purchased Foods</u>
= $ Cost of Purchased Food Used

+ Beginning Inventory of Commodity Foods
+ Commodity Foods Received during the Period of Time
<u>− Ending Inventory of Commodity Foods</u>
= $ Value (or Cost) of Commodity Foods Used

Source: Reprinted with permission from D.V. Pannell, *Cost Control for School Foodservice,* © 1996, Kentucky State Department of Education.

- Step 2: Plan cycle menus within the budget.
  — Use standardized recipes, establishing portion sizes.
  — Precost recipes.
  — Precost menus planned.
  — Postcost menus served.
- Step 3: Forecast and order by menu.
  — Order only what is needed for a week or the specified period of time.
  — Pull each recipe for the menu and make a list of ingredients needed.
- Step 4: Store food appropriately and maintain good inventory control.
  — Provide adequate storage.
  — Have no more than a seven-day inventory of purchased foods.
  — Eliminate theft.
- Step 5: Use good production procedures.
  — Use standardized recipes.
  — Batch cook when possible.
- Step 6: Serve correct-size portions.
  — Instruct servers as to portion sizes.
  — Provide portioning tools.
  — Check portion yields.
- Step 7: Handle leftovers with care.
  — Assign one staff member to storing and planning use of leftovers.
  — Store leftovers as soon as possible.
  — Use leftovers as soon as feasible.

Miscellaneous Costs

Other costs include direct and indirect costs, and these costs are being charged more and more to the school food and nutrition programs. Direct costs are items that can be specifically identified. Indirect costs are allowable costs that are necessary for the school food service to fulfill its purpose and meet its goals, but are not easily identifiable with a specific function or objective of the school food and nutrition program. Indirect costs cannot include unallowable costs such as lobbying, entertainment or fund raising. An example of an indirect cost in school nutrition programs would be electricity, however it can also include products, services, supplies and even personnel. Indirect costs can be charged school food service in a variety of ways. In the School Lunch and Breakfast Meal Cost Study, ABT Associates issued October 1994, all school districts which charged indirect costs to the school food service used a rate which was calculated or approved by the state educational agency (SEA) on the basis of a standard Cost Allocation Plan (CAP). If a rate is approved by the state agency for the school district, and the school district chooses to assess the school food service, that amount would be calculated and used in preparing the budget. For specific information about indirect costs, contact the SEA. (Source USDA: SERO). Federal regulations prohibit the use of school food service funds for capital expenditures such as expanding or building a new facility.

ESTABLISHING FINANCIAL GOALS

Planning a Meaningful Budget

A budget is a planning or goal-setting tool for financial management (see Table 7–9). Planning the budget is an effort, which requires collaboration between the district's chief financial officer, the purchasing director, and the school food and nutrition director. A budget does not guarantee that a financial goal will be met, but without a budget financial direction (or planning) is lacking. It is a written plan of how one expects the operation to perform during a specific period. It is an organized plan of operation that forecasts the amount of money that will be coming in, projects the amount of money that will be spent for each item, and predicts revenue that should be available.

Table 7–9 Example of Budget Planned from a Combination of Zero-Based and Baseline

Number of Meals	Source of Revenue	Totals	% of Revenue
BREAKFAST			
20,000	Full-price elementary students × $0.80	$16,000	0.7
15,300	Full-price secondary students × $0.80	12,240	0.5
13,500	Reduced-price students payment × $0.30	4,050	0.2
8,000	Paying-adult breakfasts × $1.25	10,000	0.4
	Federal reimbursement		
35,300	Full-price students × $0.1975	6,971	0.3
13,500	Reduced-price students × $0.7175	9,686	0.4
127,000	Free × $1.0175	129,222	5.2
	TOTAL REVENUE FOR BREAKFAST	$188,169	7.7
Lunch			
432,000	Paying elementary students × $1.50	$648,000	26.3
273,000	Paying secondary students × $1.75	477,750	19.4
29,100	Reduced-price students' payment × $40	11,640	0.5
28,700	Paying-adult lunches × $2.25	64,575	2.6
	Federal reimbursement		
705,000	Full-price students × $.1775	125,138	5.1
29,100	Reduced-price students × $1.4375	41,831	1.7
265,000	Free × $1.8375	486,937	19.7
	TOTAL REVENUE FOR LUNCH	$1,855,871	75.3
Other Revenue	à la carte sales	$174,600	7.1
	Catering	33,000	1.3
	Interest	5,010	0.2
	USDA commodities	46,769	5.9
	Other revenue	43,100	1.7
	State matching funds	19,982	0.8
	TOTAL REVENUE	$422,461	17.0
	TOTAL OTHER REVENUE	$2,466,501	100%

Expenditures	Category	Amount	% of Revenue
	Food costs—purchased	$844,134	29.9
	Food costs—USDA commodities	140,000	10.0
	School staff		
	Wages and salaries	635,930	41.9
	Fringe benefits (employer's share)	400,000	
	Central office staff		
	Salaries	147,990	6.0
	Supplies, detergents, and disposables	123,225	5.0
	Small equipment/office supplies	24,665	1.0
	Large equipment	78,928	3.2
	Other operating expense	24,665	1.0
	TOTAL EXPENDITURES	$2,419,537	98.0
PROFIT (OR LOSS)		$46,064	2.0

Advantages of a Budget

The advantages of a budget are (1) to provide goals for both the department and individuals (if goals are not established, employees and departments may lack a way to measure result); (2) to set performance standards for management; (3) to divide responsibilities among staff (everyone needs to do his or her part to meet the budget plan by controlling costs and helping to improve revenue); (4) to provide a control device to use for comparing actual income and costs with predetermined desired results; (5) to establish a yardstick; and (6) to help a manager determine whether a program can afford to make expenditures, such as purchasing equipment or attending a conference.

If the annual budget is broken down to number of serving days, the revenue and expenditures can be measured against the budget on a day-by-day or a month-by-month basis. If a problem exists, it can be spotted and corrective action taken before too much money is lost.

Factors To Consider When Preparing a Budget

To plan a meaningful budget it is important to establish departmental financial objectives. As part of the planning process, the financial expectations of the school food and nutrition program should be made clear by the top business official, the superintendent, or the school board. The method of financing school food services varies greatly from school district to school district. In some districts the income from the sale of meals pays for food, labor, supplies, and repairs. In other districts the food and nutrition program pays all costs of operation, including administrative costs, utilities, and equipment replacement. Between the two extremes will be found many other methods. That is why, before planning a budget, it is important to determine the financial obligations of the school food and nutrition program.

Other Factors To Consider When Preparing a Budget

Other factors that need to be considered when preparing a budget include the actual operating budget from the previous year, the general economic situation in the community, and changes anticipated in school facilities that could increase or decrease the number of students in school.

For the budget to be useful and serve a real purpose, it should be used as a benchmark. Table 7–10 illustrates how the budget can be broken down and used to evaluate actual revenue and expenses. For example, if revenue has fallen short of expectations (as in the planned budget), expenditures will have to be adjusted to stay within the funds available. Federal and state subsidies change annually and this will affect a budget. Changes in menu or meal prices charged and salaries and fringe benefits will affect the budget and should be considered. Also to be considered when planning a budget are the department's goals and plans (for example, facility changes, new equipment purchases, and new employee uniforms).

There are three approaches that can be used when planning the budget: baseline, zero-based, or a combination. Baseline assumes that all expenditures from the previous year were necessary and will be duplicated. The danger with using the baseline planning method is that previous errors will be built upon. Zero-based requires starting with zero and figuring all expected revenue and expenses. This method is more time consuming (Table 7–9 provides an example). A combination of the two methods is frequently used. A decision should be made: Will there be one budget for the district or one for each school? If each school food and nutrition program plans a budget, these budgets, plus central office's needs, become the district's budget.

Table 7–10 Breakdown of the Annual Budget To Be Used as a Benchmark

Category	Per Day % of Revenue	After 20 Days of Service (11% of Budget)	After 90 Days of Service (50% of Budget)	After 120 Days of Service (66% of Budget)
Breakfast revenue:				
Full-price students—elementary	$88	$1,760	$8,000	$10,560
Full-price students—secondary	68	1,346	6,120	8,078
Reduced-price student payments	22	445	2,025	2,673
Paying adults	55	1,100	5,000	6,600
Federal reimbursements:				
Full-price students	38	766	3,485	4,601
Reduced-price students	53	1,065	4,843	6,392
Free students	717	14,214	64,611	85,286
TOTAL BREAKFAST REVENUE	$1,041	$20,696	$94,084	$129,190
Percentage of total revenue	8%	7.6%	7.6%	7.9%
Lunch revenue:				
Paying students—elementary	$3,600	$71,280	$324,000	$427,680
Paying students—secondary	2,654	52,522	238,875	315.315
Reduced-price student payments	65	1,280	5,820	7,682
Paying adults	359	7,103	32,287	42,620
Federal reimbursements:				
Full-price students	695	13,765	62,569	92,591
Reduced-price students	232	4,602	20,916	27,608
Free students	2,705	53,563	243,468	321,378
TOTAL LUNCH REVENUE Percentage of total	$10,310	$204,172	$927,935	$1,224,874
revenue	75%	75.2%	75.2%	75%
OTHER REVENUE				
à la carte sales	$970	$19,206	$ 87,300	$115,236
Catering	183	3,630	18,500	21,780
Interest	28	551	2,505	3,306
USDA commodities	816	16,145	73,384	96,867
Other	239	4,740	21,550	28,446
State matching funds	11	2,198	9,991	13,188
TOTAL REVENUE FROM OTHER SOURCES	$2,347	$46,470	$211,230	$278,823
Percentage of total revenue	17%	17.2%	17.2%	17.1%
TOTAL REVENUE	$13,698	271,338	$1,233,24	$1,632,887

continues

Table 7–10 continued

Expenditures	Dollar Amount	% of Revenue	Dollar Amount	% of Revenue	Dollar Amount	% of Revenue	Dollar Amount	% of Revenue
Purchased food cost	$5,467	39.9%	$108,254		$492,067		$649,528	
Labor cost—staff								
Wages and salaries	5,755	42%	113,952		517,965		683,713	
Fringe benefits								
Central office labor								
Salaries and wages	822	6%	16,278		73,995		97,673	
Supplies and detergents,								
and disposables	684	5%	13,554		61,612		81,328	
Small equipment/office								
supplies	137	1%	2,713		12,323		16,278	
Large equipment	438	3.2%	8,682		39,464		52,092	
Other operating								
expenses	137	1%	2,713		12,332		16,278	
TOTAL EXPENDITURES	$13,440		$266,146		$1,209,758		$ 1,596,890	
Percentage of revenue		98.1%		98.1%		98.1%		98.1%
PROFIT (OR LOSS)	$258		$5,1921		$23,491		$35,997	
Percentage of revenue		.9%		1.9%		1.9%		1.9%

Steps to Planning a Budget

The steps to planning a budget are (1) forecast revenue (Table 7–9 shows how the revenue is forecasted using anticipated participation and prices) and (2) forecast expenditures. Expenditures may be more difficult to forecast than revenue (see Table 7–9). Using a combination of last year's actual expenditures plus expected increases is probably the surest approach (e.g., labor costs were $500,000 last year and a 2.5 percent raise is expected; thus labor costs for next year's budget would be $512,500).

MAKING SOUND DECISIONS USING FINANCIAL DATA

Management needs good, current, financial data by which to plan and make sound decisions. Without the data, management is making decisions that may result in deficits. A big question that a school food service director must ask is, "Is it possible to generate enough revenue to cover the costs?" This is a question that upper management needs to answer. Costs can be divided into two types, fixed and variable. Fixed costs include labor costs that do not change with numbers served and other preset costs, such as those for telephone usage and maintenance contracts. Variable costs include food and supplies that do (or should) vary in direct proportion to numbers of meals served or amount of sales. School food service management needs to know if the revenue will cover the fixed costs, as well as the variable costs, in order to make sound decisions—for example, whether to sell branded foods from other food services. There are several approaches to analyzing data before making decisions, such as determining the break-even point.

Determining and Using the Break-Even Point

One of school food service management's tools for making sound decisions is to determine for each school food service operation, as well as for the district, the break-even point (revenue needed to cover costs). This will help the school food service director tell if it is possible to break even, or to determine whether change will have to occur to make this possible.

The break-even point is that point in the service day when enough customers have been served to cover the costs of labor, food, supplies, and overhead. To determine what the break-even point is for a school or a school district's food services, the fixed cost in dollars must be determined. A simple formula is used for determining the break-even point.

Out of every dollar of sales, how much is left after variable costs are paid to pay fixed costs? Since variable costs (such as food costs) do change based on sales, those costs are expressed in percentage of revenue. To determine how much is left from every $1 of sales to pay fixed costs, the percentage of variable costs is subtracted from revenue, which is represented by 100 percent, as shown below:

100% of Revenue − Variable cost (*VC*) in %
= Contribution margin (*CM*) in %

Fixed Cost (*FC*) in $$
―――――――――――――――――――
Divided by contribution margin (*CM*) in %
= Break-even point (*BEP*) $$

For example, the break-even point at John Doe High School can be determined if the following are known:

Fixed costs: Costs of labor with fringe benefits, overhead, telephone charges, and the like, in dollars. These costs do not change from day to day dependent on how many are served.

Variable Costs: Percentage of revenue used for variable costs (food, supplies, substitute labor, etc.).

To arrive at this percentage, use data from prior months for food costs and other costs that vary according to what is served and to how many; determine the percentage of the total revenue these variable costs amount to (last year's percentages may be used until enough data are available for current year to set a trend).

The total percentages of revenue needed to cover variable costs are subtracted from the revenue of 100 percent to determine how much of the revenue is left to pay fixed costs. The difference (or what is left) is called the *contribution margin*. The fixed cost (shown in dollars) is divided by the contribution margin

(percentage changed to decimal point) to arrive at the break-even point.

Evaluating the Program Financially

The difference between bookkeeping and accounting is that accounting is management and analysis of finance, whereas bookkeeping is literately a record of the figures—and maybe stacks of computer printouts. When the data are brought together into P&L statements (with percentage of revenue), they become a good management tool.

When evaluating the department's finances, the cost of doing business needs to be examined and analyzed, which is called *cost accounting* in the business world. It is important to break down costs and make comparisons as stated above. If good planning has been done, such as during the budget preparation process, standards (limits) have been set by which a school district's food and nutrition program director is judged. When evaluating, it is important to consider each school's food and nutrition program and the district warehouse as cost centers. One does not need to be a certified public accountant to analyze data. The areas that should be evaluated are described below.

Participation

Participation is generally shown in percentage of those present who are served the meal (breakfast or lunch)—number of paid, free, and reduced-price meals in comparison to number present. Also to be considered is what percentage of those who qualify for free and reduced-price meals have been served. Compare these percentages with those of the previous year or month. If there is a decrease, the question that needs to be answered is "Why?" A decrease may occur because notification letters were not received by the parents/students or because of poor food quality. Compare participation with other school districts' participation to determine how participation in the program rates.

Sources of Revenue

Sources of revenue may be analyzed school by school by category, letting management know which schools are meeting their potential in each category. These figures should be compared with those of the previous year and month. If there is a decrease, the food service director and the managers will need to know why. Check to see whether the decreases are in state and/or federal funds or whether it is because the local school district is reducing its financial support of the program. If just a few of the schools show a decrease, the problem may be due to a reduction of participation.

Expenditures

Evaluate expenditures by checking what percentage of the revenue is being used for food (purchased and USDA) and labor costs (look at salaries and wages separate from fringe benefits). Evaluate the number of labor hours at each school by determining the productivity rate of school's staff and compare the productivity rate or meals per labor hour (MPLH) with how each school should be staffed (if a standard has been established, use it; if not, use the guidelines in Table 7–8). Determine whether the labor costs are high, what is the average cost of a labor hour, and how this compares with the competition's costs (management companies and fast-food restaurants in the area). The next step is to determine the changes needed to be competitive and reduce the costs of labor.

The cost of labor is often a problem area and deserves serious scrutiny. This is probably the most difficult cost to reduce because of union contracts and formal or informal agreements. Many school districts have not made the cuts needed—in labor hours and hourly rates of pay—to remain competitive.

Other costs that are charged to the school food and nutrition programs vary from district to district. Some school districts charge the food and nutrition program for indirect costs as well as all direct costs that can be identified. This can result in double charges.

Inventory Practices

Evaluating inventory practices includes the security, storage, receiving, and distribution of inventory and the quantity of inventory. To evaluate quantity of inventory, determine the number of days in inventory. It is desirable to keep inventory as low as possible—seven to ten days. See the section in this chapter concerning food costs for additional suggestions.

Trends That Can Be Seen

Trends help one to determine where problems are about to occur; drastic or steady increases or decreases should be questioned. For example, compare percentages of revenue spent for food and labor for the past two years. Is there a steady increase in either? If there are increases, these increases should be checked out to determine why. If the revenue increases are not keeping pace with the increases in expenditures a deficit may result. Changes or cuts are always easier to make if the director has a warning and can make the changes or cuts gradually.

Equipment Needs

Has equipment been replaced and serviced as needed, or is equipment occupying space even though the equipment does not operate? Has new equipment been added as needed? Or is the school district allowing the food service department to get behind the times with old equipment? Many school districts have not replaced equipment on an ongoing basis and in the future will need major equipment replacements.

Computerization and Use of Technology

In many school districts, the school food and nutrition programs are leading the way with use of technology—networking and using universal codes and scanners. In other districts, the school food and nutrition program is lagging far behind.

Union Contract

The union contract may need to be changed for the school food and nutrition program to maintain costs that can be covered by the revenue available in years to come. Taking steps to obtaining those changes may be hard to do. Food service directors need to provide the management negotiating team with financial data that show consequences of increases in salaries and fringe benefits, for example, how much meal prices will have to be increased if the salary or fringe benefit costs increase, what decreases in participation can be expected as a result of price increases, and how this relates to how many labor hours each school will need.

Menus

Are the food costs of the menus served within the revenue available? The food costs of the menu can be determined by pre- and post-costing menus and determining what the variance between the two amounts to (if more than two percent, corrective action is needed). Many examples of ways to reduce food costs were discussed earlier in this chapter. Nutritional analyses need to be run to determine whether the menu is meeting adequately the federal guidelines for healthy Americans. Some menus exceed those guidelines, particularly in protein, which is the most expensive item on the menu. A reduction in protein can help to bring the food cost down, as well as reduce fat.

Forecasting the Future

Although no one has a crystal ball, it is possible to some degree to predict the future on the basis of trends. Some of the areas one needs to look at for trends when planning are shown in Exhibit 7–3.

In 1998 the trends provided evidence that funding for education would continue to be tight, which means that the school food and nutrition program, as well as others, will be expected to be self-supporting, and more and more costs are likely to be charged the program. In the past a school district's budget may have paid for all district employees' fringe benefits, all replacement equipment, and all utilities. The chances that this kind of funding will continue are slim. Knowing this, the school food service director needs to identify those costs and determine how they can be covered with program revenue and what changes will need to be made.

Setting Up Internal Controls

Internal controls can cover a wide range of safeguards to prevent defrauding the school district and the school food and nutrition program. Some districts primarily use their own audit process to determine when there is a need for better accountability and more controls. An auditor from an outside firm may not be knowledgeable enough about school food and nutrition programs and food services to really check for problems. Such an audit is best done by someone who knows the regulations and procedures of the program. More information about audits may be found in Chapter 8. Above all, good audit trails should be required and checked frequently. Some of the areas where controls are needed are as follows:

Exhibit 7–3 Trends To Consider when Planning

- Federal funding increasing or decreasing
- Local general funds—cuts, increases
- Labor market—shortage or an abundance of labor
- Cost of a labor hour
- Trends in fringe benefits—e.g., cost of health insurance
- Competitions to the school food and nutrition program—e.g., district's philosophy about privatizing
- Nutritious aspects of the school food and nutrition program
- Increasing or decreasing enrollment

- Cash assets: Be certain that the schools are accounting for all revenue received.
- *Procurement:* Are competitive bids being awarded fairly? Are products specified and ordered received?
- *Inventory control:* Make certain that foods and supplies are safely and securely stored.
- *Operational efficiency:* Check productivity of staff or meals per labor hour (MPLH) two or three times a year and take corrective action when needed.
- *Adherence to district policy:* Ensure that district policy is being followed.
- *Potential theft by customers, employees, and distributors:* Are there ways of determining when theft occurs? Is there a means of stopping it?

Some of the basic control tools are cash registers or computerized point-of-sale, time and attendance records, and production records.

TAKING CORRECTIVE ACTION

There are usually three methods that can be used for correcting financial problems: increasing revenue, reducing food and supply costs (variable costs), and reducing labor costs (primarily fixed costs). The easiest is usually increasing revenue. The next easiest is reducing variable costs. The third is the hardest—reducing fixed costs, because this usually means either changing policy or reducing labor hours.

Increasing Revenue

Although the easiest way to correct a financial problem is to increase revenues, this may not actually be easy to do because it depends on how low participation is and what programs are already in operation. Some ways of increasing revenue were listed earlier in this chapter.

Reducing Food and Supply Costs (Variable Costs)

Reducing food and supply costs, or variable costs, usually means reducing waste and/or eliminating theft. Waste occurs in many ways, such as

- Overordering produce and ordering too far ahead of use
- Poor storage, resulting in a reduced food quality and possibly spoilage
- Overproducing food
- Lack of portion control
- Failure to use leftovers
- Lack of control of supplies

A concerted effort by employees to reduce food and supply waste can result in a three to five percent savings and not negatively affect food quality or service. Simply collecting all food garbage in the kitchen and from meal trays can make an impression and also give management an idea of how much of a problem food waste is.

Reducing Labor Costs (Primarily Fixed Costs)

The best time to begin reducing labor costs is before there is a problem. When comparing costs from month to month and year to year, using percentage trends can help forecast whether there will be future problems with funding and with rising costs. Labor costs are usually not easy to reduce because this usually means hurting people. It is far more desirable to use attrition to reduce positions or labor hours assigned than to have to eliminate existing positions or to reduce the hours worked by employees.

If school districts across the country were all producing at a reasonable productivity rate (see Table 7–8), the problems with high labor costs would be greatly improved. The measuring of productivity needs to be more standardized and scientific, and training in increasing productivity is desperately needed by many school food and nutrition employees. Reducing labor hours does not automatically make people more productive. It often causes low morale and further resistance to increasing productivity.

Steps for reducing percentage of revenue used for labor follow:

- Step 1: Increase productivity gradually.
- Step 2: Train employees in time and motion and in working smarter, not harder.
- Step 3: Replace old equipment with more automated equipment.
- Step 4: Evaluate using convenience foods in place of cooking from scratch if labor can be reduced.
- Step 5: Plan ways of increasing participation and sales without increasing labor hours.
- Step 6: Evaluate centralized production as a way to reduce labor hours.
- Step 7: Couple salary increases with price increases.

SUMMARY

Financial management of school food and nutrition programs will continue to be more of a challenge as budgets become tighter. School food and nutrition program directors, supervisors, managers, and staff need to be made fully aware of the goals and need to be trained in cost control management. The American School Food Service Association's *Keys to Excellence*[2] identifies financial management as a key area and indicates that the program should be administered using sound business and accounting practices. Competencies[3] needed by the school food and nutrition program directors to use sound business and accounting practices to administer the programs include establishing financial objectives and goals for the child nutrition program, directing the operation of the school's nutrition program within established guidelines for a financial management system that provides a cost-effective program of high integrity, and implementing efficient management techniques to ensure that all records and supporting documentation are maintained in accordance with federal, state, and local laws and policies.

As child nutrition programs enter the twenty-first century with the major focus of meeting the nutrition and education needs of student customers, food service leaders must implement strategies and procedures that will ensure the cost effectiveness of programs.

CASE STUDY
HOW A SCHOOL DISTRICT REDUCED LABOR COSTS BY $1 MILLION

This case study illustrates how costs can be reduced substantially by increasing productivity. The Brownsville Independent School District (BISD) is located in Brownsville, Texas, at the southernmost tip of the state, bordering Matamoros, Mexico. The food service department staff operates under a $13 million budget and employs approximately 500 people. There are 41 schools in the district (5 high, 7 middle, and 29 elementary), with an enrollment of 40,500 students. Most of the schools have on-site kitchens. Only four have food transported bulk to them from another school's kitchen. The community has a very low income level, with more than 88 percent of the student population qualifying for free or reduced-priced meals.

Problem

The BISD is under strict financial constraints and cannot financially subsidize the food service department. The department is expected to be self-supporting. New schools and renovated kitchens have been and will probably continue to be equipped with food service department revenues. The district grows at the rate of 600 to 1,000 new students a year; therefore, the department needs to plan for funds in reserves so that as schools are built, they can be equipped. In recent years, costs for labor, fringe benefits, food, and equipment have risen. Various methods of controlling costs and increasing revenues were considered.

Labor costs were taking up the greatest amount of the revenue. In checking the meals per labor hour (MPLH) it became obvious to the director, Dora Rivas, R.D., that productivity was low. Most of the employees worked an eight-hour shift—a carryover from the days when most of the food was produced from raw ingredients. At the same time there was a need to reduce the cost of labor, there was a need to increase the number of employees at service time.

Approach to Reducing Labor Costs

Reducing labor hours and costs is never easy, but the director knew it had to be tackled. Since the community depends heavily on the food service department to provide a job market for its population, the concept of laying off employees to reduce costs would have been a negative option. Instead, the department looked at various positive approaches to reducing the percentage of revenue being used for labor. It handled downsizing by using a more positive and systematic approach, which included the following:

- Adopting a new staffing formula and informing employees about what it meant
- Training managers in how to prepare work scheduling and simplify work
- Reducing paperwork
- Standardizing the menus (which meant going from six-week cycles to three-week cycles at elementary schools and one-week cycles at middle and high schools)
- Exploring ways of increasing participation and sales while maintaining labor costs, such as
  — Increasing breakfast participation (by serving breakfast in a bag, would be taken to the classroom)
  — Increasing lunch sales (Provision II—a federal regulation that allows the district to serve all students free—and installing the food court concept)
  — Increasing à la carte items and sales
  — Improving marketing/merchandising of the program

New Staffing Formula Adopted

The BISD food service department considers its menu production to be half conventional and half convenience. Since many of the food items are prepared to meet the ethnic preferences of the students, (e.g., homemade enchiladas, carne guisada, tacos, tostadas, etc.), many of the items are prepared from raw ingredients. However, many of the menu items such as hamburgers and pizzas are available in the convenience form (e.g., precooked charbroiled hamburger patties and frozen pizzas). The department does little baking and purchases pre-prepared breads, hamburger buns, tortillas, taco shells, and so forth.

The staffing formula previously used was a single-tier formula that used 14 MPLH for lunch, 19 MPLH for breakfast, and 24 MPLH for receiving schools. The department began using a multiple-tier formula[4] based on number of meals produced. This formula uses a sliding scale with the premise that the more meals a cafeteria prepares, the greater the potential for productivity. In utilizing this formula, most of the district school cafeterias would have to increase productivity from 14 MLPH to 16 to 23 MLPH.[4]

Employees Informed of New Formula

Announcement of the use of a new formula that had the potential of reducing the hours employees would work could have resulted in mass hysteria among employees fearing loss of employment. BISD approached the implementation of this new formula very cautiously and with much sensitivity to the employees and the community. The director planned cluster meetings for the employees to inform them of the department's goals to increase participation.

One of the first things BISD did to increase participation was to initiate a program entitled Special Assistance Provision II. In this program, all students receive a free meal regardless of family income. The program resulted in increased meals served, but on the downside, it resulted in a decrease in revenue (to zero) from the paying students. Employees were informed that this decrease in revenue had to be made up by a reduction in labor costs. They were assured that their jobs would not be affected immedi-

ately since the increase in number of meals served would probably make up for the loss in revenue if the labor costs were maintained or reduced. It would be the district's goal to reduce labor costs by increasing productivity. This meant that managers and staff needed to work together to achieve these goals.

As the new staffing formula was implemented, it became necessary to cut labor hours at some schools—employees were needed for fewer hours in many of the schools. The employees were given the option of (1) accepting a reduction in hours at the school to which they were assigned or (2) transferring to another school to which the hours they had been working could be maintained. They were also informed that as employees resigned, their positions would be either eliminated or changed to four-hour and five-hour positions. Surprisingly, most of the employees volunteered to accept a reduction in hours rather than leave their co-workers.

Reassignments were based on seniority if no one volunteered to a reduction in hours. A person was transferred to another school where a position was open, based on last in, first out. As food courts were established in the high schools, there developed a need for more employees at serving time, but fewer labor hours. Where staffing was changed to four-hour and five-hour employees as a result of implementation of food courts, the same options were given. The employees were informed of the new scheduling structure at their schools, and they were asked either to accept the new structure and receive a reduction in hours or to transfer to another campus where a position closer to their desired working hours was available.

The new scheduling structure was challenged by a local labor organization through a grievance procedure, and the grievance went to the school board for settlement. The school board announced that the establishing and scheduling of labor hours needed was an administrative decision, and the decision regarding labor hours needed to be handled administratively by the food service department.

Staff Development and Training

Realizing that employees do not automatically increase productivity because labor hours have been cut, the food service department trained managers in planning work schedules. If a manager believed that his or her staff could not get the work accomplished with the reduction in hours, the manager was to develop detailed work schedules to justify additional staffing.

Area supervisors, cafeteria managers, and employees were trained in how to increase productivity through work simplification. Each job function was evaluated for efficiency. Timing jobs to determine how much time was needed and constantly seeking better and faster methods of doing each job were emphasized.

Reduction in Paperwork

Managers had complained that the volume of paperwork they had to do took too much of their time. Thus, it helped when the director was able to reduce the paperwork. By initiating Special Assistance Provision II, a federal regulation, lunch applications no longer had to be processed, students did not have to be tracked by category, and meal tickets were no longer needed. (Special Assistance Provision II allows a district or school to serve all students free.) Paperwork was further reduced by implementing an automated point-of-service system whereby the meal report is computer generated. All forms filled out at the schools are continually being reevaluated.

The schools had two clerical positions to handle the paperwork (in addition to the manager), and these positions were no longer needed. The clerks were assigned to work in the kitchen.

Their titles were changed to food service clerks, and their wages were frozen at their present rates. The number of clerk positions was reduced to one clerk per school through attrition.

Menus Standardized and Simplified

The menu literally drives all cafeteria operations in BISD, and a difficult menu can make reducing labor difficult. By standardizing and simplifying the menus (inTEAM menus[5]) to a one-week cycle with food courts at the high schools and middle schools, the job of work scheduling, as well as simplifying work, was made much easier.

Results

BISD's average MPLH has gone from 14 MPLH to 17 MPLH, which has resulted in a considerable reduction in the cost of labor. The slower, more conservative approach of increasing productivity through increased participation/revenue took a period of two years to implement. The director anticipates that it could take up to three or four years to implement fully the increase in productivity as much as desired, depending on how aggressively and quickly labor costs are reduced. Thus far, the new staffing formula has resulted in significant reduction in labor costs in the overall budget. In the first year of implementation, the labor costs were maintained; however, to date, breakfast participation has increased more than 10 percent and lunch more than 15 percent. The reduction in labor costs has meant more than $1 million savings in labor. And, from all indications, the school food and nutrition program in BISD is a better program today than it was two years ago.

REFERENCES

1. D. Carr et al., *Competencies, Knowledge, and Skills of Effective District School Nutrition Directors/Supervisors* (University, MS: National Food Service Management Institute, 1996).

2. American School Food Service Association, *Keys to Excellence: Standards of Practice for Nutritional Integrity* (Alexandria, VA: 1995).

3. Carr et al., *Competencies*.

4. D. Pannell-Martin, *School Foodservice Management,* 5th ed. (Alexandria, VA: in TEAM Associates, Inc., 1999).

5. D.V. Pannell and G.B. Applebaum, *Food System Administrator's Manual* (Alexandria, VA: in TEAM Associates, Inc., 1995).

SUGGESTED READING

Barfield, J. et al. 1994. *Cost accounting: Traditions and innovations.* 2nd ed. St. Paul, MN: West Publishing Co.

Dittmer, P., and G. Griffin. 1980. *Principles of food, beverage, and labor cost controls for hotels and restaurants.* Boston: CBI Publishing Co., Inc.

Educational Foundation of the National Restaurant Association. 1992. *Cost control for foodservice managers.* Chicago: National Restaurant Association.

Escoffier, M., and S. Dennis. 1986. *Restaurant operations and controls.* Englewood Clifts, NJ: Prentice Hall.

Horngren, C., and G. Foster. 1987. *Cost accounting: A managerial emphasis.* 6th ed. Englewood Cliffs, NJ: Prentice Hall.

Horngren, C., and G. Sundem. 1987. *Introduction to management accounting.* 7th ed. Englewood Cliffs, NJ: Prentice Hall.

Kehoe, E. 1986. Educational budget preparation: Fiscal and political considerations. In *Principles of school business management,* ed. R. Wood, 149–174. Reston, VA: The Association of School Business Officials International.

Keiser, J. 1989. *Controlling and analyzing costs in foodservice operations.* New York: Macmillan Publishing.

Kotschevar, L. 1975. *Management by menu.* Chicago: National Institute for the Foodservice Industry.

McCool, A. et al. 1994. *Dimensions of noncommercial foodservice management.* New York: Van Nostrand Reinhold.

Miller, J., and D. Hayes. 1994. *Basic food and beverage cost control.* New York: John Wiley & Sons.

Ninemeier, J. 1995. *Management of food and beverage operations.* 2d ed. East Lansing, MI: The Educational Institute of the American Hotel and Motel Association.

Pannell, D. 1986. Foodservices at school. In *Principles of school business management,* ed. R. Wood, 381–414. Reston, VA: The Association of School Business Officials International.

Pannell, D. 1994. *Cost control manual for school foodservice.* Alexandria, VA: in TEAM Associates, Inc.

Schmidgall, R., and J. Damitio. 1994. *Hospitality industry financial accounting.* East Lansing, MI: The Education Institute of the American Hotel and Motel Association.

Tidwell, S. 1986. Educational accounting procedures. In *Principles of school business management,* ed. R. Wood, 107–148. Reston, VA: The Association of School Business Officials International.

York, C. 1989. Financial systems. In *Handbook of noncommercial foodservice management,* ed. J. Bakos and G. Karrick, 147–160. Gaithersburg, MD: Aspen Publishers, Inc.

CHAPTER 8

Surviving an External Review

Annette Bomar Hopgood

OUTLINE

INTRODUCTION

In fiscal year 1998 the United States government budgeted $8 billion in federal assistance to support child nutrition programs, including reimbursement for meals, the purchase of commodities, State Administrative Expense, nutrition education, and food service management training programs.[1] The responsibility of organizations receiving these public resources is, therefore, to safeguard their use toward achieving specific objectives mandated by Congress. The responsibility of professionals managing or operating child nutrition programs and of administrators of recipient organizations is to be accountable for program funds in such a manner that will ensure the public trust. Effective program managers recognize that in the public interest minimum levels of program performance are required and optimal levels are essential for program integrity.

A state or federal grantor agency's primary mechanism to ensure the integrity of public resources is the scrutiny of their use by conducting audits or reviews. For the purpose of this discussion, *integrity* represents the use of resources only as intended; as the recipient organization has agreed; and in an economical, efficient, and effective manner. A *review or audit* is the process of evaluating actual program performance at a specific time or over a period of time against predetermined expectations or standards. Minimum expectations scrutinized by a review or audit are based on current authority established by federal, state, or local governing bodies and generally accepted management practices established by professional governing bodies. Expectations are communicated through statute, regulations, policy, procedures, or guidance. Optimal performance levels include proven management practices and research within the industry that supports promising practices. Optimal performance is communicated through management indicators and standards adopted by organizations such as the American School Food Service Association's *Keys to Excellence: Standards of Prac-*

tice for Nutrition Integrity[2] and the Georgia Department of Education's *Quality Measures for Georgia's School Nutrition Program.*[3] Other indicators can be found in the National Food Service Management Institute's *Competencies for District School Nutrition Directors/Supervisors.*[4]

It is generally the responsibility of the program manager or administrator of the recipient organization to manage the organization's interests before, during, or after the review or audit. The discussion that follows will allow the reader an insight into the scope of review or audit activities that may be experienced in the management of one or more of the federal child nutrition programs. A knowledgeable program manager or administrator will find that a basic understanding of the review or audit potential can minimize negative findings and will assist the recipient organization in implementing internal controls toward the same goal.

Review and audit activity drive major program functions, including operations and training to support operations. Appendix 8–A, Selected Chronology: USDA Review Initiatives in the School Nutrition Programs, 1975–1998, reflects the significant and ongoing efforts of the federal grantor agency to refine the review and audit function within the school food and nutrition program. A review of the chronology indicates to the reader the frequency of changes in program operations that may be experienced solely as a result of the external review or audit function.

TYPES OF REVIEWS AND AUDITS

As described previously, a recipient organization will, over time, experience review or audit activity of multiple types. The purpose and benefit of each type may differ. Each type is designed to assess compliance with specific performance expectations. Many review or audit activities apply the same standards. It is possible that over a course of a fiscal year a recipient organization could experience audit or review activity of several types. For example, a recipient organization could receive in the same year an organizationwide audit required by the Uniform Single Audit Act of 1984,[5] a Coordinated Review Effort (CRE) evaluation by the state agency, known as an administrative review and required by federal regulations,[6] and an audit by the Office of Inspector General of the United States Department of Agriculture (USDA) (see discussion of each that follows). Because audit and review activity generally occurs on a cyclical basis, a grantor agency may not be able to adjust the schedule to avoid such multiple activities.

State Agency Review

Federal Regulatory Review

Description. Federal regulations require the state grantor agency to review programs operated by recipient agencies for compliance with minimum standards. In past years regulatory reviews of the School Lunch Program (SLP) and the School Breakfast Program (SBP) have been referred to by a variety of names and have included various standards (see Appendix 8–A). In November 1989, as a result of concern over duplicity of federal and state review activities in the school lunch program, Congress passed Public Law (PL) 101-147. This amendment to the 1946 National School Lunch Act[7] required a "unified accountability system" of federal and state agency administrative reviews to ensure that local School Food Authorities (SFAs) comply with federal program requirements. As a result, current state agency regulatory review activity is targeted to two areas: the critical areas of review and the general areas of review[8] and compliance with nutrient standards through menu planning, production, and service.[9]

Activity related to the first area above is referred to as the (CRE) and is mandated by Section 22 of the National School Lunch Act.[10] Independent schools or school districts, known as school food authorities (SFA),[11] are generally selected for this type of review according to a cycle of years rather than assessed need.

Administrative reviews are performed during a five-year cycle unless the state agency has secured a waiver from USDA as authorized in the statute.[12] Schools are selected as prescribed by regulations based upon (1) a numerical quota depending on the size of the SFA and (2) need as determined by their potential for noncompliance. Potential for noncompliance is determined by comparing actual meals claimed to a derived number of meals expected to be claimed. The derived number accounts for students' rate of attendance and anticipated frequency of eating meals.

Reviews of the second area of compliance with nutrient standards are referred to as healthy school meal initiative reviews and must, according to Title 7, Code of Federal Regulations (C.R.F.), Part 210.19(a)(1), be performed within a five-year cycle unless a waiver from this requirement has been granted the state agency.

Reviews of the Summer Food Service Program (SFSP),[13], the Food Distribution Program (FDP),[14] and the Child and Adult Care Food Program (CACFP)[15] are also prescribed in federal regulation, although currently the requirement to apply uniform national standards does not exist. Reclaims and follow-up in these programs may therefore differ, according to the grantor agency conducting the review. Reviews by the state or federal grantor agency may also result from a grant of other federal funds, such as Nutrition Education and Training (NET)[16] or school breakfast startup or expansion.[17] Annual reviews of contracts between SFAs and food service management companies are also specified in regulations.[18]

When a state agency fails to conduct reviews according to regulations or its own agreement with the federal agency, this performance failure can become an audit or review exception for the state agency. Refer to specific program regulations for federal requirements that will spell out the minimum review activity required of the grantor (state) agency.

Purpose and Benefits. The purpose of a state agency regulatory review of an SFA is to identify needs and subsequently to provide necessary guidance, training, and technical assistance to the SFA to achieve a minimum level of performance that is currently not in place. An improvement plan developed by the local agency with input from the state agency as needed is the primary vehicle for achieving improvement. Corrective action may, however, be required on site when certain deficiencies are found, depending on the nature of noncompliance.

State agencies receive State Administrative Expense funds[19] to perform not only the review activity but the follow-up activity required to assist the local organization in reaching compliance. The state agency is not, however, responsible for implementation of corrective action. This responsibility lies with the local agency.

A major benefit of a state agency review is to identify performance at a specific point in time that needs immediate correction or future improvement. Failure to identify and correct performance can cause audit exceptions that can extend over a period of time and result in costly reclaims of funds. Because standards differ between a review and an audit (see discussion that follows), the correction of a review finding does not guarantee that reclaims of program funds will not result from an audit covering the same or prior period of time.

Performance Standards. The standards applied during a regulatory review by a state grantor agency will depend on the program under review and the regulatory requirements placed on the state agency by the program regulations. For example, Title 7 C.F.R., Part 210(g) and Part 210.18(h), respectively, specify critical and general performance expectations in the CRE in the NSLP and SBP. Deficiencies noted during such a review are based on the local agency's actual performance in these regulatory areas. Regulatory and other federal requirements for contracts with a food service management company are also found in the USDA document, *Contracting with Food Service Management Companies: Guidance for School Food Authorities.*[20]

Current federal regulations also provide for uniform procedures by which states conduct initial and follow-up reviews and reclaim funds under the CRE.[21] Under regulations prior to the July 1,1992, effective date of CRE regulations, performance expectations and review procedures, including follow-up and reclaims, could vary from state to state. State agency procedures could also differ from those used during an administrative review by the USDA, the federal grantor agency.

State agencies currently have more latitude in determining procedures to apply to reviews of the SFSP, the FDP, and the CACFP than the SLP and SBP programs. Although performance standards are based on regulations, procedures for these reviews are not generally specified in regulation or guidance. Latitude lies in the agency's determination of which regulatory standards to review and to some degree the calculation of reclaims and follow-up resulting from noncompliance. The outside frequency of reviews is specified in federal regulations for some programs. USDA activities such as the Key Element Reporting System (KERS)[22] in the CACFP in the 1980s and the current child care integrity initiative[23] indicate that these programs are subject to future regulatory change to standardize states' use of performance standards and review procedures, similar to that done in the SLP and SBP.

Compliance with meal-planning regulations constitutes the second area for regulatory review by the state grantor agency. Because current federal statute requires that schools have a variety of options in planning meals, the review standards and procedures will vary according to the regulatory option chosen by the SFA to plan meals. Although menu-planning procedures are optional at the local level, compliance with nutrient standards and menu items offered and served as specified in federal regulations is not. Title 7, C.F.R., Part 210.10 (c), (d) and (k) contains these standards for nutrients, other dietary components, and minimum food items and/or quantities at lunch as applicable to the chosen menu-planning option. Requirements for nutrient standards at breakfast are found in Title 7, C.F.R., Part 220.8 (b), (c) and (g). State agencies currently have maximum flexibility in identifying schools for review of menu-planning practices. In conducting review follow-up activity, including the assessment of overclaims for noncompliance, state agencies must follow procedures in federal regulations at Title 7, C.R.F., Part 210.19 (a)(1). According to these same regulations, SFAs that fail to comply with nutrient standards in federal regulations must demonstrate to the state agency's satisfaction that efforts are under way to implement the standards.

Management Reviews

Description. In addition to the reviews described above, which primarily assess compliance in achieving accurate meal counts and meal or nutrient standards, program regulations require the state agency to conduct reviews where management deficiencies are evident.[24] Evidence of deficiencies specified in regulations include a declining or poor financial status, low student participation, or student rejection of foods served. Also, management reviews may be conducted by the state agency with the nonregulatory goal of working with the school or district to improve some aspect of the local program consistent with local goals, such as sanitation and safety, food preparation and quality, menu planning, student involvement, facility utilization, procurement, or nutrition education. Reviews of local operations may result from a statewide assessment of program needs required to be conducted periodically by state agencies under the NET program.[25] Management reviews conducted by the state grantor agency generally differ from regulatory reviews in that performance standards applied during the review are based on generally accepted management practices in the institutional food service industry and the research of promising practices. Regulatory noncompliance, however, will be brought to the attention of the local agency if found by a grantor agency during a management review, and corrective action will be required.

Purpose and Benefits. Findings from a management review can be a springboard to promote continuous improvement in the program under review. Just as in a regulatory review, a locally developed improvement plan is the vehicle to address program management needs. Failure to adhere to management standards will not usually result in a direct audit or review exceptions. Recommendations are made when performance does not meet industry standards, best practices, or expectations of stakeholders—students, administrators, board members, parents, and the general tax-paying public.

The benefits of a management review lie primarily in the state agency's identification of resources to assist the local agency in carrying out its own plans that will result in improvements. Resources may include formal training materials or programs, on-site technical help, or referral to existing model programs in a specific area of program management. In some cases, State Administrative Expense or Nutrition Education and Training funds may be made available to the SFA by the state agency to perform functions that could assist in implementing the continuous improvement plan, provided such can also serve as models for other local agencies. Another significant value of a state agency management review is that state personnel can share these observations and related management tools, which they have observed in reviewing other schools, districts, and institutions. The management review also provides the state agency opportunities to identify "best practices" for the purpose of showcasing or benchmarking local operations.

Performance Standards. Many states have documented performance measures or standards for local program administration and operation. Contact your state agency to determine the availability of standards within the state. National professional organizations representing the professions of institutional food service management and nutrition also have documented and published standards to promote quality operations among their members. To promote maximum utilization, performance measures should include specific, measurable indicators that can be applied by local personnel with or without the benefit of state personnel.

The American School Food Service Association has developed standards for the school food and nutrition program,[26] and competencies have been published by the National Food Service Management Institute.[27] When applied on the job, these competencies define a level of individual performance that can be translated into program performance measures. Another source of standards that can be adapted to schools is available from the National Association of College and University Food Service.[28]

Although all the areas of performance listed below may not be regulatory, they are generally recognized in the literature as vital to program quality.

- Budgeting and financial management
- Cost accounting and control
- Facility planning and utilization
- Food production and management
- Customer service
- Human resource management
- Procurement
- Sanitation
- Safety
- Student and parent involvement
- Production scheduling
- Environmental management

Other organizations exist that promote standards in discrete areas of management. For example, the National Parents and Teachers Association has developed *National Standards for Parent/Family Involvement Programs.*[29] Sanitation and food safety standards are developed, published, and administered by federal, state, and local health agencies. Accounting standards are developed and periodically updated by the Governmental Accounting Standards Board of the Financial Accounting Foundation.[30]

Other State Agency Reviews

Some state grantor agencies have been responsible for state legislation, state governing board(s) policy, or regulations whose implementation is required by local agencies and reviewed by the state grantor agency. Information about any state requirements should be readily available from the state grantor agency. Generally, nonlegislative state requirements first undergo public comment before they become effective. Local agency personnel may contact their state grantor agency about how requirements are formulated and how to provide local input into their development or revision.

Additional reviews are conducted by state agencies other than the state grantor agency, which is the state education agency in the case of the NSLP and SBP unless a waiver has been granted the state. Other state agencies include the state agency for environmental health, which is responsible for the application of food safety and sanitation standards. The state agency responsible for licensing commercial food warehouses also may conduct reviews of publicly owned warehouses operated by the school food authority or other recipients of federal financial assistance. The state fire official also may conduct reviews of facilities. Contact the state grantor agency for agency contacts regarding other review activity. Input from local operators into the development and/or revision of agency performance standards in these areas is warranted. Determine the process used in your state to generate these state agency standards, and provide input on standards that will have an impact on local operations.

Federal Agency Reviews and Audits

A variety of structures exist at the federal level to help ensure that state and local agencies entrusted with the responsibility of administering federal assistance are accountable. These include program monitoring or review by the federal grantor agency and audits conducted of the recipients of federal assistance. A wide range of audit activities includes financial audits; compliance audits with terms and requirements of a specific program; or audits to determine whether specific programs are being operated economically, efficiently, and effectively. Some common audit and review activities are discussed below.

Single Audits

A history of the Uniform Single Audit Act of 1984[31] is contained in Senate Report 98-234. According to this report, the U.S. Office of Management and Budget in 1979, responding to a General Accounting Office (GAO) report of uncoordinated and ineffective audit and reporting techniques employed by the federal government, released Attachment P to Circular A-102.[32] The attachment established a new approach to auditing of federal assistance programs. Prior to this approach audits were made on a grant-by-grant basis, resulting in overlap and duplication. Under the new single-audit approach state and local governments were to obtain a single organizationwide audit encompassing all federal grants. Because of the complex and very difficult procedures to implement nationwide the standards in Attachment P, the Committee on Governmental Affairs subsequently concluded that statutory authority was needed to achieve the uniformity nationwide, thus the enactment of the Uniform Single Audit Act of 1984.

Description. According to Senate Report 98-234, four important factors are to be considered in the audit. *First*, the audit must cover all of the funds of the entire entity being audited, not just the federal assistance funding. An exception for this condition is provided. The approach permits orderly coverage of all funds in one audit, thus avoiding disruption, duplication, and overlapping of audit efforts. Entities include state and local governments or a recipient of federal assistance from one of these governments.

Second, the audit must be conducted at least biennially but preferably annually for each entity that receives federal assistance for a fiscal year that is equal to or exceeds an expressed threshold dollar amount. The dollar threshold targets coverage to those entities receiving the majority of federal assistance. More timely audits are encouraged to provide for coverage prior to an extended period of time elapsing.

Third, the audits must be conducted by independent auditors defined by generally accepted government auditing standards and in accordance with these same standards. The Governmental Accounting Standards Boards, organized in 1984, establishes standards of financial accounting and reporting for state and local governmental entities. The board operates under the oversight (except with regard to technical decisions) of the Financial Accounting Foundation, an independent, private-sector organization. Standards are recognized as authoritative by the American Institute of Certified Public Accountants.[33] The board issues statements that direct financial accounting and reporting activities and therefore audit standards.

Fourth, the audit must include a study and evaluation of and report on the extent and condition of internal controls existing with the entity. The purpose of such investigation is to provide reasonable assurance that the entity is managing Federal programs in compliance with laws and regulations; to determine whether internal control systems are properly designed and in place to protect the integrity of funds received and whether the controls are functioning as management intended.

Purpose and Benefits. According to Senate Report 98-234 on the Uniform Single Audit Act of 1984, its purposes are (1) to improve the financial management of federal assistance programs; (2) to promote the efficient use of audit resources; (3) to help relieve state and local governments of the costs and paperwork burdens due to conflicting, redundant, and unreasonable audit; (4) to provide for the establishment of consistent and uniform requirements for financial audits of state and local governments and other recipients of federal assistance; (5) to specify standards for the financial audit requirement for federal assistance programs established after the date of enactment; (6) to have the audit requirement of the act met by each entity that received federal assistance; and (7) to have federal agencies and departments, in planning and performing any additional work and to the maximum extent feasible, rely upon and not duplicate work done pursuant to the act. Of utmost importance to the administrator of a school district is the impact of audit findings on the district's bond rating. Serious findings can impact negatively this vital area of operations.

Performance Standards. Compliance supplements are developed by the Executive Office of the President of the United States, Office of Management and Budget (OMB), and set forth major compliance requirements that should be considered in an organizationwide audit of state and local governments that receive federal assistance. Each federal assistance program has a supplement that prescribes program objectives and procedures and compliance requirements and suggested audit procedures.[34] Additionally, the supplements outline general requirements associated with the receipt of federal funds, including but not limited to civil rights, cash management, and allowable costs/cost principles.

Office of Inspector General (OIG) Audits

The Office of Inspector General (OIG) is the independent auditing arm of the USDA. OIG conducts and supervises audits and investigations relating to programs and operations of the USDA.[35] Periodically OIG surveys state agencies to determine programmatic areas that may warrant their further attention, as contained in the R.G. Poland, regional Inspector General for Audit, Office OIG, USDA, southeast region personal communication, March 13, 1997,

to Linda Schrenko, state superintendent of schools, Georgia Department of Education.

Description. OIG audits federal assistance programs administered within a USDA region or nationwide. Audits are generally focused on a narrow area of program performance. Results of audits of individual entities across the nation are often consolidated into a "roll-up audit report," which reflects trends within a federal program across states or regions. USDA's continuing efforts to improve the meal counting and claiming process in the school lunch program can be tracked to two roll-up reports. The first, in 1979, was entitled the *Twelve State Audit*[36]; the second in 1989, was entitled *Roll-Up Report* of audits of school food service programs administered by SFAs.[37]

Other programmatic areas of child nutrition programs also receiving nationwide attention through OIG audits include use of state administrative expense funds[38] and contracts for food service management companies.[39] Additionally, OIG may choose to investigate program irregularities, which are referred to USDA by state agencies under provisions of Title 7, C.F.R., Part 210.19(a)(5).

Purpose and Benefits. As a direct result of its audit and investigative activity, OIG reviews and makes recommendations on existing and proposed federal legislation and regulations. It also recommends policies and activities to promote economy and efficiency and to prevent and/or detect fraud and mismanagement in the operations of the USDA. The agency also keeps the secretary of agriculture and the Congress fully informed about problems and deficiencies relating to the administration of the USDA's programs.

Performance Standards. A review of OIG audit findings reveals latitude in the standards selected for review. Although audit standards are generally based in federal authority, an audit may include data collection or review. It is through the collection of such focused data that OIG draws conclusions about the federal administration of assistance programs and the status of federal authority over programs. OIG then reports to Congress and the Secretary of Agriculture on action required to maintain the integrity of federal assistance programs.

Food and Consumer Service Reviews

Food and Nutrition Service (FNS) is the federal grantor agency for child nutrition and food distribution programs. FNS is responsible for interpreting federal statutes; issuing program regulations, instructions, and policy memoranda establishing nationwide standards; and ensuring program integrity. FNS regional offices monitor state grantor agencies to ensure the adequacy of their administration.[40] FNS supports the states' administration of child nutrition and other programs by providing federal financial assistance for state administrative costs as authorized by Section 7, Child Nutrition Act of 1966 at Title 42, United Stated Code 1776.

FNS program integrity efforts include encouragement of state agencies to improve their management oversight and administration of targeted federal assistance programs at any point in time, and coordination with the OIG to conduct targeted audits to identify fraud and abuse in federal assistance programs.

Description. Reviews conducted by FNS under the authority of Title 7, C.F.R., Part 210.30 are generally focused on the state grantor agency and often include reviews of representative grantees, including recipients of federal child nutrition assistance. Reviews of a state agency's administration of a federal assistance program are both cyclical and based on current FNS initiatives, such as the state's administration of the new school meal initiative in 1997 (see Appendix 8–A). Review reports are transmitted to the chief state school officer or alternate state agency head and are frequently presented to state boards of education and referenced in the state's results-based budgeting and evaluation process.

Purpose and Benefits. A major benefit to the state agency under review by FNS is the ability to ascertain that its administration in programmatic areas is consistent with federal authority and to some degree the administration of the program in other states.

Performance Standards. Reviews of state and associated local agencies by FNS are based on standards found in federal regulatory authority for the program or programs under review and related policy and guidance. A typical standard reviewed by the federal agency and of interest to local child nutrition agencies is the manner by which the state agency communicates regulatory requirements to local agencies and monitors local programs consistent with regulations.

U.S. General Accounting Office Reviews

The GAO is an agency of the Congress that reviews federal programs generally at the request of congressional authorizing committees charged with passing legislation governing the federal program.[41]

Description. As charged by Congress, GAO will conduct reviews of federal, state, and local agency data and performance and will generate reports to Congress. Copies of GAO reports to Congress are available from GAO at P.O. Box 6015, Gaithersburg, Maryland 20877 or the U.S. Superintendent of Documents. Reports contain data and information collected during the specific review and significant discussion leading up to the response provided to Congress. Documentation of agency responses to inquiries is included in the report.

Purpose and Benefits. As directed by congressional committees, GAO reviews specific aspects of federal programs. Examples of such may include USDA's implementation of a specific statute, the effectiveness of program implementation compared with the intent of Congress, or a review of program performance in key areas of interest to Congress.

The benefit of a GAO review is that it is independent of any agency involved directly in administering the federal program and can scrutinize a federal agency's performance as well as the effectiveness of legislation and implementing regulations in meeting the intent of Congress. GAO reports can have significant impact on future legislative activities of Congress or on the USDA's administration of the program. Examples of reports that have been generated over the past 10 years include the December 1989 report entitled *Food Assistance—USDA's Implementation of Legislated Commodity Distribution Reforms*[42]; the March 1993 report entitled *Survey on Schools That Withdrew from the National School Lunch Program (NSLP)*[43]; the July 1996 report entitled *School Lunch Program—Cafeteria Managers' Views on Food Wasted by Students*[44]; and the August 1996 report entitled *School Lunch Program—Role and Impacts of Private Food Service Companies.*[45]

Performance Standards. Standards reviewed by the GAO are grounded in the nature of the specific request of Congress.

School Food Authority Reviews and Audits

Regulatory Review

Regulations require that local school food authorities establish internal controls to ensure the accuracy of lunch counts.[46] According to regulations, at a minimum, internal controls shall include (1) an on-site review of the lunch counting and claiming system employed by each school within the jurisdiction of the SFA, (2) a comparison of daily meal counts by category against data that will assist in the identification of lunch counts in excess of the number of lunches served each day by category to eligible children or other allowable controls, and (3) a system for following up on those lunch counts that suggest the likelihood of lunch-counting problems. Additionally, regulations require an annual review of the validity of information given by families in the receipt of free and reduced-price meals; this is known as "verification," and is required by Section 9, National School Lunch Act.[47]

Description. The annual reviews must be performed by deadlines prescribed in federal regulations or noncompliance occurs.

Purpose and Benefits. The purpose of the on-site review of meal counting and claiming procedures is to evaluate the existence and implementation of internal controls to ensure that only actual meals served are counted and that meals are properly counted and claimed in the appropriate category. Edits are locally developed or regulatory procedures conducted to reduce the potential for overpayment of federal reimbursement.

Performance Standards. Standards related to the on-site review of meal counting and claiming procedures are contained in USDA's *Accuclaim Manual: Meal Counts Count*[48] and *Eligibility Guidance for School Meals Manual.*[49] Standards related to the verification of free and reduced-priced meals and processing of free and reduced-price meal applications and nondiscrimination practices are outlined in *Eligibility Guidance for School Meals Manual* [49] and *Meal Counting and Claiming Manual.*[50]

Internal Audit

Most large school districts have internal auditing staffs that apply their own standards to determine that regulatory requirements are followed in the receipt and expenditure of federal financial and other assistance. The focus of the internal audit is to ensure that internal controls or safeguards are in place within the organization. Internal controls are those that minimize the opportunity for noncompliance to occur. See Case Study: Internal Controls.

Description. The school food authorities in large school districts may prescribe a cycle for audit staff to follow in conducting audits of federal assistance programs or, in the case of a large staff, assign audit liaisons whose responsibility is periodically to sample internal control standards and their implementation within the local agency as management intended. Internal auditors may also conduct follow-up to state and federal agency audits or reviews and supervise the implementation of corrective action.

Purpose and Benefits. The primary benefit of an internal audit is to develop or refine internal controls and promote their implementation within the local agency itself. Internal audits can detect and correct noncompliance with regulatory standards prior to the conduct of an independent external audit or review. Remember that one goal of the single audit is to determine whether internal controls exist and are implemented as management planned. The correction of a finding by an internal auditor does not guarantee that reclaims of program funds will not result from an external audit or review of the same or prior period of time. Prompt repayment of funds found internally to be overclaimed must be made to the state agency along with planned corrective action. The state agency may, depending on the nature and severity of the noncompliance, be required to report the noncompliance to the federal agency, consistent with federal regulations.[51]

Performance Standards. Internal audit standards may include all federal requirements and parallel those used by the "single audit" with the exception that auditors are not generally independent from the agency being audited because they are employed by that agency.

External Reviews

Business Reviews

With increasing pressure on recipients of federal assistance to demonstrate that their management of federal resources is optimal, the external review model can provide an independent evaluation. Such an external evaluation is sponsored by the local agency and is conducted outside any regulatory effort. This review effort usually results from a local agency's own organization of a review panel and structure that best meets its own goals. The creation of the external business review panel may be associated with a district's budget review, a district's exploration of privatization, or a district's interest in a program's performance and responsiveness to community needs, including the economical, efficient, and effective management of resources.

Description. The external review panel is generally composed of invited community members and public and private sector representatives that represent stakeholders and individuals with expertise in the institutional food service, nutrition, or other related industry. Membership may include representatives from other local government agencies, local business and industry, public and private college and university food service, health care or catering professionals, business, food service contractors, state agency personnel, or certified public accountants. Procedures for use by the panel range from being highly structured by the local agency to self-imposed procedures determined by panel members to best achieve the goals presented by the local agency. See Case Study: External Business Review for further discussion of this type of external review.

Purpose and Benefits. The purposes of the external review are prescribed by the local school board or administration and may occur as the result of a comprehensive evaluation of all programs administered by the school district or school. Child nutrition programs can benefit from the expertise of panel members from both within and outside the industry. The knowledge and experience of panel members when shared with program administrators can reveal opportunities for program management that are not currently routine for the district. Additionally, the experience of an external business review can validate that the program is operated in an economical, efficient, and effective manner. Such an assurance is important to public perception of the program and depicts the school district's interest in meeting the expectations of stakeholders.

Performance Standards. The standards for use by an external business review panel are not generally based in federal or state authority but in sound management principles or "best practices" founded in successful business and industry models. If left to the external business review panel and in accordance with the district's goals, standards generally parallel the particular expertise of its members, such as nutrition services, procurement, cost control, food production management, customer service, sanitation and safety, environmental management, or marketing.

Peer Reviews

School food authorities and other recipients of federal assistance may desire to organize a review by administrative staff of other local child nutrition programs. This may be important due to the value placed by the organization on the operational knowledge of peers.

Description. Such a review focuses on identifying and securing expertise from peers who are responsible for like operations in like schools or districts. Reviews are organized by the local organization desiring to benefit from expertise of peers or the state agency at the request of the district. Assistance from the state agency could include the identification of peers with specific skills. Funds may also be available from the state agency to assist with costs of such a review.

Purpose and Benefits. Like that of an external business review, the benefit of a peer review is the practical sharing of management practices among peers without the pressure of regulatory oversight as would be present in a review by a state or federal agency.

Performance Standards. Standards used by members of a peer review panel may be based in management and/or regulatory standards developed by the local agency sponsoring the review, the individual panel members, professional organizations, or the state agency.

Accreditation Panel Reviews

Description. Regional and state school accreditation and evaluation organizations utilize volunteer school and district personnel to apply that organization's standards for schools and district desiring to achieve accreditation recognition.[52] The purpose of accreditation and evaluation according to the New England Association of Schools and Colleges is to protect the public trust and to promote proactive self-improvement among its member organizations. Contact your local school superintendent or state education agency to determine a school's or district's involvement in the school accreditation process.

Purpose and Benefits. Each accreditation and evaluation organization develops its own purposes. Generally, purposes are to focus on improving student performance, to increase the effectiveness of the school improvement process, to provide recognition for schools having achieved validated standards, to promote staff development, to involve the school as a partner in the formation of state or regional school standards, to provide a framework for accountability, and to protect the public trust.

Performance Standards. The process of developing standards of accreditation and evaluation organizations is widely known to include member schools and districts. While standards may or may not directly relate to the child nutrition program, many standards are indirectly related to the program and provide direction for the local administrator wanting the program to track recognized standards in the education community. Examples of related standards may include length of the meal period, the sale of confections on school premises, supervision of students at mealtime, and staff development for school personnel.

PRELIMINARY ACTIVITIES

In the case of a review conducted by a federal or state grantor agency the organization under review should expect reasonable notice of planned review activity. Some schedules may be negotiable within the fiscal year if the proposed time is inconvenient because of school or staff schedules. In the case of an audit, advance notification may or may not occur. Federal regulations stipulate that federal and state officials and others acting in their capacity have the right to review records and operations at reasonable time and place, and the school food authority under review has agreed to afford access. Records must be maintained for a minimum of three years plus the current fiscal year unless there is an unresolved review or audit finding, at which time records must be maintained for an indefinite period. A state or local records retention schedule may require a period of time longer than the aforementioned federal requirement.

Reviewer Activity

Risk Analysis and/or Site Selection

While the minimum frequency of reviews or audits may be prescribed in federal or state authority, the number of and exact sites selected to be included in the review or audit may be chosen based on risk. The site's degree of risk is determined by the state agency's reviewing reported data as percentage of eligible students actually eating meals, reporting errors or irregularities including tardiness of or omissions in data, a history of noncompliance, and the general attitude of program personnel toward compliance. By targeting efforts to organizations and/or sites where risk is highest, the likelihood of finding and correcting noncompliance is heightened. Local organizations may also be selected for audit or review by the federal agency based on assessed risk.

Data Collection

In preparing for the conduct of a review or audit, the reviewing agency may collect and analyze specific data that will enable them to focus their efforts on an organization likely to be at risk and/or specific targeted areas of performance. For example, if the handling of USDA commodity foods, a cash asset, was a targeted performance area, data on commodity usage and reported commodity inventory levels may be collected and analyzed prior to site selection. If one site has large variations in usage between reporting periods or reported usage outside an acceptable range, it may be targeted for a review of its inventory, ordering practices, usage, and accuracy of production records.

The collection and analysis of data related to specific areas of program performance may be done on site after the organization is selected and before the sites are selected. Data reflective of non-compliance may also be used to determine the schedule for the organization review or audit within the cycle. The schedule may call for the organization to be reviewed early in the fiscal year to avoid a larger reclaim.

Reviewee Activity

Review of Previous Activity

Most review or audit activity will include an assessment of the agency's progress made in correcting deficiencies noted during the previous audit or review. A good starting point in a local organization's preparation for a review or audit is to review these findings and to be familiar with the organization's efforts to correct deficiencies. Additionally, peers in other local organizations that have recently been audited or reviewed may be a good source of information about any targeted efforts of the audit or review agency. For example, it may be determined that tests of compliance during one audit or review cycle are more apt to include accounting for commodities, verification of eligibility for free and reduced-price meal recipients, or documentation of severe need breakfast costs.

Internal Assessment of Compliance

In preparation for a review or audit the local organization, to the extent possible, should conduct a self-assessment of actual program performance against the standards anticipated to be applied. Such a self-assessment is best performed with a critical eye for questionable areas of program performance.

Organization and Review of Data To Be Assessed

An analysis of data is generally required before any conclusions about compliance can be made. It is advisable for the local organization to review and analyze its own data prior to a review, to determine whether data at some sites fall far outside the norm or whether data are missing or unorganized to such a degree that auditors or reviewers may have to review additional data unnecessarily in order to find what they need to conduct their test. Failure of data to be consistent and organized is one reason that reviewers observe many performance areas that they never intended to review. Any time this happens the original scope of the review or audit can expand. It is advisable, therefore, to present organized data that you have screened for accuracy, completeness, and consistency with like schools. If an internal analysis of data reveals problems such as errors in recording food inventory, it is best to correct them immediately even if the reviewer or auditor will observe your correction.

ON-SITE ACTIVITIES

Entrance Conference

To initiate the review or audit the organization under review or audit should expect an entrance conference. If this is not offered, ask for one. The conference is an opportunity to set the tone for the activities to follow. The entrance conference is the time to clarify the intended scope of the review or audit, to ask questions, and to communicate general expectations about the procedures to be followed, such as school building security, office hours, work space, and appointments with staff. It is not generally acceptable for audit work to take place outside the normal workday. The clarification of internal procedures including telephone numbers and names of key staff and the areas for which they are responsible will ensure minimal disruption of routine activities. The school food and nutrition director should apprise the review and audit staff that he or she will coordinate all contacts. Insist at the entrance conference that an exit conference be scheduled and announced so appropriate staff can attend. Record names of individuals at these conferences; secure business cards or other relevant identification. The areas cited above are discussions that are anticipated by the reviewer or auditor. The program director should always ask to be present. Staff who will be involved in the review activities and their supervisors should also be present.

Review Process

Review or audit activities will generally start at the central office of the organization under review or audit. A review of records and reports may occur at this time, which will direct future activities such as targeting of sites to visit as part of the procedures. It is important that staff be available to offer clarification and explanations as requested. When reviewers or auditors make inquiries it can be important to understand the inquiry clearly and to respond to the inquiry. It is not generally helpful to offer additional information outside the scope of the inquiry. Remember that it is the reviewer's or auditor's responsibility, not that of the agency under review, to define performance areas to be reviewed. It can be helpful for the program director to check periodically with those conducting the review or audit to confirm their findings and the general status of activity to date.

Site personnel should be briefed beforehand on the activity under way and given general directions on how they should communicate with reviewers, including recording information about significant inquiries and their responses. It is important that the director have an understanding of the scope of activity that is performed at both the central office and the chosen sites. This information may prove beneficial when findings are presented.

Positive and straightforward communications between organization staff and the reviewers or auditors can help to facilitate the goal of making an accurate statement of compliance. Tendencies on the part of organization staff to be less than cooperative may lead those in charge of review or audit activity to perceive problems when none actually exists. Employees should feel comfortable presenting factual information in order to facilitate the process.

Exit Conference

The exit conference is the time for those conducting the review or audit to present their general findings. Major findings should be presented at this time, although the final calculations of reclaims and other activities may come later. Ask that all observations of noncompliance be addressed in some detail. If organization personnel believe that findings may not be accurate they should indicate this at this time. Those in attendance at the entrance conference should also be in attendance at the exit conference. Notes of proceedings should be recorded for future reference, or proceedings could be taped with permission of those in attendance and depending on the nature of activity that has taken place to date. Confirm at the conference the anticipated date of the transmittal of the final report and the process that will follow, including general time frames for responses.

THE REPORT OF FINDINGS

The report of findings will serve as an important document in the organization's re-

sponse, follow-up, and establishment of a historical record for the organization. Confirm whether the report will first be transmitted in draft form for input or in final form. Several important actions must be taken by organization personnel when the report is received. *First*, the report is generally transmitted officially to the superintendent or head of the agency under review. Because there will be a deadline for the organization's response it will be helpful if the document is transmitted immediately to that person responsible for the response. Loss of response time resulting from a delay in its transmittal may be detrimental to those preparing a response, if required. It is important that deadlines be met or an extension be officially requested as need justifies. *Second*, check all observations that have been cited for accuracy and completeness. It is possible for errors and omissions in fact to contribute to false observations. Staff who are most familiar with an area should be responsible for reviewing observations. *Third*, confirm that the resulting recommendation or required action is related to the observation. Superfluous recommendations should be minimized by be organization's scrutiny of the relationship between the finding or observation and the recommendation. *Fourth*, clarify which recommendations require action based on federal or state authority and which recommendations are made for management consideration in program improvement. This step should be completed early in the time frame for the response; it is best clarified during the review or audit process or during the exit conference. If necessary, ask for the report to be reissued if there is a reason to believe that an area is not clear. *Finally*, it may be necessary for organization personnel to clarify the action that must take place in order to satisfy the review or audit findings. If unclear, communications should take place with the review or audit staff. In most cases the organization will have the opportunity to agree with or dispute the findings. Additionally, some federal child nutrition programs allow for an appeal of findings. If this is the case, appeal rights and procedures must be included in the report of findings. Careful attention is warranted to the deadline for filing an appeal and the appeal procedures. Failure to meet the deadline or follow procedures will generally jeopardize the right to appeal.

FOLLOW-UP ACTIVITIES AND CLOSURE

The most significant work of audit or review activity takes place after the report is agreed on. As stated earlier in this chapter, the starting point for many review or audit activities is a review of previous activity and findings. For this reason and for a healthy attitude toward compliance, it is important that the organization take follow-up seriously. A good place to start is to develop a corrective action plan that, when implemented, will provide recommendations related to required performance. Recommendations for management improvement should also be considered as related to economy, efficiency, and effectiveness of the operation. Many review activities may require the organization to file a corrective action plan prior to the review's or audit's being closed. In many cases a follow-up visit may be required to ensure that the plan is implemented. The plan at a minimum should include the specific activity to be performed, those responsible for the activity and its oversight and final evaluation, the deadline for steps to occur in completing the activity, and resources required to the completion of the corrective action, including staff development.

One of the greatest benefits of a review or audit is that program personnel may use recommendations to justify much-needed program enhancements such as automation, incorporation in the school's or district's improvement efforts, delineation of roles and responsibilities, addition of staff, and funds for capital improvements. The successful program manager will scrutinize the audit or review report for opportunities to change situations in the school or district.

A significant component of the corrective action plan will be to modify internal procedures to achieve a particular goal. This is often accomplished by consulting with state or other local staff in identifying proven procedures to address some performance area cited in the report. Examples include internal control procedures and reporting or recording-keeping forms and procedures. The corrective action plan must provide for the management of performance of employees involved in the corrective action.

Staff development and training must be provided to clarify requirements and to introduce procedures to ensure their implementation as management planned. Records of staff development activity are important in evaluating the performance of employees, which is critical to compliance. Staff development resources are available from the state agency, from internal sources, or from peers. Personnel action, including coaching or disciplinary action, may be needed in order to correct deficiencies documented in the review or audit. The report may provide the organization the resource required to address personnel issues of which the organization was aware but unable to quantify. It is essential that the corrective action plan include a process for monitoring employees for the corrective action that has been outlined.

Observation of compliance activity over a period of time is necessary to ensure that compliance is not only instigated but institutionalized throughout the organization. The supervising manager or internal auditor should be responsible for ensuring that compliance is achieved with planned activities. Observations of continuing noncompliance should be documented and shared with appropriate evaluating personnel.

When an organization has fulfilled all requirements contained in the audit report to the satisfaction of the reviewing or auditing agency, the review or audit will be closed. A letter stating that closure is achieved is important for the file of activities.

SUMMARY

Review or audit activity contains many opportunities to support an organization's continuous improvement. The needs assessment process is critical to the continuous improvement cycle. Schools are under much pressure from the public to strive toward excellence through continuous improvements. The review or audit must be seen as another element in that continuous improvement process. Much leverage can be gained for the program manager who can use the review or audit activity to improve on conditions in the school or district. Most important, the public trust is enhanced through commitment to compliance in key performance areas as outlined in the statutory goals of the public assistance program and the agreement with the grantor agency. The successful program manager will use the odious experience of an audit or review to improve on program operations. Without regard to any recommendations resulting from the application of the review or audit standards, the process of preparing for an audit can fine-tune many processes within the school or the district. The successful school food and nutrition program director will also use the experience as an excellent opportunity to celebrate with staff and the general public the many processes that are performed each and every day and that are performed consistent with expectations.

CASE STUDY
INTERNAL CONTROLS

A large school food authority identified the following program irregularities. The manager of a high school with higher-than-average student participation was absent from work for an extended period. Central office staff was assigned to substitute for the absent manager. Two factors contributed to the district's identifying noncompliance at the school. First, using production records, staff ordered food based on historical meal count data. This practice produced excess quantities for the number of meals actually served in the manager's absence. Second, the district implemented a new automated system that polled meal counts from the point of service to the central accounting office. During the absence of the manager, the counts for paid meals dropped immediately. On investigation, the district discovered that the manager owned a catering operation.

The manager was overstating paid meal counts, thus over claiming state and federal funds. Excess foods had been ordered by the manager consistent with the inflated number of meals and taken from the premises for use in the catering business. Revenue from à la carte sales was reported as revenue from paid meals. The school food authority reported to the state grantor agency and, working under its supervision, reconstructed paid meal counts using comparable school data and procedures prescribed by the USDA, FNS for use when meal count systems break down. A reclaim was established, restitution to the state agency was made, and the incident was referred to the federal agency for criminal action.

From this case study, one can see the inordinate value of internal controls and the review of their implementation. Such controls include

- Polling meal counts from the original source
- Independent party verification of meal counts
- Statements of accuracy of meal counts by cashiers and review of original-source data
- Observation of student participation on days of visits compared with reported counts
- Daily reconciliation of beginning and ending inventory, sales by item and cash receipt related to à la carte items being sold
- Review of actual versus potential income
- The establishment of participation ranges by a comparable type school and notation of exceptions
- Rotation of key management personnel
- Employee declaration of conflicting interests such as a related business operation

CASE STUDY
EXTERNAL BUSINESS REVIEW

The local school board of a major school food authority embarked on a multiyear endeavor to seek external reviews of all its business functions. These included facility planning and maintenance; grants management; and budgeting and accounting, including investments, grounds maintenance, and school food services. Business review teams were composed of public and private-sector representatives selected by the district from recommendations submitted by board members, administrators within the district and neighboring districts, professional associations, and the state agency.

This school business function study team was composed of the food service director of a state university, a nutrition professor from another state university, the state agency program director, a corporate regional manager from a private national food service management company, a site manager for a metropolitan area catering corporation, a dietitian in charge of menu planning and analysis for a major corporate health care food service, and a dietitian supervising the food service and facility operations of a major urban residential care facility. Two team members were residents of the community. The team met for six months, reviewing data, visiting schools, interviewing program staff, school principals, students, and teachers. The team members presented their report with recommendations to the local board of education. The major recommendations included but were not limited to the following:

- Use high health inspection scores as a marketing tool for the program.
- Have nutrition education visible at all times, including analysis of nutrient value of meals.

- Promote breakfast at home or school.
- Utilize the food court concept more when designing and equipping high school kitchens and cafeterias.
- Expand the number of "monotony breakers" to promote meals.
- Use terminology such as best value, combo, meal deals, and best buy on menu signs to inform students of combinations that provide the best value for their food dollars.
- To enhance the site-based management currently in place, implement staff development for school administrators on how to evaluate their nutrition manager and what expectations they should have of their managers regarding adherence to regulations and other procedures.
- Formalize in each school an improvement plan for school nutrition as a part of the school's overall improvement plan. Such a plan could address system standards of accountability as well as important objectives related to the site operation; encourage principals to include a member of the school nutrition team as part of the school's improvement committee; and include specific standards of accountability for the school nutrition program that are components of results-based evaluation for schools.

For more information on the use of business review teams, contact the Associate Superintendent for Management Services and Operations, Gwinnett County Schools, P.O. Box 343, Lawrenceville, GA 30046-0343 or call (770) 963-8651.

REFERENCES

1. Appendix, Budget of the U.S. Government, Fiscal Year 1998, page 240.

2. American School Food Service Association, *Keys to Excellence: Standards of Practice for Nutrition Integrity* (Alexandria, VA: 1995).

3. Georgia Department of Education, *Quality Measures for Georgia's School Nutrition Program* (Atlanta, GA: 1997).

4. M.B. Gregoire and J. Sneed, "Competencies for District School Nutrition Directors/Supervisors," *School Food Service Research Review* 18 no. 2 (1994): 89–100.

5. Single Audit Act of 1984, Title 31, United States Code 7501.

6. Title 7, *Code of Federal Regulations,* Part 210.18, Administrative reviews .

7. Section 22, National School Lunch Act of 1946, Title 42, United States Code 1769c.

8. Title 7, *Code of Federal Regulations,* Part 210.18(g) and (h).

9. Title 7, *Code of Federal Regulations,* Part 210.10 and 220.8.

10. Title 7, C.F.R., Part 210.18.

11. Title 7, *Code of Federal Regulations,* Part 210.2, Definitions.

12. Section 12, National School Lunch Act of 1946, Title 42, United States Code 1760.

13. Title 7, *Code of Federal Regulations,* Part 225.7, Program Monitoring and Assistance.

14. Title 7, *Code of Federal Regulations,* Part 250.19, Reviews.

15. Title 7, *Code of Federal Regulations,* Part 226.6(l) and 226.23(h).

16. Title 7, *Code of Federal Regulations,* Part 227.31(b).

17. Section 4(f) and (g), Child Nutrition Act of 1966, Title 42, United States Code 1773.

18. Title 7, *Code of Federal Regulations,* Part 210.19(a)(6).

19. Title 7, *Code of Federal Regulations,* Part 235, State Administrative Expense Funds.

20. U.S. Department of Agriculture, Food and Nutrition Service, *Contracting with Food Service Management Companies—Guidance for School Food Authorities,* June 1995.

21. Title 7, *Code of Federal Regulations,* Part 210.18(a)-(f), (l)-(r).

22. *Federal Register* 51FR31313, September 3, 1986.

23. U.S. Department of Agriculture, Food and Nutrition Services, *Child Care Management Improvement Guidance—Day Care Homes* (1997) and *Child Care Management Improvement Guidance—Child Care Centers* (1998).

24. Title 7, *Code of Federal Regulations,* Part 210.19(a)(3), Improved Management Practices.

25. Title 7, *Code of Federal Regulations,* Part 227.36, Requirements of Needs Assessment.

26. American Schoold Food Service Association, *Keys to Excellence.*

27. Gregoire and Sneed, "Competencies for District School Nutrition Directors/Supervisors."

28. The National Association of College and University Food Services, *Professional Standards Manual* (East Lansing, MI: 1995).

29. National Parents and Teachers Association, *National Standards for Parent/Family Involvement Programs* [on-line]. Available: http://www.pta.org/programs/pfistand.htm#Foreword.

30. Government Accounting Standards Board. *Facts about GASB 1997* [on-line]. Available: http://www.rutgers.edu/Accounting/raw/gasb/facts/Mission97.htm.

31. Single Audit Act of 1984, Title 31, United States Code 7501.

32. Executive Office of the President, Office of Management and Budget, *Circular A-102, Uniform Requirements for Grants to State and Local Governments, Attachment P—Audit Requirements* (October 1979).

33. American Institute of Certified Public Accountants, *About the AICPA* [on-line]. Available: http://www.aicpa.org/about/index.htm.

34. Executive Office of the President, Office of Management and Budget, *Compliance Supplement for Single Audits of State and Local Governments* (September 1990).

35. Office of Inspector General. USDA [on-line] Available: http//www.usda.gov/agencies/agencies.htm.

36. U.S. Department of Agriculture, Office of Inspector General, *Twelve State Audit,* Report number 27611-1-Ch, 1979.

37. U.S. Department of Agriculture, Office of Inspector General. Report number 270099-45-At (1987).

38. U.S. Department of Agriculture, Office of Inspector General, Report number 27601-0007-Ch, Child Nutrition Programs—State Administrative Expense Funds.

39. U.S. Department of Agriculture, Office of Inspector General, Report Number 27099-25-SF, *Contracting of Food Service Management Companies in the National School Lunch Program* (June 1989).

40. Title 7, *Code of Federal Regulations,* Part 210.30, Management Evaluations.

41. United States General Accounting Office. (1998) About GAO [on-line]. Available: http://www.gao.gov/about.gao/about/gao/htm.

42. General Accounting Office Report Number GAO/RCED-90-12.

43. General Accounting Office Report Number GAO/RCED-94-36BR.

44. General Accounting Office Report Number GAO/RCED-96-191.

45. General Accounting Office Report Number GAO/RCED-96-217.

46. Title 7, *Code of Federal Regulations,* Part 210.8(a), Internal controls.

47. Section 9, National School Lunch Act of 1947, 42 United States Code 1758.

48. U.S. Department of Agriculture, Food and Nutrition Services, Publication FNS-260, *Accuclaim Manual: Meal Counts Count.*

49. U.S. Department of Agriculture, Food and Nutrition Services. Publication FNS-274, *Eligibility Guidance for School Meals Manual.*

50. U.S. Department of Agriculture, Food and Nutrition Services. Publication FNS-270, *Meal Counting and Claiming Manual.*

51. Title 7, *Code of Federal Regulations,* Part 210.19(a)(5).

52. New England Association of Schools and Colleges, Inc., *Accreditation Standards for the Commission on Public Elementary Schools (CPES)* [on-line] Available: http://www.mec.edu/neasc/cpestan.html and *Accreditation Standards for the Commission Public Secondary Schools (CPSS)* [on-line] Available: http://www.mec.edu/neasc/cpsstan.html.

Selected Chronology

USDA Review Initiatives in the School Nutrition Programs 1975–1998

The following events reflect the various accountability systems that the United States Department of Agriculture (USDA) has developed and advanced in the school nutrition program. Changes in federal, state, and local agency procedures have been required under each new system. The sequence of activities demonstrates the serious manner in which federal, state, and local agency personnel approached each of the various methods and subsequent resources required.

1975	USDA Food and Nutrition Services (FNS) initiated Management and Technical Assistance (MTA) reviews consisting of reviews of local programs by federal and state agency review staff; the system was abandoned.
November 15, 1978	USDA, FNS announced at 43 FR 53202 in its Semiannual Agenda of Regulations plans to amend regulations for management, evaluation; and improvement designed to improve accountability; proposal became known as Program Administrative Review System (PARS); proposal raised objections primarily due to its use of statistical calculations to determine eligible reimbursement rather than actual meal counts.
Spring 1979	Office of Inspector General (OIG) of USDA issued Audit Report number 27611-1-Ch, known as the *Twelve State Audit*.
October 30, 1979	USDA proposed Assessment, Improvement and Monitoring System (AIMS) regulations at 44 FR 62453. As an alternative to PARS, AIMS was proposed to be implemented in cooperation with the state agencies to assist them

to identify operational and management problems in the administration of school nutrition programs; the AIMS intended was for state agencies to use in reviews of local programs.

November–December 1979	USDA conducted public meetings on AIMS.
December 11, 1979	American School Food Service Association (ASFSA) issued white paper on AIMS.
December 12, 1979	Congressional Subcommittee on Elementary, Secondary and Vocational Education, House Education and Labor Committee conducted hearings on AIMS.
December 13, 1979	Members of subcommittee appealed to Secretary of Agriculture Bergland to extend comment period on AIMS. Period extended to February 1, 1980.
April 28, 1979	USDA issued FNS Handbook 210, AIMS Suggested Guidance.
1984	Congress passed the Single Audit Act of 1984.
May 1987	OIG of USDA issued Roll-up Audit Report number 27099-445-At covering 13 school food authorities (SFAs) in six states and indicating that meal counts were not valid despite USDA, FNS initiatives, including AIMS.
Fall 1987	USDA initiated Strategic Planning and Management System (SPAM), an internal agency initiative to improve meal counting and claiming procedures, including an increased federal presence at the state and local agency levels.
September 9, 1988	USDA proposed in the *Federal Register* at 53 FR 35083 regulations intended to improve the accuracy of meal counting and claiming procedures through strengthened regulatory requirements and improved technical assistance to state and local agencies; initiative was known as Accuclaim.

August 1988

USDA announced Child Nutrition Federal Review Initiative (CNFRI), an agency review effort in addition to pending Accuclaim proposal.

September 1988

USDA renamed agency system from CNFRI to Federal Accountability Review Initiative (FAIR).

Fall 1988

1989 Agriculture Appropriations Act authorized $5.2 million for USDA to conduct independent verifications of school lunch claims. Conference report required USDA to use one-half for training and technical assistance.

1989

USDA announced Federal Review System (FRS), a new federal agency review initiative requiring over 100 pages of instructions and instrumentation.

March 28, 1989

USDA issued final Accuclaim regulations in the *Federal Register* at 54 FR 12575.

July 1989

USDA assembled Accuclaim Task Force of state/local personnel.

Summer 1989

USDA officials indicated that if a then-proposed "unified system" of reviews were required by Congress, there would be no public comment offered.

November 1989

Public Law 101-147, the 1989 Child Nutrition and WIC Reauthorization Bill directed USDA to develop a unified system of accountability to coordinate state and federal review efforts to ensure compliance and to minimize paperwork and burden on local school districts, and to do so through publications of regulations and the provision for public comment.

Spring 1990

USDA met with local and state agency ASFSA representatives to develop basic concept of a Coordinated Review Effort (CRE) to be proposed through regulation. USDA presented a concept. A concern by state and local personnel in attendance was that full agenda, as announced, was not conducted, including questions, answers, and significant input by state and local personnel.

December 21, 1990 — USDA proposed regulations on CRE. Over 4,000 comments were received. Original comment deadline was extended from February 19, 1991, to April 5, 1991, due to the large amount of interest.

1991 — USDA announced a new federal agency review initiative, Management Evaluation Local Level Review System (MELLRS), using a 102-page document for their use in reviewing local programs.

July 17, 1991 — USDA published final regulations on CRE at 56 FR 32920, with an effective date of July 1, 1992.

September and November 1991 and January 1992 — USDA met with task of force federal, state, and local personnel to design CRE system.

December 1991 and January 1992 — CRE was tested in several states.

February 1992 — American School Food Service Association members on Task Force report at ASFSA Legislative Conference on issues within CRE that continued to create burdens on state and local agencies.

May 1992 — State agency reviewers trained on CRE procedures.

June 1994 — USDA proposed regulations that would require nutrient-based menu planning

November 2, 1994 — PL 103-448, the Healthy Meals for Healthy Americans Act of 1994, was enacted requiring school meals to adhere to dietary guidelines, effective school year 1996–1997 and prohibiting the secretary of agriculture from requiring schools using food-based menu system from conducting or using a nutrient analysis.

January 1995

USDA proposed supplemental regulations based on provision for a food-based menu planning system in PL 103-448.

June 13, 1995

USDA published final rule on Healthy School Meal Initiative requiring state agencies to review SFAs for compliance with nutrient standards.

May 29, 1996

PL 104-149 amended the National School Lunch Act to allow use of current meal pattern or "any reasonable approach" to menu planning that would meet dietary standards and not require a nutrient analysis be conducted or used by the local schools.

1997

USDA trained state agency personnel on requirements of Healthy School Meals Initiatives for the purpose of conducting regulatory reviews.

February 1998

No regulations proposed by USDA to date to implement the "any reasonable approach" provision of PL 104-149.

March 1998

USDA, FNS headquarters announced their OIG upcoming audits of the National School Lunch Program—Meal Accountability and Claims in five of OIG's six regions. Audits are to evaluate the procedures for and the accuracy of meal reimbursements and the adequacy of FNS and state agency review of meal counts, claims, and eligibility determinations. In each region one state agency, a judgmentally selected SFA, and statistically selected schools within the SFA would be audited.

PART III

Nutrition

CHAPTER 9

Educating beyond the Plate: The Cafeteria–Classroom Connection

Amanda Dew Manning

OUTLINE

INTRODUCTION

The role of nutrition education in successful management of school food and nutrition programs is critical. Just as menu planning, purchasing, and preparation are essential management components of a successful, well-managed program, so is nutrition education. Nutrition education is the link between theory and practice. If schools plan, purchase, prepare, and serve healthy foods that children will not eat, the programs certainly do not benefit children, and the best intentions go unfulfilled. Children and their parents are demanding customers! It is not enough for the food served in schools to be healthful, it must taste great, be acceptable to the customers, and be served in an appealing, exciting environment. Students report that food *taste* is the most important factor in making a decision to eat in the school cafeteria. Other reasons reported are cost, appearance, nutritional value, and whether friends eat there.[1] Nutrition education is not just education about food; it is marketing and public relations as well. Nutrition education can increase the value of school nutrition services to parents, administrators, teachers, and students. And happy students and parents can mean that participation in school meal programs increases. A positive image of the food service program, and support from parents and students, can influence the school administration's commitment to, and support of, the school food and nutrition program as part of the total educational experience.

After studying this chapter, the student will be able to articulate the need and rationale for nutrition education in schools, identify the respective roles and responsibilities of the director and the manager in nutrition education, understand the key strategies for successful nutrition education programs, and relate professional standards of practice to one's own professional development.

THE NEED FOR NUTRITION EDUCATION

Providing healthful meals for children in school is not enough. To adopt healthy eating practices children need to learn about foods, experience eating healthful foods, learn how nutritious foods help their bodies grow and develop, and be able to develop the skills necessary to form lifelong healthy eating habits. According to the Centers for Disease Control and Prevention (CDC), healthy eating patterns in childhood and adolescence promote optimal childhood health, growth, and intellectual development; prevent immediate health problems, such as iron deficiency anemia, obesity, eating disorders, and dental caries; and may prevent long-term health problems, such as coronary heart disease, cancer, and stroke.[2] The school food and nutrition programs offer an exceptional opportunity not only to serve children nutritious meals, but also to educate them about nutrition. Because dietary factors contribute substantially to the burden of preventable illness and premature death in the United States, the national health promotion and disease prevention objectives encourage schools to provide nutrition education from preschool through grade 12.[3] The Nutrition Education and Training (NET) program, administered by the U.S. Department of Agriculture (USDA), recommends in its strategic plan that by the year 2000 nutrition education be a major component of child nutrition programs and be offered in all schools, child-care facilities, and summer sites.[4] Evidence clearly indicates that nutrition and learning go hand in hand. Well-nourished, healthy children have better attendance at school, concentrate more on their lessons, and achieve improved performance.[5,6] Goal 1 of the *National Education Goals Report* contains the following objective: children receive the nutrition and health care needed to arrive at school with healthy minds and bodies.[7] Experience shows that children often have knowledge about good nutrition, yet they do not always make healthful food choices. Therefore, it is essential that nutrition education opportunities through these and other programs concentrate not only on knowledge and attitudes, but behavior as well. The goal of any school-based nutrition education program should be to focus on helping children develop the skills and the motivation to adopt lifelong eating patterns that comply with the *Dietary Guidelines for Americans* (Figure 9–1) and the Food Guide Pyramid (Figure 9–2) published by the USDA and the Department of Health and Human Services. Many young people in the United States are making dietary choices that put them at risk for health-related problems. Establishing healthy eating patterns at an early age is critical. Poor dietary patterns that are established in childhood often follow into adulthood, and are difficult to change. According to the CDC, the consequences of poor eating habits are as follows[8]:

- Chronically undernourished children are more likely to become sick, miss class, and score lower on tests.
- Research suggests that not having breakfast can affect children's academic performance.
- Poor eating habits and inactivity are the root causes of overweight and obesity.
- Eating disorders such as anorexia and bulimia can cause severe health problems and even death.
- Poor diet and inactivity cause at least 300,000 deaths among U.S. adults each year.

Current research shows that children's diets are not what they should be. The percentage of young people who are overweight has doubled in the past 30 years. Eating disorders such as anorexia and bulimia are increasing among young people. In addition:

- More that 84 percent of young people eat too much fat, and more than 91 percent eat too much saturated fat.
- Only one young person in five eats the recommended five daily servings of fruits and vegetables. Fifty-one percent of children and adolescents eat less than one serving of fruit a day, and 29 percent eat less than one serving a day of vegetables that are not fried.

- The average calcium intake of adolescent girls is about 800 mg a day, considerably less than the recommended dietary allowance (RDA) of 1,300 mg of calcium a day.
- One student in five aged 15 to 18 regularly skips breakfast.
- Eight percent of high school girls take laxatives or vomit to lose or keep from gaining weight, and nine percent take diet pills. Harmful weight-loss practices have been reported among girls as young as nine years old.[8]

NUTRITION EDUCATION IN SCHOOLS

"Nutrition education is defined as any set of learning experiences designed to facilitate the voluntary adoption of eating and other nutrition-related behaviors conducive to health and well-being."[9(p285)]) Schools are ideal settings in which such learning experiences can take place. More than 95 percent of children in the United States, ages 5–17, are enrolled in schools.[10] School food and nutrition programs offer a "laboratory" for children to eat healthy meals—with approximately 26 million meals served each day in the school lunch program and approximately 6 million meals served in the school breakfast program—and to learn about good nutrition. Schools have skilled personnel who, with appropriate training, can contribute to the nutrition education program. Nutrition education in schools is supported by several national organizations. The American Dietetics Association (ADA) supports nutrition education for recipients of child and adolescent food and nutrition programs. The ADA's position statement on child and adolescent food and nutrition programs makes the following point:

Appropriate nutrition education to recipients of child and adolescent food and nutrition programs is recognized as a key factor in health promotion/chronic disease prevention.

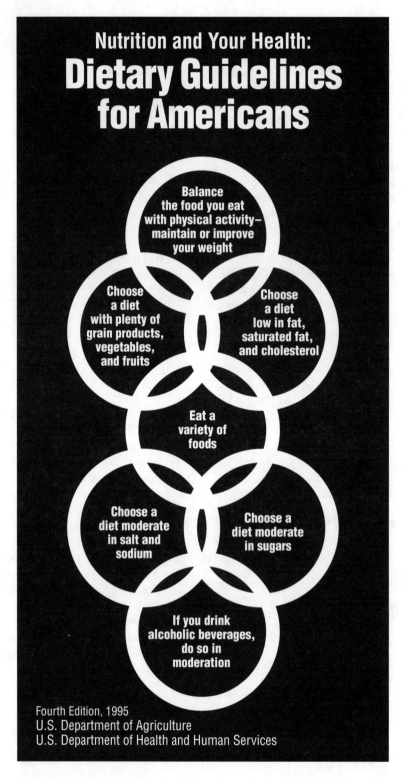

Figure 9–1 Dietary Guidelines for Americans. *Source*: Reprinted from U.S. Department of Agriculture and US Department of Health and Human Services, *Nutrition and Your Health: Dietary Guidelines for Americans, 4th ed.*, 1995.

Food Guide Pyramid
A Guide to Daily Food Choices

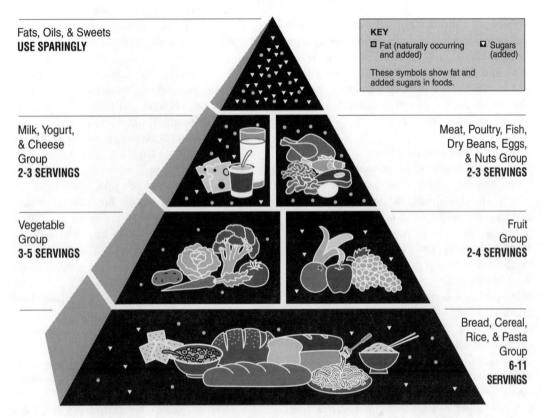

Fats, Oils, & Sweets
USE SPARINGLY

KEY
▫ Fat (naturally occurring and added)   ◪ Sugars (added)

These symbols show fat and added sugars in foods.

Milk, Yogurt, & Cheese Group
2-3 SERVINGS

Meat, Poultry, Fish, Dry Beans, Eggs, & Nuts Group
2-3 SERVINGS

Vegetable Group
3-5 SERVINGS

Fruit Group
2-4 SERVINGS

Bread, Cereal, Rice, & Pasta Group
6-11 SERVINGS

Figure 9–2 Food Guide Pyramid. *Source:* Reprinted from U.S. Department of Agriculture, *Food Guide Pyramid*, 4th ed., 1995.

As part of any comprehensive health program, nutrition should be integrated across the curriculum, in all subject areas. Delivery of nutrition education should include experiences that use integrated education resources such as the cafeteria dining area, health and physical education classes, and mathematics and writing skills designed to enhance critical thinking processes.[11]

The ADA, the Society for Nutrition Education (SNE), and the American School Food Service Association (ASFSA) issued a position statement on school-based nutrition programs and services as follows:

It is the position of the American Dietetics Association, the Society for Nutrition Education and the American School Food Service Association that comprehensive school-based nutrition programs and services be provided to all the nation's elementary and secondary students. These programs and services include: effective education in foods and nutrition; a school environment that provides opportunity and reinforcement for healthful eating and physical activity; involvement of parents and the community; and screening, counseling, and referral for nutrition problems as part of school health services.[12]

Teachers and other staff who are trained can use their educational skills to deliver age-appropriate, culturally relevant nutrition education. And finally, schools can teach students how to resist social pressures that have a negative impact on healthy eating practices, and encourage positive peer influence toward healthy eating practices.[13]

As with many other efforts in schools, a partnership of school personnel working together enhances the potential success of these efforts. The coordinated school health program offers such a model. State education and health agencies, as well as many local education agencies, are currently implementing coordinated school health programs. Eight interrelated components have been identified as being part of a coordinated school health program: (1) health education; (2) physical education; (3) nutrition services; (4) health services; (5) healthy school environment; (6) counseling, psychological, and social services; (7) health promotion for staff, and (8) parent and community involvement.[14] Each of these components has its own distinct characteristics and key elements, but they have common threads that support the health and well-being of children. Each component has linkages to each other component. Staff from each component can support each other in a cooperative and synergistic way with a common overall philosophy and goal for the entire school or district doing the implementation. Nutrition education clearly has a place in each component. For example, nutrition is a part of the health education curriculum in the school, as well as being taught in other subject areas. The integration of nutrition into other core subject areas such as math, science, and language arts makes nutrition a part of the core curriculum, and gives teachers an added incentive to teach nutri-

tion—not separately, but as part of required subjects. Nutrition fits nicely into physical education as well. Young people desiring to be better athletes certainly can benefit from accurate nutrition information to help them look, feel, and perform their best (see Figure 9–3).

The key elements of the nutrition services component of a coordinated school health program are nutritious foods; nutrition education; nutrition policies and supporting practices; screening; assessment; individual care plan; intervention; referral and follow-up; professional development; partnerships (within the school and the community), public relations and marketing; and quality criteria, evaluation, and continuous improvement.[15,16] The school food and nutrition program director is uniquely qualified to take the leadership role in implementing the nutrition services component of coordinated school health programs. The director has an ever-widening circle of influence over nutrition activities in the school and community.

A future goal for some school food and nutrition professionals, looking toward redefining programs for the new millennium, is to establish a school nutrition center where nutrition education and nutrition services are provided to students, school staff, and the community (see Figure 9–4).

A 1996 survey by the National Center for Education Statistics found that 99 percent of all public schools offer nutrition education somewhere in the curriculum, and many integrate it into the total curriculum. However, the intensity and quality of the nutrition messages was not evaluated. In addition, the survey found that approximately 90 percent of schools offer nutrition education through the school meals program. However, less than half of school meals programs offer nutrient information, serve meals to correspond with classroom activities, give tours, or provide nutrition input to newsletters. And less than one-quarter of school meals programs provide nutrition education in the classroom or conduct tasting parties.[17]

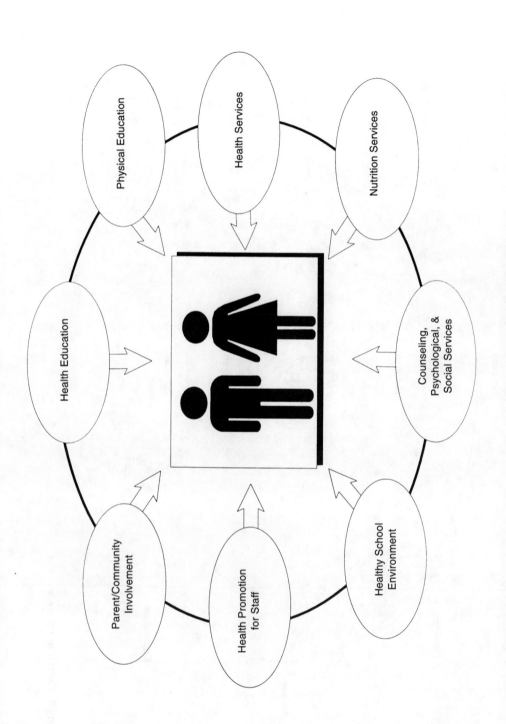

Figure 9–3 A Coordinated School Health Program. *Source:* Reprinted from A.D. Manning, Division of Adolescent and School Health, © 1994, Centers for Disease Control and Prevention.

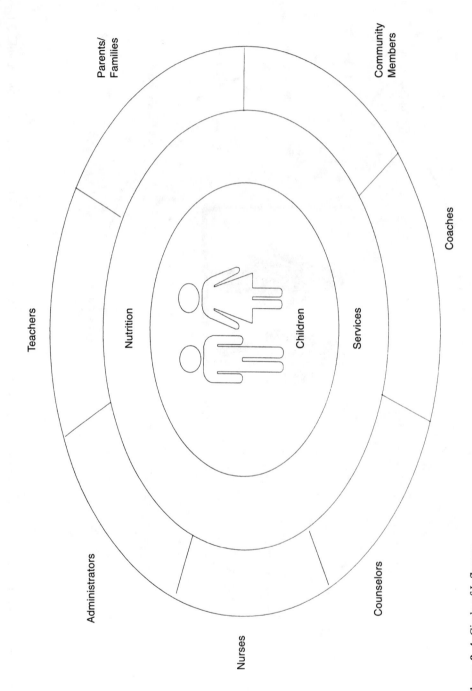

Figure 9–4 Circle of Influence.

LINKAGES BETWEEN THE CAFETERIA AND CLASSROOM

School cafeteria and classroom nutrition education activities that actively engage children can help them on the road to developing lifelong healthy eating habits. What better way to educate children about food and nutrition than in the school cafeteria? School food and nutrition professionals are uniquely equipped to provide creative nutrition education in the cafeteria—by the healthy, tasty foods they provide; by offering special promotions, activities, and events; and by forming a link with classroom teachers to make presentations in the classroom when children are studying geography, science, or history. Helping teachers introduce students to new foods by conducting a tasting party is a great way to get students interested in new foods, and to get them slowly to accept those foods in the school cafeteria. Other nutrition education ideas include cafeteria tours, nutrition contests and promotions, athletic training tables, theme days, school gardens, cooking demonstrations, suggestion boxes, and computer and video demonstrations. Classroom activities and cafeteria activities must provide consistent messages about nutrition and health. There should be mutual reinforcement of nutrition education activities being conducted throughout the school. The cafeteria becomes a *learning laboratory* where students can apply what they have learned in the classroom. In addition to the ideas above, the CDC's "Guidelines for School Health Programs To Promote Lifelong Healthy Eating" offers the following suggestions for school food and nutrition professionals to support the classroom-cafeteria link:

- Visit the classrooms and explain how school meals meet nutrition standards, including the Dietary Guidelines for Americans.
- Invite classes to visit the cafeteria kitchen and learn about preparing healthful foods.
- Involve students in planning school menus and preparing recipes.

- Decorate the cafeteria with nutrition posters and messages.
- Display nutrition information (a nutrition analysis of the meals served) about foods available and give students opportunities to practice food analysis and selection skills learned in the classroom.
- Coordinate activities with classroom teachers and other school staff.

Teachers can support cafeteria activities by teaching about nutritious foods served in the cafeteria, helping students understand the nutrition analysis of schools meals given out by the food service staff, and tie in education contests and fun activities with nutrition promotions in the cafeteria.[18]

EFFECTIVE STRATEGIES FOR SCHOOL-BASED NUTRITION EDUCATION

Children are sophisticated and getting more so every year! In an age where technology abounds, efforts to "compete" with advertising and marketing to kids offers a unique challenge. Nutrition educators must use current and proven strategies to be successful in their efforts (see Appendix 9–A). And educators must learn from competitors. The CDC's "Guidelines for School Health Programs To Promote Lifelong Healthy Eating" offer the following seven recommendations for effective school-based nutrition education programs. These guidelines are based on a review of research, theory, and current practice, and they were developed by the CDC in collaboration with experts from universities and from national, federal, and voluntary agencies. These recommendations form a foundation for ensuring a quality nutrition education program within a comprehensive school health program. The recommendations are as follows:

1. *Policy:* Adopt a coordinated school nutrition policy that promotes healthy eating through classroom lessons and a supportive school environment.

2. *Curriculum for nutrition education:* Implement nutrition education from preschool through secondary school as part of a sequential, comprehensive school health education curriculum designed to help students adopt healthy eating behaviors.

3. *Instruction for students:* Provide nutrition education through developmentally appropriate, culturally relevant, fun, participatory activities that involve social learning strategies.

4. *Integration of school food service and nutrition education:* Coordinate school food service with nutrition education and with other components of the compressive school health program to reinforce messages on healthy eating.

5. *Training for school staff:* Provide staff involved in nutrition education with adequate preservice and ongoing in-service training that focuses on teaching strategies for behavioral change.

6. *Family and community involvement:* Involve family members and the community in supporting and reinforcing nutrition education.

7. *Program evaluation:* Regularly evaluate the effectiveness of the school health program in promoting healthy eating, and change the program as appropriate to increase its effectiveness.[18]

RESPONSIBILITIES OF THE SCHOOL FOOD AND NUTRITION PROFESSIONAL

School food and nutrition professionals are in a unique position to offer healthful, tasty foods to children and to promote nutrition education. Nutrition education is a shared responsibility—between the school food and nutrition program director and the manager. However, they should not have to do the job alone. Working in partnership with administrators, teachers, and other members of the comprehensive school health program reduces the time and effort it takes to plan and provide nutrition education, and the benefits of combining expertise and pooling resources makes for a more effective program. Therefore, it is not a question of whether school food and nutrition staff should be involved in nutrition education; it is a matter of how much time each day or each week to devote to it. A director might spend one to two hours per week organizing, coordinating, and supporting activities from the district level. A manager at the school level who spends just one hour per day on nutrition education—whether talking to students coming through the line, going to a classroom, arranging for foods to be sent to the classroom for a tasting event, preparing a newsletter to send home with students, or planning with the school's comprehensive school health team—will reap great rewards. The benefits of working in partnership and providing nutrition education can bring enormous benefits to the school food and nutrition programs. For example:

- Making the cafeteria a laboratory for nutrition education increases the value of the school food and nutrition program to parents, administrators, teachers, and students.
- Nutrition education can help make the link to the school food service's role in the total education experience at school.
- Nutrition education activities can align the cafeteria with the core curriculum.
- Student participation and food consumption go up, and food waste drops.
- Students' improved eating habits are a credit to your efforts and a boost to the school community.[19]

The ultimate goal of providing nutrition education should be healthier foods that are enjoyed by students, greater participation in the programs, excellent service, positive community support, and healthier students.

THE DIRECTOR'S ROLE

Nutrition education must be valued and supported by the school district *and* the local school. At the district office, the school food and nutrition program director takes the lead responsibility for ensuring that nutrition education is recognized as an integral part of the district's instructional program. This is most likely to occur if the director does the following:

- Works with district staff to help them understand the value of educating students about nutrition and its role in good health and academic performance
- Works with district curriculum planners and staff development personnel to have nutrition education presented in a multidisciplinary manner, and to include nutrition in the district's instructional plan and staff development/continuing education activities
- Coordinates identification and dissemination of nutrition education resources with the public relations and media staff (This could include scheduling nutrition education programs over the district's satellite network.)
- Incorporates nutrition education as an integral function in the school nutrition program manager's job description and allows time in the manager's workday for this function
- Establishes a collaborative relationship at the district office with instructional, health services, and other key staff
- Forms an alliance/network with other nutrition professionals in the community to seek their support as resource persons for nutrition education, and also to promote the delivery of consistent nutrition messages—whether the child or caregiver receives these in the school setting, at the women, infants, and children (WIC) clinic, or in the 4-H club meeting
- Provides in-service for all school food and nutrition personnel on strategies for working with the total school health team, and develops and implements effective nutrition education that focuses on the cafeteria as a learning laboratory

THE MANAGER'S ROLE

The role of the school food and nutrition program manager is one of implementer and bridge builder. The manager has the day-to-day responsibility for implementing the policies and philosophy that the director and the district office administrators have established, and for building bridges to gain support and collaboration at the school level. This collaboration among school staff is essential to effectively linking the classroom and the cafeteria.

Ideally, the school principal will have an administrative policy clearly stating the importance of the school food and nutrition program to the total educational program at that school. This includes scheduling meals and allowing adequate time for children to eat those meals, having the manager attend faculty meetings, and including nutrition as part of in-service training and staff development. The manager may have to work with the principal to ensure that such a policy is in place and that it is implemented. By establishing a positive relationship with teachers and other staff, the manager can help ensure that there is support throughout the school for such a policy. With a positive working relationship established with administrators and teachers, the manager can initiate meetings to plan strategies for coordinating cafeteria and classroom. Such meetings serve to inform others about the food and nutrition program, gain buy-in, share ideas and concerns, and develop ways to work together. The results of such meetings could be the development of a schoolwide plan for nutrition education.

Managers might begin by asking the social studies teachers their schedules for studying various countries and offering to support that unit of study with theme menus, cafeteria decorations, and posters. Another way for the manager to initiate collaboration is to offer to place nutrition resource materials in the media center for all teachers to use. Managers can also offer to include teachers and other school staff in menu-planning activities.

Building bridges requires taking the initiative; establishing good, two-way communication; and being persistent. The result of taking the time and making a genuine effort to build relationships at the school level will mean greater support for the school food and nutrition program in every school.

STANDARDS OF PRACTICE FOR SCHOOL FOOD AND NUTRITION PROFESSIONALS

The ASFSA's *Keys to Excellence: Standards of Practice for Nutrition Integrity* is a self-assessment tool designed to help schools achieve nutrition integrity goals at the management and operational levels.[20] This tool provides a framework and plan of action for continuous improvement of programs. Nutrition education is a key area in this tool (see Exhibit 9–1).

The National Food Service Management Institute (NFSMI) published *Competencies, Knowledge, and Skills of Effective District School Nutrition Directors/Supervisors: Entry-Level and Beyond.*[21] This document suggests the following competencies in nutrition education for various levels of school food service personnel (See Exhibit 9–2).

The ASFSA's document *Creating Policy for Nutrition Integrity in Schools* includes as a core concept the following: "Nutrition education will be an integral part of the curriculum from preschool to twelfth grade. The school cafeteria will serve as a laboratory for applying knowledge and skills taught in the classroom."[22]

PLANNING FOR SUCCESS

The key to success is planning. Great leaders always spend time planning, and school food and nutrition program directors are leaders in school-based nutrition education. The vision that the director has for nutrition education, and the ability to communicate that vision to others, is paramount to the program's success. Also, personal commitment and a positive upbeat attitude are key to motivating others to join the nutrition education team, and stay with it! There is a wealth of material and assistance available to the director who wants to plan and implement a successful nutrition education effort (see Appendix 9–B). State child nutrition program staffs, and the nutrition education and training program staff are two state-level resources that can be helpful. The *Evaluation Guide for the Nutrition Education and Training Program* (1995)[23] and the *Needs Assessment Guide for the Nutrition Education and Training Program* (1994)[24] are two good planning documents. Community resources include the cooperative extension service, local voluntary health groups such as the American Heart Association and the American Cancer Society, college and university nutrition staff and students, dietitians, local health care providers, chefs, and others.

The success of nutrition education will not be achieved by the school food and nutrition director alone. It must be a team effort with school food and nutrition managers and other staff, teachers, administrators, parents, and students—all involved, and sharing responsibility. Time spent on upfront planning will enable nutrition education efforts to be successful, and it will put the school food and nutrition program in a very positive light with teachers, administrators, parents, and students. The following are suggested steps in planning a successful nutrition education effort in schools. (These steps are written primarily to assist the director in planning at the district level; however, they can also be helpful in planning at the school level.)

1. *Set goals and objectives:* Develop nutrition education goals and objectives that fit into the district's overall strategic

Exhibit 9–1 ASFSA's Keys to Excellence

KEY AREA: Nutrition Education

Key Achievement 2: Nutrition education is an integral part of the curriculum form pre-school through twelfth grade.

Standards of Practice	Work Needed	Plan Developed	Plan Implemented	Achieved
2.1 Nutrition education is provided at all grade levels as a component of comprehensive school health education programs and is coordinated with the school foodservice and nutrition program.				
Indicators: a. School foodservice and nutrition personnel are included as members of the nutrition/health teams that design and implement nutrition education programs.				
b. School foodservice and nutrition personnel support educational efforts implemented in the classroom, for example, tasting parties.				
2.2 Nutrition education materials and resources for all grade levels are provided for students, teachers and school foodservice and nutrition personnel.				
Indicators: a. Age appropriate/current nutrition education materials are readily accessible to teachers.				
b. Nutrition education materials are actively marketed to teachers.				

continues

Source: Reprinted with permission from American School Food Service Association, *Keys to Excellence: Standards of Practice for Nutrition Integrity,* © 1995, American School Food Service Association.

Exhibit 9–1 continued

Standards of Practice	Work Needed	Plan Developed	Plan Implemented	Achieved
c. Resource lists of nutrition education materials, including films, newsletters, videos, teaching kits, etc. are distributed to students, teachers and school foodservice and nutrition personnel.				
2.3. School foodservice and nutrition personnel assist teachers, school administrators and parents with nutrition education.				
Indicators: a. School foodservice and nutrition manager visits classroom or student clubs during the school year.				
b. Teachers are provided with a list of nutrition education opportunities through the school foodservice and nutrition program that are consistent with curriculum objectives.				
2.4. The school foodservice and nutrition program provides opportunities to reinforce classroom instruction.				
Indicators: a. School policy promotes joint nutrition learning experiences in the classroom and the cafeteria.				
b. Nutrition education materials are used in the cafeteria and on the serving line.				

continues

Exhibit 9–1 continued

Standards of Practice	Work Needed	Plan Developed	Plan Implemented	Achieved
c. Students working for the school foodservice and nutrition program gain skills in various aspects of the program.				
d. Student planned menus are used at least one time each year.				
2.5 Students are given guidance for the selection of healthful snacks.				
Indicators: a. District policy on the sale of foods outside the meals program is established and followed.				
b. Snacks offered for school activities by the school foodservice and nutrition program model and promote health eating habits.				
c. Nutrition education materials and resources about healthful snacks are provided by the school foodservice and nutrition program for the students and classroom teachers.				

continues

Exhibit 9–1 continued

Standards of Practice	Work Needed	Plan Developed	Plan Implemented	Achieved
2.6. Nutrition education incorporates principles of the Dietary Guidelines for Americans and the Food Guide Pyramid.				
Indicators: a. School foodservice and nutrition personnel provide materials to instructional staff related to the *Dietary Guidelines for Americans and Food Guide Pyramid.* b. School foodservice and nutrition personnel serve as resources in their school for nutrition activities. c. Message on menues contain information about the *Dietary Guidelines for Americans and Food Guide Pyramid.*				

Exhibit 9–2 NFSMI's Competencies in School Nutrition

FUNCTIONAL AREA 16: NUTRITION EDUCATION

16.1 Develops and implements a comprehensive nutrition education program using school food service as a learning laboratory.

16.2 Establishes role of CNP [child nutrition program] as a resource of expertise in the development and presentation of nutrition education materials and activities.

Source: D. Carr et al., *Competencies, Knowledge, and Skills of Effective School Nutrition Directors/Supervisors,* University, MS, National Food Service Management Institute, 1996.

COMPETENCY 16.1 DEVELOPS AND IMPLEMENTS A COMPREHENSIVE NUTRITION EDUCATION PROGRAM USING SCHOOL FOOD SERVICE AS A LEARNING LABORATORY.*

ENTRY-LEVEL

KNOWLEDGE STATEMENTS

Knows basic principles of nutrition as applied to developmental needs for children.

Knows basic nutrition education principles.

Knows importance of CNP personnel serving as members of the nutrition/health teams that design and implement nutrition education programs.

Knows educational goals of federally funded nutrition education programs.

SKILL STATEMENTS

Promotes healthy eating habits and provides guidelines for selecting healthful snacks through nutrition education and appropriate marketing in the school cafeteria.

Promotes activities to increase nutrition awareness among faculty, staff, and community.

BEYOND ENTRY-LEVEL

KNOWLEDGE STATEMENTS

Knows importance of including school nutrition services and nutrition education as a component of the comprehensive school health education program.

Knows effective strategies for changing customer's eating behaviors through nutrition education.

Knows importance of reinforcing classroom learning and the use of the cafeteria as a learning laboratory.

Knows principles of integrating nutrition education into the existing school curriculum.

SKILL STATEMENTS

Forms partners with the education community to support an integrated approach to education and nutrition needs.

Provides support and leadership for the development of a comprehensive nutrition curriculum, K–12.

continues

Source: Data from M. Gregoire and J. Sneed, Standards for Nutrition Integrity, *School Foodservice Research Review,* Vol. 18, pp. 106–111, © 1994, American School Food Service Association and *Competencies, Knowledge and Skills of Effective District School Nutrition Directors/Supervisors,* Functional Area 16: Nutrition Education, Competencies 16.1 and 16.2, © 1996, National Food Service Management Institute.

Exhibit 9–2 continued

COMPETENCY 16.1 DEVELOPS AND IMPLEMENTS A COMPREHENSIVE NUTRITION EDUCATION PROGRAM USING SCHOOL FOOD SERVICE AS A LEARNING LABORATORY.*

BEYOND ENTRY-LEVEL

SKILLS STATEMENTS, cont'd

Furnishes CNP expertise to the nutrition/health team in designing and implementing nutrition education programs.

Works with school officials and board of education to establish a district policy on sale and service of food outside the CNP.

Provides nutrition education programs and directs in-service training on nutrition education topics for administrators, teachers, and other staff members.

Consults with appropriate school officials about providing nutrition education guidelines to children with special dietary problems.

Involves CNP personnel as partners in classroom nutrition education activities.

Monitors school district's progress toward nutrition/health education goals.

*Competencies 16.1, 16.3, 16.4, 16.5, 16.7, 16.12, 16.13 from Gregoire & Sneed research.

COMPETENCY 16.2 ESTABLISHES ROLE OF CNP AS A RESOURCE OF EXPERTISE IN THE DEVELOPMENT AND PRESENTATION OF NUTRITION EDUCATION MATERIALS AND ACTIVITIES.*

ENTRY-LEVEL	*BEYOND ENTRY-LEVEL*
KNOWLEDGE STATEMENTS	**KNOWLEDGE STATEMENTS**
Knows techniques for development of educational materials and activities.	Knows principles of group dynamics.
Knows methods suitable for teaching children.	Knows relationship of learning to perceived benefits of interest in topic.

continues

Exhibit 9–2 continued

COMPETENCY 16.2 ESTABLISHES ROLE OF CNP AS A RESOURCE OF EXPERTISE IN THE DEVELOPMENT AND PRESENTATION OF NUTRITION EDUCATION MATERIALS AND ACTIVITIES.*

ENTRY-LEVEL

KNOWLEDGE STATEMENTS, cont'd

Knows sources for nutrition education materials for all grade levels.

SKILL STATEMENTS

Provides teachers with sources of nutrition education materials that can be provided by the CNP and are consistent with curriculum objectives.

Promotes nutrition education by providing information about menu items and snacks served at school.

Provides educational activities that help customers develop the behavorial and decision-making skills needed for making healthful food choices.

BEYOND ENTRY-LEVEL

KNOWLEDGE STATEMENTS, cont'd

Knows the educational process within the school district.

SKILL STATEMENTS

Develops and distributes resource listings of nutrition education materials to teachers, students, and parents.

Serves as a resource to instructional staff and CNP personnel for nutrition education activities.

Designs projects for the CNP that create opportunities to reinforce classroom instruction.

Coordinates the school menu and delivery of meals with nutrition education activities in the classroom.

Provides customers with accurate nutrition information and education concerning health issues related to eating habits (e.g. weight problems, eating disorders, etc.).

Develops educational experiences that teach children about school meals contribution to their health.

Encourages nutrition advisory councils and other student groups to become active participants in suggesting nutrition education objectives.

Works with instructional staff to develop a system for evaluating education materials and activities for various age/developmental levels of children.

continues

Exhibit 9–2 continued

COMPETENCY 16.2 ESTABLISHES ROLE OF CNP AS A RESOURCE OF EXPERTISE IN THE DEVELOPMENT AND PRESENTATION OF NUTRITION EDUCATION MATERIALS AND ACTIVITIES.*

BEYOND ENTRY-LEVEL

SKILLS STATEMENTS, cont'd

Evaluates effectiveness of nutrition education materials on changing customer behavior.

Communicates effectively with administrators, teachers, other school personnel, parents, students, and the community about nutrition education.

*Competencies 16.2, 16.6, 16.8, 16.9, 16.10, 16.11, 16.14 from Gregoire & Sneed research.

---

plan for the school food and nutrition program. These objectives will come as a result of examining needs and identifying problems, issues, and concerns that should be addressed.

2. *Form a team:* Bring together a team of people—teachers, administrators, parents, school nurses, students (representing schools from the district), and community members who are willing to be on the nutrition education team. Remember to include people who represent other components of comprehensive school health. Get their commitment to participate actively, and stay involved in an ongoing manner.

3. *Get buy-in:* Let the team review the goals and objectives and give input for revision. Getting buy-in is essential for success. The team will now feel ownership in the program.

4. *Decide on activities:* With the team, create an action plan for each objective. Plan the activities to meet objectives.

5. *Assign responsibility:* Let each team member take responsibility for helping to implement the activities. Be clear about who does what, and when.

6. *Identify resources:* Determine what resources are needed to fulfill the activities. Everyone on the team can help with identifying existing resources.

7. *Follow up:* Set times to meet again to review progress and do further planning as needed. Ongoing communication is key to the successful implementation of the action plan.

8. *Communicate:* Let other people in the schools and community (including the media) know about your activities. Invite their participation as often as possible.

9. *Evaluate:* Make certain the action plan includes methods for evaluation. Use the results of this evaluation to help determine whether goals and objectives were met. The results will help to improve efforts continuously.[25]

SUMMARY

Our nation's children deserve a healthy future. School food and nutrition programs can play a critical role in shaping that healthy future. Teaching children about nutrition is essential to their developing lifelong healthy eating practices. Education and health are inextricably linked—children who are not healthy cannot learn, and children who cannot learn cannot be healthy. There is no better—or more effective—way to reach children than through the school food and nutrition programs. Partnerships within the school and the community can support nutrition programs and nutrition education, making each more effective. A commitment is needed to ensure that all children have access in school to quality nutrition education in preschool through grade twelve. School food and nutrition professionals have a responsibility as the experts in their field to take a leadership role in ensuring that this vision becomes reality.

CASE STUDY
STATE–LOCAL PARTNERSHIP MEANS SUCCESS FOR ALL

Sally Anger

In 1989, the California Department of Education (CDE) launched the Child Nutrition: Shaping Healthy Choices campaign. Marilyn Briggs, Assistant Director of the Child Nutrition and Food Distribution Division, was nutrition education and training (NET) coordinator at the time. As part of NET's strategic planning, Briggs met with members of industry, food service directors, parents, superintendents, and other stakeholders on how to improve the quality of school meals.

"We realized that many factors influence the success of child nutrition programs," she said, "from offering healthy foods and applying nutrition policies, to building partnerships, teaching nutrition in classrooms, and marketing healthy food choices." One key part of the campaign at the time was to influence legislation to benefit student health. CDE collaborated with then-assemblywoman Jacqueline Speier to pass Assembly Bill 2109 in the fall of 1989. The bill required the CDE to develop nutrition guidelines that followed the California Daily Food Guide, a precursor to the Food Guide Pyramid. The guidelines applied to all foods and beverages sold on school campuses, including school meals in child nutrition programs.

"The statewide legislation created interest in the positive changes in school meals," according to Briggs. "Working with assemblywoman Speier was a win-win partnership. It provided momentum for the new initiative, and Speier was pleased to implement policy that had a direct, positive effect on children."

At the same time that Shaping Healthy Choices was getting under way, the Comprehensive School Health Program initiative was taking hold in California. In addition, the California Health Framework was being developed. "We were also working to tie into the Health Framework. A critical role for states to play is to demonstrate how different projects can fit together to improve students' eating habits," said Briggs.

Another key part of the campaign was to field-test strategies to help child nutrition programs model healthful eating practices, reinforce classroom instruction, and promote nutrition as a part of a comprehensive school health system. The NET program funded two networks of ten school districts each to test the project over three years (1990–1993). Funds were provided for hiring a nutrition education specialist for each network to coordinate and provide nutrition expertise.

From the beginning, each network district took the lead in one area of the SHAPE program, such as staff development, nutrient analysis, or nutrition education. Then they shared the successes and challenges with the other districts in their network.

The SHAPE program used a comprehensive approach to incorporate nutrition education into the state's efforts to implement the dietary guidelines. The model in Figure 9–5 evolved from the SHAPE initiative.

After field-testing the strategies and materials in additional networks, the final result was the publication of *Strategies for Success: A Resource Manual for SHAPE*,[25] a manual for child nutrition program directors to promote nutrition as an integral part of a comprehensive school health system in the school and the community.

THE SHAPE CALIFORNIA APPROACH

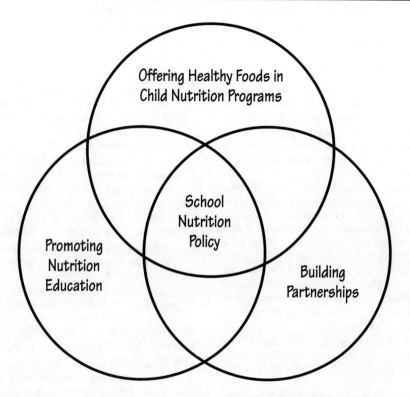

Figure 9–5 The SHAPE California Approach. *Source:* Reprinted with permission from *Strategies for Success: A Resource Manual for SHAPE,* p. 4, © 1995, California Department of Education.

The evaluation of the pilot projects also demonstrated that teachers found it easier to incorporate nutrition into the classroom if provided short and simple lessons to use. "We realized we needed a set of quick and easy lessons that could be used as a vehicle to get food service directors and teachers to work together," Briggs noted. "This led to a new partnership with health services to develop the Five a Day Power Play program."

Teachers were able to use Five a Day Power Play to tie into the educational framework in their school districts, using current teaching strategies. The partnership with health services also funded a study to evaluate the effect of the program. "We

found that as you increase the components of nutrition education, such as family and community involvement, you see an increase in the quality of the foods eaten by children," Briggs said. "Fruit and vegetable consumption increased."

When asked about strategies that states could use to promote nutrition education, Briggs commented: "A key role of the state agency is to give visibility to the exciting, new strategies being created at the local level. Sometimes it's better to discover the ideas already there and provide a vehicle for sharing them statewide. As a matter of fact, the nutrition education and training program in many states provides this vital role. Through the national NET infrastructure, the best ideas are shared nationwide."

Briggs added, "With new technology and the expansion of the NET program, the capability of nutrition educators to work together to improve children's healthy food choices will improve dramatically. It's an exciting time to be involved in child nutrition."

REFERENCES

1. AWP Research, *Nutritional Advisory Council National Survey* (Final Report to the American School Foodservice Association, Alexandria, VA, 1995), ii.
2. Centers for Disease Control and Prevention (CDC), "Guidelines for School Health Programs To Promote Lifelong Healthy Eating," *Morbidity and Mortality Weekly Report:* 45, no. RR-9 (1996): 5.
3. U.S.Public Health Service, *Healthy People 2000: National Health Promotion and Disease Prevention Objectives* (Full Report, with Commentary) (Washington, DC: U.S. Department of Health and Human Services, Public Health Service, 1991), DHHS publication no. (PHS) 91-50212.
4. R.J. Mandell, ed., *The Strategic Plan for Nutrition Education: Promoting Healthy Eating Habits for Our Children* (Washington, DC: U.S. Department of Agriculture, Food and Nutrition Service, Nutrition and Technical Services Division, 1993).
5. National Education Association of the United States, *The Relationship between Nutrition and Learning: A School Employee's Guide to Information and Action* (Washington, DC: 1989).
6. Center on Hunger, Poverty and Nutrition Policy. *Statement on the Link between Nutrition and Cognitive Development in Children* (Medford, MA: Tufts University, 1994).
7. National Education Goals Panel, *The National Education Goals Report: Building a Nation of Learners* (Washington, DC: U.S. Department of Education, 1992).
8. CDC, "Guidelines for School Health Programs."
9. J.S. Randell, ed., "The Effectiveness of Nutrition Education and Implications for Nutrition Education Policy, Programs, and Research: A Review of Research," *Journal of Nutrition Education* 27, no. 6 (1995): 285.
10. CDC, "Guidelines for School Health Programs."
11. American Dietetics Association, "Position of the American Dietetics Association: Child and Adolescent Food and Nutrition Programs." *Journal of the American Dietitics Association* 96 (1996): 913–197.
12. American Dietetics Association, "Position of ADA, SNE, and ASFSA: School-Based Nutrition Programs and Services," *Journal of the American Dietetics Assoication* 95 (1995): 367–369.
13. CDC, "Guidelines for School Health Programs."
14. D.D. Allensworth and L.J. Kolbe, "The Comprehensive School Health Program: Exploring an Expanded Concept," *Journal of School Health* 57 no. 10 (1987):409–412.
15. D. Allensworth et al., eds, *Schools and Health Our Nation's Investment* (Washington DC: Institute of Medicine, National Academy Press,1997), 174–177.
16. California Department of Education. *NETWorks: Nutrition Education and Training Program,* vols. 1 and 2 (Sacramento, CA: May l994).
17. National Center for Education Statistics, *Nutrition Education in Elementary and Secondary Schools* (Washington, DC: U.S. Department of Education, August 1996). NCES publication no. 96-852.
18. CDC, "Guidelines for School Health Programs."
19. California Department of Education, *Strategies for Success: A Resource Manual for SHAPE* (Sacramento, CA: June 1995), 334.
20. American School Food Service Association, *Keys to Excellence: Standards of Practice for Nutrition Integrity* (Alexandria, VA: 1995).
21. D. Carr et al., *Competencies, Knowledge, and Skills of Effective School Nutrition Directors/Supervisors* (University, MS: National Food Service Management Institute, 1996).
22. American School Food Service Association, *Creating Policy for Nutrition Integrity in Schools* (Alexandria, VA: 1995).
23. The Evaluation Guide for Nutrition Education and Training Program. U.S. Dept. of Agriculture, Food and Consumer Service, 1995.
24. The Needs Assessment Guide for the Nutrition Education and Training Program. U.S. Dept. of Agriculture Food and Consumer Service, 1994.
25. California Department of Education, *Strategies for Success.*

Selected School-Based Strategies To Promote Healthy Eating

The following, taken from the Centers for Disease Control and Prevention's "Guidelines for School Health Programs to Promote Life-long Healthy Eating," are appropriate activities for lower elementary school, upper elementary school, and middle and high school students. These activities are not intended to be all in-clusive. Local needs and student abilities should be taken into consideration before de-signing any nutrition education intervention. However, these activities can serve as a guide in planning. The strategies listed here are de-signed to be implemented primarily by the classroom teacher. However, the involvement of teachers, administrators, food service per-sonnel, other school staff, and parents is re-quired to be most effective. School food and nutrition professionals will benefit from using these strategies to support and enhance nutri-tion education linkages between the classroom and the cafeteria.

For Lower Elementary Students

Strategies to make the food environment more health-enhancing

- Make healthy foods (e.g., fruits, vegetables, and whole grains) widely available at school, and discourage the availability of foods high in fat, sodium, and added sugars.
- Involve parents in nutrition education through homework.
- Provide role models (e.g., teachers, par-ents, other adults, older children, and celebrities or fictional characters) for healthy eating.
- Provide cues, through posters and market-ing-style incentives, that encourage stu-dents to make healthy choices about eat-ing and physical activity.
- Use incentives, such as verbal praise or token gifts, to reinforce healthy eating and physical activity. Do not use food for re-ward or punishment of any behavior.

Strategies to enhance personal characteristics that will support healthy eating

- Make basic connections between food and health (e.g., "You need food to feel good and to grow").
- Teach the importance of balancing food intake and physical activity.
- Identify healthy snacks (e.g., fruits, veg-etables, and low-fat milk).
- Increase students' confidence in their abil-ity to make healthy eating choices by gradually building up their food selection

Source: Reprinted from National Center for Disease Control and Health Prevention Programs, *Guidelines for School Health Programs to Promote Lifelong Healthy Eating: At-A-Glance*, 1996, Centers for Disease Control and Prevention.

and preparation skills and giving them practice.

Strategies to enhance behavioral capabilities that will support healthy eating

- Provide many healthy foods for students to taste in an enjoyable social context.
- Let students prepare simple snacks.
- Have students try unfamiliar and culturally diverse foods that are low in fat, sodium, and added sugars.

For Upper Elementary Students

Strategies to make the food environment more health-enhancing

- Make healthy foods (e.g., fruits, vegetables, and whole grains) widely available at school, and discourage the availability of foods high in fat, sodium, and added sugars.
- Involve parents in nutrition education through homework.
- Provide role models (e.g., teachers, parents, other adults, adolescents, and celebrities or fictional characters) for healthy eating.
- Through class discussions and small-group exercises, provide social support for making healthy changes in eating and physical activity.
- Provide cues, through posters and marketing-style incentives that students design, that encourage students to make healthy choices about eating and physical activity.
- Use incentives, such as verbal praise or token gifts, to reinforce healthy eating and physical activity. Do not use food as a reward or punishment of any behavior.

Strategies to enhance personal characteristics that will support healthy eating

- Explain the effects that diet and physical activity have on future health as well as on

immediate concerns (e.g., current health, physical appearance, obesity, sense of well-being, and capacity for physical activity).
- Teach the principles of the Dietary Guidelines for Americans and the Food Guide Pyramid. Instill pride in choosing to eat meals and snacks that comply with these principles.
- Help students identify foods high and low in fat, saturated fat, cholesterol, sodium, added sugars, and fiber.
- Teach the importance of balancing food intake and physical activity.
- Teach the importance of eating adequate amounts of fruits, vegetables, and whole grains.
- Help students increase the value they place on health and their sense of control over food selection and preparation.
- Increase students' confidence in their ability to make healthy eating choices by gradually building up their food selection and preparation skills and giving them practice.
- Have students analyze food preferences and factors that trigger eating behaviors.

Strategies to enhance behavioral capabilities that will support healthy eating

- Provide opportunities for students to taste many healthy foods in an enjoyable social context.
- Let students prepare healthy snacks or simple meals.
- Encourage students to try unfamiliar and culturally diverse foods that are low in fat, sodium, and added sugars and that are high in fiber.
- Have students select healthy foods from a fast-food restaurant menu.
- Teach students how to recognize the fat, sodium, and fiber contents of foods by reading nutrition labels.
- Help students record and assess their food intake.

- Teach students how to use the Food Guide Pyramid to assess their diet for variety, moderation, and proportionality.
- Have students set simple goals for changes in eating and physical activity, and devise strategies for implementing these changes and monitoring progress in reaching their goals.
- When appropriate, let students practice (through role plays) encouraging parents to make healthy choices about eating and physical activity at home.
- Have students examine media and social influences on eating and physical activity; teach students how to respond to these pressures.

For Middle and High School Students

Strategies to make the food environment more health-enhancing

- Make healthy foods (e.g., fruits, vegetables, and whole grains) widely available at school, and discourage the availability of foods high in fat, sodium, and added sugars.
- Provide role models (e.g., teachers, parents, other adults, and celebrities) for healthy eating.
- Use peers as role models, and use peer-led nutrition education activities.
- Through class discussions and small-group exercises, provide social support for making healthy changes in eating and physical activity.
- Provide cues, through posters and marketing-style incentives that students design, that encourage students to make healthy choices about eating and physical activity.

Strategies to enhance personal characteristics that will support healthy eating

- Explain the effects that diet and physical activity have on future health as well as on immediate concerns (e.g., current health, physical appearance, obesity, eating disorders, sense of well-being, and capacity for physical activity).
- Have students identify reasons to adopt healthy eating and physical activity patterns.
- Teach the principles of the Dietary Guidelines for Americans. Instill in the students pride in choosing to eat meals and snacks that comply with these principles.
- Teach students how to identify foods high and low in fat, saturated fat, cholesterol, sodium, and added sugars.
- Teach students how to identify foods that are excellent sources of fiber, complex carbohydrates, calcium, iron, vitamin A, vitamin C, and folate.
- Teach the importance of balancing food intake and physical activity.
- Teach the effects of unsafe weight-loss methods and the characteristics of a safe weight-loss program.
- Help students increase the value they place on health and their sense of control over food selection and preparation.
- Increase students' confidence in their ability to eat healthily by gradually building up their skils and giving them practice.
- Help students examine what motivates persons to adopt particular eating habits. Have students keep a food diary noting what cues their own eating behavior (e.g., mood, hunger, stress, or other persons).

Strategies to enhance behavioral capabilities that will support healthy eating

- Let students plan and prepare healthy meals.
- Have students select healthy foods from restaurant and cafeteria menus.
- Teach students how to use nutrition labels to make healthy food choices.
- Teach students ways to modify recipes and prepare foods to reduce fat and sodium content and to increase fiber content.

- Help students identify incentives and reinforcements for their current eating and physical activity behaviors.
- Have students examine media and social inducements to adopt unhealthy eating and physical activity patterns, teach them how to respond to these pressures, and let them use their new knowledge to identify their own resistance strategies.
- Have students analyze environmental barriers to healthy eating and physical activity; explore strategies for overcoming these barriers.
- When appropriate, give students practice in encouraging parents to make healthy choices about eating and physical activity at home.
- Teach students to record their food intake, then have them assess and compare their diets with the standards set forth in the Dietary Guidelines for Americans and the Food Guide Pyramid. Have them assess and compare their intake of key nutrients (e.g., calcium and iron) with the intake recommended by the Public Health Service.
- Have students set goals for healthy changes in eating and physical activity, identify barriers and incentives, and assess alternative strategies for reaching their goals and decide which to follow. Show students how to monitor their progress, revise their goals if necessary, and reward themselves for successfully attaining their goals.
- Teach students how to evaluate nutrition claims from advertisements and nutrition-related news stories.

Nutrition Education Resource List

The following are sources of materials and technical assistance for nutrition and nutrition education from the national level. State departments of education and state departments of health are also good sources for obtaining information. At the local level, voluntary health promotion organizations, local dietetics associations, county cooperative extension services, local health departments, commodity food boards and organizations, and local colleges and universities may also offer materials and assistance.

American School Food Service Association (ASFSA)
1600 Duke Street, 7th Floor
Alexandria, VA 22314
(800) 877-8822, ext. 116
http://www.asfsa.org

School Food Service Foundation (SFSF)
1600 Duke Street, 7th Floor
Alexandria, VA 22314
(800) 877-8822 ext. 150
http://www.asfsa.org/foundation/

Centers for Disease Control and Prevention (CDC)
U.S. Department of Health and Human Services
Public Health Service
1600 Clifton Road, NE
Atlanta, GA 30333
(404) 639-3311
http://www.cdc.gov

Food and Nutrition Information Center (FNIC)
National Agricultural Library/ ARS/USDA
10301 Baltimore Avenue, Room 304
Beltsville, MD 20705-2351
(301) 504-5719
http://www.nal.usda.gov/fnic/
Healthy School Meals Resource System Web Site:
http://schoolmeals.nal.usda.gov:8001

*For a list of State NET Program Coordinators and State Child Nutrition Directors access the School Meals Resource System at the Web site.

National Cancer Institute (NCI)
Office of Cancer Communications
Building 31, Room 10A16
31 Center Drive MSC-2580
Bethesda, MD 20892-2580
(800)-4-CANCER (800-422-6237)
http://www.nci.nih.gov/

National Dairy Council
10233 West Higgins Road, Suite 900
Rosemont, IL 60018-5616
(800) 426-8271

*For the number of your local Dairy Council, call number listed above.

National Heart, Lung, and Blood Institute
Information Center
PO Box 30105
Bethesda, MD 20824-0105
(301) 251-1222
http://www.nhlbi.nih.gov/nhlbi/

Food and Nutrition Service
U.S. Department of Agriculture
NET Program/TEAM Nutrition*
3101 Park Center Drive
Alexandria, VA 22302
(703) 305-1624

*For a list of state NET program coordinators
and state child nutrition directors access the
school meals resource system at the Web site
given under FNIC above.

International Food Information Council
1100 Connecticut Avenue, Suite 430
Washington, DC 20036
(202) 296-6540
http://ificinfo.health.org

American Heart Association
7272 Greenville Avenue
Dallas, TX 75231-4596
(800) 242-8721
http://www.amhrt.org/

American Dietetic Association (ADA)
216 W. Jackson Boulevard, Suite 800
Chicago, IL 60606-6995
(800) 745-0775 ext. 5000
http://www.eatright.org/index.html

Society for Nutrition Education (SNE)
7101 Wisconsin Avenue, Suite 901
Bethesda, MD 20814-4805
(800) 235-6690

National Food Service Management Institute
(NFSMI)
PO Box 188
University, MS 38677-0188
(800) 321-3054
http://www.olemiss.edu/depts/nfsmi

CHAPTER 10

Menu Planning To Develop Healthy Eating Practices

Charlotte Beckett Oakley

OUTLINE

- Introduction
- Factors Influencing Menu Planning
- Challenges to Menu Planning
- Nutrition Integrity Standards for Healthy School Menus
- Federal Regulations and the *Dietary Guidelines for Americans*
- Menu-Planning Systems
  - Traditional Food-Based Menu Planning
  - Enhanced Food-Based Menu Planning
  - Nutrient Standard Menu Planning and Assisted Nutrient Standard Menu Planning
  - Any Reasonable Approach to Menu Planning
- Menu-Planning Principles
  - Customer Food Preferences
  - The Eating Occasion
  - Sensory Characteristics of Foods
  - Variety and Creativity
  - Menu-Planning Resources Available to the Program
- Menu Development Considerations
  - Menu Complexity
  - Menu Repetition
  - Offering Choices
  - Pricing the Menu
- Steps in Menu Planning
- The Menu as a Marketing Tool
- Continuous Quality Improvement of the Menu
- Application
- Summary
- Case Study: Challenge: Implementing Nutrient Standard Menu Planning
  Elaine Keaton and Karen A. Merrill
- Case Study: Challenge: Redesigning the Menu and Kitchen for Closed Campus
  Elaine Keaton and Karen A. Merrill

INTRODUCTION

The menu is more than a list of food items served to the customer. Successful menu planners know that the menu drives the program. The menu is the most influential factor in the success or failure of the program. The menu serves as the primary control for the food service operation.[1] Equipment and layout needs, purchasing decisions, staffing, and employee training are determined by the types of menu items and menu systems selected in the child nutrition program. The meal cost is primarily determined by the menu, since all food service activities requiring expenditures are affected by the menu.

Additionally, the menu teaches the customer about foods. It is desirable that student customers learn healthful eating practices early in life. Consistent and frequent experiences with nutritious meals at school provide a powerful message about good nutrition. Menus planned around the nutrition principles of the *Dietary Guidelines for Americans* (Exhibit 10–1)—variety, balance, and moderation—teach students to select nutritious, satisfying meals. As in other aspects of life, children learn best what they live.[2] A major goal of the child nutrition program is to be the laboratory that models good nutrition and provides an opportunity for the student to practice positive eating habits. It is the commitment to nutrition integrity that distinguishes the school food and

nutrition program menu from the menus of other food outlets, such as limited-menu and full-service restaurants. While the school food and nutrition menu might share common characteristics with other types of food service, the underlying principle of providing healthful meals that meet the *Dietary Guidelines* is evident in each meal offered. To that end, this chapter offers the following objectives:

- To discuss the principles of menu planning related to the nutrition integrity of the school meal
- To discuss the menu-planning options available for schools participating in the National School Lunch and Breakfast Programs
- To discuss menu-planning guidelines that consider the taste preferences of the student customer
- To discuss the various aspects of menu planning related to menu structure, including cycle menus
- To focus on the nutrition recommendations of the *Dietary Guidelines for Americans* and the Food Guide Pyramid as guidance in planning menus for school meals.

FACTORS INFLUENCING MENU PLANNING

Good school-meals menus are written with attention to numerous factors. The restaurant

---

Exhibit 10–1 Recommendations of *Dietary Guidelines for Americans*

- Eat a variety of foods.
- Balance the food you eat with physical activity—maintain or improve your weight.
- Choose a diet with plenty of grain products, fruits, and vegetables.
- Choose a diet low in fat, saturated fat, and cholesterol.
- Choose a diet moderate in sugars.
- Choose a diet moderate in salt and sodium.
- If you drink alcoholic beverages, do so in moderation.

Source: Reprinted from U.S. Department of Agriculture, *Nutrition and Your Health: Dietary Guidelines for Americans,* House and Garden Bulletin, No. 232, 1995, U.S. Government Printing Office.

industry refers to these factors as front-of-the-house and heart-of-the-house considerations.[3] Front-of-the-house considerations are those that directly involve the customer, and heart-of-the house are those that affect the day-to-day operations of the food service generally associated with the kitchen. In schools the term *front-of-the-house* refers to the serving and dining areas and the term *back-of-the-house* refers to the preparation area.

Front-of-the-house (line) menu planning considerations appropriate for child nutrition programs include the following:

- The menu includes foods that meet the nutritional needs of all the children served.
- The menu serves as the primary sales medium for the child nutrition program.
- The menu serves as the primary nutrition education tool for the child nutrition program.
- The menu content defines the operation and establishes a direction for management of the program.
- The menu attracts customers to the cafeteria and encourages them to return.
- The effective menu targets a specific market. Determine the target market before the menu is written. (Are the customers elementary or secondary students? Are the teachers and other school personnel also customers?)
- The menu construction considers the clientele's needs and desires, thus providing the type of menu that gives the food service operation its best chance for success.
- The menu balances all front-of-the-line considerations with the needs and restraint of the back-of-the-line, such as food and labor cost; equipment, space, and storage limitations; skills of preparation personnel; availability of foods; and the regulations imposed by local, state, and federal agencies.

CHALLENGES TO MENU PLANNING

In the past 20 years, the school lunch and breakfast programs have changed to reflect social and economic issues as well as findings from research establishing a link between nutrition and quality of life as well as health care costs. Not all of these changes were good. For example, during the 1980s when school meals were targeted for budget cuts, counting catsup as a vegetable as part of a reimbursable lunch was suggested.[4] Certainly any menu that had to rely on catsup as one of the vegetables/fruits for the day was a poor nutrition choice for children.

During this time, something else happened that threatened the nutrition integrity of the programs. The American family changed dramatically. Mothers joined the work force in ever-increasing numbers, and more children lived in single-parent homes. Children began to make major decisions about what was for dinner, and many children began to assume the responsibility for purchasing and preparing meals for themselves and other family members. With the new-found responsibility and freedom to make their own food decisions, children began to expect of the school the same kinds of foods they enjoyed at home and at the fast-food restaurant. The nation went all out for convenience, fast (and faster) service, and the taste of high-fat burgers, fries, and pizza. Pizza and burgers have become two top choices on the school lunch menu selected by students.

Consider the following questions, which the school food and nutrition menu planner must consider in order to meet goals of program integrity: Is it possible to operate a program with nutrition integrity when the customer has a pizza/burger mentality toward the menu at lunch as well as at dinner? How can the menu please the customers' inexperienced palates and meet the goals of good nutrition at the same time? Are burgers and pizza contradictory to good nutrition? Can the students have their pizza and eat it too? School food and nutrition programs are generally mandated by their school systems to operate on a sound financial basis. Burgers and pizza sell, as do french fries, pastries, and other foods that are traditionally high in fat, saturated fat, sodium, and/or sugars. Besides, it's not nutrition if they do not eat it. Children want what they know and like, and many are unfamiliar with the more traditional menu of meat, potatoes, and green vegetables.

Can the school food and nutrition program meet the nutrition goals of the program, please the customers' taste preferences, and run a financially sound program all at once? These are critical issues that all school food and nutrition program directors will continue to face. The challenges are great and the resources are limited. However, not all the necessary resources are costly. The most important resource available to the program is the commitment of men and women who work in child nutrition programs to the children in their schools—and to operating nutritionally and fiscally sound programs responsive to changing needs and preferences of the customers.

Designing the menu to meet all these challenges may seem to be an overwhelming task. Often cost is mentioned as the greatest barrier to providing nutritious meals that meet the recommendations of the *Dietary Guidelines for Americans.*[5] Schools that have undertaken implementing the *Dietary Guidelines* report saving money while serving more nutritious meals.[6] Good nutrition is not beyond the reach of any program. Learning to plan an acceptable menu to meet the nutrition objectives of the program is an attainable goal regardless of budgets and customer resistance. However, serving healthier school meals that customers enjoy requires a holistic approach to the menu-planning function. Much courage and patience and a sense of adventure are necessary to achieve the desired results. Enthusiasm and developing a team spirit among the school food and nutrition staff members will improve customer service and propel the program toward the goal. A generous amount of public rela-

tions directed toward the school and community and sound nutrition education programs are also keys to the lasting success of a healthier school menu enjoyed by the students.

NUTRITION INTEGRITY STANDARDS FOR HEALTHY SCHOOL MENUS

The nutrition integrity of child nutrition programs begins with a carefully planned and executed menu. The menu is a tangible reflection of the philosophy of the program and its values. A menu that meets the standards of nutrition integrity established by the school food and nutrition profession is evidence of the program's commitment to the current and future health and well-being of the children it serves. The time, efforts, and resources necessary to meet these standards are considerable and are not taken lightly or for granted. The *Keys to Excellence* support the nutrition goals of the school food and nutrition program when it states, "School meals meet the nutritional needs of all students."[7]

While the phrase *nutrition integrity* can be applied to any institutional food service operation, it has its origin in school food and nutrition.[8] Although school food and nutrition programs were begun historically to meet the child's school day food needs, many of the early programs offered limited menus. However as early as the 1920s, food service directors and academic instructors were identifying program standards that provided for meeting both food and nutrition education goals. Research of the past two decades has provided considerable information about the nutritional needs of growing children. Indeed, nutrition is a relatively new science, with much of what is known about the link between diet and health having been discovered in the last half of the twentieth century.[9]

The menus in school lunch programs, and more recently in school breakfast programs, have changed through the years to reflect the changing beliefs about what is good nutrition.[10] In 1993, the American School Food Service Association (ASFSA) and the National Food Service Management Institute (NFSMI) developed measurable nutrition integrity standards that identify levels of expected performance in school food and nutrition programs. The core concepts are shown in Exhibit 10–2.[11] All 11 core concepts are directly connected to the food items selected for the menu. Core concepts emphasize

- The importance of the nutrition principles of the *Dietary Guidelines for Americans*—variety of foods, fiber, and reducing fat, sodium, and sugar in school meals
- The need to consider student preferences in menu planning; the necessity to include

adequate calories and variety of food to support growth, development, and the maintenance of healthy body weight
- The concept of planning school meals to meet weekly nutritional goals rather than by single meals or foods
- The importance of planning extra and/or à la carte foods that meet the same nutrition standard established for the regular menu and that do not separate students who can afford them from students who cannot

Nutrition integrity standards that focus on purchasing, preparation, employee training, and nutrition education round out the process needed to ensure that the goal of healthful

---

Exhibit 10–2 Nutrition Integrity Standards for School Nutrition Programs

1. Nutrition standards, based on scientific recommendations, will be adopted to set appropriate goals. Emphasis will be placed on increasing variety of foods, dietary fiber, and reducing fat, sodium, and sugar in school meals.
2. Student preferences will be considered in menu planning. Since food must be eaten to provide nutrients, menu changes will be gradual to ensure acceptance.
3. Meals will contain adequate calories and variety of foods to support growth, development, and the maintenance of desirable body weight.
4. The nutritional value of school meals will be evaluated over a period of days, rather than a single meal or food item.
5. Purchasing practices will be developed to ensure the use of high-quality ingredients and prepared products to maximize flavor and acceptable products that meet nutrition standards.
6. Foods will be prepared in ways that ensure a balance between optimal nutrition and student acceptance.
7. Foods sold in addition to meals will be thoughtfully selected to ensure optimal nutrition quality and to foster healthful eating habits. These foods will be limited in number to prevent the separation of students who can and cannot afford additional purchases.
8. Pleasant eating environments will be provided. This includes adequate time and space to eat school meals, positive supervision, and role modeling at mealtimes.
9. Nutrition education will be an integral part of the curriculum from preschool to 12th grade. The school cafeteria will serve as a laboratory for applying critical thinking skills taught in the classroom.
10. Tools developed to train food service personnel, teachers, school administrators, and parents will be used to build teams of competent, caring individuals with common goals.
11. School food and nutrition professionals and administrative personnel will work cooperatively with legislative and other government agencies to promote policies that further the achievement of nutrition integrity in child nutrition programs.

Source: Reprinted with permission from M.B. Gregoire and J. Sneed, Standards for Nutrition Integrity, *School Foodservice Research Review*, Vol. 18, pp. 106-111, © 1994, American School Food Service Association.

school meals for all children is met. School food and nutrition authorities can measure their level of success in achieving nutrition integrity by using the core concepts, standards, and indicators established in the nutrition integrity standards and the key achievement standards of the *Keys to Excellence.*

FEDERAL REGULATION AND THE DIETARY GUIDELINES FOR AMERICANS

The results of the National Evaluation of School Nutrition Programs[12] and the *School Nutrition Dietary Assessment Study: School Food Service, Meals Offered, and Dietary Intakes* (SNDAS)[13] prompted the United States Department of Agriculture (USDA) to propose changes in the regulations for planning menus in the National School Lunch Program (NSLP) and the School Breakfast Program (SBP). The study indicated that children in America are generally consuming too much fat, saturated fat, and sodium, and too few carbohydrates. The SNDA study showed that students' average daily intake of calories from fat was 38 percent and 15 percent from saturated fat compared with the 30 percent and 10 percent of total calories from fat and saturated fat, respectively, recommended in the *Dietary Guidelines for Americans.*[14] School meals make a significant contribution to the daily food intakes of children. USDA[15] has established regulations based on congressional action that incorporates the nutrition principles of the *Dietary Guidelines for Americans* into the nutrition standard of the National School Lunch Program and School Breakfast Program. Therefore, the nutrition recommendations of the *Dietary Guidelines* are an appropriate place to start when planning school meals that meet nutrition integrity standards.

A study of school districts in one state[16] showed that, although 76 percent of the food and nutrition program directors knew of the *Dietary Guidelines*, only 59 percent could name at least two. Writing nutritionally sound menus requires the menu planner, who is usually the school food and nutrition program director, to be familiar with the *Dietary Guidelines* and the rationale that supports each recommendation. The Healthy Meals for Americans Act (Public Law 103-448), passed in 1994, required school nutrition programs to comply with the recommendations of the *Dietary Guidelines for Americans* by July 1, 1998.[17] USDA promoted the new ruling by developing the School Meals Initiative for Healthy Children (Healthy School Meals Initiative).[18]

The Healthy School Meals Initiative (SMI) supports the offering of school meals that promote health, help prevent chronic diseases, and meet specific nutritional goals. It allows the school food and nutrition program director/ manager to plan menus using the total-diet concept based on an average weekly nutrient analysis. Use of a weekly average for key nutrients allows the menu planner greater flexibility in the foods offered in the cafeteria and removes the "good" food, "bad" food stigma. In addition to the *Dietary Guidelines'* goals, the (SMI) nutrition goals include menus that have a weekly average of one-third of the recommended dietary allowances (RDAs)[19] at lunch and one-fourth of the RDAs at breakfast, and menus that provide adequate calories appropriate for each age group. The Food Guide Pyramid is a valuable menu-planning tool as it graphically presents the nutrition principles of the *Dietary Guidelines* by reflecting the number of servings that should be eaten each day from the food groups. The focus on food as a source of nutrients is promoted when the menu is planned around the food groups with attention being paid to the number and variety of servings from each of the major groups, including the breads, cereals, rice, and pasta group; the fruit group; the vegetable group; the meat group; and the milk, yogurt, and cheese group. Selections from the fats, oils, and sweets group can add flavor and increase acceptability of school meals and are appropriate as long as limited amounts are included.

MENU-PLANNING SYSTEMS

USDA has established four menu-planning systems with identical nutrient standards: traditional, food-based menu planning, enhanced food-based menu planning, Nutrient Standard Menu Planning and Assisted Nutrient Standard Menu Planning. Additionally, schools may use other approaches to planning menus, when approved by the state agency and the nutrition standards are met. The systems fit into two categories, food-based and nutrient standard-based. The USDA menu planning systems are appropriate for any school as nutrient standards are based on tested nutrition research and are related to age groups of children. Nutrition goals of the four systems include the following:

- The systems provide that not more than 30 percent of calories will derive from fat and not more than 10 percent of calories from saturated fat.
- One-third of the RDA will be provided at lunch and one-fourth of the RDA at breakfast for calories, protein, calcium, iron, vitamin A, and vitamin C.
- Other nutrients and dietary components that will be analyzed are carbohydrate, cholesterol, sodium, and dietary fiber.
- All nutrition goals are based on the weekly average of nutrients and other dietary components.

The offer-versus-serve option contained in the National School Lunch Act allows children to select fewer food items than are offered. In secondary schools, offer-versus-serve must be implemented at lunch, and elementary schools may choose to make the option available to students. Offer-versus-serve may be, but is not required, at breakfast. The goals of offer-versus-serve are to minimize plate waste and encourage more food choices.[20] Offer-versus-serve provides a challenge to the menu planner to design menus that appeal to students. When they choose less than the full menu, they are shortchanged nutritionally.

Traditional Food-Based Menu Planning

Menu systems that focus on the selection of foods from meal components is the traditional approach to meal planning. These systems designate meal components with number of servings and portion sizes from four food groups. These compose the reimbursable school lunch, that is, meat/meat alternate, vegetable/fruit, grains/breads, and milk. The breakfast components are meat/meat alternate, juice/fruit/vegetable, grains/breads, and milk. At lunch, a minimum of one food item from each of the four groups must be offered except for the vegetable/fruit components which must have two different foods. Specific quantities of these foods must also be offered. The traditional food-based menu planning system is planned to provide the meal components outlined in Table 10–1. The nutritional goals of the food-based menu planning system are the same as for all other menu-planning options as discussed under the nutrition integrity section of this chapter.

Enhanced Food-Based Menu Planning

The enhanced food-based meal pattern introduced by USDA as part of the regulations for the SMI (Table 10–2) required the same meal components under the traditional food-based option with an increase in the total amount of vegetable/fruit and grains/breads served during the week. The additional amounts of vegetable/fruit and grains/breads are required to ensure that the menu meets the recommendations of the *Dietary Guidelines for Americans* to choose more of the foods from these food categories. Diets with greater proportions of vegetable, fruits, and grain products are more likely to be higher in complex carbohydrates, including fiber, and lower in fat and saturated fat. Menu planners are encouraged to offer choices within the food components to enhance student acceptance of the meal, and the offer-versus-serve options must

Table 10–1 Food-Based Menu Meal Plans for Breakfast

Minimum Quantities for Food-Based Menus Breakfast

Meal Component	Required			Option
	Ages 1–2	*Preschool*	*Grades K–12*	*Grades 7–12*
Milk (fluid)	½ cup	¾ cup	8 fl. oz.	8 fl. oz.
(As a beverage, on cereal or both)				
Juice/fruit/vegetable	¼ cup	½ cup	½ cup	½ cup
Fruit and/or vegetable; or full-strength fruit juice or vegetable juice				

Select one serving from each of the following components or two from one component:

	Ages 1–2	*Preschool*	*Grades K–12*	*Grades 7–12*
Grains/breads (one of the following or an equivalent combination)				
Whole-grain or enriched bread	½ slice	½ slice	1 slice	1 slice
Whole-grain or enriched biscuit/ roll, muffin, etc.	½ serving	½ serving	1 serving	1 serving
Whole-grain, enriched, or fortified cereal	¼ cup or ⅓ oz.	⅓ cup or ½ oz.	¾ cup or 1 oz.	¾ cup or 1 oz.
Meat or meat alternates:				
Meat/poultry or fish	½ oz.	½ oz.	1 oz.	1 oz.
Cheese	½ oz.	½ oz.	1 oz.	1 oz.
Egg (large)	½	½	½	½
Peanut butter or other nut or seed butter	1 Tbsp.	1 Tbsp.	2 Tbsp.	2 Tbsp.
Nut and/or seeds (as listed in program guidance)[a]	2 Tbsp. ½ oz.	2 Tbsp. ½ oz.	4 Tbsp. 1 oz.	4 Tbsp. 1 oz.

[a]No more than 1 oz. of nuts and/or seeds may be served in any one meal.

Source: Reprinted from U.S. Department of Agriculture, Food and Consumer Service, *Healthy School Meals Training Manual*, p. 2-b, 1996, U.S. Government Printing Office.

be implemented in secondary schools and may be implemented in elementary schools in both food-based menu planning systems.

The nutrition standards relative to the *Dietary Guidelines* and the RDA are the same as in all other menu planning systems. Food-based menus must be analyzed to determine the nutrient content for compliance with the nutrition goals for reimbursable meals.[20] Schools may analyze the menu during the planning process. However, federal regulations require the state agency to monitor the menus through a nutrient analysis during the review process. Analyzing the menu during the planning stage ensures that nutrition goals are met. The state agency has responsibility to interpret the federal regulations and monitor programs for compliance. Therefore, schools should refer to the menu-planning guidelines that are provided by the state agency to ensure compliance with all state and federal recommendations and requirements.

Table 10–2 Food-Based Menu Meal Plan for Lunch

Minimum Quantities for Food-Based Menus Lunch

Meal Component	Required				Options
Milk (as a beverage)	6 fl. oz.	6 fl. oz.	8 fl. oz.	8 fl.oz.	8 fl. oz.
Meat or meat alternate (quantity of the edible portion as served)					
Lean meat, poultry or fish	1 oz.	11/2 oz.	2 oz.	2 oz.	11/2 oz.
Cheese	1 oz.	11/2 oz.	2 oz.	2 oz.	11/2 oz.
Large egg	½	¾	1	1	¾
Cooked dry beans or peas	¼ cup	⅜ cup	½ cup	½ cup	⅜ cup
Peanut butter or other nut or seed butters	2 Tbsp.	3 Tbsp.	4 Tbsp.	4 Tbsp.	3 Tbsp.
The following may be used to meet no more than 50% of the requirement and must be used in combination with any of the above:					
Peanuts, soynuts, tree nuts, or seeds, as listed in program guidance, or an equivalent quantity of any combination of the above meat/meat alternate (1 oz of nuts/seeds = 1 oz of cooked lean meat, poultry, or fish)	½ oz. = 50%	¾ oz. = 50%	1 oz. = 50%	1 oz. = 50%	1 oz. = 50%
Vegetables/fruits (2 or more servings of vegetables or fruits or both)	½ cup	½ cup	¾ cup plus extra ½ cup over a week[1]	1 cup	¾ cup
Grains/breads must be enriched or whole grain. A serving is a slice of bread or an equivalent serving of biscuit, rolls, etc., ½ cup of cooked rice, macaroni, noodles, other pasta products or cereal grains	5 servings per week[a] Minimum of ½ per day[b]	8 servings per week[a] Minimum of 1 per day[b]	12 servings per week[a] Minimum of 1 per day[b]	15 servings per week[a] Minimum of 1 per day[b]	10 servings per week[a] Minimum of 1 per day[b]

[a]For the purpose of this chart, a week equals five days.

[b]Up to one grains/breads serving per day may be a dessert.

Source: Reprinted from U.S. Department of Agriculture, Food and Consumer Service, *Healthy School Meals Training Manual*, p. 2-b. 1996, U.S. Government Printing Office.

Nutrient Standard Menu Planning and Assisted Nutrient Standard Menu Planning

All of the menu systems plan menus using foods; however, Nutrient Standard Menu Planning (NSMP) and assisted NSMP allow the menu planner to include any foods (except foods defined by USDA as "foods of minimal nutritional value") in any quantities to meet the weekly nutrition goals mentioned above. When using the NSMP system, menus are planned around the nutrient analysis of the menus as they are written. Menus are planned using USDA-approved computer software. Software developers provide a range of training and technical support for users of their software. When USDA first introduced the nutrient standard menu planning concept, originally called Computer-Assisted Menu Planning (COMP), it met with resistance.[21] The lack of computers and computer skills were primary concerns for many programs. NSMP was first proposed in 1994. The early adopters of NSMP reported much success and indicated lower food cost, greater flexibility in menu choices, and greater student satisfaction.[22] However, developmental costs relating to implementing NSMP must be considered in total meal cost.

In using NSMP or assisted NSMP the menu is built around the entrees defined by the menu planner, plus milk and one other food item. Additional foods and choices may be offered, and the offer-versus-serve rules apply to the NSMP and the assisted NSMP as with the food-based menu planning options. When the NSMP system is used, the menu planner conducts the nutrient analysis at the district or local level when the menus are planned. In assisted NSMP an outside consultant plans the menus based on the nutrient analysis. The outside consultant might be the state agency or a private consultant. A package of menus planned under the assisted NSMP system is available to school food authorities who wish to plan menus through nutrient analysis but lack the resources necessary to do it themselves (see Exhibit 10–3).[23] NSMP and assisted NSMP allow for creativity in planning innovative and appealing menus. For example, under NSMP and assisted NSMP, less cheese can be used on the pizza, which may improve the appearance and flavor while lowering the fat content of the pizza. Use of standardized recipes and standardized cooking techniques are essential to ensure that the meal offered to students has the same nutrient content as the planned menu. (For additional information and the details of these USDA menu-planning systems, refer to the *Healthy School Meals Training* manual.[24])

Any Reasonable Approach to Menu Planning

USDA allows other menu-planning systems for approval. Congress enacted legislation in 1995 that provides for schools to plan menus using any reasonable approach (with the approval of the state agency) as long as the menu meets the same nutrition goals as outlined in the previously discussed menu-planning options. Innovative approaches may base food choices on the Food Guide Pyramid,[25] exchange list, and other dietary plans that may have application to child nutrition programs. School food and nutrition program directors/managers who choose to plan menus under this option are looking for flexibility that allows greater opportunities to meet the regional and personal food preferences of their students, as well as to achieve a better fit to the management styles of the individual schools. School lunch and breakfast menus of the twenty-first century will reflect changes in the market base, including customer preferences. Regardless of the menu-planning system chosen by the school district, it is important to keep the basic nutrition principles in focus and to maintain a customer service orientation. Regulations for this legislation are in process.

MENU-PLANNING PRINCIPLES

In addition to the nutrition guidelines and federal regulations that the menu planner must consider, the menu planner must follow the principles of good menu planning, which include the front-of-the-line and back-of-the-line considerations discussed earlier. This section will look at the factors that affect the acceptability of foods.[26–28]

Customer Food Preferences

Menu planners who manage for excellence in the twenty-first century will strive to attain

Exhibit 10–3 Cycle-Assisted Nutrient Standard Menu

Lunch for Grades K–6			
Week 1	**5-Week Cycle Menu**		
Monday	Tuesday	Wednesday	Thursday
Chicken Nuggets	Apple Juice	Turkey and	Chilled Pineapple
Honey BBQ Sauce		Dressing	Chunks
Whole-Wheat Dinner	Spaghetti with	Supreme	
Roll	Marinara Sauce	Mashed Potatoes/	Chicken Stir-Fry
Margarine	Parmesan Cheese	Gravy	Steamed Rice
	Bread Sticks	Cranberry Sauce	
OR			OR
	OR	OR	
Hamburger/Cheese-			BBQ Pork on a
burger	Fish Fillet on Bun	Vegetable Chili	Bun
on Multi-Grain Bun	Catsup/Tartar		
Catsup, Relish, Mustard	Sauce	Whole-Wheat	Herbed Garden
Lettuce/Tomato		Dinner Roll	Pasta
	Tossed Salad	Margarine	
Oven-Fried Potato	Italian Dressing		Gingerbread w/
Wedges		Cucumber Sticks	Whipped Topping
Catsup	Seasoned Mixed	Ranch Dressing	
	Vegetables		Variety Milk
Herbed Broccoli Spears		Orange Half	
	Oatmeal-Raisin		
Chilled Applesauce	Cookie	Variety Milk	
Variety Milk	Variety Milk		

Source: Reprinted from U.S. Department of Agriculture, Food and Consumer Service, *USDA Assisted NuMenus* pp. 1–3. 1996, U.S. Government Printing Office.

the key achievement of *Keys to Excellence*, "Student preferences are considered in menu planning."[29] The menu must be well received by the students who regularly participate in the school lunch or breakfast programs and encourage nonparticipating students to give the school meal a try. Because the eating patterns of children are well established by the time they enter elementary school, the menu planner must have an understanding of the eating patterns (food culture) of the student customers. The ethnic or cultural backgrounds of students will shape their food cultures. Meeting the cultural needs of all the students in the school not only benefits the children in that culture, but the other students as well. A culturally diverse menu provides for variety that may enhance increased participation and ensure nutrition integrity without the menu planner's having to think specifically about either. Foreign grains, cheese, and vegetables are readily available in today's marketplace to add an ethnic flair to the menu. A *Tool Kit: Recipes for Healthy School Meals*[30] offers recipes for the culturally diverse menu that includes Asian, Mexican, and Italian and other Mediterranean dishes.

The ages of the students will also influence their foods preferences. Younger children may have had fewer food experiences than older children, although this is not always true. Schools throughout the United States are offering choices in menu items to all age/grade levels. Self-serve bars are popular in both elementary and secondary schools. Most children like foods that can be held in the hand. Grab-and-go breakfast and lunch menus are popular in many schools.[31] Such programs take the menu items where the customers are, rather than wait for the customers to come to the cafeteria. Special considerations in planning this type of service require foods that can be held at the proper temperature, package well, and are easy to eat on the way to class, on the school grounds, or in the classroom.

The Eating Occasion

The eating occasion determines to a large extent the types of foods offered on the menu. Special occasions such as holidays also typically include special foods. For example, Thanksgiving dinner is often associated with roasted turkey and stuffing or dressing, the Fourth of July with barbecue, and a birthday celebration with cake and ice cream. The cuisine of different cultures generally serve different foods for breakfast and lunch. Popular menus reflect the customers' expectations of what is appropriate for breakfast and what is appropriate for lunch. When introducing new menu items that may not be considered by students as traditional breakfast or lunch fare, the school food and nutrition program director/manager must market the new menu items. Creating excitement about new menu items, such as breakfast tortillas, pita, and pizza, enhances student acceptance.[32]

The special emphases on school lunch and school breakfast during National School Lunch Week and National School Breakfast Week are examples of marketing centered around specific eating occasions. Instituted by congressional resolution, the National School Lunch Week and the National School Breakfast Week promote the child nutrition programs each year through special themes, menus, and nutrition education activities.[33]

Sensory Characteristics of Food

Flavor and Aroma

The perception of flavor is a complex integration of sensations from the olfactory center in the nasal cavity; the taste buds on the tongue; tactile receptors in the mouth; and the perception of pungency, heat, cooling, and others factors when a food is placed in the mouth.[34] Flavor is a blending of taste and aroma of food. Taste is one part of flavor and involves the sensations produced when the taste buds on the tongue are stimulated. There are four primary taste sensations: sweet, sour, bitter, and salty. The aroma of a food is also essential to the perception of the flavor of the food. How a food smells is important to the student's perception of the acceptability of the flavor. For example, freshly baked yeast bread emits an aroma that travels from the kitchen to classrooms, where the students anticipate the enjoyment of eating.

Temperature of foods may also affect the flavor of foods. For example, sweet foods are generally sweeter tasting when served warm or hot, and the reverse is true of salt. Some foods contain molecules that create a sensation of coolness (i.e., menthol) and hotness (i.e., capsaicin in peppers). Serving foods at the proper temperature, therefore, will ensure that the food is served at its peak for flavor freshness.

Cooking will bring out the flavors in some foods such as baking potatoes and roasting meats. While the flavor precursors in certain foods are activated by cooking, others are obvious in the raw form such as in fresh fruits. Natural processes such as yeast fermentation create not only pleasing aromas, but wonderful flavoring compounds, too. Flavor can also be added to foods with artificial and natural flavoring ingredients. The use of herbs and spices to enhance and impart flavors to foods are also important components of the taste of school meals. Taking advantage of all of the elements of flavor development results in customer-appealing meals.

Texture

The texture of a food is important to its overall quality. Texture, consistency, and shape influence food acceptance by children. For example, children may like mashed potatoes as long as they are smooth and creamy and free of lumps. Textures that are generally liked are crisp, crunchy, tender, juicy, and firm.

Appearance

The eye appeal of a food must be pleasing to the student customer. It is very true that if foods do not look good, children will not eat them. Color, form, size, and arrangement of menu items on the plate and the serving line either attract the customers or turn them away. Children eat with their eyes first. Plan menus that have eye appeal by providing colorful, attractively arranged foods. Vary the sizes, form, and textures, also. For example, mashed potatoes, creamed chicken, and cream corn would not be a visually appealing meal. Fresh fruits and vegetables in salads and as side dishes are great menu choices to improve the appearance of meals. Golden brown crusts on meats, breads, and other baked items; molded salads from flavored gelatins; whole-grain dishes and breads; precise vegetable cuts; and many more ideas can be incorporated into the menu to enhance the presentation of the menu on the line.

Variety and Creativity

While the menu will include students' favorites on a regular basis, the school food and nutrition program director/manager incorporates variety and creativity into the menu to keep the customer interested in coming to the cafeteria. New menu items, new recipes, and new ways of presenting the menu to the customer will keep the menu fresh and fun for students. If the menu calls for a green vegetable, over time plan to use as many different green vegetables as are available; juice does not always have to be orange juice; and meals do not have to be served on the same cafeteria trays every day. Children like fun. Look for ways to create fun with the menu. Giving catchy, fun names to menu items is one way to add a little creative fun to lunch or breakfast.[35] The Howard County, Maryland school food and nutrition program director offers a "Super

Lunch" menu of fast food and a "Coach's Corner" meal designed for student athletes that is high in carbohydrates, moderate in protein, and low in fat. The program earned the USDA Best Practice Award for these and other creative innovations.[36]

Menu-Planning Resources Available to the Program

Skilled school food and nutrition personnel are among the most valuable resources to the menu-planning process. The competencies, knowledge, and skills needed by district school food and nutrition directors/supervisors[37] to plan cost-effective, nutritionally sound menus are identified in a research report available from the NFSMI. The competent menu planner develops cost-effective menus consistent with principles of good nutrition that meet all local, state, and federal guidelines and regulations; assesses consumer preference, industry trends, and current research to plan menus that encourage customer consumption; maintains nutritional integrity of the school's child nutrition program through implementation of nutrition objectives; and works with school staff, teachers, and physicians to plan menus for children with special needs.

Additional menu-planning resources are available from the NFSMI.[38] The NFSMI, a national resource center, conducts activities to improve quality and operation of child nutrition programs through research, education, and training activities; the operation of a clearinghouse for information retrieval and dissemination; and technical assistance through a national help desk. (The NFSMI is located at the University of Mississippi, Oxford, MS, and its Applied Research Division is located at The University of Southern Mississippi in Hattiesburg. NFSMI has a food service educator located at the Food and Nutrition Information Center [FNIC] in Beltsville, MD.)

The ASFSA provides valuable assistance to child nutrition programs in the nutritional and operational aspects of school food and nutrition. Training programs such as Healthy E.D.G.E. in Schools, Trimming the Fat, and Target Your Market are just a few of the resources available through ASFSA.[39]

USDA menu-planning resources include the SMI material, which provides a wealth of information on menu systems (NSMP, Assisted NSMP, and Enhanced Food-Based) designed to support the implementation of the *Dietary Guidelines* in child nutrition programs. Other SMI materials are the *Tool Kit, Assisted NSMP,* and Team Nutrition materials. The revised *Menu Planner for Healthy School Meals*[40] and the *Food Buying Guide*[41] are other essential resources needed by the school food and nutrition program directors/managers when planning the menu.

Students, however, are the most valuable resource for the menu planner. The formation of student committees and advisory groups that provide feedback and suggestions to the program are essential to the operation of customer-driven programs. Student surveys provide information about the menu that can be translated into a student-focused menu. Each cycle menu should reflect freshness and excitement. Teachers and other school personnel are customers in the cafeteria, too, and their input about menus is important to consider. Their support of the program is a key element in its overall success.

MENU DEVELOPMENT CONSIDERATIONS

Menus vary by the complexity or pattern, the interval at which they repeat, the degree of choice incorporated, and the method of pricing. Menu types include static, cycle, and single use. Static menus offer the same foods every day and are often used in restaurants. A cycle menu plans for different foods every day, is planned for a week or longer, and repeats itself. Institutional food service operations such as hospitals and schools often use cycle menus. The single-use menu is planned for some special occasion and not used again

in exactly the same form.[42] Menus may also be typed by the manner in which they are priced. Many different menu-pricing types are also used in various food service operations. Each menu type meets the specific needs of the customers or market it serves. Several different menu types may be adapted for use in the school food and nutrition setting. À la carte menus, table d-hôte menus, du jour menus, limited menus, and cycle menus all have application in school food and nutrition.[43] A combination of menu types is generally practiced in food service operations today. The characteristics of well-planned menus are the same regardless of their type. The principles of good menu planning discussed in the previous section apply to all the different menu types. The attractive presentation of high quality, well-prepared foods that meet the nutrition standards of the child nutrition program and appeal to the students is the goal of the menu regardless of the type used.

Menu Complexity

The complexity of the menu refers to the various factors that are involved in the execution of the menu. The complexity of the menu will have an impact on the management of the program. The skilled menu planner plans menus that take maximum advantage of the resources available to the program. Equipment, serving times, number of production staff available, and the skill levels of these individuals are considered during the planning process. The menu is influenced by and influences all front-of-the line and back-of-the line decisions.

Some menu patterns are more complex than are others; for example, the food-based menu patterns require more meal components than do the menus planned using the NSMP options. Choices within the menu components also increase the complexity of the menu. Although NSMP may result in menus with only three components (entree, milk, and one other item), the processes followed to develop the menu are more complex than those used to plan menus around the four meal components (meat/meat alternate, vegetables/fruits, grains/breads, and milk).

Equipment and Facilities

The menu plan must balance the use of existing equipment. For example, planning several menus that require the use of the convection oven beyond its capacity within the preparation time will hold up production and overuse the equipment. The menu must be one that can be produced in the available work space. The production staff are the best sources of information on the usage of equipment. Involving them in menu planning will prevent equipment usage errors.

In addition to production space and equipment, the menu must be planned around the storage and service equipment and space available. If several choices of chilled items, such as salads and desserts, are on the menu plan for the day, it may be difficult to hold all of these items at the appropriate temperature for service. The menu plan must also consider the number of pans, serving utensils, and tableware, which includes trays, plates, bowls, flatware, and beverage containers. If available, serving carts and kiosks and disposable dinnerware will expand the serving capacity of the menu as it becomes more complex.

Food Service Production Staff

The planned menu must be one that can be produced with a fair distribution of the workload among the food service production staff. Planning a mix of foods that require prepreparation and those that require little will avoid unnecessary last-minute preparation, and will distribute the production staff's workload evenly throughout the day. The skill levels of the staff are considered when the menu is planned to ensure that the staff is able to produce the menu as planned. Training is required when existing skills are challenged by the menu or by the addition of new menu items or preparation techniques.

Food Availability

The menu planner knows the market and incorporates new and varied foods into the menu when they are available. The seasonality of fruits and vegetables and the factors associated with their purchase are considered when the menu is planned. Alternate menu items are included when products are not available at a price the menu planner can afford.

Financial Considerations

The menu will affect the budget for all aspects of the operation. A menu that can be executed in an efficient manner saves labor costs. Some school districts report cost savings when the NSMP system is used, since the protein requirement is met by serving a smaller portion of meat than is allowed on the food-based options. Similarly, school districts are concerned about the cost of the additional vegetables/fruits and grains/breads required on the enhanced food-based system. A careful mix of higher-priced items with lower-priced ones will help balance the impact of serving the higher-priced item, as will serving the higher-priced items less often.

The right mix of prepared products and from-scratch items to match the available labor is determined by the menu planner who plans the menu to take advantage of the best prices on the market. For example, some fresh produce is priced lower during the peak growing season. Menus that take advantage of locally grown produce not only save cost, but support the local economy. A menu that uses available equipment eliminates the expense of purchasing additional equipment.

Menu Repetition

Calculating the nutrient content of the menu for key nutrients is easier when menus are planned in a cycle of several weeks that repeats on a scheduled basis. The nutrient analysis of a cycle menu is valid as long as the menu does not change. When menu items must be substituted, the nutrient analysis is re-

Suggestions for Maximizing the Budget through the Menu-Planning Process

- Plan the menu to take advantage of the most cost-effective purchasing systems available to the program.
- Menus are planned, with the most appropriate market forms of meats, fruits, and fresh vegetables specified when purchasing.
- Appropriate substitutions are planned and printed on the menu to avoid costly substitutions during rush times when best decisions might not be possible.
- The menu planner is thoroughly familiar with the current cost of all the items that are needed to produce the menu.
- Menus are written with enough flexibility to take advantage of unexpected cost savings.
- Some prepared products are expensive when compared with the cost of on-site production of the same menu item. Similarly, seasoning mixes are less expensive when prepared on site.
- The menu can be planned to limit plate waste and unserved foods on the line by offering choices and listening to the requests of the customers.
- The menu is planned to maximize available labor.
- The menu takes full advantage of the commodity food products available to the program.

calculated based on the guidelines established by the federal regulations and the state agency. Generally, if the substitute item is similar in nutrient content (i.e., whole-wheat bread for multigrain roll or canned peaches for canned pears) or the substitution decision is made within a prescribed time from the day it is served the menu does not have to be reanalyzed. All planned menu changes include a new nutrient analysis, as does the purchase of different brands or market forms of a food on the menu, and the use of new recipes for existing menu items. The cycle menu may be written at the district level and customized to meet the student preferences at the school level. A separate nutrient analysis is completed for each version of the menu without having to start from scratch each time.

Cycle menus offer the advantage of cost controls through standardized procedures for production and service. When the menu is repeated and menu items are prepared over and over by the production staff, procedures can become standardized, resulting in more efficient use of time by the production staff. Labor costs go down when the staff works more efficiently since it takes less time to do a familiar task, and more work can be accomplished in less time by fewer individuals. Not only do staff become more efficient in producing the menu, they become more skilled in producing a quality product when standardized procedures are followed.

Cycle menus also offer the advantage of cost controls through forecasting and purchasing procedures that are standardized for the cycle menu. Forecasting involves projecting or predicting the amount of food items that need to be prepared on any given day to meet customer demands. Forecasting has a direct impact on the amount of food products and ingredients that are purchased. Since the cycle menu is planned well in advance of production and because the quantities produced are based on previous production records for each menu, the successful menu planner is able to purchase only those products that are needed in the appropriate quantities. Unnecessary inventory is a luxury the typical child nutrition program cannot afford. At the same time that the cycle aids in forecasting and purchasing to avoid unnecessary purchases, the cycle aids in the forecasting and purchasing of ample food products and ingredients to meet production demands.

The repeat intervals and number of days in each menu can vary. Menu cycles may extend for one week and repeat at the beginning of the next week. Such menus are predictable to the customers and to the staff. When the menu repeats too often, the customers may become bored with the foods offered. Short-cycle menus may lend themselves to low participation on days that offer less popular meals. However, if the cycle is too long, the staff may need to be more skilled in preparation techniques and the number of different items in the inventory may increase. Predictability in the menu makes forecasting easier and may be important to customer satisfaction. Today's student customer demands and expects certain foods on the school menu. The list of students' favorite foods is small. Participation in the program depends on the availability of these favorite foods. Students are more likely to accept new foods when they are offered with familiar ones. The cycle menu provides the repetition nutrition experts say is necessary for the acceptance of a new food.

Flexibility is planned into the best cycle menus. Quality cycle menus allow opportunities for manager's specials, seasonal fruits, and the use of unexpected leftovers. Special promotions and menu items built around special school events can be worked into existing menus. Flexible cycle menus also allow for emergency situations such as delivery delays, natural disasters, power failures, and any other condition that might alter the production or service of the school meal.

A combination of the basic cycle menu and daily specials, salad, and other food bars, as well as pizza and hamburger lines that are offered each day, is possible. Additionally, the menu can be written so that there are cycles for each of the food bars; sandwich and fast food-type menus can cycle separately. Various combinations of the different cycles provide opportunities for the program to provide the foods the customers really want without the boredom that might occur if all the elements of the menu were on the same cycle. The nutrition goals for all menus produced and served to the students are the same. When multiple options are available to students, the nutrient analysis may be more complex than when there are fewer selections. Entering the various salad and food bars as recipes makes the task of nutrient analysis manageable.

Single-Use Menus

Special school or community events, theme days, and unique menus are examples of single-use menus. For example, the ASFSA each year publishes a special menu for National School Lunch Week and National School Breakfast Week. Schools are encouraged to promote these special events by serving the theme menus in place of the regular planned menu. School-related theme menus can focus on athletic events, homecoming activities, awards dinners, prom week, and many others. Other ideas for single-use menus come from special promotions such as the Five-A-Day Program and National Nutrition Month. Holidays are traditionally a time for the school food and nutrition program to serve special menus.

Although single-use menus take time to write, promote, and execute, there are advantages of the single-use menu, including the following:

- The single-use menu allows the school food and nutrition program to become an important participant in the overall school program.
- The single-use menu that promotes theme menus such as American Education Week or National Nutrition Month, contributes to the community spirit of the school, generates excitement about coming to the cafeteria, and allows for the creative expression of the food service staff. Special menus can be recycled and used again. Maintaining a file of special menus along with the production schedules, purchasing orders, recipes, and any other information used during the special event will save

planning future similar special events or promotions.

Static or Restaurant-Style Menus

The à la carte menu offers foods priced separately and are generally available to increase sales for the program. Whether eating in a school cafeteria or a white-cloth restaurant, the customer generally pays more for a meal chosen from an à la carte menu. Not all school food authorities allow à la carte menu sales, since they can interfere with the selection of the regular meal that has been carefully planned to meet the nutritional needs of the students. Some schools offer a limited number of individually priced items to supplement the school meal. This is particularly popular for students with large appetites who may want extra milk or an extra entree. Schools that do not participate in the National School Lunch Program or the National School Breakfast Programs may rely heavily on popular à la carte menu items regardless of their nutritional value.

The table d-hôte menu is opposite in structure and pricing to the à la carte menu. The table d-hôte menu offers a full meal at a single price. This pricing structure is used in school food and nutrition programs participating in the federal programs. Program regulations require that the meal be priced as a unit; however, the customer is not required under the offer-versus-serve provision to take the full meal. Restaurants and some schools offer table d-hôte menus with choices within menu categories. For example, customers generally choose from several entrees, vegetables, salads, or desserts. The fast-food industry offers a less sophisticated version of table d-hôte menus in meal deals such as McDonald's Happy Meal and Wendy's Biggie Combo dinners. Children enjoy the familiarity of packaged meals. Advantages to the food service staff include faster service to customers, which results in faster-moving lines. Since packaged meals are popular with students, it is easier for the school food and nutrition program direc-

tor/manager to forecast the number of portions needed, and there is less waste due to overproduction.

The du jour menu means the menu of the day. In school food and nutrition programs the menu may change every day or some menu items may be served every day, while other selections vary from day to day. Creating daily menu specials as du jour items adds interest and excitement to the program. Du jour items need not be advertised if the element of surprise appeals to the children in a school. If du jour menus repeat on the same day of each week, the menu may be too predictable to be interesting enough to entice older students into the cafeteria. A variation of the du jour theme would be to designate a certain day of the week as ethnic cuisine day and vary the ethnicity of the menu each week. Students learn to anticipate the meal without becoming bored with the menu. If the program supports the production of more than one type of cuisine each day, then the menu for each cuisine could vary for added variety, nutritionally and culturally. Du jour menus also provide the advantage of the utilization of carry-over foods and bargain food purchases. The unexpected availability of a food items may also prompt the school food and nutrition program director/manager to offer a du jour menu selection.

Offering Choices

Regardless of the menu-planning option selected by the menu planner or the school food authority, choices of food items within and across food components should be made available to ensure that students have an opportunity to select a variety of delicious, nutritious foods. Offering choices is the literal translation of the recommendation of the *Dietary Guidelines* to "eat a variety of foods." Choices within food components or categories will ensure that the students will find a food that is familiar and also encourage students to try a new food.

Many school menus are limited menus offering the required food items and few if any choices. However, more and more schools are finding ways to restructure the programs to allow for more choices and greater variety in the meals served. Some school food and nutrition program directors/managers report that the students in their schools prefer limited menus over menus that offer choices. Younger children may feel overwhelmed if there are too many choices on the cafeteria line, and some secondary school students may not want to take the time to decide what to select. Student preferences vary from schools to school. A menu is successful when students select a nutritious school meal from the choices offered.

Limited-choice menus are just that—they provide minimal decision making by the students. For example, the menu may offer a choice of two entrees, three vegetables/fruits, and two grains/breads, and a choice of milk. While the offering of a choice of milk is required, the menu planner makes the decision to offer choices for the other meal components. At first glance, it may seem easier to offer choices in a food-based menu planning environment than in an NSMP environment; however, it is equally simple to extend the concept of choices to NSMP and assisted NSMP. Excellent nutrient standard-based menus include choices of the required entree, milk, and other item. For example, the school food authority using NSMP may offer an entree that is listed on the menu as a hamburger (which includes the meat patty, bun, and lettuce and tomato) and a chef's salad with crackers. The students select the entire entree of their choice as one component of the meal. Milk and one other item must be added for the meal to be reimbursable.

Full-choice menus allow choices within all meal components. Menus also may be planned to allow customers to select from a choice of full meals, such as blue-plate specials, box lunches/breakfasts, yogurt or cheese and fruit plates, and any creative combinations built around local and regional favorites. Creating clever meal deals with catchy names and attractive packaging grab the customer's atten-

tion. Added incentives can include offering one free item with the purchase of the full meal. Younger children may enjoy receiving a small prize in each packaged meal or earning points that can be applied toward a special treat for the entire class, such as a pizza party for the class that has the greatest participation in the promotion. Special meals may offer cost savings to the operation as foods are bundled and less popular items are sold along with more popular ones, thus decreasing the amount of leftover foods on the line. Also, once customers have the food they may be more likely to try new foods served along with familiar favorites. If the packaged meal is attractive enough to the customers, participation in the program could increase. Bundling in the fast food industry has increased the amount of "bundled items" sold.

Some school menus are structured around certain menu items that are served every day with variable choices. For example, tossed salad and fresh fruit are served every day with two or more other vegetable/fruit choices that change daily. Even these constants may be varied by offering differing food combinations and a variety of dressing. Such menus offer consistency and predictability that may appeal to some students. However, the menu planner should encourage variety in meal selection by the students by offering a wide range of other choices in the meal component to enhance the overall nutritional adequacy of the students' meals over time. Additional, menu planning and production are simplified when menu items are constant. The nutrition staff is familiar with the preparation of the food items, thus decreasing the time needed. Forecasting the number of servings needed each day is based on previous production and sales records.

The advantages of offering choices include the following:

- Increased food selection
- Less plate waste as students are more likely to eat foods they like

- A shift in the responsibility for selecting a nutritious meal to the student and away from the menu planner
- Introduction of new and interesting foods to students that expand their food knowledge and experiences
- More attractive presentation of meals with the addition of a variety of foods and food preparation techniques
- Interest and excitement for the mealtime experience, and others

Choice within the menu also offers a challenge to the menu planner and the production staff. The more complex the menu becomes, the more complex the production will be. More food items require a carefully planned production schedule. This may translate to more staff training. The nutrient analysis of the menu is also more extensive when items are added to the menu. Personnel may be reluctant to add choice or increase the number of existing choice for this reason. However, once the items are entered into the recipe database, the analysis can easily be completed.

Some schools have the perception that it takes longer to move customers through the serving line when a choice has to be made. Posting and announcing the menu ahead of time, talking about the menu to younger children before they come to the cafeteria, preplating foods, and self-serve bars are a few suggestions that help keep the line moving. Whatever the disadvantages to a particular program, offering choices should be considered by the menu planner. Once obstacles to offering choices are identified, strategies to overcome each one can be developed. In the final analysis, menus that feature choices can bring fun and excitement to the school food and nutrition program and meals that the students look forward to eating.

Pricing the Menu

Various price structures exist for school meals. Pricing of school meals and the method of establishing the price of the lunch and breakfast vary across the country. School food and nutrition program directors provide information to their administrative supervisor or to the local school board related to costs and budgets needed. The local board of education generally approves the sale price of meals based on a recommendation from staff. In most instances prices are set at the beginning of the school year. As stated earlier, schools participating in the National School Lunch Program or The School Breakfast Program are required to have meals priced as a unit. General pricing principles include establishing the cost of the meals based on the cost of food, labor, and the availability of USDA-donated commodities. Menus that are labor intense, rely little on commodities, or rely heavily on high-priced prepared products (each product should be evaluated individually for cost effectiveness) may lead to prices that are higher than menus that take greater advantage of commodities, control labor, and select prepared products carefully for the degree of value added. Establishing a fair and reasonable price for the meal is important to student participation in the program. It is to the advantage of the program to keep the sale price within the reach of the paying student. Studies have shown a direct relationship between level of meal price increase and participation decline.

In addition to meals priced as a unit, school food authorities may approve the sale of additional food items along with the regular meal. Extra food sales (selected from foods offered as part of the reimbursable meal) and the sale of à la carte items not part of the reimbursable meal are regulated by the state agency. Not all states allow the sale of extra foods and/or à la carte food items. Menu planners must be thoroughly familiar with the requirement of the state agencies that administer the child nutrition programs in their states. There is much discussion among child nutrition professionals on the place that à la carte sales have in the programs. The sale of extra food items that are part of the reimbursable meal is generally viewed as a means of enhancing student satisfaction, especially for students that need more calories than the regular meal provides (i.e., student athletes, children experiencing growth spurts). However, à la carte sales are generally instituted as a means of increasing revenue. The food items selected for sale to the student customer should be selected to make a positive nutrition contribution to the menu available to the customers.

As a means of supporting the nutritional integrity of the school meal program, it is generally recommended that only those foods that make a significant nutritional contribution to the daily food needs of children be available in the school. Despite this sound recommendation, flavored beverages and soft drinks, candies, salty snack foods, snack cakes, and other items of low-nutritional quality are often sold as à la carte items. The sale of such items may be in competition with the school meal program. The *Code of Federal Regulations* (7 C.F.R. Chapter 2, 210.11) defines competitive foods to mean any food sold in competition with the program to children in food service areas during the lunch periods. The regulations specifically prohibit the sale of foods of minimal nutrition value in food service areas during the lunch period. School food and nutrition programs participating in the National School Lunch and Breakfast Programs must follow guidelines established by the state agency related to sale of competitive foods. Foods of minimal nutritional value may not be part of the reimbursable meal. State agencies may establish competitive food rules that limit serving certain foods as described by the agency during specified times during the school day or at all.

On the other hand, many programs offer higher nutrient-dense foods on the à la carte menu. When foods are sold separate from the reimbursable meal, they are not included in the nutrient analysis even though they are part of the student's meal. When à la carte food items are available to students, the nutrition needs are better met when all foods served in the cafeteria follow the same nutrition standard and contribute positively to the nutrient intake of the students.

Foods of Minimal Nutritional Value as Identified by USDA

- Soda water
- Water ices (water ices that contain fruit or fruit juices are not included)
- Chewing gum
- Certain candies
  —Hard candy (e.g., sourballs, fruit balls, candy sticks, lollipops, starlight mints, after-dinner mints, sugar wafers, rock candy, cinnamon candies, breath mints, jawbreakers, cough drops)
  —Jellies and gums (e.g., gumdrops, jelly beans, jellied and fruit-flavored slices)
  —Marshmallow candies
  —Fondants (e.g., candy corn and soft mints)
  —Licorice
  —Spun candy
  —Candy-coated popcorn

STEPS IN MENU PLANNING

Once the menu-planning system and type of menu have been selected and the principles of good menu planning are understood, the school food and nutrition program director/manager is ready to write the menu. *Healthy School Meals Training*[44] refers to these steps as the "ABCs of menu planning":

- Collect menu resources.
- Select the grade or age group.
- Determine number of choices.
- Evaluate the starting point.
- Determine a time period.
- Select the entree or main course.
- Select the other menu item(s).

- Provide fluid milk choices.
- Meet nutrition goals.
- Evaluate.

In food-based menu systems, the entree or main item is considered the center of the plate; however, the concept of what an entree is has changed. Grains and vegetable entrees are finding their way to the center of the plate traditionally occupied by meat, poultry, and fish dishes. Once the entree is selected, other foods that complement the flavor and other sensory characteristics of the entree are planned.

THE MENU AS A MARKETING TOOL

The menu is the most visual evidence of the mission of the child nutrition program. As discussed earlier in this chapter, the menu is the tangible commitment of the program to the food and nutrition needs of the children it serves. When the principles of good menu planning are followed and foods are properly prepared, high-quality foods are presented to the customers. Such meals will sell themselves. Seasonal menus, signature menu items, consistent portion control, special menus that focus on school and community events, in-house branding of foods, and nutrient disclosure (for students who are interested in the nutritional aspects of the program) are additional menu-planning ideas that will help the menu sell the child nutrition program.[45]

The cafeteria is a great place to involve the whole school in special events that promote the school food and nutrition staff as an integral part of the school system and increase the participation in the program at the same time. For example, in Xenia, Ohio,[46] the school food and nutrition staff invited students to spend a week at the beach! A beach party kit provided banners and beach-theme decorations. The cafeteria staff dressed in beach wear, and foods such as "Caribbean chicken patty" and "surfboard taters" were served. On one day, all but 20 children ate the beach party lunch!

CONTINUOUS QUALITY IMPROVEMENT OF THE MENU

Menu evaluation in school food and nutrition is a necessary continuing process that assesses customer satisfaction and food acceptability, profitability, and nutrition integrity. Food acceptability can be measured by using plate waste studies, sales data, customer surveys, and simple observation.[47]

The *Keys to Excellence: Standards of Practice for Nutrition Integrity*[48] provides standards of practice and indicators for the continuous review, evaluation, and improvement of child nutrition programs.[49] The *Keys to Excellence* indicators for nutrition standards include those related to menu planning:

- Menus are planned to meet the National School Lunch Program requirements.
- Planned menus are followed with only appropriate menu substitutions.
- Choices of food items within each menu category are provided.
- Menus are analyzed for nutrient content.
- Planned menus and standardized recipes are followed to ensure the nutrient accuracy of the meals served.

Before the menu is put into production, the menu planner makes an assessment of the menu to determine whether the menu is planned so that the following apply:

- Ingredients and food products are available at a price that fits the school food and nutrition program budget.
- Equipment is adequate to prepare the menu.
- Adequate time is available to prepare the menu.
- Food service employees have the necessary knowledge and skills needed to prepare and serve the menu.
- Unnecessary repetition of ingredients in food items is avoided.
- High-fat foods are balanced with lower-fat choices, strongly flavored foods are lim-

ited, textures of foods vary in the meal, a variety of food flavors are planned, and all foods flavors are compatible.

- Flavoring ingredients are pleasing to the customers.
- A variety of colors are planned.
- The presentation of the food is attractive.

APPLICATION

Dietary Guidelines for Americans recommendations include the following, which should be considered in menu planning.

Eat a Variety of Foods. Planning a menu that offers variety in food choices over time improves the nutritional quality of the meals served in the cafeteria. Foods from all the food groups and many different foods from within each food group ensure variety in the nutrients available to the student customer. No one food is a perfect food, containing all the nutrients children need for good health, growth, and development. Variety in foods offered makes eating more enjoyable. Offering choices within food groups is a good way to encourage children to select foods from all menu categories, especially the least favorite vegetable group. In addition to the nutrients known to be in foods, scientist are discovering other substances that are needed for health and may prevent chronic diseases. When planning the menu for variety, keep in mind that certain nutrients such as calcium and iron are critical nutrients for growing children and are found in abundance in few foods. Therefore, the menu contains a reliable source of calcium such as dairy products and iron from lean meats, cooked dry beans and lentils, leafy green vegetables, whole grains, and fortified cereals to ensure adequacy.

The *Healthy School Meal Training* manual offers the following suggestions for planning variety in school meals:

- Plan a different meat or meat alternate or a different combination of meat or meat alternates for each day in the week.

- Follow a plan for providing a good variety of meats and meat alternates in the main dishes.
- Include raw or cooked vegetables in salads.
- Plan to use raw or cooked fruits in fruit cups and desserts.
- Use a different combination of two or more servings of vegetables and fruits each day. Include all forms of vegetables and fruits: fresh, canned, frozen, and dried.
- Plan to use a different kind of bread or bread alternate each day. Include a variety of enriched rice, macaroni, noodles, and other pasta products.
- Offer schoolmade loaf breads or hot breads, such as rolls, sandwich buns, muffins, biscuits, or cornbread as often as possible.

Balance the Food You Eat with Physical Activity. Although it is the menu planner's responsibility to plan the menu and not the physical education program, both food intake and physical activity play a role in the growing rate of obesity in children. Lower-fat meals may help prevent obesity in children, but fat restrictions below the recommendation of not more than 30 percent of total calories are advised with caution and should be prescribed by a qualified medical professional. Fat restriction for children less than two years of age is not recommended. Teaching children to eat grains, vegetables, fruits, and lower-fat dairy and other protein-rich foods is recommended. The combination of a healthful diet, physical activity, and the effects of normal growth in overweight children is the desirable approach to helping children achieve a healthy body weight. SMI suggestions for planning menus that promote healthy weight in children include the following:

- Serve plenty of fruits and vegetables.
- Serve more pasta, rice, breads, and cereals without fats and sugars added in preparation.

- Serve less fat and fewer high-fat foods.
- Serve desserts and sweets in moderation.

Choose a Diet with Plenty of Grain Products, Vegetables, and Fruits. Surveys show that many children do not eat adequate amounts of fruits and vegetables. The results of the *California Dietary Practices Survey of Children, Ages 9–11*[50] reported that only one-third of the children surveyed knew the recommended number of servings of fruits and vegetables and less than one-fourth ate five servings a day as recommended. Grains, fruits, and vegetables provide vitamins (vitamin A from carotene, vitamin C, vitamin B_6, and folate), minerals, and fiber; and they are a valuable source of calories in the form of carbohydrates. As the school menu incorporates fewer calories from fat, carbohydrate calories are key to providing a meal that meets the caloric requirements of the students served.

Whole grains, fruits, and vegetables are sources of soluble and insoluble fiber. Both types of fiber are part of a healthful diet and have been studied for their role in the prevention of certain chronic diseases. The benefits of fiber in the maintenance of a healthy digestive system is well documented.[51] SMI suggestions for menu planning to meet the recommendations of the guideline include the following:

- Offer vegetables higher in fiber, such as cooked dry beans, broccoli, tomatoes, leafy greens, carrots, and potatoes with skin.
- Offer raw vegetable salads.
- Offer vegetarian baked beans.
- Offer whole or cut-up fresh fruits higher in fiber such as those with edible skins— apples, pears, nectarines, peaches—and those with edible seeds such as berries and bananas.
- Offer quick breads, muffins, crackers, or cookies made with whole grains or whole-grain flours such as cornmeal, wheat flour, oats, bulgur, and brown rice.
- Serve a variety of pasta salads.

- Offer whole-grain breads and cereals at breakfast and for snacks.

Choose a Diet Low in Fat, Saturated Fat, and Cholesterol. It is generally accepted that a diet that is lower in total fat, saturated fat, and cholesterol is related to a lower risk of heart disease. Since the risk of heart disease, and other chronic diseases, can be diminished by lifestyle factors that include healthy eating habits, it seems appropriate to begin early in life. Planning school meals with this in mind allows children an opportunity to learn and practice healthy eating habits. By age five a diet that contains no more than 30 percent of calories from fat is appropriate.[52] Lowering fat in school menus gradually helps ensure greater student acceptance.[53]

Follow the suggestions below to meet the recommendations of the *Dietary Guidelines* for total fat, saturated fat, and cholesterol:

- Offer lean meats, fish, poultry, cooked dry beans, peas, and lentils.
- Choose entrees without added fat.
- Offer reduced-fat or nonfat salad dressing.
- Balance higher-fat foods in menus with items lower in fat. For example, offer baked french fries or baked potatoes instead of deep-fried french fries with chicken nuggets or burgers.
- Replace higher-fat grain products such as croissants, doughnuts, and sweet rolls with lower-fat grain products such as bagels, English muffins, and pita bread.
- Serve jam, jelly, or honey instead of butter or margarine on breads and rolls.
- Increase the variety of low-fat grain products such as noodles, brown rice, barley, and bulgur.
- Encourage low-fat (2 percent and 1 percent) and skim milk choices.

Choose a Diet Moderate in Sugars. Sugar and sugary foods offer the menu planner an opportunity to increase the calorie content of meals that have been modified for lower fat. Remember, when the fat goes out, so do calories. When the energy needs of the children are high, calories from sugar provide a tasty alternative for fat. Unlike fats, sugars have not been linked to the etiology of chronic diseases. Sometimes teachers and parents may object to sugar and sugar-containing foods being on the school menu. Often hyperactivity and dental health are cited as reasons not to include sugars in the school meal. Research does not support the notion that sugar causes or aggravates hyperactivity in children, nor does sugar lead to dental caries in children if proper dental hygiene is followed.

Sugars add flavor and interest to the school meal, which may also suffer when fat is modified. When used in moderation, sugar is an acceptable part of healthier school meals. However, many foods high in sugars may be low in other nutrients, such as the vitamins and minerals needed for good health. Various forms of sugars are used in processed foods. Look for these forms of sugar on food labels: sucrose or table sugar, confectioner's sugar, brown sugar, raw sugar, turbinado sugar, glucose or dextrose, fructose or fruit sugar, high-fructose corn syrup, molasses, honey, maltose concentrate, lactose or milk sugar, syrups, corn sweetener, and fruit juice concentrates. SMI suggestions for sugar include the following:

- Use fruits packed in light syrup.
- Use healthful grain desserts.
- Use fresh or frozen fruit desserts.

Choose a Diet Moderate in Salt and Sodium. Sodium is an essential nutrient for adults and children; however, most Americans eat more salt and sodium than they need. Sodium is associated with high blood pressure in some people. Children like the taste of highly salted processed foods such as processed meats, cheeses, most snack foods, packaged mixes, and ready-to-eat cereal. Lower the salt in the school menu gradually for greater student acceptance. Less salt and other sodium-containing ingredients means less flavor.

Any flavor loss due to modification of recipes to lower sodium will require the addition of alternate flavors, such as the use of fresh, dried, or frozen herbs and/or spices. Alternate methods of cooking such as dry sauté for lean meats and the addition of flavorful vegetable stocks to menu items also enhance flavors of foods that have been modified to reduce the salt/sodium content. Menu-planning tips for reducing salt and other sodium-containing ingredients from Healthy School Meals Training include the following:

- Check the sodium content of ready-made foods such as soups, meats, and main dishes and select those lower in sodium. Take advantage of the nutrition facts label found on most food products or the nutrient profile provided by the manufacturer.
- Choose entrees that use herbs and spices as flavor enhancers.
- Prepare foods with lower sodium products and review the recipe for ways to reduce sodium and use herbs and spices.
- Serve salted snacks such as crackers, pretzels, or nuts in smaller amounts.
- Serve smaller amounts of condiments such as mustard, catsup, relish, and salad dressing.
- Offer salt-free seasonings as an alternative to the saltshaker.

The last of the *Dietary Guidelines* is, "If you drink alcoholic beverages, do so in moderation." This guideline has no direct application in school food and nutrition programs, as neither alcoholic beverages nor alcohol as an ingredient in cooking are allowed as part of the school nutrition program. However, the school food and nutrition program promotes a healthy lifestyle for all students. Alcoholic beverages involve risks to health and other serious problems for children and adolescents. The guideline provides a link for the school food and nutrition program to support other school programs that promote an alcohol- and drug-free lifestyle.

Janet H. Bantly, R.D. (ASFSA President, 1996–1997), said, "All children—poor, middle class, or affluent—have nutritional needs. As we approach the beginning of a new century, it is time to call on policy makers, school administrators, and staff to help us focus on each individual child's needs. We must not let the day-to-day battle for survival obliterate our role in providing for the health and learning of a child."[55(p9)]

Successful implementation of the *Dietary Guidelines* requires the menu planner to develop a strategy or plan of action. Implementation strategies include the following considerations:

- Remember that children are the primary focus for changes in the meals served in the school lunch and breakfast programs. Keep in mind the nutritional needs and taste preferences of the students when writing menus to meet the recommendations in the *Dietary Guidelines*.
- Make changes gradually and concentrate on one guideline at a time. For example, if a menu or recipe is modified for the fat content, cut sodium or sugar in another. Working on one goal at a time will cause less confusion and resistance to the changes made.
- Provide good-tasting, high-quality food choices.
- Serve foods that children are familiar with and like, along with new, unfamiliar foods to improve acceptance.
- Serve small free tastings of modified or new food choices before they are added to the menu.
- Enlist the support for healthier school meals from the entire school food and nutrition staff, school administrators, teachers, and parents.
- Celebrate success. Set small goals and work to achieve them. Move on to the next goal. The *Healthy People 2000: National Health Promotion*

and Disease Prevention Objectives[54] for the nation established the goal of at least 90 percent of the schools in America offering school meals that meet the nutrition recommendation of the *Dietary Guidelines for Americans* of no more than 30 percent of total calories from fat and no more than 10 percent of total calories from saturated fat by the year 2000. Menu planning that includes low-fat milk, cheese, cottage cheese, mayonnaise, and salad dressing, and meatless entrees to balance higher-fat foods such as ground beef allow greater opportunity to meet the weekly fat goals of the *Dietary Guidelines*. Offering choices and a variety of high-quality foods prepared and served in a pleasant environment are essential to the achievement of this objective. Nutrition education efforts that target lifestyle changes of the student customers and creative marketing are also required if the changes made in the programs' menus are to have lasting effects on the nutritional well-being of children.

- Refer to Chapter 9 for ways to coordinate the school food and nutrition program with the instructional program.

SUMMARY

The school food and nutrition director begins the process of meeting customers' needs and wants with the menu. Offering a variety of choices all focused on meeting nutritional needs and customer preferences is the beginning. Believing this, the director follows through with standards and practices for all other parts of the system — purchasing, production, service, and evaluation — to ensure that the menu is served to the customer as envisioned in the planning process. Leadership for excellence in menu planning ensures the highest quality of meals served to provide satisfied customers.

In every sense, the menu drives the program. All operational areas related to the school food and nutrition program are directed by the menu and the foods that are its basis. Everything from purchasing to staff training are affected by the menu. Menu planning is one of the most important functions carried out by the school food and nutrition program director/manager. It is a time-consuming and detailed activity, requiring knowledge and skills related to foods, customer satisfaction, and financial and operational considerations. In the regulatory environment of the school food and nutrition program, the menu planner is challenged to meet federal and state requirements for reimbursement, while meeting food preferences of students and other customers to ensure that the goals of the program are met and participation remains high.

The menu is the program's best communication tool, relaying the good nutrition message to all who are in the school setting. A well-designed and properly orchestrated menu pleases student customers and meets their expectations for flavor and appearance of foods

that are familiar to them. A well-written menu will also challenge the student diner and encourage the development of a wider range of culturally acceptable foods as part of the overall educational experience. The menu communicates the school food and nutrition program's commitment to good nutrition to the rest of the school and the community.

For many school food and nutrition programs, it has been difficult to integrate the nutrition program into the mainstream of the educational system. Now more than ever, it is critical that school food and nutrition directors/managers be proactive in setting high standards for school meal menus that are planned and offered to students: Menus that not only meet the nutrition goals of the program, regardless of the menu planning option used, but also allow the program to operate in a cost-effective manner. Achieving the proper balance in managing the school food and nutrition program to meet the demands of the students, the ever-increasing demands of school administrations for self-supported school food and nutrition programs, and a commitment to offering healthful food choices is not easy. However, achieving this balance is possible, and the menu planning process is where it all begins.

CASE STUDY
CHALLENGE: IMPLEMENTING NUTRIENT STANDARD MENU PLANNING

Elaine Keaton and Karen A. Merrill

The Albuquerque Public School (APS) system is on the cutting edge of menu development. As with any improvement effort, a long-range plan must be in place and improvements made gradually. Our first efforts toward implementing the *Dietary Guidelines for Americans* (DGA) focused on meals served in elementary and middle schools, as the high schools at that time had an open campus. In the second Case Study, the APS undertook the challenge of re-engineering the menus in the high schools.

Since the early 1980s, when the first set of *Dietary Guidelines* was published, APS has carefully planned menus with nutrient content as a key factor. Cutting the fat, serving nutrient-rich foods, and limiting simple carbohydrates have all played important roles in the APS menus. The school nutrition action project (SNAP) was just the beginning of healthier students at APS. SNAP was developed by a committee of parents and teachers. The food service director acted as an advisor. SNAP was roughly based on the early version of the DGA. The following SNAP guidelines were the basis for our menus:

- Eat a variety of foods.
- Increase the use of whole, natural foods, such as grains, fruits, and vegetables.
- Reduce the use of artificial additives, preservatives, and food coloring.
- Reduce fat, saturated fat, and cholesterol.
- Reduce the amount of refined white flour and sugar.
- Reduce the amount of sodium.

APS food services believed that every small change would help to safeguard the health of the children. The concept of SNAP was to involve students, teachers, parents, and food service personnel in the creation of nutritious school meals. Student involvement helped to build enthusiasm, encourage participation, and decrease waste.

By the early 1990s the nutrition coordinator began analyzing menus for nutrient content. Since these factors have been employed for over a decade, converting to nutrient standard menu planning (NSMP) in the mid-1990s was a snap! The first step to NSMP was to survey a random sample of students. This survey asked the student questions such as:

- What are your favorite menu items?
- How often would you like to have these items served? Popular main dishes and side dishes (fruits, vegetables and desserts) were listed.
- Which food establishments do you visit? Fast-food places such as Taco Bell, McDonald's, and Pizza Hut were listed.
- The students were asked to rank factors that played an important role in their dining environment. A few of the factors were price, promotions, speed of service, and food quality.

Once all surveys were collected the students' favorite foods were ranked. After foods were ranked, a four-week cycle menu was completed with the students' favorite dishes in mind. The purpose of the cycle menu was to limit the work involved in analyzing the menu, to create unity throughout the district, to streamline ordering and inventory, and to simplify food storage and preparation. Supervisors, managers, cooks, and bakers all had a chance to make menu suggestions. Once the menu was perfected and finalized, recipe development and modification began.

The nutrition coordinator for the district began the menu modification by targeting the cafeteria managers and kitchen employees.

Cooking classes taught by the nutrition coordinator demonstrated how to modify recipes for fat. In most bakery recipes applesauce or prune pureé was substituted for part of the fat (margarine, butter, etc.) The challenges to cut fat from main dishes were substantial, as the most popular items with students were pizza and Mexican foods. In order to decrease fat in these naturally high-fat items some low-fat cheese was substituted for regular cheese, frying was eliminated (for example, corn tortillas for enchiladas are normally fried), meats were drained, and in many cases butter or margarine was decreased and sometimes eliminated. To compensate for the flavor lost from decreased fat, a variety of spices were added to recipes.

Not all main dishes could be modified to low-fat dishes. To leap this hurdle high-fat dishes were incorporated into a week's menu of lower-fat offerings. In addition, fruit was offered as a dessert and more vegetables and grain products were offered on the menu.

Standardized recipes were developed for the new low-fat products. The recipes were utilized at all schools and the central kitchen, which provides food for 76 satellite schools. The importance of standardized recipes was stressed. Cooks and bakers became aware that they could no longer add that little extra butter. Standardized recipes created unity and consistency of product throughout the school district. It would not matter where school breakfast or lunch was eaten, every school would have the same great-tasting meal.

In the midst of all the menu changes, the food service department was busy evaluating a computer program that could be operated districtwide. The department wanted a computer program that would address all needs: nutrient analysis, cost accounting, meal accounting, and inventory and production planning. Important considerations for the computer program included ease of use, cost of hardware and software, installation, and support.

The final step was implementing nutrient analysis of the menu. Initially, the nutrition coordinator analyzed recipes and entered nutrient data on prepared products. Analysis of the menu items for each cycle week was then completed. Menus were adjusted and reanalyzed to meet the nutritional goals and nutrient standards for NSMP.

NSMP was readjusting the mind-set of managers from using food-based patterns to the realization that practically any food item can fit into a healthy breakfast or lunch.

CASE STUDY
CHALLENGE: REDESIGNING THE MENU AND KITCHEN FOR CLOSED CAMPUS

Elaine Keaton and Karen A. Merrill

Eleven high schools are in the Albuquerque Public School (APS) district. Before closed campus was adopted, all high schools had an open campus with one lunch period of 50 to 60 minutes. When the lunch bell rang, a mass exodus off campus occurred.

During the 1995–1996 school year, the superintendent announced the decision to close campus for high school students. The closed campus would affect one grade level for the next four years, until the entire student body would be required to remain on campus for lunch. Several principals challenged the closed campus by rearranging the schedule. In these schools, sessions were begun and concluded earlier, with lunch as the final period. Only students who took the bus or participated in after-school programs (i.e., sports, clubs) were required to remain on campus. This schedule was a great challenge, as the menu had to draw students into the cafeteria or participation could drop significantly.

For the remaining schools with a traditional schedule, many changes from the food service department were required to accommodate closed campus, as cafeterias were not built to serve the entire student body at one time. In addition, the menu did not have a wide variety of choices that today's students demand. A menu survey was conducted so that students would have input in the menu planning. The food service director viewed the closing of campus as an opportunity to streamline the cafeteria operation. A lot of training was necessary for the high school managers. These managers were accustomed to running their own "fast food" store, that is, all grab-and-go or snack foods.

Previous to the 1996–1997 school year, high school cafeteria managers had some freedom to create their own menus. Managers essentially ran their own restaurants, catering to likes of the students. The main meal at the high school cafeteria was either a reimbursable/traditional lunch or a reimbursable combo meal; however, reimbursable meal sales were limited. Most sales were from à la carte items in the snack bars. Training was implemented to teach managers menu planning (based on NSMP), purchasing and ordering (based on a one-week cycle menu with numerous built-in choices).

A consultant was hired to guide the department in making needed changes. The consultant spent time at each high school, after which suggestions were presented. Several individuals from the food service department, the director of special projects, and principals had the opportunity to tour schools in the Corpus Christi and Brownsville districts of Texas. The opportunity to visit cafeterias in other school districts generated ideas for remodeling changes at APS. Some of the remodeling included the following: kitchen equipment was updated; serving areas were remodeled in a food court system to accommodate more students; the seating areas were colorfully painted and decorated; and cafeterias were given catchy names, and banners and signs were displayed.

The first step APS took toward closed campus was to do a pilot study involving two high schools. From the pilot study it was discovered that in order to run a cafeteria with a closed campus effectively the following changes must be made:

- Standardization of recipes and menus throughout the high school cafeterias
- Creation of a one-week cycle menu with many choices
- Creation of a restaurant atmosphere, including remodeling the cafeteria, eliminating compartment trays and providing effective service
- Control of trash

We began the standardization process by creating a one-week cycle menu, since the menu drives all other operational functions. The menu had to be created first in order to determine necessary equipment, serving stations, and kitchen layout. The new menu was designed to be served in the food court system. The nutrition coordinator created the menu with input from high school managers, cooks, and bakers. This menu consisted of many choices, including traditional hot entrees, hamburgers, submarine sandwiches, salads, pizza, and Mexican entrees. Careful menu planning helped to eliminate unnecessary trash caused by convenience foods and excessive use of containers for different food items. Adequate trash receptacles eliminated littering on the campus. Receptacles were discreetly hidden by the use of covered enclosures.

The improvements made by the food service department created school spirit. Principals began investing school funds to help with the improvement of their cafeterias. Overall, closed campus has resulted in many positive changes, with the main one being the streamlined cycle menu that provides food acceptable to the students.

REFERENCES

1. M.C. Spears, *Foodservice Organizations: A Managerial and Systems Approach*, 3rd ed. (Englewood Cliffs, NJ: Merrill/Prentice Hall, 1995).

2. U.S. Department of Agriculture (USDA), *Nutrition and Your Health: Dietary Guidelines for Americans*, 4th ed. Home and Garden Bulletin No. 232 (Washington, DC: U.S. Government Printing Office, 1995).

3. J.B. Knight and L.H. Kotschevar, *Quantity Food Production: Planning and Management*, 2nd ed. (Boston: CBI Publishing Co., 1989).

4. D. VanEgmond-Pannell, *School Food and Nutrition*, 3rd ed. (Westport, CT: AVI Publishing Co., 1985).

5. P. Birkenshaw, "Nutrition Integrity in School Menu Planning," *School Business Affairs*, 1994, 7–8.

6. P. Stevenson, "Nutrition Integrity in Action: Planning for Success," *School Business Affairs*, 1994, 9–14.

7. American School Food Service Association (ASFSA), *Keys to Excellence: Standards of Practice for Nutrition Integrity* (Alexandria, VA: 1995).

8. Birkenshaw, "Nutrition Integrity."

9. National Research Council, *The Recommended Dietary Allowances*, 9th ed. (Washington, DC: National Academy Press; 1989).

10. J. Martin, "The National School Lunch Program—A Continuing Commitment. *Journal of the American Dietetic Association* 96 (1996): 857–858.

11. M.B. Gregoire and J. Sneed, "Standards for Nutrition Integrity," *School Food Service Research Review* 18 (1994): 106–111.

12. J. Radzikowski and S. Gale, "The National Evaluation of School Nutrition Programs: Conclusions," *American Journal of Nutrition* 10 (1984): 454–461.

13. J. Burghardt et al., *The School Nutrition Dietary Assessment Study: School Food Service, Meals Offered, and Dietary Intakes* (Alexandria, VA: United States Department of Agriculture/Food Nutrition Service, Office of Analysis and Evaluation; 1993).

14. USDA, *Dietary Guidelines for Americans*.

15. National School Lunch Program and School Breakfast Program, "School Meal Initiatives for Healthy Children" (7 C.F.R. 210, 220). *Federal Register*, June 13, 1995;60:31188–31222.

16. S.L. Hurd et al., "Evaluation of Implementation of the U.S. Dietary Guidelines into the Child Nutrition Programs in Texas," *Journal of the American Dietetic Association* 96 (1996): 904–906.

17. Martin, "The National School Lunch Program."

18. USDA Food and Consumer Service, *Healthy School Meals Training* (Washington, DC: U.S. Government Printing Office, 1996).

19. National Research Council, *Recommended Dietary Allowances*.

20. USDA, *Healthy School Meals Training*.

21. Birkenshaw, "Nutrition Integrity."

22. R.E. Thaler-Carter, "In the Spotlight: Denise I. Stilley," *School Foodservice and Nutrition* 20 (1996): 56.

23. USDA Food and Consumer Service, *Assisted NuMenus* (Washington, DC: U.S. Government Printing Office, 1996).

24. USDA, *Healthy School Meals Training*.

25. USDA, Human Nutrition Information Service, *USDA's Food Guide Pyramid* (Hyattsville, MD, 1992).

26. M. Bennion, *Introductory Foods*, 10th ed. (Englewood Cliffs, NJ: Merrill/Prentice Hall, 1995).

27. M. McWilliams, *Fundamentals of Meal Management*, 2nd. ed. (Redondo, CA: Plycon Press, 1993).

28. USDA, Food and Consumer Service, *A Tool Kit: Recipes for Healthy School Meals* (Washington, DC: US Government Printing Office, 1996).

29. ASFSA, *Keys to Excellence.*

30. USDA, *A Tool Kit.*

31. S. Morrison, "Build a Better Student Body," *School Foodservice and Nutrition* 20 (1996): 34–38.

32. P.L. Fitzgerald, "Breakfast Bonanza," *School Foodservice and Nutrition* 20 (1996): 63–70.

33. ASFSA, "Think Smart, Think Breakfast," *School Foodservice and Nutrition* 20 (1996): 25–31.

34. Institute of Food Technologists' Expert Panel on Food Safety and Nutrition, "Food Flavors," *Food Technology* 43 (1989): 99.

35. P. Jenkins, "Start the Year Off Right?" *School Foodservice and Nutrition* 20 (1996): 50.

36. "Profile of Success: Mary Klatko," *School Foodservice and Nutrition* 20 (1996): 16–20.

37. D.H. Carr et al., eds. *Competencies, Knowledge and Skills of Effective District School Nutrition Directors/Supervisors* (University, MS: National Food Service Management Institute, 1996).

38. National Food Service Management Institute, the University of Mississippi, PO Drawer 188, University, MS 38677. Phone: (601) 232-7658.

39. American School Food Service Association Emporium, Alexandria, VA. Phone: (800) 728-0728.

40. USDA Food and Consumer Service, *Menu Planning Guide for School Food Service* (Washington, DC: U.S. Government Printing Office, 1983).

41. USDA Food and Consumer Service, *Food Buying Guide for Child Nutrition Programs* (Aid No. 331) (Washington, DC: U.S. Government Printing Office, 1984; Revised 1990).

42. Spears, *Foodservice Organization.*

43. Knight and Kotschevar, *Quantity Food Production.*

44. USDA, *Healthy School Meals Training.*

45. M.D. Donovan, ed., *The New Professional Chef*, 6th ed. (New York: Van Nostrand Reinhold, 1996).

46. Fitzgerald, "Breakfast Bonanza."

47. Spears, *Foodservice Organization.*

48. ASFSA, *Keys to Excellence.*

49. S. Terry and T. Cline, "A New Set of Standards," *School Foodservice and Nutrition* 18 (1994): 79–84.

50. California Department of Health Services, *The California Dietary Practices Survey of Children, Ages 9–11: Focus on Fruits and Vegetables* (Sacramento, CA: 1993).

51. E.N. Whitney and S.R. Rolfes, *Understanding Nutrition*, 7th ed. (Minneapolis MN: West Publishing Company, 1996).

52. USDA, *Nutrition and Your Health.*

53. Hurd et al., "Evaluation of the U.S. Dietary Guidelines."

54. U.S. Department of Health and Human Services, *Healthy People 2000: National Health Promotion and Disease Prevention Objectives* (DHHS [PHS] Publication No. 91-50213) (Washington, DC: U.S. Government Printing Office, 1990).

55. J.H. Bantly, "Focus on the Child," *School Foodservice and Nutrition* 20 (1996): 9.

CHAPTER 11

Healthy Meals for Healthy Preschool Children

Jeanette P. Phillips, Helene Kent, and Charlotte B. Oakley

OUTLINE

INTRODUCTION

The preschool child experiences more than food and nutrition education in the child care setting, whether center or child care home. The child experiences nurturing, assumes responsibility, and learns interpersonal and other socialization skills.

> Eating experiences condition our entire attitude to the world, and again not so much because of how nutritious is the food we are given, but with what feelings and attitudes it is given. Around eating, for example, attitudes are learned, or not learned, which are the preconditions for all academic achievement, such as the ability to control oneself, to wait, to work now for future rewards. . . . That how one is being fed, and how one eats, has a larger impact on the personality than any other human experience.[1(pp16–17)]

The Child and Adult Care Food Program is the fastest growing federally funded food assistance program. Until recently, parents have been the primary gatekeepers of the young child's nutritional status. With more caregivers in the workforce and a rapidly growing eating-out trend by families, it has become more acceptable for parents to share the gatekeeper responsibility with other adults outside the home. Since the first pilot child care food program was funded by Congress in the 1960s, the nation has experienced dynamic social and economic changes. Research findings are continuing to support the need for concerted attention to the child during the preschool years. It has long been known that the first few years of a child's life have a major impact on long-term health and well-being.

National reports, including the *Healthy People 2000-National Health Promotion and Disease Prevention Objectives*[2] and the congressional *Goals for Education Challenge 2000*,[3]

reflect the national concern to provide preschool children with situations that promote growth and development, including learning readiness. These goals are supported by many child care programs that implement quality standards for performance.

Preschool and kindergarten programs help children develop mental, social, and physical skills. Such programs are wise investments in children, especially those from disadvantaged homes. The problems of "at risk" children and their parents are more than a school problem. Unless there is effective local coordination of health and social services linked to educational programs, some children will not be ready for the first grade in the year 2000.[3]

The child's basic physical and emotional structure is in place by age five.[4] School food and nutrition program directors have an important role and a vested interest in seeing that the food and nutrition opportunities provided young children in their communities are of the highest quality. The director's role will vary, depending on the school district's involvement in the operation of child care programs. Some directors have a direct role because the school district will sponsor and operate child care centers. School food authorities may serve as child care sponsors, vendors, and/or partners in providing quality child care. In each case, the school food and nutrition program director should assume a partnership role with the other community leaders in advocating effective programs and assisting in establishing standards. Young children enrolled in child care centers that provide quality food and nutrition experiences are more likely to participate in the school meal program when they enter kindergarten or first grade. These children have had an opportunity to develop positive eating behaviors during their most teachable time of life.

The eating habits and attitudes about food that children develop during their preschool years often last throughout their lives. One of the most effective times for having an impact on a child's long-term health potential is during the developmental years. Physical activity and the development of healthy eating patterns will help ensure nutritional well-being at all ages. The goal is to produce healthful and acceptable meals delivered in an environment that promotes healthy living and readiness to learn.

Many children are enrolled part-time or full-time in child care, and the number will continue to increase.[5] The child care environment may be either a child care home, where a few children are cared for in the provider's home, or a child care center that may enroll from a few children to several hundred. Many children spend long hours in child care and consume one-half to three-fourths of their daily food intake while in child care. The role of the child care provider is important in ensuring that children eat healthful meals and develop lifelong healthy eating habits. Child care providers have unlimited potential for helping to improve the health and well-being of our youngest citizens. Consequently, it is very important that training for child care providers emphasizes the importance of the caregiver's role in helping children develop healthy eating habits. For some children, she or he may be the only person who is able to give special attention to this aspect of their development.[6]

Food and nutrition professionals seeking excellence in child care programs strive for cost-effective program management. The purpose of this chapter is to create an awareness of the opportunities available to the school food and nutrition directors and other nutrition professionals, such as registered dietitians, to affect eating and learning behaviors of children as a community advocate or a program administrator. Food and nutrition personnel will find help in providing meals and snacks that meet preschool children's nutritional needs; offer a variety of nutritious foods; and teach eating habits that promote pleasurable eating, reduce chronic disease risks, and support a lifetime of good health.[7] The specific objectives of this chapter are to do the following:

- Provide an overview of the federally funded child care programs.
- Discuss nutritional needs and nutritional status of young children.
- Discuss the impact of the eating environment on the development of socialization skills and food preferences of young children.
- Identify standards that promote effective child care programs.
- Identify training needs to assist child care staff in the planning, preparation, and service of meals and snacks that meet children's nutritional and socialization needs.
- Assist in the evaluation of the quality of food and nutrition services presently being provided.
- Identify the role of the provider and the dietitian in the child care setting.

OVERVIEW OF CHILD CARE PROGRAMS

Nearly 60 percent of the 15 million preschool children whose mothers work outside the home are enrolled in child care centers or child care homes. Substantial numbers of children whose mothers are not employed outside the home use supplemental care in child care programs. More than 70 percent of preschool children enrolled in child care are in full-time programs, averaging 8 to 10 hours daily care.[8] Approximately one-fourth of these children are enrolled in the federally funded Child and Adult Care Food Program (CACFP), which provides reimbursement for meals based on family income eligibility standards.

Nutrition professionals have a unique opportunity to maximize the potential of all young children, regardless of race, national origin, special needs, or economic status, by routinely providing nutritious meals and snacks. Children need to be offered a variety of nutritious foods that are served in a pleasant atmosphere where they practice positive eating and social skills. In this setting young children can also be taught food habits that prevent disease and support a lifetime of good health.[9]

Child care in the United States is a patchwork of different arrangements that include child care centers, regulated child care homes, nonregulated child care homes, and other placements such as care in the child's home by a relative or other caregiver.[10] Child care facilities may be operated by nonprofit groups as a service to the community or for profit by individuals or corporations (see Exhibit 11–1).[11] Some business groups and companies provide subsidized child care for their employees. The availability of high-quality child care is a fringe benefit for many of America's working parents. The need for quality child care will continue to escalate as more mothers enter the work force and more children are raised in single-parent households.

Providing healthful meals and snacks to children during the day (and sometimes the evening as well) in a pleasant eating environment is a major responsibility for the child care facility. Child care programs have joined the family table as a gatekeeper of the food supply and serve as a nutrition learning laboratory for increasing numbers of young children.[10] Foods consumed in the child care setting and the environment in which they are served have a major impact on whether children's immediate nutritional needs are met and health-promoting eating patterns are developed.

Child and Adult Care Food Program

The Child and Adult Care Food Program was permanently authorized by Congress in 1975 as part of the National School Lunch Act.[12] (Public Law 101-147 changed the name of the child care food program to child and adult care food program.) The legislation prescribes criteria to ensure nutritious meals and snacks for all children. The program is administered by the U.S. Department of Agriculture (USDA), which provides federal funds and USDA commodities or cash equivalents to

---

Exhibit 11–1 Federally Assisted Programs for Preschool Children and Local Administrators

Federally Assisted Program	Local Administrator
Child and Adult Care Food Program	Licensed child care centers, family day-care homes, Head Start programs
Sets criteria and provides funding for nutritious meals and snacks and nutrition education in child care settings	
Head Start Program	
Provides comprehensive health, educational, nutrition, social and other services to low-income preschool children and their families	Local Head Start program
Special Supplemental Food Program for Women, Infants, and Children (WIC)	Health agencies, social services, community action agencies
Provides supplemental food and nutrition education as an adjunct to health care to low-income pregnant, postpartum, and breast-feeding women and to infants and children at nutritional risk	

Source: Reprinted from G.C. Frank-Spohrer, *Community Nutrition: Applying Epidemiology to Contemporary Practice*, p. 250, © 1996, Aspen Publishers, Inc.

child care centers, adult day-care centers, and regulated child care homes that serve snacks and meals to children and adults. The program provides reimbursement for meals served to children aged 13 years or younger in child care homes and child care centers.

Programs operating under the CACFP receive financial assistance by way of the state agency responsible for its administration. Child care home providers participate in the CACFP through a sponsoring organization approved by the state agency. Sponsors employ staff who are responsible for meeting prescribed requirements of record keeping, management, monitoring, and provider training. The Personal Responsibility and Work Opportunity Reconciliation Act of 1996[13] made significant changes in program eligibility requirements that resulted in a decreased number of child care homes participating in the CACFP.

In 1997 there were 28,865 child care centers and 186,932 regulated child care homes participating in the CACFP. Almost a third of the children served by the CACFP are cared for in child care homes, 25 percent in Head Start centers, and the remaining 44 percent in other child care centers. Approximately 22 percent are under two years of age and 60 percent are aged three to four years. One-fourth of the children enrolled receive three to four meals each day. There were 2,575,492 children enrolled in the CACFP in March 1997. Sixty-four percent of the children served met the family income eligibility guidelines for free meals, seven percent of the children met the reduced-price meal category guidelines, and twenty-eight percent of the children did not qualify for either free or reduced-priced meals. Child care homes serve a higher percentage of free meals than child care centers.[14]

Head Start

Head Start is a national program which provides comprehensive developmental services for America's low-income, preschool children ages three to five years and social services for their families.[15] Specific services for children focus on education, socioemotional development, physical and mental health, and nutrition. The children who participate are eligible for a broad range of medical, dental, mental health, and nutrition programs. Nutrition education is emphasized and integrated into the curriculum. Parent and community involvement, the cornerstone of the program, has made it one of the most successful preschool programs in the country. In 1998 approximately 1,400 community-based nonprofit organizations and school systems developed unique and innovative programs to meet specific needs.

The major components of Head Start are education, health, parent involvement, and social services. Nutrition services are an integral part of the Head Start program. Head Start programs are required to participate in the CACFP, which enhances the quality of nutrition education activities and food service operations. As participants in the CACFP, Head Start programs adhere to the same nutrition standards and meal patterns of other child care programs (see Tables 11–1 and 11–2).

The success of the Head Start program, which began in 1965, prompted the Congress to establish the Early Head Start program in 1994 to reach low-income pregnant women and families with infants and toddlers. This expansion was based on research evidence that the period from birth to age three years is critical to healthy growth and development and later success in school and life. The purpose of the Early Head Start program is to enhance children's physical, social, emotional, and cognitive development; enable parents to be better caregivers of and teachers to their children; and help parents meet their own goals, including that of economic independence.

The services provided by Early Head Start programs are designed to reinforce and respond to the unique strengths and needs of each child and family. Services include the following:

Table 11–1 Child and Adult Care Food Program Infant Meal Pattern

Meal	Birth through Three months	Four through Seven months	Eight through Eleven months
Breakfast	4–6 fl. oz. breast milk or iron-fortified infant formula *Meals containing only breast milk are not reimbursable*	4–8 fl. oz. breast milk or iron-fortified infant formula 0–3 Tbsp infant cereal (optional)	6–8 fl. oz. breast milk, iron-fortified infant formula, or whole milk 2–4 Tbsp infant cereal 1–4 Tbsp fruit and/or vegetable
Lunch or supper	4–6 fl. oz. breast milk or iron-fortified infant formula *Meals containing only breast milk are not reimbursable*	4–8 fl. oz. breast milk or iron-fortified infant formula 0–3 Tbsp infant cereal (optional) 0–3 Tbsp fruit and/or vegetable (optional)	6–8 fl. oz. breast milk, iron-fortified infant formula, or whole milk 2–4 Tbsp infant cereal or 1–4 Tbsp meat, fish, poultry, egg yolk, cooked dry beans, or dry peas, or ½–2 oz. cheese or 1–4 oz. cottage chees, cheese food, or cheese spread 1–4 Tbsp fruit and/or vegetable
Supplement	4–6 fl. oz. breast milk or iron fortified infant formula *Meals containing only breast milk are not reimbursable*	4–6 fl. oz. breast milk or iron-fortified infant formula	2–4 fl. oz. breast milk, iron-fortified infant formula, whole milk or fruit juice 0–½ slice bread or 0–2 crackers (optional)

- Meals containing **breast milk** may be claimed when the infant is 4 months old or older and when the center or day-care home provider provides at least one other required meal component.
- **Formula** served must be iron-fortified infant formula. The formula must be intended as the sole source of food for normal, healthy infants, and must be served in the liquid state at the manufacturer's recommended dilution.
- **Infant cereal** must be iron-fortified, dry infant cereal. Infant cereal is often mixed with breast milk, formula or milk.
- **Fruit juice** must be full strength.
- **Bread or crackers** must be made from whole-grain or enriched meal or flour.
- **Nuts, seeds, or nut butters** are not allowed as a meat alternate.
- **Whole milk** may be served at eight months of age as long as the infant is consuming approximately one-third of his or her calories as a balance mixture of cereal, fruits, vegetables, and other foods. (A policy change in the near future will not allow whole milk to be served to children less than one year old. Contact your state agency or sponsor for information.)

Source: Reprinted from U.S. Department of Agriculture, Food and Nutrition Service, Midwest Region Child Nutrition Programs, *"What's in a Meal?" A Resource Manual for Providing Nutritious Meals in the Child and Adult Care Food Program,* January 1999, U.S. Government Printing Office.

Table 11–2 CACFP Meal Pattern Requirements for Three- to Five-Year-Old Children

Breakfast	AM Snack	Lunch	PM Snack	Supper
Bread or bread alternate (including cereal)	(select 2–4) Milk, fluid Juice or fruit or vegetable	Meat or meat alternate	(select 2–4) Milk, fluid Juice or fruit or vegetable	Meat or meat alternate
Juice or fruit or vegetable	Bread or bread alternate	Vegetable and/or fruits (2 or more) Bread or bread alternate	Bread or bread alternate	Vegetable and/or fruits (2 or more) Bread or bread alternate
Milk, fluid	Meat or meat alternate	Milk, fluid	Meat or meat alternate	Milk, fluid

Source: Reprinted from U.S. Department of Agriculture, Food and Nutrition Service, *Child and Adult Care Food Program—Nutrition Guidance for Child Care Centers,* September 1995, U.S. Government Printing Office.

- Quality early education in and out of the home
- Home visits, especially for families with newborns and other infants
- Parent education, including parent-child activities
- Comprehensive health services, including services to pregnant women
- Nutrition
- Ongoing support for parents

Staff development and training are provided to staff at all levels and in all program areas, including nutrition and food service operations. The child development associate program gives professional and nonprofessional employees the opportunity to pursue academic degrees or certification in early childhood education. Bilingual specialization in available to meet the needs of a diverse population of Head Start staff. Outreach and training activities also assist parents in increasing their parenting skills and knowledge of child development.

The Head Start programs are administered by the U.S. Department of Health and Human Services (DHHS) Administration of Children, Youth, and Families. The CACFP is administered by the USDA Food and Nutrition Services (FNS). The coordination of services of these two programs demonstrates a collective, collaborative national approach to meeting the needs of infants and young children and their families.

Special Supplemental Nutrition Program for Women, Infants, and Children

The Special Supplemental Nutrition Program for Women, Infants, and Children (WIC) is designed to serve pregnant, postpartum, and lactating women, and infants and children up to the age of five years. The purpose of WIC is to provide supplemental foods and nutrition education. Additionally, WIC is to be an adjunct to other health care services. WIC has consistently proven to be one of the most effective federally funded nutrition programs.[16] National standards are established by USDA to ensure that adequate nutrition services are provided to the clientele. The administering state agency provides a plan for nutrition education, including training to persons delivering nutrition education. The nutrition education is evaluated annually at the state level and includes the views of the participants concerning its effectiveness. Child care providers who participate in the CACFP can support the goals of the WIC program by reinforcing the nutrition education messages provided through the WIC program. The WIC and Head Start programs have professional requirements for supervising personnel.

The overwhelming success of the WIC program in ensuring positive outcomes for pregnancy and early infancy can largely be attributed to prenatal care and access to supplemental foods and formulas. This success is supported by the program's national standards, professional requirements for supervising personnel, and requirements for nutrition education and evaluation. WIC, like no other program, creates a sustainable framework through a systems approach for meeting the health and nutrition needs of pregnant and postpartum women, infants, and children (Figure 11–1). The CACFP allows nutrition professionals an opportunity to ensure continuity of nutrition services for young children and to sustain the success achieved in the WIC program.

Other Child Care Programs

Many states and local communities have enrichment programs to enhance learning readiness for prekindergarten students. These programs are often outside the regular school program, and meals and snacks are available through the CACFP. In other cases these enrichment programs are integrated into the school, and meals are provided through the National School Lunch Program (NSLP) or School Breakfast Program (SBP) along with those meals for kindergarten through grade 12 students. Federal reimbursement for snacks served in school to prekindergarten children is currently available under the CACFP. However, school food and nutrition leaders are attempting to secure a legislative provision to allow for the payment of snacks under the school meals program. Private programs that operate outside the federally sponsored CACFP and school food and nutrition environment also offer meals and snacks for young children. Ideally these programs provide the same high-quality meal service and nutrition education opportunities.

NUTRITION NEEDS AND NUTRITIONAL STATUS OF YOUNG CHILDREN

Nutritional Status

Most of the children in the United States are well nourished, and overweight in young children is the exception rather than the rule. The *Healthy People 2000* objectives address certain areas of concern related to nutrients, such as iron, that is problematic for some children.[17] Children from low-income households are most likely to suffer from malnourishment

Systems Model for Healthy Mothers and Infants

The WIC Program

Input	Controls	Outcomes
Prenatal Care	Standards	Healthy Mothers
	TRANSFER	
Supplemental foods		Healthy Infants
Nutrition Education		Healthy Children
Professional Personnel		

←←←←←←←←←←←←←←←Evaluation →→→→→→→→→→→→→→→

Figure 11–1 Systems Model for Healthy Mothers and Infants

and growth retardation due to inadequate energy intake and nutrient deficiencies. Hunger is a way of life for many of America's young children and the child care food programs provide a much needed safety net to protect young children, millions of whom live in poverty.[17,18]

Nutrition Needs

The nutrient needs of infants and children aged one to three, four to six, and seven to ten years are defined in the recommended dietary allowances (RDA).[19] The RDAs are designed to promote the maintenance of good nutrition for healthy people and are expressed as average daily intakes over time to provide for individual variations among people (Table 11–3). The nutrition principles of the *Dietary Guidelines for Americans*[20] help reduce the risk factors associated with chronic diseases, including heart disease and cancer. The *Dietary Guidelines* are designed to help caregivers of children over two years of age to choose diets that will meet nutrient requirements, promote health, support active lifestyles, and reduce risk of chronic disease. The recommendations for total calories from fat, saturated fat, and cholesterol are based on research findings dealing with adults and chronic disease. These recommendations may not be appropriate for very young children; however, by the time children reach school age they should be following a diet that is based on the *Dietary Guidelines*. Overzealous applications of the fat-related guidelines may lead to undernutrition and poor growth and development of the young child. The Food Guide Pyramid[21] translates the *Dietary Guidelines* into the kinds and amounts of food to eat each day.

The menus plans for the CACFP are designed to meet two-thirds of the child's RDAs for key nutrients and calories. Meals and snacks in the child care program should meet meal pattern requirements and reflect the nutrition principles of the *Dietary Guidelines* as illustrated in the Food Guide Pyramid.

Meals served by institutions participating in the CACFP shall consist of a combination of foods that meet minimum nutritional requirements prescribed by the Secretary on the basis of tested nutritional research.[22]

The CACFP regulations contain meal and snack patterns with appropriate accommodations for the age of children, the number of hours at the center or program site, and any cultural or ethnic differences in food habits. A child in a part-day program (four to seven hours per day) should receive food that provides at least one-third of the RDAs, while those in a full-day program (eight hours or more per day) should receive at least one-half to two-thirds.

Children have an opportunity to learn and practice healthy eating habits when served meals and snacks consistent with the *Dietary Guidelines*. Meals and snacks should be planned so that they are appetizing; give consideration to the children's cultural food patterns and to the size of their appetites; and provide appropriate numbers of servings of dairy products, meat and/or meat alternates, vegetables, fruit, and grain products.[23]

The CACFP infant meal plan specifies breakfast, snack, lunch, and supper—these are just guidelines. Infants six months of age or under should not be expected to comply with a rigid feeding schedule. It is best to feed infants on demand. Between four and seven months of age, infants begin to show signs of developmental readiness for semisolid foods. The portions for solids listed on the infant meal pattern are optional for this age group. The decision to introduce solid foods should be made in consultation with the parents. If infants are fed solid foods before they are developmentally ready, choking may occur.

Early feeding may inappropriately replace breast milk or formula that is nutritionally complete for young infants. It is best to serve infants breast milk or iron-fortified infant for-

Table 11–3 Recommended Dietary Allowance

AGE (yrs)	Weight (kg)	Weight (lb)	Height (cm)	Height (in)	ENERGY (kcal)	PROTEIN (g)	VITAMIN A (µg)	VITAMIN D (µg)	VITAMIN E (mg a-TE)	VITAMIN K (µg)	VITAMIN C (mg)	THIAMINE (mg)	RIBOFLAVIN (mg)	NIACIN (mg NE)	VITAMIN B6 (mg)	FOLATE (µg)	VITAMIN B12 (µg)	CALCIUM (mg)	PHOSPHORUS (mg)	MAGNESIUM (mg)	IRON (mg)	ZINC (mg)	IODINE (µg)	SELENIUM (µg)
Infants																								
0.0–0.5	6	13	60	24	650	13	375	7.5	3	5	30	0.3	0.4	5	0.3	25	0.3	400	300	40	6	5	40	10
0.5–1.0	9	20	71	28	850	14	375	10	4	10	35	0.4	0.5	6	0.6	35	0.5	600	500	60	10	5	50	15
Children																								
1–3	13	29	90	35	1300	16	400	10	6	15	40	0.7	0.8	9	1.0	50	0.7	800	800	80	10	10	70	20
4–6	20	44	112	44	1800	24	500	10	7	20	45	0.9	1.1	12	1.1	75	1.0	800	800	120	10	10	90	20
7–10	28	62	132	52	2000	28	700	10	7	30	45	1.0	1.2	13	1.4	100	1.4	800	800	170	10	10	120	30
Males																								
11–14	45	99	157	62	2500	45	1000	10	10	45	50	1.3	1.5	17	1.7	150	2.0	1200	1200	270	12	15	150	40
15–18	66	145	176	69	3000	59	1000	10	20	65	60	1.5	1.8	20	2.0	200	2.0	1200	1200	400	12	15	150	50
19–24	72	160	177	70	2900	58	1000	10	10	70	60	1.5	1.7	19	2.0	200	2.0	1200	1200	350	10	15	150	70
25–50	79	174	176	70	2900	63	1000	5	10	80	60	1.5	1.7	19	2.0	200	2.0	800	800	350	10	15	150	70
50+	77	170	173	68	2300	63	1000	5	10	80	60	1.2	1.4	15	2.0	200	2.0	800	800	350	10	15	150	70
Females																								
11–14	46	101	157	62	2200	46	800	10	8	45	50	1.1	1.3	15	1.4	150	2.0	1200	1200	280	15	12	150	45
15–18	55	120	163	64	2200	44	800	10	8	55	60	1.1	1.3	15	1.5	180	2.0	1200	1200	300	15	12	150	50
19–24	58	128	164	65	2200	46	800	10	8	60	60	1.1	1.3	15	1.6	180	2.0	1200	1200	280	15	12	150	55
25–50	63	138	163	64	2200	50	800	5	8	65	60	1.1	1.3	15	1.6	180	2.0	800	800	280	15	12	150	55
50+	65	143	160	63	1900	50	800	5	8	65	60	1.0	1.2	13	1.6	180	2.0	800	800	280	10	12	150	55
Pregnant					(+)300	60	800	10	10	65	70	1.5	1.6	17	2.2	400	2.2	1200	1200	320	30	15	175	65
Lactating																								
1st 6 mo.					(+)500	65	1300	10	12	65	95	1.6	1.8	20	2.1	280	2.6	1200	1200	355	15	19	200	75
2nd 6 mo.					(+)500	62	1300	10	11	65	90	1.6	1.7	20	2.1	260	2.6	1200	1200	340	15	16	200	75

Source: Reprinted with permission from *Recommended Dietary Allowances: 10th Edition.* Copyright 1989 by the National Academy of Sciences. Courtesy of the National Academy Press, Washington, D.C.

Note: α-TE = α-tocopherol equivalents; 1 mg d-α-tocopherol = 1α-TE.

mula for at least the first year. After the first year, whole milk can be introduced. Whole milk provides essential fatty acids that are required for normal brain development, healthy skin and hair, normal eye development, and resistance to infection and disease.[24] It is recommended that whole milk be used until two years of age, after which 2 percent milk can be introduced.[25]

Introduce new semisolid foods gradually. Introduce one new food at a time and wait about a week to introduce the next new food, because this will help identify any food allergies that might develop. The texture of foods must meet the different developmental stages. Prepare the food in a way that is easy to eat. Infants and young children must have constant adult supervision during mealtimes. Choking may occur as children begin to feed themselves. Adults need to be available to help avoid choking and assist children with any other feeding needs. Holding an infant during bottle feeding will help prevent choking and will also lessen the likelihood that tooth decay (nursing bottle tooth decay) may develop due to the pooling of formula or milk in the infant's mouth that may occur when the infant is fed from a propped bottle. When babies are put to bed with a bottle, they are likely to suck for long periods of time, which can change the shape of the jawline.[26]

Healthy People 2000 includes the following objective: "Increase to at least 75% the proportion of parents and caregivers who use feeding practices that prevent nursing bottle tooth decay."[27]

IMPACT OF THE EATING ENVIRONMENT ON THE DEVELOPMENT OF SOCIALIZATION SKILLS AND FOOD PREFERENCES

Adults who work with young children need to understand the developmental needs of children and how to model their own behavior to accommodate those needs. Developing appropriate eating skills and behaviors is an important part of the child's total social development. Creating an environment that fosters healthy and happy eating occasions requires planning that takes into considerations the child's readiness to accept new and different foods and experiences. The social skills learned during mealtime can be applied to other social interactions that children experience each day.

Create an Eating Environment Conducive to the Development of Socialization Skills

- Establish a calm atmosphere for eating.
- Have adults serve as role models and eat with children.
- Encourage quiet conversation and positive behavior.
- Provide enough time for children to eat.
- Provide chairs, tables, and utensils that are comfortable and of appropriate size.
- Involve children in the meal service.

Establish a Calm Atmosphere for Eating. The atmosphere at mealtime has an impact on the development of children's attitudes about food and eating. The mealtime atmosphere is affected by the physical setting, the timing of meals, how children are transitioned to the meal, the table and its setup, the participation of the adult caregiver, and the noises or movements around the room. Children are better able to focus on the meal, to eat, and to learn about the foods they are eating if the atmosphere is calm and relaxed. Children eat better when they have a chance for quiet time between the meal and play or other activities. They are also more receptive to learning about the foods, and fewer spills and other accidents are likely to occur when the environment is relaxed and the children are ready to participate. Soft music, reading a story, and singing with the children are ways to make the transition from active time to mealtime.

Have Adults Serve as Role Models and Eat with Children. The caregiver usually sets the tone for the meal. Adults need to sit with the children and eat the same meal as the children while modeling good eating behaviors. Adults who have a positive attitude toward food and the mealtime experience will have more success in teaching these skills to children. Adults should taste all foods and not show personal food preferences.

Mealtime also provides an opportunity for nutrition education. The caregiver should talk to the children about the foods being eaten, discuss what the foods are, how they are grown, where they come from, how they help the body grow. At this age children are developmentally ready to learn about colors, textures, tastes, and the differences and similarities of foods they are eating. Caregivers can make positive, encouraging statements when discussing the food and the meal, while avoiding any negative, directive, or pressuring statements. Watching adults eat influences children's own eating choices, encourages children to try the foods, and helps children develop healthy attitudes toward the food and the mealtime experience.

Adults seated at the table should eat the same foods and drink the same beverage served to the children. They should eat at least a small amount of each food provided to the children to model positive eating behavior; however, when adults must eat foods that are different from what is served to the children, they should consider eating their own food away from the children. Children and adults should be seated during the meal, and excessive getting up and down should be avoided. Children will often stop eating when the caregiver leaves the table. Serving the meal family style, and placing all the food on the table decreases the need for getting up and down to get more food.

Encourage Quiet Conversation and Positive Behavior. Children should be encouraged to make positive comments about the food. Give a smile or a positive comment when children eat their food. Refocus children who are distracted or who are distracting others. Adults can guide children to display acceptable behavior at mealtime. Give the child choices that encourage him or her to join in the mealtime in an appropriate manner. When children indicate that they do not care for a certain food, the caregiver can positively redirect the conversation to change the subject and discuss topics other than the food. However, a child's food preferences should be respected and the future opportunities to explore and experience the food considered. Offering a wide variety of foods over time will help ensure a nutritionally adequate and balanced diet and will enhance the likelihood that children are served foods that meet their taste preferences.

Provide Chairs, Tables, and Utensils That Are Comfortable and of Appropriate Size. Children need to feel comfortable when learning about foods and developing their eating skills. Learning to eat is a skill just as difficult as reading. Like reading, learning to eat requires a great deal of practice and will likely involve many mistakes. Children are often slow and messy as they learn to handle new tools and acquire new skills. The caregiver can ensure a pleasant mealtime with minimal stress by accepting the slower eating pace of the children and the inevitable spills that occur as a normal part of learning to eat. The caregiver should provide children with eating utensils that are easy to handle. Placing the table over a hard, easy-to-clean flooring surface, and making sure cleanup materials are readily accessible makes cleaning up easier. Allow the children to participate in the cleanup of spills as part of the mealtime routine. Adults should consider this a natural part of the day's activities and not a punishment. Taking care of their own spills and helping clear the table following a meal teaches the children social responsibility. Always offering more food or beverage to replace what was spilled, regardless of the circumstances surrounding the mishap, further enhances the development of social responsibility. Children learn to trust the world to meet their needs, while assuming responsibility for their near environment.

Involve Children in the Meal Service. Use a variety of appropriate ways to motivate children to try different foods and to increase mealtime enjoyment. When children participate in some aspect of the meal service, they take more ownership in it and are more likely to eat the meal. Growing, selecting, preparing, and experimenting with foods open a whole world of wonders and discoveries for young children. Children can be included in meal planning, grocery shopping, meal preparation, setting the table, passing the food, cleaning up spills, mealtime conversation, and cleaning up after the meal.

Children need to have their decisions concerning foods respected. The more different food children experience, the greater the variety of foods they are likely to learn to like and eat. Eating a large variety of foods provides the best opportunity for children to get the nutrients they need for optimum growth and development. Children learn to eat a variety of foods by observing others eating, by exploring new foods using all their senses, by comparing unknown foods with foods they are familiar with, and by being in an environment that supports learning. As stated earlier, learning to eat unfamiliar foods is like learning any new skill and requires repetition, reinforcement, and encouragement. Introducing new foods in a manner that encourages children to accept them requires persistence and patience. Persons of any age can be reluctant to try new foods when they are first presented, and it may take some time before acceptance occurs. It is unreasonable to expect children to agree instantly to taste and eat new foods.

Clearly defining mealtime responsibility is important to developing healthy eating habits. According to Ellen Satter,[28,29] adults are responsible for choosing and presenting nutritious foods to children in a positive and supportive fashion, and children are responsible for how much and whether or not they eat what is presented to them. Children need to learn to listen to and respond to their bodies' hunger and fullness cues to develop healthy eating habits. Making a child eat, overencouraging a child, or withholding food from a child may interfere with the child's ability to learn to regulate his or her own eating. Eating in response to something other than internal hunger and fullness cues may lead to eating problems later in life.

Parents should be advised if a child is an ongoing problem eater or if growth appears to be a problem. Children should not be reprimanded for refusing to taste or eat all the food on their plates. Instead, let the children know when the next meal will be served so they can make final decisions about whether to eat more. Food left on plates should be thrown away without comment. Although no one wishes to see food wasted, plate waste is a normal part of eating, especially when new foods are served or when children are new to the child care setting or classroom.

Children sometimes need help learning what a reasonable portion size is, particularly when the meal is served family style. USDA Instruction 226.20 outlines requirements that CACFP should follow in serving meal family style (see Exhibit 11–2).[30]

The caregiver is wise to remember that young children often go through food jags where they will eat the same foods over and over again, often to the exclusion of other foods. Children may also eat a lot during periods of rapid growth and eat very little at other times. While these eating extremes may cause concern, it is important that adults avoid overencouraging, pressuring, or forcing children to eat. Forcing or bribing children to eat can cause children to dislike food and develop un-

Exhibit 11–2 Requirements That CACFP Should Follow When Serving a Meal Family Style

---

ACTION BY: Regional Directors
                    Special Nutrition Programs

SOURCE CITATION: Section 226.20

Family Style Meal Service in the Child and Adult Care Food Program

The Child and Adult Care Program (CACFP) has long been recognized for its nutritional goals of providing nutritious meals to children and helping them establish good eating habits at a young age. Family style meal service provides a further opportunity to enhance these goals by encouraging a pleasant eating environment that will support and promote mealtime as a learning experience.

Family style is a type of meal service which allows children to serve themselves from common platters of food with assistance from supervising adults setting the example. In *A Planning Guide for Food Service in Child Care Centers (FNS-64)*, the chapter, "Making Mealtime a Happy Time," provides guidance for family style meal service in the CACFP. Family style meal service encourages supervising adults to set a personal example and provide educational activities that are centered around foods. This approach allows children to identify, and be introduced to new foods, new tastes, and new menus, while developing a positive attitude toward nutritious foods, sharing in group eating situations, and developing good eating habits.

Unlike cafeteria lines, unitized meals, and pre-set service, the family style method affords some latitude in the size of initial servings because replenishment is immediately available at each table. Even when a complete family style service is not possible or practical, it may be useful to offer a component or components in a family style manner particularly when smaller children are being served or when a new food item is being introduced. This latitude must be exercised in compliance with the following practices, at a minimum:

(1) A sufficient amount of prepared food must be placed on each table to provide the full required portions of each of the food components for all children at the table, and to accommodate supervising adult(s) if they eat with the children.

DISTRIBUTION	MANUAL MAINTENANCE INSTRUCTIONS	RESPONSIBLE FOR	Page
5, 6, 11, 12	Remove FNS Instruction 783-9, Rev. 1, from Manual. Insert this Instruction.	PREPARATION AND MAINTENANCE: CND-100	5-3-9

FNS Instruction 783-9
REV. #2

(2) The family style meal service allows children to make choices in selecting foods and the size of the initial servings. Children should initially be offered the full required portion of each meal component.
(3) During the course of the meal, it is the responsibility of the supervising adults to actively encourage each child to accept service of the full required portion for each food component of the meal pattern. For example, if a child initially refuses a food component, or initially does not accept the full required portion of a meal component, the supervising adult should offer the food component to the child again.
(4) Institutions which use family style meal service may not claim second meals for reimbursement.
(5) Meals served which follow the guidelines laid out in this Instruction are eligible for reimbursement.

Source: Reprinted from U.S. Department of Agriculture, *Family-Style Meal Service in the Child and Adult Care Food Program*, USDA Instruction 226.20, U.S. Government Printing Office.

healthy attitudes about food that carry over into adulthood. Using food as a reward or punishment sets up perceptions of food as something other than a source of nourishment.[31,32]

Bettleheim has presented an enlightening perspective on feeding the young child.[33] Remembering that a majority of children participating in the CACFP come from low socioeconomic homes, Bettleheim's perspective has meaning for professionals involved with the federally assisted programs. According to Bettleheim, teachers and cooks fail to realize that children develop a sense of food security by wasting food and asking for more. When food is left on the plate and more is always offered at future meals, the child learns that adequate food will always be available—"that despite waste, enough is left, that we can feel that this is a good world, worthwhile to come to terms with its demands."

Food battles might result when adults go beyond encouraging children to eat and try to make eating decisions for children. Children are then less likely to eat well and enjoy a variety of foods. Most food battles can be avoided if children are encouraged but not pressured to eat. Encouraging children to eat does not mean that adults need to respond to all of the children's food demands. Always giving children what they want when they want it can deprive them of opportunities to explore and evaluate a variety of nutritious foods.

Franks-Spohrer[34] has reported that young children provide reliable and consistent information related to their food preferences. Several techniques have been identified as useful to the child care staff in determining the likes and dislikes of three- and four-year-old children. The reader who wishes to conduct similar research may consider the following techniques:

- *Facial hedonic scale:* Children are asked to rate preference for a sample of food by circling the face that reflects how they feel about a food.
- *Ranking scale:* A group of foods is offered to the children, who are asked to taste and select the ones they like best. The process is repeated after the preferred foods are

removed to determine a list of food preferences.
- *Plate waste method:* Children are served a measured portion of food; the amount remaining is measured to determine the amount consumed as an indication of how well the children liked the food.
- *Informal tasting with small bites:* Combining tasting of foods with other learning activities will also help children develop important associations about foods and science and health.

FACTORS THAT INFLUENCE THE MEAL SERVICE IN THE CHILD CARE SETTING

Standards To Promote Healthy Meals

Nutrition standards for child care programs have been published by a number of government and professional organizations, including DHHS for the Head Start program,[35] USDA/FNS for the CACFP,[36] American Public Health Association and American Academy of Pediatrics for home child care,[37] and the Society for Nutrition Education for child care.[38] These standards established by professional groups should be used regardless of the source of funding for the child care center because nutritional needs of children and the role of the child care center are similar regardless of family income or the source of funding. The reader is encouraged to consult these references for details on the specific recommendations and regulations of each of these groups. The goal of the *Healthy People 2000—National Health Promotion and Disease Prevention Objectives,* objective No. 217,[39] is to increase to at least 90 percent the proportion of child food services with menus that are consistent with the *Dietary Guidelines for Americans.*

The position of the American Dietetic Association (ADA), Nutrition Standards for Child Care Programs, states, "It is the position of the ADA that all child care programs should achieve recommended standards for meeting children's nutrition and education needs in a safe, sanitary, supportive environment that promotes healthy growth and development."[40(p323)] The ADA position outlines standards that support those established by the professional and governmental agencies previously identified. The ADA nutrition standards cover six major areas: (1) menu planning, (2) meal preparation and service, (3) nutrition consultation and guidance provided by a qualified nutrition professional, (4) nutrition education and training for the child care staff and the children, (5) a physical and emotional environment that is conducive to developing healthy eating behaviors, and (6) compliance with local and state regulation.

All menus should be nutritionally adequate and consistent with the nutrition recommendations of the *Dietary Guidelines for Americans*. Meals and snacks should follow recommended patterns with appropriate accommodations for ages of the children, number of hours they spend at the center or child care home, and cultural or ethnic differences in food habits. The addition of fat, sugar, and sources of sodium should be minimized in food preparation. The food service staff should be trained in culinary techniques that rely on the natural flavors of foods without the addition of excessive amounts of fat, sugar, and sources of sodium. Basic menu planning and the preparation and service of healthful food prepared to the taste preferences of children are discussed in greater detail in Chapters 10 and 15. As in other child nutrition programs, the food service staff responsible for menu planning should consider the following:

- Include plenty of fresh fruits, fresh or frozen vegetables, and whole-grain products.
- Provide foods in quantities that balance energy and nutrition needs with the children's small appetites.
- Prepare and serve foods that are consistent with best practices for food safety and sanitation.

Every child care facility can benefit from the services of a qualified nutrition profes-

sional such as a registered dietitian. Registered dietitians are trained in food service management, which includes planning and evaluating menus to ensure that they are nutritionally adequate and consistent with the *Dietary Guidelines for Americans*. The registered dietitian can guide food service personnel to apply these recommendations appropriately with consideration for the ages of the children in the child care center or child care home. Furthermore, the registered dietitian has the expertise necessary to train and supervise child care personnel in the principles of food preparation and safe and sanitary food handling. A well-trained food service staff has the confidence needed to create the right physical and emotional environment needed for children to accept and enjoy mealtime. When the child care center or child care home follows the standards discussed here and is in compliance with local and state regulations related to wholesomeness of food, food preparation facilities, food safety, and sanitation, the overall quality of the care provided is ensured.[40]

Menu Guidelines

The *Dietary Guidelines for Americans*, developed by the USDA and the DHHS[41] provides guidelines for diets for healthy Americans over two years of age. These guidelines are as follows:

- Eat a variety of foods to get the energy, vitamins, protein, minerals, and fiber you need for good health.
- Balance the food you eat with physical activity—maintain or improve your weight.
- Choose a diet with plenty of grain products, vegetables, and fruits.
- Choose a diet low in fat, saturated fat, and cholesterol.
- Choose a diet moderate in sugars.
- Choose a diet moderate in salt and sodium.
- If you drink alcoholic beverages, do so in moderation.

The Food Guide Pyramid[42] is a graphic illustration of the *Dietary Guidelines for Ameri-*

cans (Figure 11–2). The pyramid recommends the number of servings of foods from each group that should be eaten daily. Serving a variety of foods helps ensure that children will not become bored with the foods offered and will learn healthy food habits. The pyramid is an effective nutrition education tool to use with the child care staff and with the children.

Guidelines for Infants

As previously discussed in this chapter, meals served to children under 12 months of age must follow the infant meal pattern developed by the CACFP to ensure the health and nutrition of children. It is not appropriate to apply the nutrition recommendations in the *Dietary Guidelines for Americans* to children under two years of age with regard to fat, saturated fat, and cholesterol intake. Ranges are given for each food portion to serve to infants. The reader and the child caregiver should be careful to note that the amounts listed in Table 11–1 and Table 11–2 are the *minimum* portions required to meet the meal pattern requirements. Infants may need greater amounts than indicated on the chart to maintain proper growth and optimum development according to individual needs. Foods served should always be of developmentally appropriate texture and consistency.

It is especially important to work closely with the parents when feeding infants in the child care setting. It is the parents' responsibility to decide when new foods are introduced to the infant. Establishing a cooperative and collaborative relationship with parents is important in ensuring that the infant's feeding and nutritional needs are met in the most appropriate and beneficial manner.[43,44]

Menu Planning

Nutritious meals require balance, variety, and moderation. Menus should contain a wide variety of foods based on the Food Guide Pyramid and the *Dietary Guidelines*. Variety improves the nutritional quality of the meal and increases the likelihood of having foods available that the children like. The CACFP meal pattern as shown in Tables 11–1 and 11–2 is the beginning point for planning the menu. The CACFP food charts provide valuable guidance about meal components and amounts for preparing children's meals. Keep in mind that the meal pattern lists *minimum* portions. Children may desire to eat more food than specified in the meal patterns. In these instances, providers need to serve larger portions to children whose individual activity and metabolic level require additional food.

The menu should

- Contain

    A variety of whole grains and pasta products

    Fresh and processed fruits, fruit juices, and vegetables

    Lean meats, trimmed of visible fat

- Incorporate beans and lentils into meatless meals
- Limit serving highly processed or convenience foods, such as hot dogs and bologna
- Select desserts carefully as they often contain only sugar, fat, and calories
- Include

    Vitamin C-rich foods daily

    Vitamin A-rich foods at least every other day

    Iron-rich foods, such as lean meats, spinach, dried beans, tuna, and eggs

    Milk with all meals

    100% fruit juice

- Provide adequate calories for growth and development by including nutrient-dense foods (foods that are a good source of a nutrient[s] relative to the calories provided)

Source: Reprinted from Food and Consumer Service, *Child and Adult Care Food Program, Nutrition Guidance for Child Care Homes*, 1995, U.S. Department of Agriculture.

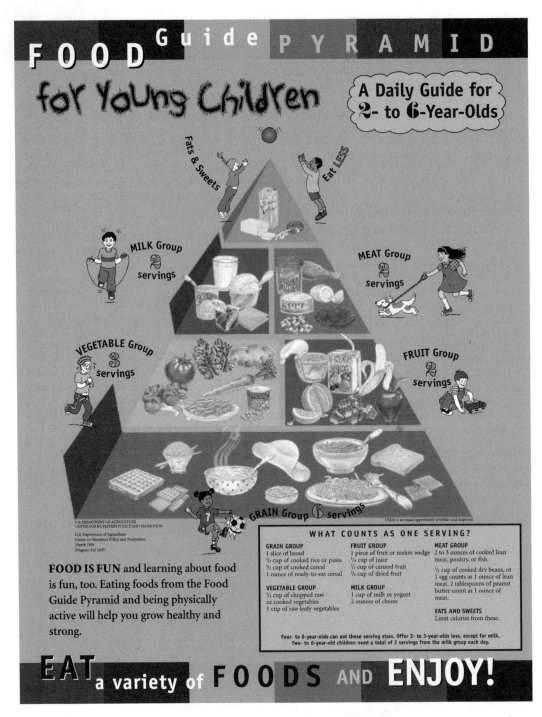

continues

Figure 11–2 Food Guide Pyramid for Young Children. *Source:* Reprinted from Center for Nutrition Policy and Promotion, *USDA's Food Guide Pyramid for Young Children*, Program Aid 1650, March 1999, U.S. Department of Agriculture.

Figure 11–2 continued

PLAN FOR YOUR YOUNG CHILD... The Pyramid Way

Use this chart to get an idea of the foods your child eats over a week. Pencil in the foods eaten each day and pencil in the corresponding triangular shape. (For example, if a slice of toast is eaten at breakfast, write in "toast" and fill in one Grain group pyramid.) The number of pyramids shown for each food group is the number of servings to be eaten each day. At the end of the week, if you see only a few blank pyramids...keep up the good work. If you notice several blank pyramids, offer foods from the missing food groups in the days to come.

	SUNDAY	MONDAY	TUESDAY	WEDNESDAY	THURSDAY	FRIDAY	SATURDAY
Milk	△△	△△	△△	△△	△△	△△	△△
Meat	△△	△△	△△	△△	△△	△△	△△
Vegetable	△△△	△△△	△△△	△△△	△△△	△△△	△△△
Fruit	△△	△△	△△	△△	△△	△△	△△
Grain	△△△	△△△	△△△	△△△	△△△	△△△	△△△
	△△△	△△△	△△△	△△△	△△△	△△△	△△△
Breakfast							
Snack							
Lunch							
Snack							
Dinner							

It is important that menus served to children provide adequate calories and nutrients to ensure growth and development. Menus should contain nutrient-dense foods to meet energy and nutrient needs without contributing to obesity among the children. The amount of fat in children's diets should be based on their age and energy needs. A sufficient amount of all food items should be prepared. Allow children to choose foods to satisfy their hunger because they are the best judges of how much and what to eat. A well-planned menu will help ensure children receive nutritious and attractive meals.

Two major decisions must be made regarding how menus are planned—how frequently the menu is planned and the process and factors considered in planning the menu. *First, determine the frequency of the menu*. That is, will the menu change weekly or will the menu be repeated over a number of weeks? Cycle menus are recommended. Cycle menus are a set of planned menus that are repeated in the same order for a period of time, such as four weeks or six weeks. The menu is different every day during the cycle, but the entire menu is repeated when the time period elapses. A cycle menu should be planned to offer variety and flexibility with substitutions. Cycle menus should be adjusted to replace foods not available and to observe holidays, special occasions, and birthdays. See Chapter 15 for a complete description of cycle menus.

Second, determine the process and considerations in planning the menu. The menu-planning process begins by selecting main dishes for the menu-planning period and then selecting foods that complement them. In selecting menu items, consideration must be given to including foods that vary in color, texture, shape, flavor, and temperature. Plan for different foods every day as much as feasible; avoid including the same food on the same day of the week. Vary preparation methods and avoid such things as creamed chicken and creamed potatoes or all white foods or all soft foods. Preparation of frequently used foods such as potatoes should be varied. Include seasonal

foods when they are available. Plan theme menus to celebrate holidays, cultural events, and special occasions. See Table 11–4[46] for an example of menus planned for use in the CACFP child care center or family child care home. These meals and snacks meet the nutrition recommendations and apply the suggestions for good menu planning in the child care environment discussed in this chapter. Centers and homes might wish to consider sharing copies of menus with parents as a way of enlisting the parents as partners in reinforcing the good nutrition habits learned in child care.

Guidelines for Menu Planning in the Child Care Setting

- Plan menus for at least a week ahead of time.
- Plan menus for a week or more to help avoid repeating the same foods too often.
- Plan menus ahead and help save money by buying foods in season and buying in bulk.
- Plan menus in advance and organize the shopping list to help save time in shopping.
- Plan menus in advance so that quality purchasing and good food preparation techniques can be used to prepare healthier meals.[45]

In addition to considering the age and developmental stage of the children when planning the menu, menu planners must consider any special nutritional or feeding needs or diets of the children in their care. For information about planning meals for children with special needs, see Chapter 12. As discussed earlier, infants have special feeding needs that must be followed. The texture of food as well as the shape and size of bites should be based on the needs of the child. The caregiver needs enough information on feeding infants and children with special needs to provide assurance that

Table 11–4 Menus for CACFP

Meal Pattern	Monday	Tuesday	Wednesday	Thursday	Friday
Breakfast					
Juice or fruit or vegetable	Orange juice	Tomato juice	Grape juice[a]	Grapefruit sections	Cantaloupe cubes
Grains/bread	Oatmeal with raisins	Cheese toast	Cornflakes with banana slices	Scrambled eggs / Biscuit	Cinnamon raisin bagel / Honey
Milk, fluid	Milk[b]	Milk	Milk	Milk	Milk
Lunch or supper					
Meat or meat alternate	Apple turkey pita pockets	Beef patty	Peanut butter sandwich on whole-wheat bread / Chicken vegetable soup	Tuna salad	Red and white beans / Couscous[c]
Vegetable and/or fruit	Steamed baby carrots	Lettuce and tomato	Peach slices	Celery sticks / Apple wedges	Chopped tomatoes / Pear slices
Grains/bread		Baked potato wedges / Hamburger bun		Wheat crackers	
Milk, fluid	Milk	Milk	Milk	Milk	Milk
Snack: select two of the following:					
Meat or meat alternate	Toasted angel food cake[d]			Low-fat strawberry yogurt	Pizza sauce for dipping
Juice or fruit or vegetable	Pineapple chunks	Watermelon chunks			Green pepper rings
Grains/bread			Blueberry muffin	Graham crackers	Soft bread sticks
Milk, fluid	Milk / Water	Milk / Water	Milk / Water	Water	Water

[a]Fortified with vitamin C.
[b]Use whole milk for ages 1 and 2; low-fat milks may be used for ages 3–5.
[c]Couscous is an instant, tiny pea-shaped pasta of Mediterranean origin.
[d]Does not contribute to the meal pattern requirement.
This menu is planned in accordance with the nutrition recommendations of the *Dietary Guidelines for Americans.*

Source: Reprinted with permission from the National Food Service Management Institute, *What's Cooking?* Vol. 2, p. 2, © 1996, National Food Service Management Institute.

food servings are appropriate for the individual child or infant. Avoid serving infants and children up to the age of four foods that may be a choking hazard. Foods that may lead to choking in young children include foods such as raw fruits and vegetables, hot dogs, hard candy, peanuts, grapes, popcorn, nuts and seeds, tough meats, thick layers of peanut butter, and raisins and other dried fruits. If these foods are offered to children, they should be modified to avoid a choking hazard; for example, slice grapes or hot dogs in half lengthwise.[47]

It is important to consider the preferences of children in planning menus; however, it is also important to balance their preferences with the need to offer a variety including new foods. The menu-planning process should involve the children, parents, and staff in planning and evaluating their acceptance. The mass-media advertising influences children's desire to try new and different foods. Some of these are nutritious and others are not. The menu planner should evaluate the product advertised and determine whether and how it fits into the meal pattern and the center budget. Some of these foods can be included in the menu occasionally and used as an opportunity to teach children about making wise food choices.

Menus are a major determinant of cost-effective food and nutrition programs. The menu should be precosted at the time it is planned so that the meal service stays within the budget. By following the menu as planned, while allowing an adequate amount of food to meet the nutritional needs and hunger levels of the children, the personnel can operate the program in a cost-effective manner.

Careful attention to the CACFP meal patterns and other regulations related to record keeping and reporting will ensure that the center or home is reimbursed for the meals and snacks served to the children enrolled in the child care program. Reimbursement funds paid to the child care program through the state agency are dependent on meals and snacks meeting the prescribed meal patterns and the keeping of accurate production and serving records. While these funds may not cover all of the food service–related cost of operating the child care program, they are a significant source of revenue for many programs. Therefore, participation in the CACFP exerts a strong influence on the menu-planning process.

Other considerations to keep in mind when planning the menu include the availability of storeroom space, existing inventory levels, any equipment limitations, the culinary skills of the food and nutrition program staff, time available to prepare food, and storage requirements for prepared foods. If the food production area of the child care center is used for other programs, such as after-school care or adult day care, the center food and nutrition program manager may need to organize and secure the storage and inventory of foods and supplies to ensure that adequate and planned foods are available when needed.

Similarly, child care home providers must take into account the size of their kitchen and the availability of storage space. Storage spaces (separate from the family's) for groceries and supplies used in the preparation and service of meals and snacks to the children enrolled in the family child care program are needed to ensure that adequate foods are available to the children at all times. A closet or cabinet can be dedicated to the foods and serving supplies used for the children. When the foods intended for the children in child care cannot be stored in a separate refrigerator, a section or portion of the family refrigerator can be designated for this purpose.

Procurement

Purchasing of foods for the child care setting can be very different from purchasing for other types of child nutrition programs. Because the numbers and sizes of servings are quite small in family child care homes, when compared with school lunch and breakfast programs, much of the purchasing for child care often takes place at the local grocery store or food market. Child care home providers may shop for child care groceries and supplies along with the regular family shopping. Provider training must address the need for accountability of foods and supplies in reporting costs and use. Separate storage space for foods and supplies intended for the children in child care helps the caregiver maintain accurate records and helps ensure the availability of foods and supplies when needed. When possible, the family child care provider may shop on different occasions for the family and the child care meals.

Larger centers may serve adequate numbers of children or have adequate storage space to justify purchasing from vendors and having foods delivered to the center. Sponsors may also facilitate the purchase of foods in quantities that increase purchasing power for the centers and homes under their sponsorship. Or they may join a purchasing cooperative operated by one or more school districts. For information about cooperatives, the sponsor should contact the state child nutrition agency. When the sponsor purchases foods in bulk, divides, and delivers them to the participating centers and/or homes, care must be taken to ensure the sanitation and safety in each step of the process. The state agency rules and state laws that regulate purchasing in child nutrition programs apply to centers and sponsors of child care homes participating in the CACFP. The reader is encouraged to refer to Chapter 13 for a complete discussion on the purchasing procedures and purchasing guidelines for school and child nutrition programs.

When purchasing foods for the child care home or center, many of the same rules of purchasing for the school meals program apply. The first rule is that the best quality allowable under the budget should be purchased. For example, only the freshest produce is purchased and served to the children in child care. The child care center or child care home staff responsible for the purchasing of foods understands the principles of purchasing and is familiar with the standards of quality of all foods

purchased. When purchasing takes place at the grocery store, the child care provider is trained to use information on food labels to help make wise nutrition choices. According to law, all food labels must include the common name of the product; the name and address of the manufacturer, packer, or distributor; the net contents in terms of weight, measure, or count; the ingredients in order of predominance by weight from greatest to least; nutrition information; and the serving size.

The nutrition facts panel on the food label provides information on the nutrient content of a food. Under the Nutrition Labeling and Education Act (NLEA),[48] nutrition information must be listed for total calories, calories from fat, total fat, saturated fat, cholesterol, sodium, total carbohydrate, dietary fiber, sugars, protein, vitamin A, vitamin C, calcium, and iron. Additional nutrient information may also be listed on the label, such as fiber content and other essential vitamins and minerals. The child caregiver can learn about the nutritional qualities on almost all food products. However, the labels of foods for children under two years of age may not carry information about saturated fat, polyunsaturated fat, monounsaturated fat, cholesterol, calories from fat, or calories from saturated fat in keeping with the nutrition recommendations that caution parents and other caregivers about restricting the fat intakes of children under two. Remember that fat is important during the first years of life to ensure adequate growth and development. Additionally, labels for foods for children under four years of age may not include the percentage daily values for total fat, saturated fat, cholesterol, sodium, potassium, total carbohydrate, and dietary fiber. The nutrition facts label will list the nutrients and the total quantitative amounts. However, these labels may include percentage daily values for protein, vitamins, and minerals and the calorie conversion information given as a footnote.

The NLEA provides uniform definitions for terms that describe a food's nutrient content, such as "light," "low-fat," and "high-fiber," to ensure that these terms mean the same for any product on which they appear. The purchaser can also look for terms such as "whole-grain" or "enriched" or "fortified" when selecting breads and other grain products. Other products are also fortified with nutrients, such as orange juice fortified with calcium and skim milk fortified with vitamins A and D. The term *refined* on the label can be a signal to the child care provider that nutrients may have been lost during processing. (For more information on the NLEA, refer to the *Federal Register*, January 6, 1993.)

Another example of using the label to make a wise nutrition choice is to look for "full strength" on fruit juice products. Fruit drinks are beverages that contain some full-strength juice along with added water and possibly other ingredients. Some state agencies and sponsors credit only full-strength juices; however, others may credit fruit drinks that contain 50 percent fruit juice when twice the required amount is served. The center or child care home provider can receive information of serving juices from their state agency or sponsor.

Equally important in the provider training is proper handling and storage to ensure product quality and food safety of all foods purchased and brought into the child care center or home.

- Examine foods to make sure they are free from soil, signs of contamination (i.e., broken or damaged containers), signs of spoilage (i.e., off-odors; wilting, browning, or bruising of fresh produce).
- Never accept frozen foods if partially thawed or containers show evidence that the product has been thawed and refrozen.
- Check temperatures of all foods, especially meat, poultry, fish, dairy foods, and all frozen products to ensure their safety.
- All dry foods are properly stored in tightly covered containers to prevent rodent and insect infestation. The same rules of food safety that apply in the school food service are applicable to the child care setting as well. (The reader is encouraged to refer

to Chapter 18 for a complete discussion on the safe handling and storage of all food products.)

Food Preparation and Safety

The goal of food preparation and service in the child care setting is to serve high-quality, nutritious meals that are acceptable to the children and are prepared under the safest and most sanitary conditions possible. Maintaining quality during preparation requires the application of the basic principles of food preparation discussed in Chapter 15. Special attention is given to the preservation of nutrients that are destroyed when foods are not handled properly. Some positive practices include checking expiration dates on packages, storing foods at the proper temperatures, cooking vegetables until tender-crisp, and steaming and microwaving as appropriate. Child care provider staff should understand and practice serving food at its peak of freshness. If necessary to hold foods the appropriate temperature should be maintained.

The needs in this area will vary depending on whether the site is a child care center or child care home. The child care center's needs will reflect the size of the center, staffing patterns, the availability of equipment, and storage space. It is also possible that the child care center will contract with another organization for the production of meals and snacks. When meals and foods items are prepared off-premises by a contractor or other organization, it is the child care center director's or sponsor's responsibility to ensure that the facilities, delivery equipment, and all personnel who come in contact with the foods meet the strictest safety and sanitation standards. Frequent, unannounced visits to the food preparation site are necessary to determine that the highest food safety and sanitation standards are met at all times. Contractors should be required to follow all local, state, and federal laws related to food handling, and the implementation of a Hazard Analysis Critical Control Points

(HACCP) program should be in evidence. Inspection of the entire operation from purchasing specification and purchasing practices to receiving and storage of raw materials are part of the center director's or sponsor's responsibility. All facilities, including receiving, storage, preparation, and holding areas, present potential problems. Remember to check the cleanliness and temperatures of transportation equipment, including trucks or vans used to deliver finished food products to the child care center or home. All the rules of safe food handling apply just as in on-site preparation facilities. When contractors do not live up to the standards of safe food handling, the child care center or sponsor must look for alternative sources of food production.

Provider training must ensure that all persons engaged in the child care center know and practice requirements for safe handling and serving of foods. There is renewed emphasis placed on food safety in food service with major outbreaks of food poisoning occurring in food service establishments. USDA's CD-ROM training package entitled *Serving It Safe*[49] is one example of an excellent food safety training course for food service personnel. The food safety needs of child care homes are prescribed in state licensing requirements. It is important to recognize the diversity of situations and the need for a variety of training. Local and state regulations must be followed by both center and child care home staff.

The goal of safe food handling and serving practices is accomplished by following certain guidelines, including the following:

- Follow proper handwashing procedures. The importance of handwashing for young children and child care staff cannot be overemphasized. Transmission of disease is an important concern in child care. The use of simple but correct handwashing techniques is the most important way to reduce transmission of illness in this setting. Wash hands thoroughly with soap and water before handling foods or utensils. Repeat after every staff or child visit to the restroom, changing diapers, touching the hair or face, leaving the kitchen area, wiping up spills, and any other time contamination of the hands occurs.
- Wash hands, utensils, and work surfaces thoroughly after contact with raw eggs, fish, meats, or poultry. Cross-contamination can occur when this practice is not followed.
- Persons with infected cuts or sores, colds, or other communicable diseases must not be assigned tasks that require them to touch foods or utensils or other surfaces that come in contact with food.
- Wash all fresh produce that will be served raw, such as lettuce, celery, carrots, apples, and peaches.
- Cook all foods properly, following standardized procedures and recipe directions.
- Monitor the internal temperature of all cooked products using a stem thermometer.
- Discard any stored food products or prepared foods that may be questionable.

Meal Service

As discussed earlier, the meal service provides an opportunity to meet two needs for the preschool child: (1) to have immediate food and nutrition needs met and (2) to learn how to make wise food choices and expand their knowledge about food and nutrition. The role of the provider in meal service also includes providing appropriately sized utensils for children to handle so that they can participate in the service of the meal. The meal service environment should allow the children to choose foods to eat. Serving style may be family style or buffet. If family style, the table is set with plates, glasses, and flatware at each place and the food is passed in small bowls or baskets from which the children serve themselves. Small pitchers are used so that children can pour their own beverage. (Note: some states require that milk be served in an individual serving container or from the original milk carton.

Providers and sponsors must check with the state agency for procedure.) If food is served buffet style, food is placed in serving dishes on a table or counter of appropriate height, and older children serve themselves. Both styles help young children to make choices and feel independent when they choose and are allowed to serve themselves. Quality meal service always observes the highest standards of sanitation in every aspect of the meal service.

- Sanitize tables before and after meal service.
- See that chidden and caregivers wash their hands before mealtime.
- Provide/use tongs, spoons, scoops, etc. to serve food.
- Teach children to pass and serve food in a sanitary manner that involves their touching only that portion being selected. The children can choose which piece of food they want by looking at it. Children should take what foods they touch. They should not touch the food or the insides of the serving containers. Remember this will require practice and is a natural part of learning.
- Teach children to cover coughs/sneezes with the insides of their elbows, never into the food. Hands should be washed again if they become contaminated during the meal service, for example, after coughing or sneezing into hands.
- Keep foods covered during the meal service and at all other times.
- Modify meal service style during certain periods, such as the flu season, to discontinue children serving themselves.
- Provide appropriate child-size furniture, serving bowls, and utensils to further facilitate eating. Serving utensils, plates, and glasses should be easy to use and have broad bases so that fewer spills occur.
- Space the meals to meet children's needs, usually serving meals and snacks about two hours apart. Have a reasonable time frame for meals with regular starting and ending times. Children should have plenty of time to eat and socialize and should not be rushed. About 20 to 30 minutes should give children enough time to eat but not so much that they get bored or disruptive.
- Integrate nutrition education into the child care setting: The school food and nutrition professional helps the caregiver understand the importance of and develop skills in integrating nutrition education into the overall plan in centers and homes. The caregiver must be provided with training, including the resources needed to be effective in nutrition education. Some of the activities that should become a regular part of the caregiver's day include discussing menu items with children during the meal service and incorporating healthy foods and nutrition experiences into the child care setting that will result in nutrition-conscious child care staff, families, and children.

Adults are responsible for providing learning experiences to help children understand the importance of making nutritious food choices. The learning experiences should be appropriate for children's developmental ages. Very young children can explore foods and learn how they help the body grow. As they develop, they can learn the categories of food and the number of servings they should have from each category every day to help them grow and develop. Older children can learn more about nutrients. Provide opportunities for children to experiment with foods using all their senses. When children learn to explore and to evaluate foods using their own senses, they will be able to use these skills throughout their lives. There are many well-designed nutrition education curriculums developed to assist in teaching nutrition to children.

The provider's role in helping children learn to eat new foods: Adults need to develop a way of interacting that is child responsive if they are to be successful in helping children develop healthy eating habits. It is important to clearly define mealtime responsibility. As previously noted, according to Ellyn Satter,[50,51] adults are responsible for choosing and presenting nutritious foods to children in a positive and supportive fashion, and children are responsible for how much and whether or not they eat what is presented to them.

Many times children do not learn to eat new foods because adults assume that the children will not eat them. In order to learn to like new foods, children must first be served new foods. How the food is presented and the adult's attitude influences how receptive the children will be to the new food. If the adult assumes that the children will try and enjoy the new foods, they will be more likely to do so. Talk to children about a new food during a quiet time before the meal. Discuss the new taste, color, shape, and aroma children will experience when they taste the new food. Emphasize similarities between the new food and other familiar foods. Allow opportunities for the children to explore the new food using their senses. Provide children with several noneating experiences before offering the food to taste. Offer familiar foods along with new foods to give children the opportunity to compare the known with the unknown. Serve the new food first to a child who is adventurous and eats most foods as children will usually follow other children's leads and will try the food. Adults should eat the new food themselves and let the children see how much they enjoy it. It is important for the adult to model the behavior for the children to imitate. Try preparing the new food in several different ways. Wait several weeks, then serve the new food again. Finally, always give a smile or a positive comment when children taste a new food.

Staff Training

Child care centers participating in the CACFP are required to provide orientation and ongoing training for all caregivers.[52] Specific information needed by all employees in child care facilities include basic concepts of nutrition, including nutrition issues in the child care setting, interpretation and application of nutrition information and resources, cultural beliefs and practices, and the food acceptability of preschoolers, procurement and production techniques with attention to specifications, labels, storage cost, nutrient retention, and standardized production.[53]

Effective staff training for CACFP personnel is essential to the assurance that the program meets the food and nutrition needs of the children. Training based on the needs of caregivers will result in more effective programs and satisfied personnel. Adults learn best when they understand why they are learning certain information or skills, when they are told and shown how to do new tasks, when they are shown the task, when they have opportunity to practice the task, and when they receive positive feedback on how they are doing. Setting aside time for training is an important part of the management of the child care program. Center directors or sponsors and child care home sponsors provide the training needed for the food service staff.

All food service staff should be trained in food and nutrition menu planning, creating a positive environment that promotes the development of good eating habits, and serving as role models in developing good eating habits that children can emulate. Training must provide caregivers information about how they can evaluate their own program. In the child care center, teachers and teachers' aides benefit from the food service training, since these are the caregivers that are most likely to eat with and serve the children. Teachers have a tremendous impact on the behaviors of young children and need to be prepared to teach desirable social and food-related behaviors.

Food-preparation techniques that save time are critical to the busy food service staff. Many child care centers and homes rely on the food service staff to fulfill more than food service responsibilities. Sometimes the caregiver is the cook and the person responsible for cleaning up, which is generally the case in the child care home. Teachers and teachers' aides may have food-preparation tasks to perform as well. Many state agencies have developed a training plan for child care personnel.

Resources for training are available from the state and sponsoring agencies. Community colleges and universities often offer education and training opportunities in child care, nutrition, and food and nutrition program. Often dietetics and nutrition programs in colleges and universities have students knowledgeable about foods and nutrition topics who are available to the child care center or home to provide training sessions for the staff. Dietetic interns can be valuable members of the center staff to plan and prepare meals while they meet the special-interest requirement of their supervised practice programs. Contact your local college or university for more information on the availability of these resources. The local health department nutritionist and the county extension service home economist are others sources of valuable and reliable food and nutrition information. The food and nutrition professionals who work in these federally funded programs may also be available to present training sessions and provide educational materials for use in training the staff. The services of a registered dietitian is also recommended when the center or sponsoring agency does not have a registered dietitian on staff. Contact the local or state dietetics association for the names of consultants.

APPLICATION

A number of recommendations that have the potential to positively influence children's eating patterns and nutritional status are as follows:

- Promote partnerships and coordination among government programs, the private sector, and the school to support the family structure, which is pivotal for teaching

decision making and self-management of health and nutrition.
- Develop family-school partnerships for teenagers to combat negative peer influences and help parents and adolescents adopt positive health and eating behaviors.
- Reform the welfare system to reward work, bolster parents' academic and job skills, and ensure a decent standard of living that will enable families to provide adequate food and foster healthful eating patterns.
- Reduce fragmentation and lack of coordination among food assistance, public health, social service, and education programs that serve the same target populations.
- Form partnerships with the media to help children improve their eating habits by promoting food choices consistent with recommendations made in *Dietary Guidelines for Americans.*[54]

According to *Caring for our Children—National Health and Safety Performance Standards: Guidelines for Out-of-Home Child Care Programs,*[55] there are three guiding principles for food and nutrition services in child care settings: (1) Food should help to meet the child's daily nutritional needs and reflect individual and cultural differences. Foods should provide an opportunity for learning, and activities should complement and supplement those of the home and the community. The facility can assist the child and family to understand the association between nutrition and health and various ways to meet the nutritional needs. (2) A nutrition specialist or food and nutrition program expert is a vital member of the facility's planning team to ensure implementation of an efficient and cost-effective food service. (3) To prevent food-borne illness, proper equipment and food handling are essential.

The school food and nutrition professional as a stakeholder of children's nutrition in the community needs an understanding of the importance of healthful meals for children in preschool programs and the impact these have on the school food and nutrition program. In this chapter, an overview of the federally assisted programs has been described to assist in meeting this need. Although the CACFP operates under a different set of regulations, the nutrition standards and program goals are similar to those in schools. By describing the role of the caregiver in child care programs, the school food and nutrition professional will be in a position to be proactive in the community in advocating quality programs and assisting in providing training and resources.

Standards outlined in *Keys to Excellence*[56] are generally applicable to the child care setting and may be used to assess the needs of child care centers. The nutrition professional should be an active partner with other stakeholders in the community to ensure quality care in the child care setting. One important role that the school food and nutrition professional can play is to identify the competencies needed by the decision maker for child care programs. An important goal of any school food and nutrition professional should be to have the school food and nutrition program become the community nutrition program. Being proactive in advocating for child care programs is an important step in that direction.

SUMMARY

Helping children make the transition from child care in the preschool setting to the school environment requires the help of the entire community. The African proverb "it takes a village to raise a child" is true today more than ever before. Community groups needing to be involved include parents, schools, community resources, federal and state agencies that administer programs dealing with child welfare issues, national organizations such as the American School Food Service Association, the American Dietetic Association, the American Academy of Pediatrics, and many educational and social associations.

The CACFP is itself a bridge or facilitator for the transition of children into school and provides the foundation for healthy eating that is continued in school food and nutrition programs. Children who have experienced a wide variety of nutritious food choices in the child care setting are ready to make good food choices at school. The transition from child care meals to school meals is natural and less traumatic when both child care and school programs follow the same guiding principles of planning and preparing healthful meals for children. The young child entering kindergarten should find the same nutritious food choices at school that he or she learned to enjoy in the child care center or child care home. Schools are responsible for the continuum of nutrition care of children. When schools do not meet the high standards of menu planning offered in the child care center, then the welfare of the children has not been adequately considered. When child care and schools follow the basic nutrition requirements established for the programs and plan meals that meet the nutrition recommendations in the *Dietary Guidelines for Americans*, the welfare of the nation's children has been served. Effective child care programs will make a major contribution to helping children to be ready to learn when they enter kindergarten and/or first grade. Child care provides an exciting opportunity for the school food and nutrition professional to be recognized as an important stakeholder in the growth and development of children.

CASE STUDY
STATE AGENCY TURNS A MONITORING VISIT INTO A
TECHNICAL ASSISTANCE OPPORTUNITY

Helene Kent

Introduction

The State Child and Adult Care Food Program (CACFP) in Colorado provides each newly approved child care center with a training visit within 12 weeks of operation. Each visit is carefully planned to meet the needs of center staff, as there are limited numbers of state agency staff to meet the needs of the nearly 300 child care centers statewide. It is important that the staff associated with CACFP understand program requirements and know how to operate the food program according to program rules. The visit also provides an opportunity to begin the training and technical assistance needed by the center to achieve all of the CACFP program goals.

Kim Green, a state-level CACFP nutrition consultant, is responsible for conducting program reviews in 90 centers each year. As time is limited, Kim must carefully plan each contact for maximum assistance to the center staff. Kim's job is to see that CACFP record keeping is accurate and consistent with program requirements and to review menus, food preparation, procurement, and service practices, ensuring that health, safety, and nutrition standards are being met. Kim also observes the mealtime environment, as the child care experience offers an opportunity for young children to establish positive eating and social habits.

Problem

Kim's problem is determining how to conduct a training review effectively and provide technical assistance to staff working in a child care center.

Strategies for Achieving the Goal

Kim Refreshes Her Knowledge of the Center

Kim recently visited Rainbow Haven Child Care Center, which serves 20 three- to six-year-old children. The center had three teaching staff, including Diane Logan, who is the director and also does the cooking. The center had been participating in CACFP for three months, so this was the first on-site visit by a state CACFP representative. Diane had attended the new center training where she had met Kim. Diane had also spoken to Kim several times on the phone when she was completing the CACFP enrollment paperwork.

Kim Considers the Purpose and How To Prepare the Director for the Visit

Kim was aware that a visit from the CACFP program staff can be stressful to a new center director, so she called Diane before the visit. Kim outlined what would happen during the site visit and what would be reviewed. She also stressed that this was a training visit, not a program review, since the center was new to CACFP. The visit would be used to discuss CACFP requirements and to answer questions. Kim sent Diane a letter after they spoke that clearly outlined the content of the upcoming visit. A checklist was also sent to help Diane prepare for the visit.

Observations during the Visit, Discussions of Findings, and Plan for Follow-up

The day of the site visit, Kim reviewed records and watched the preparation and serving of food in the center. She made notes and had the following summary of findings. Diane did a very good job of ensuring that all the paperwork was done correctly. She also made sure that the food offered to the children met the food pattern requirement and that there were sufficient quantities. The food was handled and prepared in a sanitary fashion. However, the same breakfast, lunch, and snack menus were repeated every two weeks. The food, although wholesome, was repetitive and bland, and did not follow USDA *Dietary Guidelines* related to variety. The menus also had few vitamin A- and C-rich fruits and vegetables listed. The center staff put the food on the plates for children and did not allow children to serve themselves. Mealtime was chaotic, with lots of noise and children playing at the tables and not eating. The teachers did not eat the same food as the children, although Diane was willing to provide meals and snacks to staff. The teachers also sat together at a table near the doorway and often did not notice when a child was requesting additional food.

Kim and Diane spent an hour in an exit interview to discuss the observed issues. Kim complimented Diane for the many positive elements of the food program that were in place. They spent time discussing the areas that could be strengthened. Kim had identified two main areas that needed to be addressed, improving the quality of menus and enhancing the mealtime environment so the children would eat better, learn to eat new foods, and enjoy their mealtime social experience more. Diane's commitments to helping children eat well was evident as they talked. Diane agreed that the mealtime atmosphere could be improved and asked Kim for help in identifying changes. She expressed concern about changing the menus because she believed that the children would not eat unfamiliar foods. Kim spent time addressing her concerns, and although Diane was not completely convinced, she indicated willingness to try some changes suggested by Kim. She agreed to read materials that Kim would mail and to send a six-week cycle menu to Kim in two months. Kim promised a return visit in three months.

As a follow-up to the visit, Kim sent Diane tools to increase her knowledge of menu planning and enhancing the mealtime environment. Kim chose handouts, a workbook, and two videos developed for child care staff on these subjects. The materials were specific to the topics and were developed to meet the needs of child care center staff. The materials were succinct, easy to use, specific, attractive, and designed for the adult learner. Kim prepared a packet of materials and sent them to Diane within a week of the site visit. She then called Diane two weeks later to see if she had any questions.

Four weeks after the site visit Kim received the six-week cycle menu developed by Diane. It was well done and included a variety of foods chosen for young children. A mixture of new and familiar foods was listed. Kim was complimentary about the menus and made a few suggestions when she called to discuss the menus. Diane told Kim that the children were eating the food provided and enjoyed it. She had more questions on how to encourage children to eat new foods, which they discussed.

The other area that Diane reported on was her progress in developing a more positive mealtime atmosphere. Diane had identified how important it was to have staff more involved in the children's mealtime, so she had prepared an in-service using materials provided by Kim. At the end of the in-service, the teachers agreed that sitting with the children would be helpful and that eating the same foods as the children would be important. They also discussed how to enhance learning during the meal. One of the staff was apprehensive about allowing the children to try family-style meal service because she was concerned about the mess. The staff agreed to implement only some components of family-style meal service at this time and then evaluate how it was working.

Outcomes

Kim returned to the center in three months and the changes were noticeable. Teachers were sitting with children and helping them as needed. Conversations were happening at each table. Children were serving themselves and passing foods to their neighbors. The children and the adults seemed much happier with the mealtime. Children were given additional foods when they requested it. Staff were pleased with the changes and remarked that the children were eating better. Diane told Kim about some challenges of the transition and they discussed possible solutions.

Kim and Diane reviewed the changes made over the last few months that had improved the menus offered to the children and had also made mealtime more pleasant. Kim had provided Diane and her staff with information about feeding children and helpful strategies that would work in their child care setting. Kim listened to Diane and gave her education materials, ideas, and advice tailored to her needs. Kim drew on her knowledge of nutrition, adult education, behavior change strategies, and consultation techniques so that she could assist Diane. Diane was willing to look at how to enhance the food program in her center and to implement new methods of feeding children. The result was a child care program that focused on providing healthful and acceptable meals delivered in an environment that promoted healthy living and readiness to learn, which helps to ensure the well-being of children.

REFERENCES

1. Bettleheim, *Food To Nurture the Mind* (Washington, DC: Children's Foundation, 1970), 16–17.

2. U.S. Department of Health and Human Services (DHHS), *Healthy People 2000: National Health Promotion and Disease Prevention Objectives.* (DHHS) (PHS) Publication No. 91-50213 (Washington, DC: U.S. Government Printing Office; 1990).

3. *Goals for Education Challenge 2000*, Southern Regional Education Board (Atlanta, GA, 1988).

4. P.L. Pipes and C.M. Trahms, *Nutrition in Infancy and Childhood* (St. Louis, MO: Mosby–Year Book, 1993).

5. B. Willer et al., *The Demand and Supply of Child Care in 1990* (Washington, DC: National Association for the Education of Young Children, 1991).

6. *Promoting Wellness: A Nutrition, Health and Safety Manual for Family Child Care Providers* (Atlanta, GA: Save the Children, Child Care Support Center, January 1994).

7. M.E. Briley and C.R. Gray, "Nutrition Standards in Child Care Today," *Topics in Clinical Nutrition* 9 (1994): 20–29.

8. Willer et al., *Demand and Supply of Child Care in 1990.*

9. Briley and Gray, "Nutrition Standards in Child Care Today."

10. M.E. Briley and C.R. Gray, "Nutrition Standards in Child Care Programs: Technical Support Paper," *Journal of the American Dietetic Association* 94 (1994): 324–328.

11. G.C. Franks-Spohrer, *Community Nutrition: Applying Epidemeology to Contemporary Practice* (Gaithersburg, MD: Aspen Publishers, Inc., 1996).

12. P.L. 95-627, amendment to the National School Lunch Act.

13. P.L. 104-193, the Personal Responsibility and Work Opportunity Reconciliation Act of 1996, *Federal Register,* 1996.

14. U.S. Department of Agriculture (USDA), U.S. Summary, June 1997.

15. U.S. Department Health and Human Services. Head Start Program Performances Standards. Washington, DC:US Government Printing Office; 1994.

16. USDA, "National WIC Evaluation: Evaluation of the Special Supplemental Food Program for Women, Infants, and Children," *American Journal of Clinical Nutrition* (suppl 48) (1988).

17. DHHS, *Healthy People 2000.*

18. American Dietetic Association (ADA),. "Position of the American Dietetic Association: Nutrition Standards for Child Care Programs." *Journal of the American Dietetic Association* 94 (1994): 323.

19. National Research Council, *The Recommended Dietary Allowances*, 10th ed. (Washington, DC: National Academy Press, 1989).

20. USDA and U.S. Department of Health and Human Services, *Nutrition and Your Health: Dietary Guidelines for Americans*, 4th ed. Home and Garden Bulletin No. 232. (Washington, DC: U.S. Government Printing Office, 1995).

21. USDA, Human Nutrition Information Service, *USDA's Food Guide Pyramid* (Hyattsville, MD: 1992).

22. P.L. 103-448, amendment to the National School Lunch Act, Sect. 17.

23. USDA, DHHS, *Dietary Guidelines.*

24. USDA, Food and Nutrition Service, *Nutritional Needs of Infants*. P 81, FNS-288.

25. ADA, "Position of the American Dietetic Association."

26. E.N. Whitney and S. Rolfes, *Understanding Nutrition* (Minneapolis, MN: West Publishing Co., 1997).

27. DHHS, *Healthy People 2000*.

28. E. Satter, *Child of Mine: Feeding with Love and Good Sense* (Palo Alto, CA: Bull Publishing Co., 1986).

29. E. Satter, *How To Get Your Kid to Eat—But Not Too Much* (Palo Alto, CA: Bull Publishing Co., 1987).

30. USDA, Family-Style Meal Service in CACFP. USDA Instruction 226.20.

31. Satter, *Child of Mine*.

32. Satter, *How To Get Your Kid To Eat*.

33. Bettleheim, *Food To Nurture the Mind*.

34. Franks-Spohrer, *Community Nutrition*.

35. DHHS, *Head Start Program*.

36. P.L. 95-627.

37. American Academy of Pediatrics and American Public Health Association, *Caring for Our Children—National Health and Safety Performance Standards: Guidelines for Out-of-Home Child Care Programs* (Maternal and Child Health Bureau, National Center for Education in Maternal and Child Health, APHA/American Academy of Pediatrics, 1992).

38. Society for Nutrition Education. *Position Paper on Nutrition in Child Care Settings* (Minneapolis, MN: 1990).

39. DHHS, *Healthy People 2000*.

40. ADA, "Position of the American Dietetic Association."

41. USDA, DHHS, *Dietary Guidelines*.

42. USDA, Human Nutrition Information Service, *Food Guide Pyramid*.

43. USDA, Food and Consumer Service, Midwest Region Child Nutrition Programs, *"What's in a Meal?" A Resource Manual for Providing Nutritious Meals in the Child and Adult Care Food Program* (Chicago: 1994).

44. USDA, Food and Consumer Service, *Child and Adult Care Food Program—Nutrition Guidance for Child Care Centers* (Washington, DC: U.S. Government Printing Office, September 1995).

45. National Food Service Management Institute, *CARE Connection* (University, MS: 1997).

46. Oakley, CB. *What's Cooking?* (University, MS: National Food Service Management Institute; 1997).

47. C.B. Oakley et al. Evaluation of Menus Planned in Child Care Centers Participating in the Child and Adult Care Food Program. *Journal of the American Dietetic Association* 95 (1995):765–768.

48. Nutrition Education and Labeling Act, *Federal Register*, No. PB-93-139905, January 6, 1993.

49. USDA, Food and Nutrition Services, *Serving It Safe*. FCS-295. (Washington, DC: 1996).

50. Satter, *Child of Mine*.

51. Satter, *How To Get Your Kid To Eat*.

52. USDA, Family-Style Meal Service.

53. D. Fredricks, "Staff Development to Fuel Excellence," *Poppy Seed*, 1994.

54. S.J. Crockett and L. Sims, "Environmental Influences on Children's Eating," *Journal of Nutrition Education* 27 (1995): 235–249.

55. American Academy of Pediatrics; American Public Health Association, *Caring for Our Children*.

56. American School Food Service Association, *Keys to Excellence* (Alexandria, VA: 1995).

CHAPTER 12

Nutrition Management for Children with Special Food and Nutrition Needs

Janet W. Horsley and Wanda L. Shockey

OUTLINE

- Introduction: An Overview of Children with Special Food and Nutrition Needs
- National and State Surveys
- Regulations and Legislation
- Challenges for Child Nutrition Programs: Implementing the Regulations
    Menu Modifications and the Diet Prescription
    Equipment Needs
    Teamwork To Develop a Nutrition Plan
    Creating a Positive Eating Environment
    Food Safety and Sanitation
    School Policy and Decision Making
- Costs
- Training Needs and Resources
- Application
- Summary
- Case Study: Management of Special Dietary Needs for Students without Disabilities
    Wanda L. Shockey
- Appendix 12–A: Nutrition Training and Resource Materials

INTRODUCTION: AN OVERVIEW OF CHILDREN WITH SPECIAL FOOD AND NUTRITION NEEDS

Proper nutrition is necessary for the growth and development of all children. Children with special health care needs have additional physical and emotional stresses that put them at increased risk for nutrition-related health problems that may have an impact on learning and school performance. Dietary modifications, therapeutic feeding regimens, and a supportive eating environment will help a child with special needs to receive optimal nutrition. Child nutrition programs face the challenge of identifying and serving these high-risk children in day care and school programs. The purpose of this chapter is to provide information and guidance to assist in the planning and management of nutrition services that are accessible to all children, including those with special health care needs. This chapter addresses the following objectives:

- Define the population of children with special health care needs and describe the nutrition service needs of these children at school or child care programs.
- Review the legislation that promotes equal access and appropriate nutrition-related accommodations for children with disabilities in child nutrition programs.
- Review programmatic, administrative, and fiscal considerations when implementing an inclusive child nutrition program.
- Discuss nutrition training needs and identify resource materials.

Federal programs define children with special health care needs as those children "who have or are at increased risk for chronic physical, developmental, behavioral, or emotional conditions and who require health and related services of a type or amount beyond that required by children generally."[1] This definition includes children who are chronically ill, medically fragile, or technology dependent. It is estimated that between 10 percent to 15 percent of the childhood population in the United States has a chronic condition disease or disability.[2]

This population of children is a high-risk group for nutrition-related health problems. Consequently, nutrition problems associated with chronic illnesses and disabilities are many. It is estimated that up to 40 percent of children with special health care needs have a nutrition-related problem.[3] Other studies have shown higher prevalence of nutrition problems, particularly for younger children with developmental disabilities for whom a reported prevalence rate is as high as 92 percent for one nutrition risk criterion and 67 percent for children with more risk criteria.[4] Potential nutrition problems for these children include altered energy and nutrient needs, feeding delays and oral motor problems, chronic constipation or diarrhea, and drug-nutrient interactions.[5–7]

Recent advances in health care technology and medicine have contributed to increased survival rates of low-birth-weight infants, children with chronic illnesses and congenital anomalies, and survivors of trauma.[8] Higher survival rates have led to increases in the number of children with temporary or long-term health care needs, including technology assistance.[9] Medical advances and changes in legislation to ensure inclusion in public schools have caused an increase in the number of students with special health care needs who are in education settings. School food and nutrition programs provide one of many supportive services for children with special needs.

Studies have documented that healthy nutrition practices can make a difference for school-age children, and that school food and nutrition programs make a difference. Reports have indicated that children who participate in the school breakfast program have significantly higher scores on standard achievement tests, reduced absenteeism, and lower tardiness rates, compared with their peers who do not participate.[10] Participants in the school lunch program have been shown to have "superior" nutrient intakes, as compared to a nonparticipant.[10] Therefore, these programs seem beneficial for all participating children. These health and educational benefits are particularly important for the vulnerable population of children with special needs to support their school attendance and provide them with the energy and nutrients to participate actively in the classroom and their therapy programs.

NATIONAL AND STATE SURVEYS

National and state surveys of school food and nutrition staff and special educators document the need for increased training and support for school systems to attend to the necessary health care services and to make food and nutrition services more accessible and better integrated in the school day for children with special feeding needs.[11–14] State survey results, such as Montana's technical assistance document, *Serving Students with Special Health Care Needs,* show an increasing incidence of high-risk students who require daily or intermittent management of health care services.[15] Montana's survey achieved a 66 percent response rate from school districts and special education cooperatives. Ninety percent of the respondents expressed the need for state guidelines, 91 percent indicated that preservice training did not prepare staff for serving this student population, and 62 percent reported the need for inservice training.[15]

A statewide survey of school division special education directors in Virginia identified 2,456 children with special health care needs. The most common diagnoses identified included seizure disorder, cerebral palsy, Down syndrome, congenital heart disease, and diabetes, all of which have nutrition implications. The author reported that 37 percent of this sample was noted to require special foods at mealtime, 32 percent required special feeding procedures (i.e., tube feedings, special feeding equipment, supervision at mealtime, etc.), and

eight children were found to be on homebound education services due to nutrition or feeding problems. Only 10 percent of the respondents reported using the services of a registered dietitian as a consultant in menu planning and meal modifications for children with special needs.[16]

Likewise, in a statewide survey of food service administrators in the Mississippi public school system, except those schools exclusively serving children with special health care needs, 1,728 children were identified as requiring special diets. The most common meal modifications of the school lunch program included omission or substitution of menu items, recipe modifications requiring a change of ingredients, and textural modifications of foods.[17]

In a national survey of school food and nutrition managers, district school nutrition directors/supervisors, and district special education directors the most frequently reported conditions of children requiring dietary modifications were food allergies and intolerances, diabetes, and conditions in which feeding problems were associated. Less than 25 percent of the respondents reported using a registered dietitian as a consultant in meal planning and preparation. This research study identified six significant barriers that impede the provision of specialized nutrition services for children with chronic conditions and disabilities. These barriers are listed in Exhibit 12–1.[18]

Cumulatively these studies show the need for health and specialized nutrition services, and document the barriers and problems that challenge child nutrition programs to provide appropriate and nourishing meals for all children. Furthermore, these studies illustrate the importance of keeping statistics on the number of children requiring special diets, their diagnoses, and the types of diets required to forecast program needs and influence legislation related to child nutrition at the state and national level to better serve children with special needs.

Exhibit 12–1   Barriers to Specialized Nutrition Services in Schools

- Limited knowledge and skills
- Limited communication among school nutrition personnel, teachers, administrators, and parents
- Limited integration of nutrition with special education
- Lack of clarification of responsibility, including funding
- Liability concerns
- Limited use of dietitian consultants

Source: Reprinted with permission from K. Yadrick and J. Sneed, *Providing for the Special Food and Nutrition Needs of Children,* © 1993, National Food Service Management Institute.

REGULATIONS AND LEGISLATION

Child nutrition programs operate under the National School Lunch Act of 1946 and the Child Nutrition Act of 1966. In 1975, Public Law 94-142, the Education of All Handicapped Children Act, and supportive state legislation related to children with disabilities mandated the provision of free and appropriate education for all children with disabilities. As a result of this legislation, many children with special needs are in public schools and are participating in the National School Lunch and School Breakfast Programs. In 1986 special education services were mandated for preschool age children that expanded the population of children receiving meals at school. Additional protections for these children and support for their health and related needs have been established through subsequent legislation including the 1982 Amendments to the Rehabilitation Act of 1973 and the Americans with Disabilities Act of 1990.[19,20] Exhibit 12–2 outlines the important legislation pertinent to child nutrition programs.

In response to these legislative mandates, the United States Department of Agriculture (USDA) developed regulations and policy guidelines that provide for equal access to school meals for all children. Subsequent legislation, Public Law 103-448, the Healthy Meals for Healthy Americans Act of 1994 included a mandate to develop a school program guidance manual, *Accommodating Children with Special Needs in School Nutrition Programs.* This guidance was developed by the USDA in consultation with the U.S. Department of Education and the U.S. Department of Justice to be a resource for school staff to implement policy guidelines related to meal substitutions for medical and other special reasons.[21]

CHALLENGES FOR CHILD NUTRITION PROGRAMS: IMPLEMENTING THE REGULATIONS

When one envisions food and nutrition services in day-care settings and schools, it brings to mind a mental picture of children around a table in a common room or cafeteria enjoying the socialization and nourishment of their meal or snack. The process of designing and delivering meals becomes more complex and may take a few extra steps to develop and serve developmentally appropriate, safe, and nutritious meals for children with special needs in a positive eating environment. When developing food and nutrition programs to serve all children, including children with special needs, there are many program considerations. These include serving as part of the interdisciplinary health care team; securing diet prescriptions for meal modifications; purchasing necessary equipment for food preparation or feeding; monitoring of growth; developing a nutrition plan for students with special needs; providing an inclusive, safe, and successful eating environment; and reinforcing food safety and sanitation.

Exhibit 12–2 Regulations Related to Children with Special Needs

1975 Public Law 94-142, The Education of All Handicapped Children Act mandates that children with disabilities have free and appropriate education in the least restrictive environment.

1982 Amendments to the Rehabilitation Act of 1973, Section 504, mandates equal access to services for children with disabilities participating in federally funded programs. This act requires child nutrition programs to provide meal modifications for children who are unable to eat meals because of their disabilities. Schools and institutions must have medical certification from a physician for children requesting accommodations.

1982 7 C.F.R. (*Code of Federal Regulations*), Part 15, provides instructions for school food service operations funded by USDA to provide meals at no extra charge to children requiring modified diets.

1986 Public Law 99-457, IDEA (Individuals with Disabilities Education Act) mandated that by 1991 all states provide early intervention services for infants and toddlers from birth through age two years and special education services for preschoolers ages three years through five years who meet eligibility criteria. This law resulted in the development of preschool programs for children with special needs in schools, so that food and nutrition service personnel had to begin to address a younger group of high-risk children.

1990 Americans with Disabilities Act protects all individuals with disabilities from discrimination.

1994 Public Law 103-448, The Healthy Meals for Healthy Americans Act of 1994 mandates the development of guidance by USDA to interpret program considerations for providing meal modifications and strategies for school food service to facilitate coordination within the school system and the community.

Source: Adapted with permission from J.W. Horsley, Nutrition Issues Facing Children with Special Health Care Needs in Early Intervention and at School, *NUTRITION FOCUS for Children with Special Health Care Needs,* Vol. 9, No. 3, p. 2, © 1994, Center on Human Development and Disability, University of Washington.

Menu Modifications and the Diet Prescription

Requests for menu modifications fall into three categories: (1) students with disabilities who have a prescription from a medical authority (service required); (2) students without disabilities who have a request by a medical authority (service optional); and (3) students with special preferences (optional, within existing menu choices). USDA regulations and guidance provide parameters for schools. However, clear and comprehensive local policies and procedures will be required to ensure that regulatory requirements are met and that optional services are provided in a consistent and nondiscriminatory manner.

As specified in the USDA regulations, child nutrition programs must make food substitutions or accommodations for students with disabilities. However, menu modifications must be based on a prescription from a licensed physician for all children with a documented disability. As outlined in Exhibit 12–3, a child is considered to be disabled if he or she has "a physical or mental impairment which substantially limits one or more major life activity, has a record of such an impairment, or is regarded as having such an impairment."[21]

For other children with chronic conditions, such as food intolerances or elevated cholesterol levels, who are not considered "disabled," substitutions and meal modifications may be made on a case-by-case basis, according to established local policies and procedures. These modifications must be based on a prescription from a recognized medical authority. The recognized medical authority is a physician, physician's assistant, registered nurse, nurse practitioner, or other specialist recognized by the state agency.[21] The diet prescription must document the following elements: the child's

Exhibit 12–3 Definition of Disability

According to the Rehabilitation Act of 1973 and the Americans with Disabilities Act of 1990, the term "physical or mental impairment," includes, but is not limited to:

- orthopedic, visual, speech, and hearing impairments
- cerebral palsy
- epilepsy
- muscular dystrophy
- multiple sclerosis
- cancer
- heart disease
- metabolic disease such as diabetes or phenylketonuria
- food anaphylaxis or severe food allergy
- mental retardation
- emotional illness
- drug addiction and alcoholism

Source: Reprinted from U.S. Department of Agriculture, Food and Consumer Services, *Accommodating Children with Special Dietary Needs in School Nutrition Programs: Guidance for School Food Service Staff,* 1995, U.S. Government Printing Office.

---

disability and an explanation of why the disability restricts the diet (if applicable); the major life activity affected by the disability (if applicable); and the food or foods to be omitted, as well as the food or choice of foods to be substituted.[21,22] An example of a diet prescription form is provided in Exhibit 12–4.

Menu and meal modifications may vary depending on the needs of the individual child. Possible dietary manipulations may be to increase calories for a child who is underweight and requires a high-calorie diet to support health and growth; to restrict calories for a child who has a low metabolic rate and is at risk for obesity; to restrict certain products that contain ingredients that may not be tolerated by a child with a metabolic disorder; or to change the texture of foods to ground, chopped, or puréed consistencies for the child who has feeding problems or oral-motor dysfunction. Table 12–1 illustrates modifications of a regular menu for special diets.[22] Many of these modifications can be made within the meal pattern requirements. If schools have a variety of menu choices and offer-versus-serve implementation, many students can meet their needs by making appropriate selections, thus promoting independence and contributing to a more normal and inclusive environment. A meal that requires significant changes in the nutrient content or meal pattern is reimbursable provided a diet prescription from the appropriate medical authority documents these changes and is on file in the agency.[23]

Student requests based on preferences instead of medical statements do not meet the strict definition of "special health care needs." However, increasing numbers of students and/or parents/guardians are making requests based on their self-perceived health needs. It is important to establish policies regarding how such requests (e.g., vegetarian, low fat, etc.) will be handled. Local policy may provide for special accommodations in these circumstances; however, the school must ensure that the meal pattern and/or nutrient standards are met or meals cannot be claimed for reimbursement.

Equipment Needs

Important considerations in the development of nutrition services for children with special health care needs are the equipment needs re-

Exhibit 12–4 Eating/Feeding Evaluation: Children with Special Needs

Student's Name				
School Name				
Student's Age	Grade level		Classroom	
Does the student have a disability?			Yes	No
If Yes, describe the major life activities affected by the disability.				
If Yes, does the student have special nutritional or feeding needs? If Yes, complete this form and have it signed by a physician.			Yes	No
If the student is not disabled, does he/she have special nutritional or feeding needs?		Yes		No
If Yes, complete this form and have it signed by the appropriate medical authority.				
If the student does not require special meal considerations and is able to eat a regular diet, the parent can sign at the bottom and return the form to the school food service.				
List any dietary restrictions or special diet.				
List any allergies or food intolerances to avoid.				
List foods to be substituted.				
List foods that need the following change in texture. If all foods need to be prepared in this manner, indicate "All." Cut up or chopped to bite size pieces:				
Finely ground:				
Puréed:				
List special equipment or utensils needed.				
Indicate any other comments regarding the student's eating or feeding patterns.				
Parent's Signature			Date	
Physician's or Medical Authority's Signature			Date	

Source: Reprinted from U.S. Department of Agriculture, Food and Consumer Services, *Accommodating Children with Special Needs in School Nutrition Programs: Guidance for School Food Service Staff,* 1995, U.S. Government Printing Office.

lated to food preparation, feeding skill development, and nutrition monitoring. Food preparation equipment may be needed to modify textures of foods for children with oral-motor deficits. Potential food preparation purchases may include a baby food grinder, food processor, blender, or vertical cutter mixer. Special feeding equipment may also be required for

Table 12–1 Lunch Menu Modifications

Menu	Low-Calorie/ Diabetic	High-Calorie	Chopped	Ground	Puréed
Chicken breast	Baked; not fried; pull off skin	No change	Chop into bite-size pieces	Creamed chicken = grind meat and add cream soup	Purée chicken meat with chicken broth or cream soup
French fries	Baked potato	No change	Mashed potatoes	Mashed potatoes	Purée mashed potatoes with gravy or low-fat milk added for correct consistency/calories
Green beans	No change	Add one pat margarine	Chop into bite-size pieces	Well cooked; mashed	Purée with cream soup, chicken broth, or vegetable juices
Biscuit	Serve plain	Add one pat margarine; jelly or honey	Cut into quarters or bite-size pieces	Substitute rice, or finely chopped noodles or mashed potatoes	Substitute mashed potatoes puréed with gravy or low-fat milk for correct consistency/calories
Canned pears	Canned in natural juices	Canned in syrup	Cut in cubes	Chopped and mashed	Puréed with pear juice
Milk	Low fat	Whole	Whole or low fat	Whole or low fat	Whole or low fat

Source: Adapted with permission from Child Nutrition Programs, Ideas for Modifying Texture of Items for Special Diets, *CARE: Special Nutrition for Kids,* © 1995, Alabama Department of Education.

children developing independent feeding skills.[24,25] Special feeding equipment may include specialized cups, such as a spouted cup, a two-handled cup or a cut-out cup; modified utensils, such as plastic-coated spoons, or utensils with built-up or curved handles; and adapted plates with divided sections or sloping sides. Figure 12–1 illustrates examples of special feeding equipment.

Finally, measuring equipment may need to be purchased to monitor the nutritional status of children with dietary or feeding concerns through routine growth measurements. A standard scale and stadiometer may be available in many schools and agencies, but may not be sufficient to measure children in wheelchairs or with orthopedic problems that impair their ability to stand independently. Wheelchair, table or chair scales, and length boards may be purchased to accommodate these children, or the agency may choose to communicate with a specialty clinic, where the child is monitored to obtain growth measurements.[26] All measurements should be plotted on standard National Centers for Health Statistics (NCHS) pediatric growth charts or diagnostic-specific growth charts to determine the child's progress.

Teamwork To Develop a Nutrition Plan

When addressing the nutritional needs of a particular child, careful planning is essential.

Cups

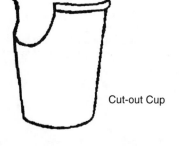

The cut-out cup is used to prevent a child from hitting his or her nose on the rim of the cup. This helps to keep the head from tipping back and prevents choking.

Cut-out Cup

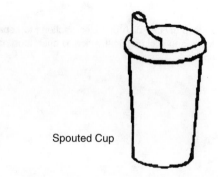

A spouted lid is used to promote lip closure on the spout and to prevent fluid from spilling while drinking.

Spouted Cup

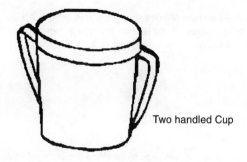

A two-handled cup is used for the child who cannot hold and balance a cup in his or her hand. The extra handle adds stability.

Two handled Cup

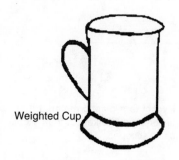

A weighted cup is used for the child who has trouble keeping the cup upright when returning it to the table or tray.

Weighted Cup

continues

Figure 12–1 Examples of Special Feeding Equipment. *Source:* Adapted with permission from Child Nutrition Programs, Ideas for Modifying Texture of Items for Special Diets, *CARE: Special Nutrition for Kids,* © 1995, Alabama Department of Education.

Figure 12–1 continued

Dishes or Plates

A dish with a sloping or built-up side helps the child to have a surface to scoop against to get food on the spoon.

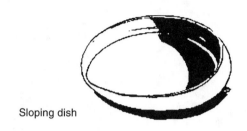

Sloping dish

A deep divided dish provides sections to separate foods and walls against which to push food on the spoon.

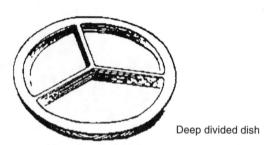

Deep divided dish

Food guards provide a metal frame which can be placed around a plate to provide a raised side against which to scoop food.

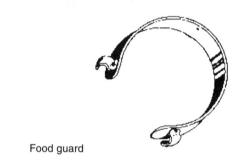

Food guard

Weighted dishes help to stabilize the plate so that it will not move while scooping food.

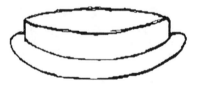

Weighted dish

Dycem is a plastic material that can be placed under a plate to keep it from slipping while food is being scooped.

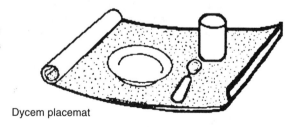

Dycem placemat

continues

Figure 12–1 continued

Spoons, Forks, and Knives

Built-up handles can be made with soft rubber or plastic material to help a child who cannot grip the utensil.

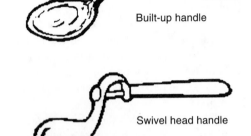

Built-up handle

A spoon with a swivel head helps a child who cannot hold the spoon in the proper position to balance food on the spoon.

Swivel head handle

Curved handle spoon

Spoons and forks with curved handles help a child with poor muscle control or limited wrist movement to pick up food and bring it to his or her mouth.

Plastic-coated spoons help to protect a child who has a bite reflex that causes him or her to bite down on the utensil when it enters the mouth.

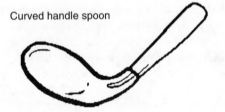

Plastic coated spoon

The rocker knife/fork is used for one-hand cutting and eating.

Rocker knife/fork

The universal cuff is a strap that is used to hold the fork or spoon in the hand when a child has little or no grasp.

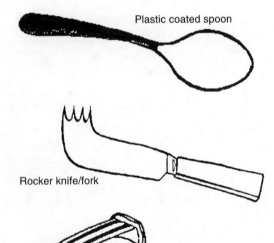

Universal cuff

Several tools are available to use as management plans for children with special needs. An individualized health care plan (IHCP) is needed for each student requiring individualized intervention to enable participation in the education program.[27–32] Depending on the needs of the child, it may be part of the 504 Accommodation Plan, the Individualized Education Plan (IEP), or it may be used alone. In the day-care setting nutrition plans may be developed using elements of the plans described in this section.

The IHCP team includes the school nurse, school administrator, teacher, parent, student (if appropriate), a representative from the food and nutrition program, and the child's nutritionist, and other health care professionals to address the student's needs. The school nurse is generally responsible for the role of the team coordinator.[33] By working collaboratively the multidisciplinary team can ensure that the student's special health care needs are met in a medically safe and educationally appropriate environment. The *Guidelines for the Delineation of Roles and Responsibilities for the Safe Delivery of Specialized Health Care in the Educational Setting*[34] can be used in the provision of feeding requirements as part of daily living activities. These guidelines must adhere to each state nurse's practice act and are helpful in designating appropriate personnel to perform tasks defined in the IHCP.[35] The IHCP can be a component of the special education IEP or the 504 Accommodation Plan, or it may stand alone as a document to meet the needs of the student with a disability who requires limited assistance and is included in the regular classroom (see Figure 12–2).

In 1994 the National Association of School Nurses, Inc., addressed the problem of nutrition status not being included in the IEP.[36] They recommended the incorporation of the Individualized IHCP as a part of the IEP in the special education process and cited school

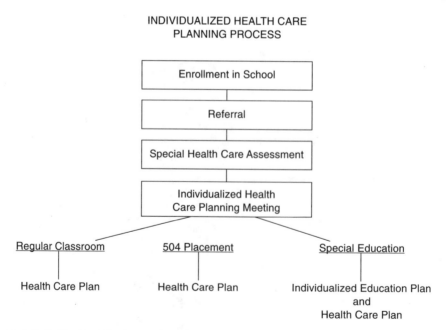

INDIVIDUALIZED HEALTH CARE PLANNING PROCESS

Enrollment in School

Referral

Special Health Care Assessment

Individualized Health Care Planning Meeting

Regular Classroom — Health Care Plan

504 Placement — Health Care Plan

Special Education — Individualized Education Plan and Health Care Plan

Figure 12–2 Individualized Health Care Planning Process. *Source:* Reprinted with permission from Individualized Health Care Planning Process, *Serving Students with Special Health Care Needs*, p. 10, © 1993, Montana Office of Public Instruction.

nurses as key personnel in the coordination of the health care team. The nurse's role in the documentation of the health care plan includes nutrition status issues to be addressed by the team nutritionist.

The IEP is utilized when developing health-related services for children in special education programs. Every child in special education is required to have an IEP. The nutrition component may be incorporated in the plan or may be addressed through the IHCP, as noted above. It provides a plan to document resources that enable a student with special needs to benefit from the education curriculum.[37,38] Historically, the IEP has not been well utilized to plan nutrition programs for students with special needs, even though it is believed to be a best practice. In a 1986 survey of special education directors in Virginia only 33 percent of the 78 respondents reported that there was some type of nutrition component in the IEP. Further investigation of the nutrition content of these plans revealed that in the majority of cases the IEP focused on feeding therapy and independent feeding skills, but did not address growth or nutritional status issues.[39] In addition, a 1993 national survey of school food and nutrition managers, district directors/supervisors, and district special education directors documented that the number of IEPs that contained a dietary objective was far fewer than the number of children identified with conditions that may require meal modifications or nutrition services.[40]

Like the IHCP, the IEP is developed by an interdisciplinary committee. The committee is composed of the child's teacher; another representative from the local school division who is qualified to supervise special education; the child's parent(s); the child (if appropriate); and other specialists identified to address the child's needs. When nutrition plans are developed, a representative from the child nutrition program and the child's nutritionist should be members or this team.[41-44] It is required that the parent(s) sign the IEP and consent to the plan before services are delivered. This plan is to be reviewed and revised annually but may be reviewed anytime during the year at the request of the parent or a member of the school staff. Exhibit 12–5 outlines the content of the IEP.

The content of the IEP is to be focused on the child, and therefore the objectives should be student oriented. The plan should reflect what the child will achieve as a result of the resources and services provided by the school.

Similarly, the 504 Accommodation Plan is a tool used for planning nutrition services. It is designed for the child who is not in special education, but does have special dietary needs. The 504 Accommodation Plan may be developed to address the nutrition accommodations during the school day with goals and objectives similar to those of the IEP.[45]

Potential nutrition-related goals for an IHCP, IEP, or 504 Plan include developing or refining self-feeding skills; improving oral-motor function; improving mealtime behavior; identifying

---

Exhibit 12–5 Content of the Individualized Education Plan (IEP)

- Statement of the child's present level of educational performance
- Statement of the annual goals, including short-term instructional objectives related to the specific goals
- Statement of the specific education instruction and related services for the child
- Statement of the extent to which the child may participate in a regular educational program
- Projected dates for initiation and duration of services for each objective
- Appropriate objective criteria and evaluation procedures and schedules for determining at least annually whether the objectives are achieved

and communicating nutrition needs; improving food preparation skills; improving growth rates; and maintaining laboratory data (e.g., serum glucose, phenylalanine levels) within normal limits.[46,47] An example of an IEP nutrition goal and supporting objectives is provided in Exhibit 12–6.

Creating a Positive Eating Environment

A successful eating environment is one in which children are comfortable and can enjoy their meals while socializing with their peers. Most children will eat in a cafeteria, and this should be encouraged in order to optimize the social aspect of the eating environment. However, some children will require additional assistance and may need a quiet, less distracting environment in order to attend to the task of eating. For these children, a screen may be placed in the cafeteria or common eating room, or children may be positioned so that they are not focusing on the full room of students to decrease distractions or provide some additional privacy. Cafeterias need to provide space to accommodate wheelchairs, have appropriate seating arrangements for children with special equipment, and have adequate lighting for children with visual impairments.[48]

Aside from the physical layout of the cafeteria, consideration must be given to the length of mealtime. Many children feel rushed to complete their meal within the limited time period, and children with special needs may be particularly slow at mealtime due to feeding delays, lethargy, or poor appetites. If their mealtime is consistently compromised, these children may need extra time in the cafeteria or may need assistance in getting to the cafeteria early to accommodate their needs.[49] These modifications may be incorporated in the IEP, 504 Plan, or IHCP. Specific considerations for a positive eating environment are outlined in Exhibit 12–7.[50]

Food Safety and Sanitation

Safety and sanitation issues are a priority for every child nutrition program. The child nutrition program manager is responsible for following state sanitation regulations related to storing, transporting, preparing, and serving all foods. Due to their nutritional risk and medical status, children with special health care needs may be more vulnerable to germs, infections, and food-borne illnesses. Therefore, care should be taken to ensure food safety and sanitation. Besides the use of proper hand washing and personal hygiene, particular attention

---

Exhibit 12–6 Sample IEP Goals and Objectives

Timmy is a nine-year-old boy with spastic cerebral palsy and a seizure disorder. He has delayed feeding skills and is significantly underweight. His school meals are puréed and he is assisted by an aide at mealtime. His IEP includes a nutrition component to address the need for weight gain.

GOAL: Timmy will gain weight and continue to grow taller during the school year.

OBJECTIVE 1. Timmy will drink four ounces of a high-calorie, high-protein nutrition supplement at least three days per week with his school breakfast.

OBJECTIVE 2: Timmy will eat his school lunch supplemented with high-calorie additives (e.g., margarine, powdered milk, instant breakfast milkshake, etc.) at least three days per week.

Source: Reprinted with permission from J.W. Horsley et al., Case Study: Cerebral Palsy, *Nutrition Management of School Age Children with Special Needs: A Resource Manual for School Personnel, Families and Health Professionals, 2nd ed.*, pp. 58–59, © 1996, Virginia Department of Education and Virginia Department of Health.

Exhibit 12–7 Components of a Positive Eating Environment

Scheduling:
- Allow ample time for the child to eat.
- Let the child begin to eat before others enter the cafeteria if distractions are a problem.

Space:
- Plan the appropriate space to accommodate wheelchairs:

  Doorways 32 inches wide

  Aisles 34 inches wide

  Tables 5 feet 6 inches apart

  30 inches above the floor

  12-inch clearance underneath from the outer edge toward the interior of the table
- Make serving line easily accessible (including aisle width and self-serving table height).
- Allot adequate space for feeding aides.

Location:
- Provide ramps as needed to ensure cafeteria accessibility.
- Seat child who is easily distracted away from heavy traffic areas.
- Screen off sections of the room for distractible children.

Lighting:
- Provide adequate lighting for students who are visually impaired.
- Use lighting to create a warm atmosphere.

Self-Help Devices:
- Offer compartmentalized plates to help children in scooping food.
- Provide utensils with modified handles as needed.
- Facilitate proper positioning with tables and chairs.
- Provide braille-typed menus to visually impaired children.
- Provide trays on rolling stands or with attachments to wheelchairs.

Food:
- Serve all food items at proper temperature.
- Offer appropriate portion sizes.
- Prepare food attractively for the student—even if it is pureed.
- Position food on plate/tray clockwise for the child with visual impairment.

Student /Staff:
- Treat the students with special needs as "normally" as possible.
- Model appropriate behavior for the benefit of the other students.

Source: Reprinted with permission from U.S. Department of Agriculture, Southeast Regional Office, and the University of Alabama at Birmingham, *Meeting Their Needs: Training Manual for Child Nutrition Personnel Serving Children with Special Needs,* pp. 53–54, © 1993.

---

should be paid to keeping foods at the correct temperature (i.e., hot foods should be kept above 140 degrees Fahrenheit and cold foods should be kept below 40 degrees Fahrenheit[51]) to prevent the development of bacteria and food-borne pathogens. This is a significant concern when foods are transported from the kitchen to the feeding site. Temperature charts are useful to document appropriate temperatures at mealtime.[52] A second important consideration is the need to have all serving utensils and special feeding equipment sanitized in the kitchen. If a kitchen is not on site, procedures need to be in place to ensure that all feeding equipment is sanitized appropriately.[52,53]

School Policy and Decision Making

In order to address the nutritional needs of individual students with special dietary or feeding concerns with equity and cost effectiveness, local school policies regarding requests for dietary modifications and procedures for dealing with new issues and questions are essential. Local policies and procedures are needed to address the provision of meal modifications, as well as purchasing foods, equipment, or nutrition services associated with modified school meals.[54] In general, schools are required to make meals accessible for all students, and this philosophy is reflected in the USDA regulations. While the USDA regulations and guidance materials are useful for answering the majority of questions related to dietary changes, there are areas where it is left to the school system to determine on a case-by-case basis how certain situations will be handled. The outcome of these decisions will have an immediate impact on the child who has a dietary need and will also affect future children, once a precedent has been established. Issues where the obligation to provide accommodations is left to the school administration include requests for dietary modifications for a child who is not considered to be disabled and requests for children with temporary or short-term disabilities.[55] In addition, the direct and indirect costs of providing modified meals are present in every case. In order to save both administrative time and cost, policy development and planning related to special meal requests which exceed the regulations are critical for each school district.[56]

COSTS

The cost of meal modifications, labor, and equipment to provide nutrition services for children with special needs in child nutrition programs is variable. Factors that influence the range of costs include salaries and personnel costs, types of food substitutions and special feeding equipment, and the number of children requiring nutrition and feeding services in a particular agency.[57] A study conducted by the National Food Service Management Institute documents the types and ranges of expenses for eight school districts from three states in the southeast and southwest. In this study, data collection occurred for six days in fifteen schools within eight different school districts. The median enrollment in the schools was 666 students, and the median number of meals served during the study period to children requiring dietary modifications was six. A summary of the labor, food, and equipment costs is provided in Exhibit 12–8.[57] The indirect costs are calculated based on staff time spent to obtain and interpret diet orders, purchase food products and equipment, train staff, and monitor school attendance for targeted children. The direct labor costs are calculated for nutrition consultation to a district office for meal preparation at targeted schools. Based on the salaries of the staff and consultants involved in the activities described above, these costs are variable.

Food and equipment costs show a range of values, as well. Typical food purchases included sugar-free foods and low-sodium substitutes. One district purchased in excess of $700 per month of commercial nutrition supplements for 15 students; however, this was an exception in this study, and the median food cost was much lower. For individual schools, the food cost for modified diets with food substitutions was very similar and slightly less than that of regular meals. Equipment costs were for food preparation equipment, including blenders and food processors, with a median cost of $125 per year. Based on the findings from this study, the cost of preparing and serving special meals, although differing between schools, is not a significant expense for the average school system.[57]

Regardless of the costs for labor, food, and equipment, each school district should establish purchasing policies that address these areas of expense. In general, the school food authority should be able to absorb these costs.

Exhibit 12–8 Costs Associated with Providing Specialized Meals at School

School District	School
Labor Costs Based on Staff Time:	*Labor Costs Based on Staff Time:*
Indirect Cost Range : 1–55 hours/month	Indirect Cost Range: 2 minutes–3 hours/child
Indirect Cost Median: 12 hours/month	Indirect Cost Median: 6 hours/month or 1 hour/child
Direct Cost: 4 hours/ child*	
* only one district reported	Median Direct Cost:
	Textural Modifications of Meals: 1 hour/child
	Special Meal Preparation:
	5 minutes for breakfast
	8 minutes for lunch
Direct Food and Equipment Costs:	*Direct Food and Equipment Costs:*
Median Food Cost: $20 /month	Cost Differential between regular and modified meals:
Median Equipment Cost: $125/year	Breakfast: $.05 less than the cost of a regular meal
	Lunch: $.01 less than the cost of a regular meal

Source: Reprinted with permission from M.T. Conklin and M.F. Nettles, *Costs Associated with Providing School Meals for Children with Special Needs,* © 1994, National Food Service Management Institute.

However, when there is difficulty in covering unusual expenses, alternative sources should be explored. Potential resources include special education funds (provided the meal modifications and/or nutrition services are specified in the IEP), Medicaid, Medicare, special grants, or community resources (e.g., voluntary health organizations, or civic organizations).[58]

TRAINING NEEDS AND RESOURCES

Training in the area of children with special feeding and dietary needs is an identified area of continuing education for child nutrition programs. In the Mississippi survey of food service administrators in public schools, training needs were reported in many areas. In this survey, food service administrators ranked their greatest training needs. The top categories included menu modifications for specific disorders (i.e., chronic renal disease, phenylketonuria, food allergies, and diabetes), calculating macronutrients in daily menus, and textural modifications.[59] Likewise, a national survey of school nutrition managers, district school nutrition directors/supervisors, and district special education directors identified the highest rated training needs to be understanding liability issues; calculating macronutrient content of menus; modification of recipes to lower fat, cholesterol, and sodium; and understanding the physical and emotional needs of children with disabilities and chronic conditions.[60]

Responding to these identified training needs, the USDA and the National Food Service Management Institute have taken leadership in the area of implementing training programs and developing resources. Since 1992 national, regional, and state conferences have been organized. In the southeast several training manuals and instructive video tapes have been developed by child nutrition programs and Nutrition Education and Training (NET) programs with USDA funding.[61] Examples of training materials and resources are outlined at the end of this chapter.

In 1995, the USDA issued a request for proposals for special dietary and medical needs grants. These grants offered funding on a competitive basis to state educational agencies for distribution to schools and institutions to assist them with nonrecurring costs associated with accommodating the special dietary needs of children with disabilities in child nutrition programs. With these funds, many states have had opportunities to enhance their services for this population of children.

Human resources and direct services for children with special needs will vary from state to state. In some states registered dietitians working in pediatric specialty clinics have coordinated with schools and community agencies to provide nutrition consultation, screening, and/or assessment services. These services may be sponsored by the Title V, Children with Special Health Care Needs Program in the state health department[62] or contracted for through special funding.[63] Other resources for nutrition consultation or technical assistance include state public health nutrition and maternal and child health programs, university-affiliated programs; practice groups within the American Dietetic Association, including the Pediatric Nutrition Practice Group, School Nutrition Services Practice Group, and Dietitians in Developmental and Psychiatric Disorders; and pediatric dietitians in local hospitals. Potential funding sources for these services may be explored through Medicaid/Medical Assistance Programs, private insurance, private pay, or the Special Supplemental Feeding Program for Women, Infants and Children (WIC).[64–66]

APPLICATION

A well-developed and an inclusive child nutrition program will include the multiple steps illustrated in Figure 12–3.[67] Teamwork between school staff and parents and clear policy making and planning are key components of successful nutrition management for children with special dietary and feeding needs. This figure shows the administrative processes to consider when addressing special nutrition needs. The primary policy and planning steps at the top of the figure include parent notification of school procedures, establishment of services from a registered dietitian, clarification of funding issues, and training of school personnel. All four steps need to be addressed in order to administer a school food and nutrition program that is responsive to students with special needs. Issues addressed in the vertical boxes illustrate the flow of actions to be taken in response to a request for a meal modification.[67]

Providing meals for children with special feeding and dietary needs in child nutrition programs offers new opportunities for school food and nutrition personnel, educators, and registered dietitians. Child day-care centers, state departments of education, school districts, and local school systems will need the expertise of the registered dietitian for meal modifications and menu planning. In addition, education and school food and nutrition personnel will be challenged to work as a team in a coordinated fashion with health care providers and families in the identification of children requiring special meals or feeding procedures, the development of appropriate nutrition plans for these children, and the delivery of modified meals. In order to comply with USDA regulations, and to reinforce a positive and supportive nutrition program, there will be an ongoing need for training of food service, school and day care staff regarding feeding and nutrition issues for children and youth with disabilities. This area of child nutri-

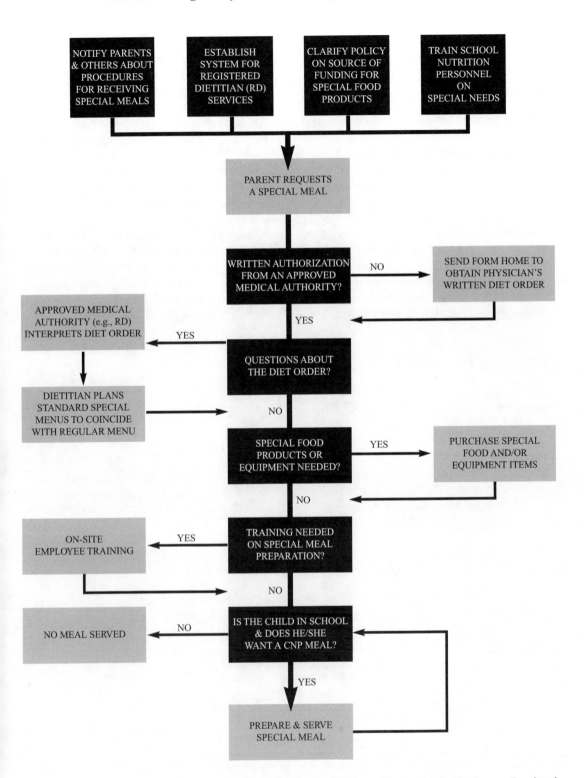

Figure 12–3 Steps Involved in Managing Nutrition Services for Children with Special Needs. *Source:* Reprinted with permission from M.T. Conklin et al., Managing Nutrition for Children with Special Needs, *NFSMI Insight*, Vol. 1, No. 1, p. 3, © 1994, National Food Service Management Institute.

tion will continue to offer many challenges, as well as many opportunities.

SUMMARY

Children with disabilities, chronic illnesses, and developmental delays are at increased risk for nutrition-related health problems. Meeting the nutritional needs of this population requires teamwork and collaboration between child nutrition program personnel, health care providers, and families. Successful management will require attention to federal regulations, the delivery of modified meals in compliance with diet prescriptions, the development of individualized nutrition plans, the design of accessible and positive mealtime environments, knowledge of food safety and san-

itation issues, budgetary planning for food substitutions and special equipment needs, and, ongoing staff development and education. The importance of these principles is reinforced in two important documents for school food and nutrition program managers and directors. Competency 7.4 in the National Food Service Management Institute's *Competencies* and standard of care 1.9 in the *Keys to Excellence* describe the skills, knowledge, and indicators that are foundations of an inclusive child nutrition program.[68,69]

The provision of special diets and feeding procedures will support the growth, health, and academic achievement of young children and students with special needs. Achieving this outcome is a challenge and an opportunity for all child nutrition program personnel.

CASE STUDY
MANAGEMENT OF SPECIAL DIETARY NEEDS FOR STUDENTS WITHOUT DISABILITIES

Wanda L. Shockey

Ms. Smith, the new food and nutrition manager at Solo Elementary School, has a high school diploma and two years work experience as a food service assistant. Ms. Johnson, a parent, brought Ms. Smith a physician's list of foods to be excluded from her daughter Candy's school breakfasts and lunches. The medical statement indicated that Candy has mild allergic reactions to corn, barley, and chocolate. No medical claim of disability, life-threatening reaction, or major life activity affected by the allergy is contained in the statement.

Ms. Smith explained to Ms. Johnson that Candy will need to bring her breakfast and lunch each day because schools are not required by federal regulations to make substitutions for children with food allergies or intolerance unless the reaction is considered life threatening. The parent was upset because she had personal knowledge that a student at the Apollo Middle School in the same school district was being served a special meal at breakfast and lunch due to allergies. She called the superintendent and a school board member to complain about the difference in service for her child and another child in the district.

The superintendent called Mrs. March, the school food and nutrition program director. Mrs. March explained that there are departmental policies and procedures in place for handling special dietary requests for students with disabilities, but no policy exists for those requests for students without disabilities. Each manager makes decisions on a case-by-case basis. The superintendent asked Mrs. March to respond to the parent.

Immediate, short-term, and long-term management actions by the school food and nutrition program director will address the current problem and prevent future problems of this nature.

Immediate Actions by the Food and Nutrition Program Director

1. Reassured the parent that the school district wants to be a partner with families to meet children's special dietary needs, to the extent that adequate resources exist. Informed her that a system would be established within a week to omit designated foods from Candy's school meals and that a policy would be developed to make further accommodations if determined feasible.

2. Identified the items that contain corn, barley, or chocolate on a cycle of school breakfast and lunch menus.

3. Met with the parent, teacher, and food service manager to discuss ways the problem foods can be avoided by the student. Agreements made during the conference:

   • The parent will discuss the menu with Candy and teach her which foods will be omitted. She will mark the items she wants Candy to avoid on the school menu and return a copy to the teacher and the manager.

   • The teacher will remind Candy of the items to avoid each day.

   • The manager will post a copy of the menu with a picture of Candy on the kitchen bulletin board and instruct the serving staff to omit designated menu items. The last person on the serving line will check Candy's tray to be certain it does not contain a menu item she cannot have.

   • The parent will send supplemental

food on any day the menu does not contain adequate food after problem items have been eliminated.

Short-Term Actions by the Food and Nutrition Program Director

A multidisciplinary team was composed of a school nurse, registered dietitian, school business official, food and nutrition program director, principal, teacher, and food service manager. The team discussed the feasibility of delivering special dietary services prescribed by a medical authority for students without disabilities. The team concluded that expansion of current policy to include services for these students was desirable and feasible. The team agreed to become the policy development team. The policy had these key components:

- Delineation of roles and responsibilities of parents, students, and school personnel
- Identification/referral process for students without disabilities who have special dietary needs

- Criteria for development of an individual health care plan where appropriate
- Substitution of foods available in the normal marketplace for foods excluded by a physician or other recognized medical authority
- Plan for communicating new policy to staff, parents, and students

The team recommended that the school district's board of education adopt a policy providing that all students, with or without disabilities, who have special dietary prescriptions from a recognized medical authority, be provided substitutions as determined appropriate by a registered dietitian or registered nurse. The board of education voted to adopt the policy with the proviso that (1) a cost evaluation system of expenses and staff time be in place prior to implementation, and (2) the impact of the new policy be reviewed at the end of one year. Pending the outcome of these considerations, recommendations for continuance or revision will made to the board.

REFERENCES

1. Maternal and Child Health Bureau, Division of Services for Children with Special Health Care Needs, Department of Health and Human Services, Rockville, MD, August 13, 1995: 1 [Letter].

2. M.T. Baer et al., "Children with Special Health Care Needs," in *Call to Action: Better Nutrition for Mothers, Children and Families,* ed. C.O. Sharbaugh (Washington, DC: National Center for Education in Maternal and Child Health, 1991), 191–208.

3. J. Hine et al., "Early Nutrition Intervention Services for Children with Special Health Care Needs," *Journal of the American Dietetic Association* 89, no. 11 (1989): 1636–1639.

4. C.T. Bayerl et al., "Nutrition Issues of Children in Early Intervention Programs: Primary Care Team Approach," *Seminars in Pediatric Gastrointestinal Nutrition* 4, no. 1 (1993): 11–15.

5. M. Bax, "Nutrition and Disability," *Developmental Medicine and Child Neurology* 35, no. 12 (1993): 1035–1036.

6. E.M. Blyler and B.L. Lucas, "Position of the American Dietetic Association: Nutrition in Comprehensive Program Planning for Persons with Developmental Dis-

abilities," *Journal of the American Dietetic Association* 92, no. 5 (1992): 613–615.

7. M.T. Baer et al., "Providing Early Nutrition Intervention Services: Preparation of Dietitians, Nutritionists, and Other Team Members," *Infants and Young Children* 3, no. 4 (1991): 56–66.

8. J. Gittler and M. Colton, *Alternatives to Hospitalization for Technology Dependent Children: Program Needs* (Iowa City, IA: National Maternal and Child Health Resource Center, University of Iowa, 1987).

9. U.S. Congress, Office of Technology Assessment, *Technology-Dependent Children: Hospital v. Home Care—A Technical Memorandum* (OTA-TM-H-38) (Washington, DC: U.S. Government Printing Office, 1987).

10. Center on Hunger, Poverty and Nutrition Policy, *Statement on the Link Between Nutrition and Cognitive Development in Children,* 2nd ed. (Medford, MA: Tufts University School of Nutrition, 1995), 9–11.

11. Montana Office of Public Instruction, *Serving Students with Special Health Care Needs* (Helena, MT: 1993).

12. J.W. Horsley, "Nutrition Services for Children with Special Needs within the Public School System," *Topics in Clinical Nutrition* 3, no. 3 (1988): 55–60.

13. L.T. Gandy et al., "Serving Children with Special Health Care Needs: Nutrition Services and Employee Training Needs in the School Lunch Program," *Journal of the American Dietetic Association* 91, no. 12 (1991): 1585–1586.

14. K. Yadrick and J. Sneed, *Providing for the Special Food and Nutrition Needs of Children* (University, MS: National Food Service Management Institute, September 1993).

15. Montana Office of Public Instruction, *Serving Students*.

16. Horsley, "Nutrition Services for Children."

17. Gandy et al., "Serving Children with Special Health Care Needs."

18. Yadrick and Sneed, *Providing for the Special Food.*

19. R.P. Reeder et al., "Making a Difference with Special Needs Students," *School Food Service Journal* (1994): 66–68.

20. J.W. Horsley, "Nutrition Issues Facing Children with Special Health Care Needs in Early Intervention Programs and at School," *Nutrition FOCUS for Children with Special Health Care Needs* 9, no. 3 (1993): 1–8.

21. U.S. Department of Agriculture, Food and Consumer Service, *Accommodating Children with Special Dietary Needs in School Nutrition Programs: Guidance for School Food Service Staff* (Alexandria, VA: 1995).

22. Alabama Department of Education, Child Nutrition Programs, *CARE: Special Nutrition for Kids* (Montgomery, AL: 1995).

23. USDA, *Accommodating Children.*

24. Horsley, "*Nutrition Issues.*"

25. Alabama Department of Education, *CARE: Special Nutrition.*

26. Horsley, "Nutrition Issues."

27. Montana Office of Public Instruction, *Serving Students*.

28. Arkansas Department of Education, Special Education Section, *Resource Guide: Developing School Policies on Children with Special Health Care Needs* (Plantation, FL: South Atlantic Regional Resource Center [SARRC], 1996).

29. State of Connecticut Department of Education, *Serving Students with Special Health Care Needs* (Hartford, CT: Publications Office, State of Connecticut Department of Education, 1992).

30. Utah State Office of Education and Mountain Plains Regional Resource Center, *Guidelines for Serving Students with Special Health Care Needs* (Salt Lake City, UT: 1992).

31. V.G. Chauvin, *Students with Special Health Care Needs: A Manual for School Nurses* (Scarborough, ME: National Association of School Nurses, Inc., 1994).

32. American Federation of Teachers, Council for Exceptional Children, National Association of School Nurses, and National Education Association, *Guidelines for the Delineation of Roles and Responsibilities for the Safe Delivery of Specialized Health Care in the Educational Setting* (Joint Task Force for the Management of Children with Special Health Care Needs: 1990).

33. Chauvin, *Students with Special Health Care Needs*.

34. American Federation of Teachers, *Guidelines*.

35. Utah State Office of Education, *Guidelines*.

36. Chauvin, *Students with Special Health Care Needs*.

37. Horsley, "Nutrition Issues."

38. H.H. Cloud, "Role of School Food Service in Providing Nutrition for Children with Special Needs, *Topics in Clinical Nutrition* 9, no. 4 (1994): 47–53.

39. Horsley, "Nutrition Services."

40. Yadrick and Sneed, *Providing for the Special Food.*

41. J.W. Horsley et al., *Nutrition Management of School Age Children with Special Needs: A Resource Manual for School Personnel, Families and Health Professionals*, 2nd ed. (Richmond, VA: Virginia Department of Education and Virginia Department of Health, 1996).

42. N. Wellman et al., *Feeding for the Future: Exceptional Nutrition in the IEP* (Miami, FL: Florida Department of Education, Nutrition Education and Training Program, and Florida International University, 1995).

43. K.A. Cross-McClintic et al., "School-Based Nutrition Services Positively Affect Children with Special Health Care Needs and their Families," *Journal of the American Dietetic Association* 94, no. 11 (1994): 1307–1309.

44. B. Cross et al., "Nutrition Management of Children with Special Needs," *School Food Service Journal* (1992): 57–59.

45. Horsley et al., *Nutrition Management*.

46. Horsley, "Nutrition Issues."

47. Horsley et al., *Nutrition Management*.

48. U.S. Department of Agriculture, Southeast Regional Office, the University of Alabama at Birmingham, *Meeting Their Needs: Training Manual for Child Nutrition Program Personnel Serving Children with Special Needs* (Atlanta, GA: 1995).

49. Cloud, "Role of School Food Service."

50. USDA, *Meeting Their Needs*.

51. U.S. Department of Agriculture, Food and Consumer Service (FCS-295), *Serving It Safe: A Manager's Tool Kit* (Washington, DC: 1996), 47.

52. Alabama Department of Education, *CARE*.

53. Cross et al., "Nutriton Management."

54. M.T. Conklin et al., "Managing Nutrition Services for Children with Special Needs," *NFSMI Insight*, 1, no. 1 (1994): 3–4.

55. USDA, *Accommodating Children.*

56. Conklin et al., "Managing Nutrition."

57. M.T. Conklin and M.F. Nettles, *Costs Associated with Providing School Meals for Children with Special Food and Nutrition Needs* (University, MS: National Food Service Management Institute, 1994).

58. USDA, *Accommodating Children.*

59. Gandy et al., "Serving Children."

60. Yadrick and Sneed, *Providing for Special Food.*

61. Cloud, "Role of School Food Service."

62. Horsley, "Nutrition Issues."

63. L. Lichtenwalter et al., "Providing Nutrition Services to Children with Special Needs in a Community Setting," *Topics in Clinical Nutrition* 8, no. 4 (1993): 75–78.

64. Baer et al., "Providing Early Nutrition."

65. Horsley, "Nutrition Issues."

66. E.R. Allen and J.W. Horsley, "School Nutrition Services for Handicapped and Chronically Ill Children," *Journal of Nutrition Education* 23 (1991): 260C–260D.

67. Conklin et al., "Managing Nutrition."

68. D. Carr et al., *Competencies, Knowledge, and Skills of Effective District School Nutrition Directors/Supervisors* (University, MS: National Food Service Management Institute, 1996), 103.

69. American School Food Service Association, *Keys to Excellence: Standards of Practice for Nutrition Integrity* (Alexandria, VA, 1995), 12.

Nutrition Training and Resource Materials

- Conklin MT, Nettles MF, Martin J. Managing nutrition services for children with special needs. *NFSMI Insight.* 1994; 1:1–6.
- Cross B. *Conference Proceedings: Nutrition Management for Children with Special Needs in Child Nutrition Programs.* University, MS: National Food Service Management Institute; 1993.
- Horsley JW, Allen ER, Daniel PW. *Nutrition Management of School Age Children with Special Needs: A Resource Manual for School Personnel, Families, and Health Professionals.* 2nd ed. Richmond, VA: Virginia Department of Education and Virginia Department of Health; 1996.
- National Food Service Management Institute. *Annotated Bibliography: Nutrition Management for Children with Special Needs in Child Nutrition Programs.* University, MS; 1993.
- Alabama Department of Education, Child Nutrition Programs. *CARE: Special Nutrition for Kids.* Montgomery, AL; 1995.
- Rokusek C, Heinrichs E, eds. *Nutrition and Feeding for Persons with Special Needs.* 2nd ed. Pierre, SD: South Dakota Department of Education and Cultural Affairs, Child and Adult Nutrition Services; 1992.
- U.S. Department of Agriculture, Southeast Regional Office, and the University of Alabama at Birmingham. *Meeting Their Needs: Training Manual for Child Nutrition Program Personnel Serving Children with Special Needs.* Atlanta, GA; 1993.
- Wellman N, Sinofsky J, Crawford L, Frazee C, Rarback S, Murphy A, Parham P. *Feeding for the Future: Exceptional Nutrition in the IEP.* Miami, FL: Florida Department of Education, Nutrition Education and Training Program, and Florida International University; 1995.
- Breault J., Gould, R. *Special Foods for Special Kids.* Topeka, KS: Department of Hotel, Restaurant, Institution Management and Dietetics at Kansas State University, Department of Communications, Kansas State University College of Agriculture, and Kansas State Board of Education, Nutrition Services; 1995.
- Minnesota Department of Children, Families and Learning. Nutrition management for Children with Special Needs. St. Paul, MN: Minnesota Children; 1996.
- Internet:
    American Dietetic Association:
        http://www.eatright.org
    Food and Nutrition Information Service:
        http://www.nal/usda.gov/fnic/
    National Food Service Management Institute:
        http://olemiss.edu/depts/nfsmi/special.html
    The Food Allergy Network
        http://www.foodallergy.org/
    The National Maternal and Child Health Clearinghouse
        http://www.circsol.com/mch/

PART IV

Operations

CHAPTER 13

Procurement

Marlene Gunn

OUTLINE

INTRODUCTION

Purchasing has a greater impact on the quality of food served to children than any other school food and nutrition management function. Effective purchasing practices support the two major goals of the child nutrition programs as outlined in the National School Lunch Act: (1) to protect the health and well-being of the nation's children by serving nutritious meals and (2) to expand the market for nutritious agricultural commodities. Management of the purchasing systems for food, equipment, services, and supplies also has a major impact on the cost effectiveness of the school food and nutrition program. Establishing vendor relationships that ensure service, consistency, and quality is key to achieving effective purchasing.

Today, purchasers for school food and nutrition programs operate in seller-dominated markets. The vendor pool may be dominated by two or three major companies. Small independent companies find it difficult to compete for school food and nutrition program business. Change in procurement practices must occur if food and supply costs are to be controlled and the *Dietary Guidelines for Americans* are to be successfully implemented. If acceptable quality food products are not purchased, there is nothing the food service assistant can do to correct the problem during food preparation. Effective procurement systems will support the highest quality product and service a school district can afford and provide for consistency, as well as price.

In order to manage a school food and nutrition program for excellence in the twenty-first century, there must be a strong linkage among purchasing, nutrition integrity, and financial success. Six principles provide a basis for developing strong purchasing programs that support nutrition and financial goals of child nutrition programs.

1. Food procurement for child nutrition programs occurs in a dynamic environment that influences availability, cost, acceptability, and nutritive value of foods.
2. Food procurement in this dynamic environment requires continual evaluation of program needs, products, and food procurement methods.
3. Food procurement is inextricably linked to the nutrition quality of meals served and implementation of the *Dietary Guidelines for Americans.*
4. Food procurement is integrally related to the financial management of child nutrition programs.
5. Food procurement decisions are based on scientific information, government regulations, cost, product quality, customer demands, and environmental constraints in order to provide nutritious and acceptable meals to America's children.
6. Food procurement for child nutrition programs is performed in an ethical manner by qualified professionals.[1]

Purchasing standards identified in *Keys to Excellence* provide direction for developing purchasing programs to support

- practices that ensure the use of high quality ingredients and prepared products
- ethical procurement practices that provide the best quality products and services for resources available.[2]

Social and economic conditions will force change in school food and nutrition purchasing in the twenty-first century. The purpose of this chapter is to provide information for the school business official and the school food and nutrition director to consider in developing and implementing a procurement system reflective of program goals and societal changes. In most school districts, the school business official and the school food and nutrition director are partners in establishing and implementing procurement systems that meet the needs of all constituents in the school district.

This chapter is not written for the novice purchaser, but rather for individuals who understand the basics of purchasing and want to fine-tune their procurement strategies. The specific objectives of the chapter are as follows:

- Establish a framework for conducting cost-effective school food and nutrition purchasing in a dynamic market.
- Review the legal background and requirements for public purchasing.
- Identify and discuss steps in developing a purchasing system.
- Describe strategies for developing and using critical path planning for cost-effective purchasing.
- Compare the use of food descriptions versus specifications.
- Examine receiving procedures as the final act of effective purchasing.
- Describe how effective procurement systems apply to the purchasing of services and equipment.

LAWS, REGULATIONS, PROCUREMENT CODES, AND ETHICS

The use of the term *public purchasing* indicates that funds being expended were derived from tax collections. Public purchasers' activities are more visible than those purchases made by private firms. Public purchasing and most of the federal and state laws can be summarized by four key phrases:

1. Maintain open and free competition.
2. Maintain comparability of products and price comparisons.
3. Document the decision-making process.
4. Develop a procurement plan that is approved by the governing board.[3]

The federal government, all state governments, and many local governing bodies have laws, regulations, model procurement codes, or other guidance that must be followed when making expenditures of tax dollars. School food authorities participating in the federally assisted school food and nutrition programs must have a working knowledge of legal requirements outlined in the law, regulations, Federal Management Circulars, and policy.[4] Many of these laws or regulations discuss ethical behavior when conducting business. Practices that result in personal gain or even the appearance of personal gain are considered unethical. The reputation of the school food and nutrition program and the individual can be done irreparable harm by unethical conduct.

School food and nutrition purchasers are not expected to be experts in food law but should know the laws in general, their purpose, and where to find additional information. Purchasing for the child nutrition programs is conducted in a regulatory environment. As a minimum the food purchaser needs to be familiar with the following legal documents.[5]

Federal Regulatory Environment

Federal Management Circular A 102 attachment 0 and 7 C.F.R. 210 and 3016 are related to purchasing under a federal grant and apply to purchases with child nutrition programs funds.

The Food, Drug and Cosmetic Act controls the labeling of food products. The implementing regulations contain the federal standards of identity for food. The 1990 amendment (Nutrition Labeling and Education Act) has a significant impact on food labels.

The Agricultural Marketing Act created the standards for processed fruits and vegetables. The U.S. Department of Agriculture (USDA) operates a voluntary grading service and maintains the quality grade standards for processed fruits and vegetables.

The Meat Inspection Act and the Poultry Products Inspection Act provided for the inspection program that ensures that meat products sold in interstate commerce are wholesome. All meat crossing state lines is labeled with an inspection mark. It also contains the number of the establishment where the product was manufactured.

The Tariff Act of 1930 covers labeling of imported foods. This act is administered by the U.S. Customs Service.

The Sherman, Clayton, Robinson-Patman, and Federal Trade Commission Acts are related to antitrust. The purpose of these acts is to maintain open and free competition in the marketplace.

The Perishable Agricultural Commodities Act provides for the voluntary inspection and regulation of fresh fruits and vegetables.

PLANNING

Purchasing is often forgotten in the daily crisis of managing a food service operation until it, too, is a crisis. At the point that purchasing becomes a crisis it is too late to correct the problem. In most operations it is necessary to deal with the symptom and therefore the crisis continues to occur. Adequate planning allows the school food and nutrition professional to deal with the problem and develop systems that avoid the daily crisis. Written procedures are needed for the purchasing process to maintain continuity and effective planning.

In the manufacturing industry, getting the right product to the right place at the right time is called critical path planning. Critical path planning techniques can be applied to school food and nutrition programs. The objective of purchasing for these programs is to get an acceptable product to the right place (site or warehouse) at the right time. Annually develop a critical path plan for all requests for prices (milk, bread, small equipment, fresh produce, etc.). A critical path plan for a request for pricing for milk and milk products is presented in Table 13–1.

The date indicated as "week of" means the task is completed during that week. Staff members assigned to complete a task can place it on their personal calendar. Advance scheduling of a task avoids delaying until there is not adequate time to do a quality job.

Table 13–1 Critical Path Plan for Milk and Milk Products

Task	Date	Information Used To Develop Plans
Develop product list	Week of March 19	School starts August 14
Estimate quantities	Week of March 19	School board approval required
Conduct prebid conference	April 16	School board meets second Tuesday of each month
Revise document and product list	Week of April 24	Board agenda items due two weeks prior to meeting date
Issue price requests	May 23	
Open bids or prices	June 13	
Complete bid evaluation	June 27	
Approval if necessary	July 11	
Notify vendors of bid award	July 18	
First delivery	August 13	

Source: Reprinted with permission from M. Gunn, *First Choice, A Purchasing Systems Manual for School Food Service*, Vol. 4, p. 48, © 1995, National Food Service Management Institute.

The critical path for dry/frozen/refrigerated foods, paper products, kitchen supplies, and miscellaneous cleaning supplies will be the most difficult to plan. The number of products and the number of tasks to complete in the critical path is greater than for any other requests for pricing. Table 13–2 presents a sample critical path for this request for pricing.

A critical path is planned by inserting the first delivery date and working backward. Another aspect of planning for the purchasing task involves providing site managers, order processors, and vendors with clear instructions related to dates for order placement. An order placement calendar developed for each school year is an effective communication tool. Decisions on whether orders will be placed and deliveries received during weeks when there is a school holiday can be reflected on the calendar. Having sites place back-to-school orders before they leave for the summer is also a good idea. The order placement calendar reflects all of these decisions.

PURCHASING SYSTEM

The purchasing cycle begins with menu planning and ends with food preparation. An effective purchasing system must have policies or procedures that provide structure and control for many activities. The purchasing system consists of

- Research and define product movement policies and procedures.
- Develop the product list and procedures for adding or deleting products.
- Estimate quantities of each product to be purchased.
- Develop food descriptions that define the product characteristics necessary to meet menu and budget requirements. Research the quality indicators for each product.
- Screen brands for approval.
- Define the methods to apply when obtaining prices.
- Receive products.

Table 13–2 Critical Path for Dry/Frozen/Refrigerated Foods, Paper, and Kitchen Supplies

Task	Time Lapse Before Next Step	Date To Be Completed
Develop product list	One month	
Estimate quantities	Six weeks	
Mail draft of a product list to potential vendors	Three weeks	
Conduct first prebid conference	Three months	
Screen products and brands for approval	One week	
Mail draft of a product list to potential vendors	Three weeks	
Conduct final prebid conference	Two weeks	
Revise instructions and product list	Two days	
Issue request for pricing	Three weeks	
Open bids or price quotes	Two weeks	
Evaluate vendor offers	Two weeks	
Notify vendors of successful offer	Three weeks	
First delivery		

Source: Reprinted with permission from M. Gunn, *First Choice, A Purchasing Systems Manual for School Food Service*, Vol. 4, p. 48, © 1995, National Food Service Management Institute.

Product Movement and Product Movement Policy

Product movement procedures are a key element of a cost-effective purchasing system. Product movement is influenced by decisions related to warehouse versus site delivery, order placement, and size of inventory. The school food and nutrition program decision maker has two options to consider in determining a product movement policy: (1) Will the district operate or lease a warehouse or (2) will the district have products delivered direct to the meal preparation site? In many school districts a warehouse is in operation. The food purchaser will find it helpful to complete a warehouse cost study to determine the value of this operation. A form for conducting a warehouse cost study is presented as Appendix 13–A at the end of this chapter. Vendors will often encourage a school district to operate a warehouse. Vendors can reduce the number of stops their trucks must make and decrease their cost of doing business. The costs of products are seldom reduced enough to cover the school district cost of warehouse operations. Food service vendors are specialists in warehouse operations and devote 100 percent of their time to this task. School districts specialize in educating children and can only devote a small percentage of their time to warehouse operations.

Just-in-time (JIT) product movement is the system of purchasing of food as close to preparation time as possible. The quality of service provided by the distribution community makes it possible for most locations to receive a weekly delivery of groceries and supplies. The advantages of JIT delivery are reduced inventory, cost, and paperwork. If direct-to-site delivery (JIT) is the selected product movement method, site storage capacity evaluation is essential. Once a decision is made about storage capacity at the sites, the frequency of site deliveries must be decided. The larger the size of the order delivered the lower the price. Once the frequency of delivery is established, a dollar value of inventory for each site can be established. The smaller the site inventories the more food and supply costs will be controlled. An adequate inventory level is one that covers the meals to be served between deliveries plus two days' safety stock. Milk/milk products, bread/bread products, ice cream, and fresh produce are generally delivered direct to the site. In some school districts a portion of the dry/frozen/refrigerated foods and kitchen supplies are delivered direct to the site and the remainder is delivered from a school district warehouse. When this situation exists the school district is risking a dilution of both site and warehouse deliveries to a point that neither the school district warehouse nor the vendor has a cost-effective delivery size. A split delivery system often develops as the school district makes an effort to deal with the flow of USDA–donated foods.

Often site storage capacity is inadequate to deal with the surges in delivery of donated foods. The surges in volume of donated foods can be mitigated by use of the services of a commercial distributor. If the state agency food distribution delivery system uses a commercial distributor, the payment of excess time storage fees is often less than the cost of school district warehouse operation. If donated foods are delivered from a state-operated warehouse to the school district, consider use of a commercial distributor for receipt and delivery to sites. The donated foods can be delivered to the commercial distributor by the state agency. The commercial distributor then delivers the donated foods to the site with the school district–purchased foods. If the school district volume is not adequate to use direct diversion (delivery in truckloads direct to a school distict) or the state does not pay for storage from state funds, this suggestion will result in the payment of two fees. The first fee is paid to the state and the second fee is paid to the commercial distributor. The two fees are normally less than the cost of school district warehouse operation. Joining or forming a purchasing cooperative of several school districts can result in enough volume of donated foods to use the direct-diversion option.

Product movement, a key element in a cost-effective procurement program, is facilitated when the school district has a written product movement policy. Elements of such a policy are as follows[6]:

- A product movement method defined: warehouse, or JIT.
- Products classified by product movement type.
- Par stocks are identified for repeated-use items.
- Standing orders are placed for many par stock items.
- Twice-a-year order dates are placed for low-volume items.
- Lead times are given that avoid orders in transition.
- There is effective use of technology (computers, communication) to improve product movement.
- Order calendars are used that convey the delivery plan.

Developing the Product List

Historical records are the best source of information for use in developing the product list. Accounting software normally prints reports of items purchased. If reports are not available from the accounting software, the vendors who had the contract in the previous time period may assist with obtaining this historical information. The majority of vendors can produce a usage report. The usage report provides a list of items and the quantity purchased. The software used by some vendors requires advance notice of the need for this information. Some vendor software is programmed to delete this information at the end of a business period (four or five weeks) if it has not been told to archive the information. If no other sources provide the historical information, it will be necessary to develop a list from the invoices for a given period of time. Prior to issu-

ing each request for prices, the staff responsible for menu planning and purchasing can review the list and make necessary modifications.

A procedure for changes in the product list is necessary for control of quality and cost. Adequate market research allows management to make informed decisions about changes in the menu. Development of food descriptions that control quality requires that staff have sufficient lead time to study the quality indicators before obtaining pricing for new items.

The life cycle phase when new products will be considered for purchase is an important part of product list procedures.

All products have four phases in their life cycle. The four phases are presented below.

1. Launch—product cost is high and there is no competition.
2. Growth—product cost begins to decrease and sales growth is rapid.
3. Maturity—product cost continues to decrease as competition increases.
4. Final—the product becomes established and cost and competition stabilizes or it is withdrawn from the market.

The lowest price will be paid for products if they are purchased during the maturity phase. The menu planner's search for new products to relieve the boredom of customers who eat in the same place each day often results in purchasing these products during the high-cost launch phase. A new product will be just as new to students whether purchased in the first year or the third year after introduction. On the other hand, if every school food and nutrition purchaser waited until maturity to purchase, manufacturers would have no motivation to develop new products for school food and nutrition programs. School districts need to develop procedures that are consistent with their program goals and cash resources.

Estimating Quantities

Reliable information on the quantity of each item to be purchased is essential to obtaining a reasonable price. Historical information modified by management decisions is the most reliable method of estimating quantities. All of the methods discussed under product lists also provide quantity estimates and can be used to obtain the historical information.

Several variables affect quantity estimates. The variables are the school district calendar, fluctuations in the number of meals served, and the delivery schedule for donated foods. The effective period of pricing (monthly, quarterly, semiannually, or annually) determines the impact of the variables. The length of the contract (effective period for pricing) determines the difficulty of estimating quantities. Annual quantities are affected only by the number of meals served. The number of days in a school year is normally stable. Management must balance the potential for the higher cost of long-term contracts against the difficulty of estimating quantities for short periods of time. The potential for higher cost can be decreased by a pricing system that allows for escalation based on the food market.

Quantities are more difficult to estimate for short periods of time. Requests for pricing are normally based on calendar months. The number of days meals will be served in a calendar month varies from year to year, based on the school calendar. The historical information will have to be modified to reflect the difference in the number of serving days in a calendar month. The amounts and types of donated foods received are somewhat stable from year to year. The delivery period for donated foods is not predictable and will affect the quantities used for short periods of time (monthly, quarterly, semiannually). Although improvements continue to be made in the delivery schedule for donated foods, the complexity of the delivery system at the federal, state, and local levels creates many uncontrollable variables. The delivery system (commercial distributors, school district warehouse, or site delivery) used by the school district determines how the donated foods' delivery will affect the quantity estimates. The donated foods represent a small percentage of the total food purchases. There-

fore, they do not cause major disruption in the estimates of total food needs. Quantities that are accurate at plus or minus 10 percent are generally considered acceptable.

Good communication between school district and vendor staff will solve most quantity-estimating errors. A knowledge of the number of inventory turns (frequency) the vendor requires for all products will improve communication. Items that the vendor sells to its general customer mix are managed differently from those stocked exclusively for the school district. Failure to provide accurate quantities or to honor the quantities presented to vendors can have a long-range detrimental impact on pricing.

Product Knowledge and Purchase Description

Developing and maintaining knowledge of products requires commitment. It is important to maintain a current product reference library. The reference list at the end of this chapter contains excellent suggestions for printed materials. The printed reference library is supplemented by the many resources available on the Internet.

Products used to produce and serve school food and nutrition menus are constantly changing. The food description is a significant factor in determining the quality of food served to children. The term *product or food description*

Purchasing Reference Library

Standards and Labeling Policy Book, USDA, 1995. Superintendent of Documents.

Code of Federal Regulations, Title 9, Part 200 to the end, *Animal and Animal Products, 1995.* Superintendent of Documents.

The Packer 1995 Produce Availability and Merchandising Guide, 1995. Available from The Packer.

Quantity Food Purchasing, 4th ed., Kotschevar and Donnelly

Frozen Food Book of Knowledge, 1995: National Frozen Food Association

The Almanac of the Canning and Freezing Industry. 1995. Available from Edward F. Judges Co.

Choice Plus—A Food and Ingredient Manual. 1996. USSDA.

M.C. Spears, *Foodservice Procurement: Purchasing for Profit*

Adapted from *First Choice: A Purchasing System Manual for School Food Service.*[7]

means a list or description of quality indicators measurable at the receiving site or through random testing of samples. A specification is a statement that contains a detailed description or enumerates particulars of a product. Various authors list different elements for a food specification. The list below presents the opinion of several authors on characteristics of a specification.

- Name of product
- Federal grade
- Size information for container and product
- Unit on which price will be based (bid units)
- Quality indicators: product type dictates the quality indicators (e.g., type, style, pack, syrup density, specific gravity, age, exact cutting instructions, weight range, composition, condition upon receipt of product, fat content, cut of meat used, market class, variety, degree of ripeness or maturity, geographical origin, temperature during delivery and upon receipt, sugar ratio, milk fat content, milk solids and bacteria count, brand names, trim or yield, preservation or processing method, trade association standards, chemical standards)
- Packaging procedures and type of package
- Test or inspection procedures

The question is, how is the school food and nutrition purchaser to know all those details on more than 300 items? Some of the best specifications are written by food technologists employed by the Agricultural Marketing Service (AMS) of USDA. All school food and nutrition programs participating in the USDA–donated foods program can obtain copies of these specifications from their state food distribution agency. Presented in Exhibits 13–1 and 13–2 are two examples.

As these examples indicate, there are many quality factors. Many of these factors can be measured only by sophisticated inspection methods. The monitoring of many of these quality indicators requires the presence of an inspector on the processing line and the raw ingredient receiving dock. For many decades school food and nutrition program staff have used the term *specification* to mean a description of quality indicators that are measurable in a site receiving area or through random testing of samples. The term *food description* best describes the words used in school food and nutrition program purchasing to communicate with vendors. Limit food descriptions to those quality indicators measurable during the screening process. The use of food descriptions in combination with approved brands and code numbers allows school food and nutrition program staff to achieve comparability.

Some food products have a greater impact on the quality of food served to our customers than others. A general rule is *80 percent of the dollars are spent on 20 percent of the products.* When allocating time resources to the development of food descriptions, focus on those products that fall in this high-dollar category. Adequately researched descriptions for this category of food items will have the greatest impact on both the cost and nutrition integrity of the meals served. School districts do not have unlimited time for development of food descriptions, which is a time-consuming task. Plan to control the integrity of food descriptions once developed. Unless adequate resources are assigned to purchasing, the devel-

Exhibit 13–1 Specifications for Mixed Vegetables

Name of Product: Mixed Vegetables, Frozen
Pack Size: 30-pound bulk, or 12/2½-pound or 6/5-pound
Grade: Grade B or better
A. Salient Characteristics
1. The frozen mixed vegetables shall have been produced in the United States, shall have been packed from vegetables from the current crop year or later in accordance with good commercial practice, and shall meet the following additional requirements:
   a. The frozen mixed vegetables shall meet the requirements of U.S. Grade B or better, as defined in United States Standards for Grades of frozen mixed vegetables, currently effective. The product shall consist of the following mix:
      (1) Not more than 40 percent by weight of carrots (diced style ⅜- to ½-inch cubes);
      (2) Not more than 40 percent by weight of corn (sweet golden or yellow corn kernel); and
      (3) Not more than 40 percent by weight of green peas (early or sweet style).
   b. For mixed vegetables packed in 2½-pound containers, the average net weight shall be not less than 2½ pounds and no individual container shall be less than 2 pounds 6.7 ounces. For 5-pound containers the average net weight shall not be less than 5 pounds and no individual container shall be less than 4 pounds 13.9 ounces. For 30-pound containers the average net weight shall be not less than 30 pounds and no individual container shall be less than 29 pounds, 5 ounces.

B. Container/ Packaging
1. Frozen product shall be packed in primary containers of food grade quality in compliance with the Food Additives Regulations of the Federal Food and Drug Administration. The containers shall be completely sealed (tack sealing acceptable). Thirty-pound containers shall be polyethylene type. However, these containers closed with a tying device or folded in a commercially acceptable manner shall be considered completely sealed. Kraft paper containers without polyethylene liners are not acceptable.
2. Shipping cases shall be packed with twelve 2_-pound , six 5-pound, or one 30-pound bulk container each as may be applicable. The construction and sealing of shipping cases shall be adequate to withstand normal refrigerated shipping and cold storage and shall meet one of the following requirements: (1) corrugated fiberboard construction, rated at a minimum of 250 pounds per square inch bursting strength, or (2) shipping cases for product packed in the paperboard containers shall be of corrugated fiberboard construction, rated at a minimum of 200 pounds per square inch bursting strength, (3) shipping container should be marked with name and address of packer, the month and year packed, and the last five digits of the contract number.

Source: Reprinted from U.S. Department of Agriculture, Food and Nutrition Service, *FNS Instruction 716-1, Specifications for Donated Foods,* 1992, U.S. Government Printing Office.

---

opment of error-free food descriptions is an impossible goal.

For the purpose of writing product descriptions, foods may be grouped as one ingredient, one ingredient plus seasonings, and multiple-ingredient products. A large majority of the items purchased can be classified as a one-ingredient product. Examples of these products are sugar, flour, salt, fresh produce, and milk. The food descriptions for these items consist of the name of the product, the intended use of the product, any pack size requirements, and any special characteristics. Examples of special characteristics are the requirements for the addition of iodine to salt, or the fat content of milk. The variation in quality among the various brands of these products is limited and has an insignificant impact on the

Exhibit 13–2 Specifications for Chicken Patties

Item: Chicken patties, nugget-shaped, breaded, frozen
Pack size available: 40-pound carton (about 852 nugget-shaped patties or 142 two-ounce servings)
Grade: Made from ready-to-cook fowl of U.S. Procurement Grade II or better

A. Salient Characteristics

1. The meat and skin which will be used to make the nugget-shaped patties shall be from ready-to-cook fowl, raised in the United States, of U.S. Procurement Grade II (7 CFR Part 70) or better, of not more than 5 pounds. The nugget-shaped patties shall not be processed earlier than 30 calendar days prior to the date of contract.

2. Ready-to-cook chickens, meat, and skin shall be free of rancidity and foreign or off-odors, and show no evidence of mishandling or deterioration. They shall have a bright and desirable color and show no evidence of freezer burn or dehydration, thawing, or refreezing. The deboned chicken, meat, and skin shall be free of excessive weepage or moisture (liquid or frozen form). The frozen ready-to-cook chickens, meat, and skin shall have been adequately packaged to safely protect the product during storage. These products shall have been identified in a manner so the quality and the time in storage can be determined.

3. The finished nugget-shaped patties shall be in good condition at time of shipment. At time of shipment and during transportation, frozen nugget-shaped patties must be held at an environmental temperature of not higher than 0° F (-18 degrees C), except that during loading the nugget-shaped patties may not exceed 10° F (-12° C). Frozen nugget-shaped patties showing any evidence of defrosting, refreezing, or freezer deterioration may be rejected.

4. The temperature of the meat and skin which will be used to make the nugget-shaped patties must not exceed 55° F (13° C) at any time during blending, grinding, and between these processing steps up to the cooking operation. Meat and skin exceeding this temperature will be rejected. Carbon dioxide may be used for cooling and controlling temperatures.

5. Formulation of raw chicken portion
   a. The following proportions of raw fowl meat, raw fowl skin, and other ingredients shall be used in preparing the chicken portion of the nugget-shaped patties.

White meat (minimum)	32.6 %
Dark meat (maximum)	34.6 %
Mechanically deboned meat (maximum)	16.0 %
Skin (maximum)	7.0 %
Water (maximum)	8.0 %
Isolate soy protein (maximum)	1.0 %
Salt (maximum)	0.5 %
Sodium phosphates (maximum)	<u>0.3 %</u>
	100 %

   (1) Sodium phosphates are limited to those listed in 9 CFR Part 381.
   (2) White meat may replace dark meat. Hand-deboned white meat or dark meat may be substituted for mechanically deboned meat or skin.
   (3) These percentages are for formulating the raw chicken portion of the nugget-shaped patties only. The ingredient statement on the label must include all ingredients used in the finished nugget-shaped patties, including the batter and breading.
   b. Fowl meat—Tendons, bones, cartilages, large blood vessels, bruises, blood clots, and discoloration shall be removed. Giblets shall not be used and no cooked poultry shall be used except a maximum of 2 percent of the batch may be reworked product, if used by the next production shift (no later than 72 hours).

continues

Exhibit 13–2 continued

> c. Mechanically deboned fowl meat—Kidneys and necks cannot be used. Thigh and drumstick bones cannot be used. (This applies to the form of intact muscle portions left by other deboning techniques)
>
> d. Fowl skin—Skin must be separated from the fowl meat before formulating and grinding. Skin that is bruised or which contains pinfeathers, feather particles, or hair must be excluded.
>
> e. Fowl fat—Fat in the fowl meat and skin may be used. Abdominal fat from heavy flow (4½ pounds or more with necks and giblets) must be excluded.
>
> 6. Preparation for blending. Meat and skin shall be prepared for blending by grinding as outlined in the current announcement. Skin must be initially ground separately from the meat using a plate with holes ⅛ inch (3.18 mm) in diameter.
>
> 7. Blending
>
>   a. Sodium phosphates and salt must be mixed with the water and added as solution to the other ingredients in the formula during blending. The sodium phosphates must be thoroughly mixed with the water prior to the addition of the salt to the solution.
>
>   b. Ground meat, mechanically deboned meat, ground skin, and isolated soy protein must be mechanically blended uniformly with the solution of sodium phosphates and salt.
>
> 8. Forming. The ground and blended formulated raw mixture shall be mechanically formed into institutionally acceptable nugget-shaped patties of uniform size. The nugget-shaped patties shall be ⅜ inch (9.5 mm) to ⁷⁄₁₆ inch (11.1 mm) in thickness.
>
> 9. Batter/Breading
>
>   a. Following forming, the raw nugget-shaped patties shall be batter/breaded in a manner that will produce a uniformly covered finished product.
>
>   b. The amount of batter/breading shall not exceed 22 percent of the weight of the raw batter/breaded nugget shaped patties prior to pre-browning or frying.
>
>   c. The batter/breading will be a commercial flour-based product which may include spices, seasonings, and other ingredients as needed to produce the desired texture, flavor, and color. The flour will be enriched. Ingredients will include iodized salt added at a level not to exceed 9% by weight of the dry batter and exceed 3% by weight of the dry batter and breading combined. Food additives and ingredients shall be used in accordance with 9 CFR Part 381.
>
> *Source:* Reprinted from U.S. Department of Agriculture, Food and Nutrition Service, *FNS Instruction 716–1, Specifications for Donated Foods,* 1992, U.S. Government Printing Office.

quality or nutritional content of meals. The manufacturing processes for these items are stable and therefore the descriptions seldom change.

An indication on request for pricing that the vendor may choose the brand to bid is a cost-effective decision. Vendors can use their knowledge of manufacturers/processors to offer the brand that provides the best price. Many words could be used to allow vendor choice. The words most commonly used are *distributor's choice.* Approximately 50 percent of the items

on a typical school district's request for pricing will be classified as a one-ingredient product, and the brand approval type will be distributor's choice. Table 13–3 shows examples of the way a one-ingredient food might look on a request for pricing.

Another group of products contains one ingredient plus seasonings, such as salt, sugar, or fruit juice. The canned and frozen fruits and vegetables fall in this category. As an example, green beans contain green beans and salt. The majority of products in this category have a

Table 13–3   One-Ingredient Format Example

Item Number	Description	Brands Approved	Bid Unit	Quantity	Unit Price	Extended Price
0001	Salt: For table use; iodized; maximum 25 lb per bag How packed? Brand quoted?	Distributor's choice	10 lb			
0002	Apples, fresh: to be packed to U.S. or Washington State Fancy grade standard; Red Delicious 100 count	Distributor's choice	Box			

standard of identity and grade standard developed by the federal government in cooperation with manufacturers/processors. The standard of identity defines what ingredients are allowed if a food is labeled by a specific name. The Food and Drug Administration (FDA) develops the standards of identity for all foods except meat. The standards of identity for meat are developed by the USDA. The standards of identity can be found in the *Code of Federal Regulations (CFR)*.

The grade standards define the quality characteristics of a food. The grade standards for all foods are developed by the USDA and can also be found in the *Code of Federal Regulations*. The grade standards are also available on the Internet, and copies can be obtained on computer disk from the Agriculture Marketing Service (AMS) at USDA. Commercial item descriptions (CIDS) have been written by the food quality assurance staff, AMS, USDA. CIDS are developed for products for which a standard of identity or grade standard does not exist. The CIDS are available on the Internet, in printed form, and on computer disk. The descriptions for these products would include the name of the product, the form (slices, dices, halves), the grade standard, and the pack requirements. Products in this category that do not have a grade standard or standard of identity will require more detailed descriptions and specific brand approvals. Examples are the frozen vegetable blends. Each manufacturer/processor of a frozen vegetable blend such as

an Oriental vegetable blend will include different vegetables and a differing percentage of each vegetable.

Approximately 15 vendor buying groups have developed labels that are used exclusively by their members to market and sell many food products. These private labels have been used extensively for canned and frozen fruits and vegetables. The products packed under these private labels are packed to the U.S. grade standards but are not actually graded by federal inspectors. These buying groups invest many resources in maintaining the quality of the product packed under their label. School districts can depend on the integrity of the private label to control the quality of canned and frozen fruits and vegetables. Tables 13–4 and 13–5 present the private label and the grade standard reference.

The private label groups use a specific color or distinctive logo for each of the quality levels. Request a copy of the color designations or logos for each of the quality levels from all potential vendors. It may be necessary to approve brands from manufacturers who do not pack their product under a private label. The term used to describe this type of brand approval is often *private label plus*. Approval of a label other than those from the private label groups is verified through a grade report. The processed products branch of the Agricultural Marketing Service at the USDA will provide an unofficial grade report of a sample product for a very reasonable fee. Approximately 20

Table 13–4   Private Labels and U.S. Grade Standard Reference for Fruits

Grade Standard	Private Label
U.S. Grade A or U.S. Fancy	First quality private label
U.S. Grade B or U.S. Choice*	Second quality private label
U.S. Grade C or Standard	Third quality private label

*The majority of private label groups pack "choice" grade of peaches, pears, and fruit cocktail under the first quality label.

Source: Reprinted from U.S. Department of Agriculture, Food and Consumer Service, *Choice Plus, A Reference Guide for Food and Ingredients*, Program Aid FCS-297, p. 17, 1995, U.S. Government Printing Office.

percent of the items on a school district request for pricing can be approved as private label. Table 13–6 provides examples of how this type of brand approval would appear on a request for pricing.

The third group of foods is the most complex to manage. The term often used to describe this highly processed group of foods is *multiple ingredients*. The meat/meat alternate and bread/bread alternate components of the meal are often this type of item. The food descriptions for this group are difficult to develop and maintain. Determining the equality of the brands available is time consuming and involves several steps. Steps in developing descriptions for multiple-ingredient foods are as follows.

- Determine whether standards of identity exist for this food product.
- Obtain copies of Standards of Identity for the food product and become familiar with content.
- Obtain copies of labels for this product from all potential manufacturers.

- Compare labels to the Standard of Identity in order to develop an understanding of the terminology.
- Review the ingredient legend on the labels and obtain definitions for the major ingredients.
- Write a draft of the product description.
- Request a review of the description from such persons as a food technologist associated with one of the manufacturers or a peer.
- Make revisions as needed and develop the working description.

Brand Approval Process

Two options for brand approval are available. The working description can be issued with no reference to brands, or a proprietary description can be issued with all acceptable brands listed. A common practice in purchasing is to list one brand as a point of reference, followed by the words *or equal.* This practice can lead to higher cost of food products, for it

Table 13–5   Private Labels and U.S. Grade Standard Reference for Vegetables

Grade Standard	Private Label
U.S. Grade A or U.S. Fancy	First quality private label
U.S. Grade B or U.S. Extra Standard	Second quality private label
U.S. Grade C or U.S. Standard	Third quality private label

Source: Reprinted from U.S. Department of Agriculture, Food and Consumer Service, *Choice Plus, A Reference Guide for Food and Ingredients,* Program Aid FCS-297, p. 17, 1995, U.S. Government Printing Office.

Table 13–6 One-Ingredient Plus Seasonings' Format Example

Item Number	Description	Brands Approved	Bid Unit	Quantity	Unit Price	Extended Price
0001	Peaches, canned: slices; to be packed to U.S. Grade B Standard (first quality label); clingstone; extra light syrup; 6/10	Private label	Case			
0002	Broccoli, frozen: cut; to be packed to U.S. Grade A Standard; 12/2$^1/_2$ lb only.	Private label plus ABC brand	Case			
0003	Vegetable blend, frozen: mixture to contain cut broccoli, cauliflower florets, crinkle cut carrots; 12/2 lb only	ABC brand, PQR brand, XYZ brand	Case			

signals to the vendor a brand preference. Brand preferences result in higher cost for the majority of food products. Equal quality is available from a wide range of manufacturers. Most school districts purchase what is available in the marketplace. The volume of an item purchased by a school district is seldom large enough for a manufacturer to custom-produce products. The amount of "off invoice" (sheltered income) that the distributor receives from manufacturers often determines the brands that are available for purchase. The school district must maintain a current knowledge of product characteristics and of what is available in the marketplace.

There is a direct relationship between the number of brands approved and the price paid for products. The greater the number of brands approved the greater the competition. Updating the brands approved each time a request for pricing is issued also has a positive impact on the competition. If the option of using a working description with no brand is used, it will be necessary to determine the equality of brands and compliance with descriptions for all brands offered. This determination will have to occur in a short period of time.

Normally the time between viewing prices offered and making an award recommendation is limited to two or three weeks. This time limit is imposed to limit the length of time a vendor has to hold prices firm. The longer prices must be held firm the greater the risk to the vendor, and therefore higher prices will result. If a proprietary description with all brands listed is the option chosen, then the school district staff knowledge will be expanded by the knowledge of a food technologist at the manufacturer. Open and free competition is increased when vendors are encouraged to call attention to inequalities between brands.

When using proprietary descriptions with approved brands, carefully planned and executed processes are used to ensure that all vendors have an opportunity to present their brands. The steps in the process are presented below.

Step 1—Hold information-gathering meeting with all potential vendors.

Step 2—Screen all brands suggested for approval.

Step 3—Notify vendors of the results of screening. Allow vendors whose brands were not approved to submit another product. The district should develop a policy on the number of times a screening may be repeated.

Step 4—Issue a final draft of the product list with all approved brands.

Step 5—Conduct a final prebid conference with all potential vendors. Encourage any discrepancies in the equality of brands approved to be brought forward for discussion.

Screening Brands for Approval

A three-part screen of brands will reduce the amount of time devoted to this task. The three parts are a paper screen, an appearance screen, and a student acceptance screen. (See Appendix 13–B for the sample protocol.) The paper screen is composed of a comparison of the label information, and nutritional information. Table 13–7 presents a brand comparison based on the label and the nutritional information. This paper screen is cost effective for the school district and the vendor. When the brands are compared with the working description, any brands that do not meet requirements will be eliminated before testing. The paper screen will save staff time and manufacturers the cost of samples.

The appearance screen evaluates the visual characteristics of a product. As an example, the diameter of sandwich meat is compared with the size of the bread the product will be served on. The type of packaging and the appropriateness for the school district storage conditions represent another visual evaluation. The preparation instructions provided by the manufacturer are checked. A determination of whether the school sites have appropriate equipment for preparing the product is made. Table 13–8 lists the criteria for evaluation of preparation instructions.[8]

The student acceptance screen is the final part of the brand screening process. Products screened for acceptability will endure the test of time. Vendors will encourage the practice of

rating products as number one, two, or three because it can be used as a marketing tool. This practice can be very costly for a school food and nutrition program. Any brand that is acceptable and comparable is approved. General guidelines for student taste screens are as follows.

- Testing is more reliable if a special group of students is not selected. (Acceptability research indicates that many products will receive acceptable ratings because the students are "special.") Serve products as a part of a regular meal service. Only those students who choose the product to be screened complete a rating scale.
- Only one brand of a product is tested at a single meal service.
- When testing different brands of a product always serve the same accompanying items. A brand served with a favorite item will always rate higher than a brand served with a less popular accompaniment.
- The brand is prepared according to manufacturer's directions and in the equipment available at the majority of sites.
- Sales representatives of the brand are not present at the testing. The student's opinion of the product, not the personality of the sales representative, is what is being sought.

To maintain open and free competition, it is necessary to notify a vendor if its brand is not rated acceptable. Most manufacturers can offer many products that meet the quality indicators of the description. Always remember that the more brands approved the lower the price paid for the product.

Choosing the Process for Obtaining Prices

The environment in which the distribution of food occurs is constantly changing. Studying the marketplace environment is the most important part of choosing a method for obtaining prices. School food and nutrition pro-

Table 13–7 Brand Comparison from Label and Nutritional Data Sheets

Working description: chicken nuggets, frozen: breaded; ready to serve after reheating; chicken breast with rib meat to be first ingredient; to be CN labeled to provide 2 oz meat/meat alternate (or a school district might specify grams of protein); dried whole egg solids to be no higher than third position in the meat block; No VPP; maximum 15 grams fat.

Characteristics	Brand A	Brand B	Brand C	Brand D
Mfg. code #	3535	49110	2377	3245
Est. #	P9141	P7091A	P1325	P184
CN Label #	018584	014048	021893	029095
Pack	10#/320 pieces	10.13#/324 pieces	10.31#/250 pieces	10#
Serving size	6 = 2 oz meat/ meat alternate or 12 grams of protein	6 = 2 oz. meat/ meat alternate or 13.2 grams of protein	5 = 2 oz Meat/ meat alternate or 14 grams of protein	4 = 2 oz meat/ meat alternate or 16.3 grams of protein
1st ingredient	Boneless chicken breast w/rib meat	Chicken breast w/rib meat	Chicken breast w/rib meat	Chicken breast w/rib meat
2nd ingredient	Water	Water	Water	Water
3rd ingredient	Dried whole egg	Dried whole egg	Dried whole egg	Vegetable protein product (isolated soy)
4th ingredient	Sodium phosphate	Salt	Seasoning	Dried whole egg
5th ingredient	Salt	Sodium phosphate	Sodium phosphate	Salt
Total calories	210	261	230	230
Total fat	15 grams	17.4 grams	15 grams	12.5 grams
Saturated fat	3 grams		3 grams	
Carbohydrate	7 grams	13.5 grams	10 grams	10.4 grams
Protein	12 grams	13.2 grams	14 grams	16.3 grams
Sodium	500 mg	630 mg	360 mg	596 mg
Nutrient data source	Analytical data rounded	Not known	Not known	Not known

Note: information on additional nutrients and copies of the label attached.

Source: Reprinted with permission from M. Gunn, *First Choice, A Purchasing Systems Manual for School Food Service,* pp. 88–90, © 1995, National Food Service Management Institute.

---

grams represent only a small percentage of the total market to which a distributor can sell. Understanding how the more dominant market shares conduct business is valuable information when making a decision about pricing structure.

It is necessary to make two decisions about the system for obtaining prices: (1) Will the distributors be given a guarantee of the number of cases per delivery? (2) What pricing mechanism (firm price or escalating) will be used? In the first decision, will the distributor be given a guarantee of the number of cases to be delivered per delivery drop? Information on the distributor cost for each delivery is proprietary and therefore not generally available. In 1995 the number frequently quoted and generally accepted is a fixed cost of $60.00 and a vari-

Table 13–8 Evaluation of Preparation Instructions

Product	Ham/Buffet Style	Pizza, Frozen	Oven-Baked French Fried Potatoes
Manufacturer/brand	Oak USA	Spruce	Aspen
Code number	12030	78952	32478
Type of storage	Refrigerated		Frozen
Length of storage			
Thawing		Do not thaw	Do not thaw
Equipment		Convection/conventional oven	Convection or Standard Oven
Cooking time/ temperature	Cook at 325 degrees to an internal temperature of 160 degrees	Convection—350 degrees for 11 to 18 minutes; Conventional—400 degrees for 15 to 24 minutes; internal temperature 150 degrees	Preheat the oven. For one pan cook 10 minutes; add a minute for each additional pan. If the oven has a vent, open it to release excess steam.
Special instructions	Slice and place in a roasting pan with ½ cup water, cover with foil	Cheese substitute products generally are cooked at 25 degrees lower temperature.	
Length of holding		Best if served within 30 minutes; discard after two hours.	
Where instructions were found	Fact sheet	In the box	On the box

Source: Reprinted with permission from National Food Service Management Institute, *New Generation Foods, Breakfast Lunch Training,* pp. 7–8, © 1997, National Food Service Management Institute.

able cost of $2.00 per case. This generally converts to about $6.00 per case for 10 or more cases and drops to $1.50 for 300 or more cases. The general rule to apply when making a decision about drop size guarantees is that the larger the number of cases expected per delivery drop the lower the cost. Making the decision to allow each item to be awarded on the basis of the price of that item provides no guarantee of delivery drop size. This method is often referred to as line item award. Table 13–9 is an example of line item award.[9]

The first decision relates to the number of cases per delivery. In order to obtain the best pricing, a distributor can be given a delivery drop guarantee by grouping items and basing the buy decision on the bottom-line price of all

items. This method of guaranteeing a vendor drop size is referred to as "bottom line," "aggregate," or "all or nothing." The decision as to number of items to place in a group for bottom-line award must be based on the vendors serving the market area. Failure to consider the vendors serving the market can result in restriction of competition and failure to maximize competition.

Common groups of items are normally based on vendors serving the market. The commonality of the items may or may not be considered. The product movement policies of the school district have a major impact on the grouping of items. The largest expenditure of dollars will be for food. Requests for pricing for food are commonly grouped as milk and

Table 13–9 Vendor Award Method: Line Item

Product Name	Potential Vendor A	Potential Vendor B	Potential Vendor C
Peaches	$20.36 (low quote)	$22.94	$23.41
Pears	$22.49	$23.95	$22.46 (low quote)
Sugar	$19.06	$18.75 (low quote)	$21.45

Source: Reprinted with permission from M. Gunn *First Choice, A Purchasing Systems Manual for School Food Service*, p. 97, © 1995, National Food Service Management Institute.

milk products, bread and bread products, ice cream, fresh produce, low-volume annual items, and dry/frozen/refrigerated meats/vegetables/fruits/other food items.

Low-volume annual items are those products that each site purchases only once or twice annually. Some examples of low volume annual items are seasonings and food color. The largest group included in this list are the dry/frozen/refrigerated foods. This group may be subdivided based on the product movement policies of the school district and the vendors serving the market.

Paper items and miscellaneous kitchen supplies represent a high number of items. Miscellaneous kitchen supplies include such items as handwashing soap, glass cleaner, and other cleaning supplies. Cleaning supplies for use in automatic dish- and ware-washing equipment are normally included in a separate request for pricing. Special instructions and descriptions are required for these items. The vendors providing these supplies are frequently specialists. Often paper and miscellaneous kitchen supplies are included in the request for pricing for food items. Paper specialists serving the market area may make it necessary to group paper and miscellaneous kitchen supplies separately. Significant savings may be realized by combining some items such as paper towels, office supplies, garbage bags, and other paper items with the school district's request for pricing.

School food and nutrition program directors need to determine what each vendor offers for sale because vendors serving the market determine how items are grouped for the purpose of

obtaining prices. Specialty vendors will constitute the largest group from which the school district will purchase. Specialty vendors sell only certain items, which are often determined by the type of delivery equipment required, the storage required, product knowledge, and the source of supply. Specialty vendors will be found offering for sale only milk and milk products, bread and bread products, paper supplies, pest control services, dish machine and ware-washing chemicals, equipment, meat products, foods that require dry storage, fresh produce, insurance, or many other combinations.

The full- or broad-line food service vendor's objective is to offer for sale all of the items necessary to operate a program. The typical full- or broad-line food service vendor may carry as many as 7,000 items in inventory. This vendor offers all dry/frozen/refrigerated foods, paper and miscellaneous cleaning supplies, dish machine and ware-washing chemicals, small and large equipment, milk and milk products, bread and bread products, and fresh produce. Fresh produce requires special refrigeration equipment for storage and delivery. The full- or broad-line vendor may choose not to offer fresh produce. Milk and milk products and bread and bread products consume high cubic footage in the warehouse and on delivery vehicles. Full- or broad-line vendors often decide to provide these items only to low-volume customers. Open and free competition must be maintained in order to obtain the best pricing and comply with federal purchasing guidelines.

The vendors serving the market must be considered when grouping items for the purpose of obtaining prices. The greater the number of vendors offering prices, the better the pricing the school district will receive. The school district must balance the cost of processing requisitions and purchase orders, receiving deliveries, and processing invoices with the number of groups of items. It is necessary to utilize quantities of each item to be purchased to determine the lowest overall total. Table 13–10 presents an example of a bottom-line award in order to guarantee a vendor a certain delivery drop size.[9]

The second decision relates to the price being offered. The simplest form of pricing is a firm price for a specified period of time (bid period). When a firm price is requested, the vendor must assume the risk for changes in the market. The longer the price must remain firm the higher the cost will be. A more cost-effective approach for a school food and nutrition program is a pricing system that protects the vendor from changes in the market.

A large share of the distributor's business is based on cost of the product plus a percentage. Most national restaurant chains and a large percentage of the health care market uses this approach to pricing. In using this approach the vendors profit and operating cost return goes up as the cost of the product increases. If the cost of the product (free on board [FOB] distributor's warehouse) is $10.00 and the percentage is 10 percent of cost then the invoice cost of this product would be $11.00. If the FOB cost of this product increases to $11.00 then the invoice cost would increase to $12.10.

Although cost plus a percentage of cost is not an allowable method for schools operating under the National School Lunch Program and The School Breakfast Program there is an allowable alternative. The alternative is reimbursable cost plus a fixed fee for service. When this pricing structure is used, the request for pricing is in two parts. The first part is the FOB distributor's dock cost for the product. The second part is the distributor's fee. The distributor's fee must include the cost of warehousing, delivery, the cost of money for inventory, selling or customer service cost, and the profit margin. The basic difference in this approach is that the fee is fixed for the duration of the contract.

Under the reimbursable cost plus a fixed fee for service, product cost of $10.00 and a fee of $1.00 would have an invoice cost of $11.00. If the product increased in cost to $11.00 and the fee remains fixed at $1.00 the invoice cost increased to $12.00. This approach requires that distributors adjust their thought processes to the risk associated with increases in operating cost. With cost plus a percentage the distributor has some built-in increases in revenue to cover increases in operating cost; with reimbursable cost the fee is fixed, therefore they

Table 13–10 Vendor Award Method: Bottom Line

Product Name	Quantity	Potential Unit Price	Vendor A Extended	Potential Unit Price	Vendor B Extended	Potential Unit Price	Vendor C Extended
Peaches	25 cs	$20.19	$504.75	$22.02	$550.50	$21.50	$537.50
Pears	10 cs	$20.94	$209.40	20.48	$204.80	$21.50	$215.00
Sugar	15 bags	$15.98	239.70	$16.63	$249.45	$14.10	211.50
Bottom line total			$953.85 (low quote)		$1,004.75		$964.00

Source: Reprinted with permission from M. Gunn, *First Choice, A Purchasing Systems Manual for School Food Service*, p. 97, © 1995, National Food Service Management Institute.

must quote a higher fee to cover increases in operating cost.

Most purchasers attempt to audit the FOB cost of the product. In the early 1980s when this approach began developing it was possible to audit the invoices from the manufacturer to the distributor and determine that the distributor was charging only the cost of the product. In the late 1980s freight was deregulated and off-invoice rebates (commonly called sheltered income) to distributors grew to represent large dollars. It became cost prohibitive to conduct audits to determine the distributor's cost.

It is particularly important that public purchasers perform audits of a distributor's cost since they are reimbursing the distributor for the FOB cost of product. Since freight deregulation and the growth of sheltered income have resulted in prohibitive costs for conducting audits, reimbursable cost plus a fixed fee is not a viable alternative for school food and nutrition programs. A modification of this system to use third-party market bulletins to determine increases and decreases in the cost of product is a reasonable alternative to conducting an audit. There are many reliable third-party market reports available to the operator to track the cost of product. This modification would require that the price at the time of the initial pricing be firm for a specified period of time and that the vendor petition for increases and the school food and nutrition program staff petition for decreases. A reasonable period of time to hold the price firm is three to six months. The pricing proposals can contain an emergency clause for providing some relief to the distributor and the school food and nutrition program. The majority of the time the price of product will remain stable; however, since a perishable agricultural product is being purchased, wide swings in market cost can occur. The first step in applying this approach to pricing is to study the various market reports available. The major advantage of this pricing structure is that long-term contracts can be developed. Annual contracts with multiple-year renewals allow the school food and nutrition program to develop

partnerships with their business partners (distributors and manufacturers).

Receiving

The most important ingredient in a successful purchasing system is an effective receiving system. The objective of the receiving system is to achieve control of the product delivered. Excellent product movement policies, well-written food descriptions, effective screening of approved brands, and cost-effective purchasing systems can be lost at the point where the product is received. The school food and nutrition program director is responsible for establishing controls to ensure that items received are consistent with items ordered. Critical to receiving success is adequate training, communication, and facilities for the site receiver.

Evaluation of the receiving area at the sites is the first step in changing the receiving process. Many sites are old, and the receiving area cannot be changed. The food purchaser should seek ways to improve the receiving area and especially during renovation of an existing facility or construction of a new facility. To learn about the quality of the receiving area ask the following questions.

- Does the truck have to back across a playground, into heavy traffic, or up a hill? Could the access be designed so that the truck does not have to back, but could drive straight to the receiving door?
- Do any of the food items have to be carried up steps? How many doors does the delivery truck have? Can a portable conveyor be used during the unloading process?
- Is access to the receiving area limited during certain times of the day?

School food and nutrition staff need to be advocates for improved receiving areas during the site selection process. A positive learning experience is to observe the delivery of groceries to some of the national chain restaurants in your location. Distributors now have sophisticated computer equipment on trucks and can obtain information on how long a delivery to a given site requires. The length of time for unloading can now be factored into the price paid for product.

Equipment needed in the receiving area needs to be evaluated. Are scales necessary in the receiving area of a school food and nutrition program today? The products purchased determine the need for scales. In the majority of sites no items are purchased that require weighing by the school food and nutrition program. Even catch weight (inconsistent weight) items are preweighed by the manufacturer and the weight is recorded on the box. Weight tolerances are clearly defined in federal regulations and the weight is a part of the label. Reputable manufacturers would not risk a felony conviction for mislabeling a product. Fresh produce requires weighing only when billed as cost per pound. As an example, fresh cabbage is ordered by the sack. The weight of a sack of cabbage will vary based on the amount of rain at the growing site, the age of the product, and the amount of humidity in the storage facility. If fresh produce is weighed, it will be necessary to develop a list of acceptable tolerances. There is also a trend to purchase fresh produce in the "value added or fresh cut" form. The weights on these products are standard and are controlled by labeling laws. A large percentage of fresh produce is purchased by count.

Some equipment necessary in a receiving area includes:

- Thermometers appropriate for taking the temperature of chilled and frozen products
- A stable writing surface, which can be a fold-down shelf at the receiving door or (if space permits) a small desk or table
- A two-wheel cart or dolly for moving product into the appropriate storage area

Written procedures for receiving, including a receiving report along with appropriate training, must be provided to the site receiving staff. Procedures should include handling of discrepancies, shortages, and general condition of products received. Some writers indicate that the receiving report should also note the quality of service received. This allows the school district to recognize quality service as well as report poor service. Chapter 14 discusses the receiving report in relation to the production system. The report allows the site receiver to determine quickly that the brand and code number of the product selected is the product being delivered.

For those items that carried the brand-approval type of distributor's choice the receiving task is not very complicated. It is only necessary for receiving staff to verify that the correct amount of the product is received. Since the brand-approval type selected indicated that the school district had no preferences for these products, it does not matter what brand is delivered.

The private-labeling program of the selected distributor is a part of site-receiving staff training. Recognizing from memory the label colors or logo and the grade of the product is an important receiving skill. It is important that staff know what items are approved under the private-labeling program of the distributor and the grade for each product contained in the product description. In addition to training in this area it is helpful if the receiving report lists the grade for each product.

Those products that are approved by manufacturers' brand and code numbers require the most attention during the receiving process. Reading the labels on meat products is an important part of training for receiving staff. It is important that they understand the numbers found on a meat label. The numbers on a meat label are as follows:

- Product code—the number assigned by the manufacturer to identify a specific product.
- Establishment number—the number found in the federal government sanitation inspection circle and is specific to a manufacturing facility. This number helps to

ensure that the correct brand is being received.

- Code date—can be identified because it is rubber- or machine-stamped on the label or box rather than being printed on the label. This is the number that identifies the date, time, and production line on which a product was manufactured. This is the critical number to a manufacturer when a problem with the quality or safety of a product is identified.
- CN Label number—this number is very important in the approval process for brands which requires a CN-labeled product. This number is of little use in the ordering and receiving process. Distributors do not carry this number in their databases. Recognition of this number increases understanding of food products.

The receiving report identifies the name of the product, the brand, and code number. Employees carefully check these items against the receiving report. These items normally represent a large percentage of the dollars in any order.

Checking frozen product for evidence of freezer burn or thawing is a major quality issue. Any product with these problems is not accepted. The temperature of chilled products is checked and recorded. The code dates for such items as fresh-cut produce, bread, and chilled meats are verified and recorded on the receiving report.

A product feedback system is established for the site staff to report to purchasing any concerns about product. Often a lengthy form is designed to provide information on a product. These lengthy forms create a barrier to communication. The site receiver is the employee on the firing line, and a complicated form results in inadequate feedback. Simple feedback systems such as a phone call to a designated voice mail box, electronic mail to a designated address, a phone call to a person, or a special card with no questions but simply a line in which to write are effective. A staff member on the purchasing staff is assigned to conduct follow-up on any feedback received from site receivers. Providing feedback to the receiver who took the time to provide information will encourage more frequent use of the feedback system.

PURCHASING SERVICES

A school food and nutrition program requires the purchase of many services. Some of the services required are pest control, telecommunication, courier, marketing, equipment maintenance, computer software maintenance, staff training, insurance, legal, auditing, consulting, and garbage removal. The school district policies will determine which of these services are provided by in-house staff and which are provided by external vendors. An example is courier service. An employee of the school district often provides this service. This employee may provide courier service between schools of the district for food service and other departments or they could provide this service only for food service.

A request for proposal (RFP) is often the most appropriate purchase method for service contracts. An RFP allows the evaluation of many variables in addition to cost. When developing a request for proposal the variables must be identified and a point value assigned to each variable. Selection criteria for food service equipment maintenance are presented as an example in Table 13–11.

It is advisable to utilize an RFP selection committee to determine a contract award. Each individual on the selection committee scores the responses to the RFP separately, and the scores are averaged to determine the award.

Another approach to determine the award is to rank RFP panel scores or discard the low and high score in order to negate the effect of a panel member who gives all very high or very low scores. The calculation of budget points is not normally supplied to the selection committee until the subjective scores for other criteria have been recorded. The points for budget are determined by awarding the lowest price quote

Table 13–11 Selection Criteria for Equipment Maintenance RFP

Selection Criteria	Maximum Points	Points For This Response
Years company has been in food service maintenance business	10	
Years experience of technical staff	20	
Brands of equipment owned by school district compared to factory authorized service agent brands for this company	10	
Length of time to obtain parts for brands of equipment where they are not a factory authorized service agent	10	
Response time on emergency calls	15	
Membership in Commercial Food Equipment Service Association, Inc. (CFESA)	5	
Budget—routine maintenance bottom line	10	
Budget—hourly rate for emergency service	10	
Budget—percentage discount off manufacturers list price for replacement parts	10	
Total points	100	

the maximum number of points. All other responses receive a percentage of the points allowed. If the budget for routine maintenance contained in the response was $4,000.00, then in this example 10 points would be assigned to that response. If another response offered a price of $5,000.00 the calculation of points would be as follows: $4,000 divided by $5,000.00 equals 80 percent. Eighty percent of 10 points equals eight points. In the example for equipment maintenance, it will also be necessary to make similar budget calculations for the hourly rate for emergency service and the percentage discount off the manufacturer's list price for replacement parts.

If the service being purchased is bid as a bottom-line request for prices there would be only one budget calculation.

PURCHASING EQUIPMENT

Equipment purchased to support the food preparation of the school district can generally be classified as large equipment and small equipment. In some states the price determines whether it is classified as large or small equipment. This price is normally used to determine when the equipment is to be included in the

general fixed assets inventory of the school district. Equipment costing over $2,500, for example, may be considered large equipment. A procedure is needed in each school district for determining the dollar amount used to classify large and small equipment. A general rule often followed is that if it is fixed (installed permanently) it is considered large equipment. Large equipment purchases are made as a part of new construction, renovation projects, or to replace existing equipment. The small equipment category includes portable equipment designed for multiple use, such as forks, pans, serving utensils, brushes, garbage cans, or carts.

The design of a new facility is a major responsibility for a school food and nutrition program director. For further discussion of equipment purchasing and facility design, see Chapters 14 and 17. The design of a new facility has a long-range impact on the effectiveness of program operation from both a food quality and cost control standpoint. Staffing of the site and product movement should be given primary consideration. Determining the menu system to be used in the facility is the first major decision to be made. All other decisions should be based on the menu system. Effective use of all the team players will be necessary to produce an effective facility. The members of the new construction team are as follows:

- End user group: school board, superintendent, principal, School/and Nutrition Program food director, food service manager, purchasing staff, and food service employees
- Design group: architect, food service consultant, specifier, and draftsman
- Construction group: construction manager, general contractor, kitchen equipment contractor, fabricator, equipment manufacturer
- Follow-up group: school food and nutrition manager, food service employees, manufacturer's agent, and service agent.

The phases in a new construction project are

- Project concept: Define the operating profile, the menu, the hours of service, number of customers, cost objectives, growth requirements, and special requirements such as health/safety or aesthetics.
- Preliminary design: Perform a space configuration study. Provide flow diagrams (the movement of food from receiving through service and the movement of customers from entry to exit), equipment layout, utility requirements, and budget estimates.
- Final design: Provide specifications for equipment to be purchased and fabricated, utility drawings and specifications, contract documents, and terms and conditions.
- Bidding: Evaluate bids, determine and negotiate changes, and award contract.
- Contract implementation: Check construction and equipment installation. Do a final walk-through; provide change orders and corrections as needed.
- Start-up: Provide operator training, equipment use and care manuals, warranty service.

In many school districts the director of the school food and nutrition program will not be consulted until the new project is in the final design phase. One of the advocacy roles the school food and nutrition director assumes is related to new construction and site selection. In the seller's market in which food is purchased, long-term delivery costs must be considered when selecting sites for new schools. Access to the receiving area will have a long-term impact on the cost paid for food. The site should provide access for delivery trucks without having to cross playground areas or bus loading and unloading areas.

The extent of a renovation project will determine which of the phases of new construction will be necessary. A renovation project could be as simple as replacement of an existing piece of equipment or as extensive as a new construction project. Unless the school food and nutrition program director is working in a school district with a rapidly growing student population, equipment purchasing skills will be necessary on an infrequent basis. Costly mistakes can be avoided by employing the appropriate professionals from the design group to provide advice and assistance when equipment is being replaced. The National Food Service Management Institute recently published a guide to help school food and nutrition program directors navigate the process of purchasing food service equipment.[10,12]

ACTIONS TO AVOID

Any action that eliminates competition is to be avoided. Purchasing products that link product to equipment is very expensive. It is common to find a request for pricing that requires a milk company to provide the equipment for cooling the milk. This "free" piece of equipment is very expensive when the additional cost added to the product cost is considered. Other examples of equipment are free beverage equipment that requires use of a specific brand of juice, handwashing soap that requires a specific dispenser, paper towels that require a special dispenser, and napkins that will fit only one dispenser.

Adult brand prejudice is the most costly practice among purchasers for school food and nutrition programs. Purchasers' lack of knowledge of how products are manufactured, control of brands available in a market by the distributors, and adult food and taste preferences often cause a restriction of competition and thus higher purchase cost. Often students are blamed for this adult brand prejudice because of inadequate screening procedures for product. Students react to change, rather than to the acceptability of a product. Screening of products is conducted in a manner to avoid a reaction to change. Introducing a new brand in the middle of the school year will often result in a negative acceptability rating.

There is a direct relationship between the number of brands approved and the price paid for product. The lower the number of acceptable brands the higher the cost. The purchasing system is designed to decrease the impact of adult brand prejudice.

Vendor favoritism is another costly purchasing practice. Awarding business on the basis of favoritism decreases competition and results in higher cost. Selling product is a business, and if vendors are aware of practices of favoritism, such as always awarding the business to the same company, they will not work as hard for school food and nutrition program business.

SUMMARY

Establishing and implementing an effective purchasing system requires a strategic decision that has an impact on the nutritional integrity, student acceptance, and financial success of the child nutrition programs. The twenty-first century projections for the application of technology in developing new foods, the impact of the global market, and the continuing quest for meeting the nutritional needs of students with meals they enjoy give the school nutrition purchaser a real challenge. There is no easy list of strategies of how to conduct cost-effective purchasing for a school food and nutrition program. A most important factor in successful purchasing is having a professional school food and nutrition director who understands the linkage between purchasing and program goals. Hiring decisions for program directors are often based on the school board assessment of a person's ability to manage effectively the logistical and financial aspects of this portion of a director's job. The knowledge and skills required of school food and nutrition directors in the twenty-first century will entail up-to-date knowledge of laws and regulations as well as skills in managing the marketplace.[11]

Purchasing is practiced in a dynamic environment. Items produced by manufacturers change constantly. The ownership and, therefore, the service level of distributors is in a constant state of flux. The needs of the school food and nutrition programs will continue as school food and nutrition professionals seek excellence in program operation for students. Many issues have an impact on effective purchasing, requiring constant efforts to seek and understand the bigger picture. The school food and nutrition director, in partnership with the school district purchasing office and the food industry, must continue seeking creative approaches to purchasing and must apply quality measures to the process to determine that nutritional and financial goals are being met. The challenge can be arduous but rewarding. The children served each day deserve the best that can be purchased with the funds available.

CASE STUDY
THE QUEST FOR BETTER PRICES

Janet Beer and Carol McLeod

The Challenge

In the late 1980s school districts were still trying to recover from the federal budget cuts experienced in 1981. As costs escalated during this period it became increasingly difficult to maintain program quality within the revenues available. A major portion of the budgeted funds is used to purchase food and kitchen supplies. This portion of the budget can be controlled by changes in management systems. In addition to the need to control or reduce costs, school districts that purchased in less than truckload quantities (approximately 40,000 pounds) were having difficulty purchasing new products available on the market. The products stocked by vendors were being determined by the larger school districts in the vendor's market area.

Actions

In 1989 Tigard-Tualatin, Newberg, and McMinnville school districts formed a purchasing cooperative. These school districts are located in the state of Oregon. The Newberg and McMinnville school districts have the same food and nutrition program director. The goal was to share the workload and to see whether lower prices would result from the combined purchasing. Having gained information and product descriptions gleaned from Portland public schools and another three-district purchasing cooperative, the new cooperative (co-op) began issuing combined requirement bids twice a year. Each district estimated the quantities they would buy for the specified six-month period. The combined estimates were sent out for formal bids to local distributors. Bids were awarded to multiple vendors based on low bid on each item. Each district paid half of the expense of processing the bid. From that point on each district acted independently, having its school board approve the bid, sending in orders, and receiving and paying for products. Lower prices were received and some reductions in administrative time devoted to the purchasing task were realized.

At the end of the first year the two districts were approached by another small co-op in the area that had been jointly bidding for dairy and bread products. A new co-op group was formed that now served seven districts. Following the same bid format outlined above, the seven districts issued a formal bid with combined estimated usage for a one-year time period. The award was again on the individual line items, and was given to multiple vendors. Administrative costs were shared equally by the seven districts. Districts independently approved the bid award, purchased, and paid for products. The increase in estimated usage again resulted in lower prices and improved quality of products.

Success of the co-op was shared, and other districts asked to join in the third year. Twenty-two districts were now involved, and administration of the co-op became more complicated. The time needed to process the combined bid expanded. Brokers and suppliers became more interested in being awarded portions of the bid. Brokers and manufacturers' representatives wanted more time to show products and to interact with co-op members. A formal structure for the co-op was developed during the third year of operation. As in any volunteer organization, a small number of people were doing the actual work involved with processing of the bid. Even so, the core group believed that the benefit to their individual districts in reduced prices and improved product quality justified the time spent in managing the bid process.

The decision was made to expand membership aggressively. The leadership of the co-op believed that even larger estimated quantities would mean still lower prices, and there would be additional members to help with the processing of the bid. Postcards were mailed to all the districts and business managers in the state. The leadership made a presentation at the Oregon School Food Service Association annual meeting and made personal phone calls inviting districts to join. The State Department of Education Child Nutrition Division, recognizing from marketbasket cost comparisons that the co-op prices were lower than many districts were paying independently, began encouraging districts to join. The growth resulted in 76 members for the 1994–1995 school year. These school district represented 177,000 students. For the 1995–1996 and the 1996–1997 school years the co-op had 89 member districts and represented more than 200,000 students, or approximately 40 percent of the students in the state.

Leadership and Organization Structure

Groups are enriched if they have a variety of leaders; each leader brings different skills and knowledge to the organization. But like all volunteer organizations, it was difficult to persuade people to assume the responsibility of leading the co-op. The chairperson and co-chairperson are food service directors of member districts, in addition to the responsibilities of leading this co-op.

Quality leadership is critical, and the individuals need to feel rewarded. Therefore a leadership plan was developed and approved by the member districts. A progressive plan of a member being first treasurer, then the co-chair, and finally the chair was developed and implemented. In the middle of the second year it was recognized that this rapid turnover of leadership was not in the co-op's best interest. As the chair and co-chair worked on managing the co-op purchasing they had developed both a definite philosophy and strong working rela-

tionships with the distributors, brokers, and manufacturers' representatives. This philosophy and relationships could not simply be passed on to the next individual. The decision was made that the leadership would retain their positions for a minimum of three years or until the year 2000. The co-op members would assess the next evolution at that time.

In addition to the volunteer leaders, a paid employee was essential to process the bid information. Initially the co-op hired a registered dietitian for this position. However, the majority of the work was clerical, and the following year a food service secretary who worked part-time for one of the member districts was hired to work as the bid clerk. The bid clerk performs all the clerical work of the co-op. She has computerized the processing of the bid and developed a program to fax all co-op members automatically. This allows the leadership to send information overnight to all members at minimal expense. The co-op hopes eventually to have the capability to E-mail all members.

As the group grew larger, developing links with national manufacturers gave the co-op the opportunity to negotiate for better-quality products at lower prices. The chair and the co-chair have been sent to several national-level meetings to develop and maintain working relationships with the manufacturers' representatives. There is recognition by the group as a whole that the leaders spend many hours on co-op issues. The support staff in their districts also spends time on these issues. In recognition of the time involved, and the expense of incidental supplies used, the decision was made to help offset the expense to the leaders' districts with a payment of $500 to $1,000 to each of their districts. Payment is based on a minimum of $500 for 50 members, increasing by $100 for an additional 10 members to a maximum of $1,000.

Beginning with the 1995–1996 bid, all members are required to attend one meeting per year. This meeting gives the co-op chairs an opportunity to explain the direction for the coming bid. It also gives the member districts an opportunity to provide feedback on how the current bid is functioning, as well as provide input on where the leadership is directing future bids.

Financial

The co-op is not a separate public agency. The formal issuance of awards is done by each individual district's school board. Each school district is responsible for ordering, receiving, and paying for its own food and supplies. All liability and legal responsibility remain with the individual districts. All co-op fees are collected prior to the beginning of the bid cycle. If there is excess revenue in the co-op account, at the close of the bid processing period it is returned to the member districts. No funds are carried over from year to year.

A budget is estimated for the expenses of a bid cycle and approved by the members at the annual mandatory meeting. The total estimate is divided by the number of members, and that sum becomes the membership fee for that bid cycle. The co-op members recently decided the fee for the 1997–1998 bid will also be adjusted according to the districts' student membership. All fees must be collected before the bid is issued. Table 13–12 presents the budget for the 1997–1998 school year.

Product Selection

The goal of the co-op is to allow all interested vendors to have an opportunity to participate in the bid process. A "show and tell" day is scheduled each fall to give brokers and manufacturers' representatives an opportunity to show their new products. Vendors are charged $100 per table to participate in the co-op "show and tell" food show. After the vendor "show and tell" day is concluded the product description committee meets. The majority of the products are bid on a distributors' choice basis. Distributors' choice means that any manufacturer's product that meets the product description is acceptable. Some products termed *manufacturer defined* are specified by noting the acceptable manufacturers and their identifying product code numbers. Manufacturer defined products are tested and selected by students. The co-op believes that products are not tested as a double blind, against another product, or by food service directors. Products are selected in the same environment we serve them, by students, on the normal lunch tray, at

Table 13–12 Projected Budget 1997–1998 (Based on 75 Member Districts)

Income	
Member fees	$13,125
Show and tell	$ 4,400
Total	$17,425
Administrative Expense	
Clerk	$4,000
Printing	1,800
Advertising	125
Postage	900
PO Box	60
Conferences (four)	6,000
Supplies	250
Phone and fax	300
Show and tell	500
Fee to chair/co-chair	2,500
Miscellaneous	990
Total	$17,425

mealtime. Once students are seated and eating, they are given two slips of paper. One has a smiley face, the other a frowny face. They are asked to turn in whichever slip represents what they thought of the lunch just served (and hopefully eaten). Products receiving 80 percent smiley faces are approved. Products that fail can be retested in a different school on vendor request.

Bid Organization

Once the product descriptions are finalized, a bid packet is sent to each co-op member. The packet includes the product descriptions with a space for the district to estimate its annual usage for the coming bid cycle. It also includes the co-op agreement and fee information for the coming bid cycle. This agreement identifies the district's obligations on joining the co-op. Districts agree to purchase the quantities they estimate or to let the vendor know in advance if they choose not to purchase estimated items and why. The bid is a requirements bid (our best guess), not a demand bid (a firm offer to buy a specific amount). Districts have historically been able to purchase additional amounts if needed.

The estimates are compiled into a grand total. The bid is then advertised and mailed to all interested vendors. During the first two weeks after the bid is mailed, vendors may submit items that they believe to be "equal or alternates" to the items in the bid. All alternates and equals are tested during the third week, and a bid addendum is issued identifying any additional acceptable items.

As part of the formal bid process vendors are asked to identify the fee (dollar amount per case) they will place on all items purchased by co-op members that were not described in the formal bid document. The fee quoted by vendors is a tier, with higher fees for lower-value items. In the Northwest, non–bid items typically may be priced at up to 25 percent over cost. The co-op averages from 8 percent to 12 percent over cost for non–bid items.

The bid is opened five weeks after it is issued. At that time prices are compiled and a committee reviews them. Historically a variety of awards was offered to members. The A award was based on lowest-priced item meeting the product description with no consideration to minimum delivery requirements or geographical restriction. This category of award was used by the larger districts with warehouses willing to purchase from multiple vendors. The second award category, the B award, was selected by comparing prices between just two distributors. Many districts liked having two sources for their food and supplies. This category of award was selected by approximately 25 percent of the membership. The final category of award, the C award, was given to the distributor who had the lowest bottom-line extended total, and was therefore a sole or prime distributor. The majority of the member districts selected the C award. All award choices were mailed to the members. The award choices were then presented by the individual districts' food service director or business manager to the district's school board for approval.

During the bid cycle distributors are allowed to escalate and deescalate bid prices if their costs from their suppliers have increased or decreased. After the bid cycle begins, price audits are conducted. Members submit invoices they question, and the co-op chairpersons meet with the distributors to review the manufacturers' invoices to determine whether the appropriate price has been charged.

Outcomes

The major advantage of belonging to the co-op is the reduction in product pricing. The State Department of Education Child Nutrition Division conducted a study comparing the current pricing of a small district with the co-op prices. The co-op prices were significantly lower. Breakfast meal costs would have been 37 percent less, and lunch meal costs would have been 17 percent less if the school districts had belonged to the co-op. Only three items that were compared cost more through the co-op. The remainder of the items were 5 percent to 95 percent less expensive. In addition to being less expensive, bid products are more likely to be available when the number of brands and items a distributor is required to stock are reduced. Other advantages of co-op membership include the improved quality and the availability of the products on the bid. Also, the co-op has reduced the workload for all the member districts as well as the vendors and distributors. Sharing the work has made purchasing more fun for all of us. There have been many comments from business and industry members that they feel they are getting a very fair chance to sell to the co-op members.

The co-op has developed into an informal network. For many districts, especially the smaller ones, this is the first time they have been able to meet regularly with their peers. Discussions are rarely limited to purchasing issues. Employee supervision and selection, student management challenges, fiscal issues, and nutrition issues are frequent topics. All members benefit from the hundreds of years of collective experience the group encompasses.

Next Steps

Feedback obtained through the co-op's annual meeting is that members are pleased with the advantages of buying cooperatively. Consideration is being given to expanding the program. Last spring the co-op tried its first venture in purchasing small equipment as a group. Plans are developing to attempt purchasing large equipment once or twice a year. Each of these additional purchasing programs will charge a small fee to involved districts to cover their expenses. The co-op is beginning to influence the commodity-processing decisions that are made by the state. Two co-op members serve on the state commodity advisory committee.

The co-op is considering supplying nutrient information of bid items to member districts for an additional charge. The informal network of the co-op will greatly assist members in understanding and adapting to any new regulations and programs. Members attending the 1996 annual conference of the American School Food Service Association were given an assignment. Members attending the conference reviewed nutrient analysis software. The goal of the members was to recommend software for use by all co-op members.

Beginning with the 1997–1998 school-year bid cycle only the sole distributor award will be issued. The majority of members already purchase this way. They believe that there are cost savings to developing a partnership with a primary distributor. One bid document with multiple styles of awards was difficult for distributors to implement. Distributors and manufacturers were unsure of what portion of the estimates they might receive in the variety of award categories. The leadership thought it was time for the co-op to develop long-term relationships and partnerships with vendors and distributors. The bid will contain an extension clause that potentially will allow the award to be valid for up to five years. The leadership has met with all distributors that will be potential bidders for the 1997–1998 bid to discuss the change in format.

Another change being considered is category management within the product list. Category management involves grouping products, such as potatoes, and bidding them as a bundle to the manufacturer. The objective of this change is to give a single manufacturer a large volume and mix of products, so the manufacturer can reduce the margin needed to make its profit and lower pricing to the co-op. The leadership has met with representatives from various manufacturers of the proposed category-managed products (potatoes, cereals, beef, chicken, and turkey) and has received favorable feedback.

Keys to Success

After eight years experience we have identified three points critical to the success of a purchasing cooperative:

1. Remember that it is a process. It will continue to evolve, grow, and change.
2. Get a good bid clerk. Computerize as many functions as possible.
3. Understand that the goal is to work with vendors and distributors. If we make their life easier, they will make ours easier, and everyone wins!

REFERENCES

1. J. Sneed et al., *Impact of Food Procurement on the Implementation of the Dietary Guidelines for Americans in Child Nutrition Programs*, Conference Proceedings (University, MS: National Food Service Management Institute, 1992), 182–184.

2. American School Food Service Association, *Keys to Excellence: Standards of Practice for Nutrition Integrity* (Alexandria, VA: 1995), 26–28.

3. United States Department of Agriculture Food and Consumer Service, *Choice Plus: a Reference Guide for Food and Ingredients* (Washington, DC: USDA Program Aid FCS-297,1996), 17.

4. Office of the Federal Register, National Archives and Records Administration, *Code of Federal Regulations,* Volume 7, Agriculture, Parts 210–299, and Volume 9, Part 200 to the end (Washington, DC: 1997).

5. M. Gunn, *First Choice: A Purchasing Systems Manual for School Food Service* (University, MS: University of Mississippi, National Food Service Management Institute, 1995), 7, 10, 14–18, 33–42, 48, 51–52, 75–76.

6. United States Department of Agriculture Food and Nutrition Service, *FNS Instruction 716-1, Specifications for Donated Foods* (Washington, DC: 1992).

7. Gunn, *First Choice*, 88–90.

8. National Food Service Management Institute, *New Generation Foods, Breakfast Lunch Training* (University, MS: University of Mississippi, 1997), 7–8.

9. Gunn, *First Choice*, 97.

10. J. Parenteau, *Study on Food Cost* (Salem, OR: Oregon Department of Education, 1994).

11. D.H. Carr et al., eds., *Competencies, Knowledge and Skills of Effective District School Nutrition Directors/Supervisors* (University, MS: National Food Service Management Institute, 1996).

12. National Food Service Management Institute. *A Guide for Purchasing Foodservice Equipment (*University, MS: Author, 1998).

Self-Assessment of Warehouse Cost

When other departments share a warehouse, some cost is pro-rated. Square footage of space occupied by each department is one way to pro-rate cost. Count only the storage space each department takes. Assume all departments use equally the common areas, such as receiving office space, and other general use space. Determine the space food sevice uses as a percentage of total space. Apply this percentage against any cost category such as pest control and utilities. Other deparments probably won't share some cost such as refrigerators and freezers; therefore, include 100% of those cost.

Example: 10,000 square foot warehouse and food service occupies 5,000 square feet.

10,000 divided by 5,000 = .50 or 50%

Annual utility cost for the warehouse is $950

$950 × .50 = $475 − food service share of utility cost

1. Warehouse occupancy	
Warehouse occupancy costs money in lease costs or investment income, if the district owns the warehouse. A good rule of thumb is $5 per square foot. You might check local warehouse lease cost in your area.	
Formula: $5 × _____ sq. ft. =	$
Maintenance of refrigerators and freezers costs money. Use last year's cost as a good guide.	
Formula: last year's cost =	$
The average life of refrigerators and freezers is somewhere between 5 and 10 years, subject to personal opinion and previous experience.	
Formula: Current purchase cost of refrigerators and freezers = $_____ divided by _____ (number of years useful life) = annual cost =	$
Estimate pest control service for the warehouse, based on the previous year's cost	
Formula: Previous year's cost =	$

continues

Estimate utilities (electricity, gas, water, garbage fee etc.), based on the previous year's cost.	
Formula: Previous year's cost =	$
Total cost of warehouse occupancy	$
2. Delivery equipment	
The normal life cycle of trucks for warehouse delivery is five years. Use a different life cycle for the cost of the delivery equipment, if you prefer. Refrigerated trucks (dry and frozen compartments) and non-refrigerated trucks have a replacemnt cost. The replacement cost should be included in the cost of the warehouse operation.	
Formula: Cost to replace trucks $_____ divided by 5 or other year's annual cost =	
Estimate fuel, oil, grease, and tires based on previous year's cost.	
Formula: Previous year's cost =	$
Estimate repairs to vehicles and refrigeration units from previous year's cost. Consider increasing this cost 10% a year as the vehicles and refrigeration units get older.	
Formula: Previous year's cost =	$
Base cost of vehicle insurance, and annual cost, on the current annual premium. The type of insurance and the cost you are required to pay will vary by state.	
Formula: Current annual premiums =	$
Cost of motor vehicle license and/or tag. The type of license and tag required and the cost will vary by state. The previous cost of the motor vehicle license and tag is a good estimate.	
Formula: Previous annual payment =	$
Total cost of delivery equipment	$
3. Salary and Fringe Benefits	
Consider salaries for all warehouse personnel regardless of the fund which makes the payment. Food service may pay some personnel directly or you may pay a pro-rated share of the total payroll. The square footage calculation discussed earlier is and equitable approach to pro-rating salary cost. If the warehouse and delivery personnel also make food deliveries such as those in bulk or pre-plated from a central preparation system, determine what portion of their time is devoted to the warehouse operation.	
Formula: Pro-rated share of salaries	$
Formula: Pro-rated share of fringe benefits =	$
Total cost of salary and fringe benefits	$

continues

4. Inventory investment	
Inventory can be a hidden cost—money invested in the inventory could be in the bank earning interest. Once an item is purchased it is the propery of the school district. The risk of the loss of the inventory becomes a cost to the school district. Calculate the cost of inventory investment by multiplying the average dollar value of the inventory by the interest rate.	
Example: $100,000 (last year's average monthly inventory at month's end × .045 (current interest rate) = $4,500	
Formula: $_____ (average month and inventory) × _____ (current interest rate) = $_____ cost of investment in inventory.	
Assigning a cost to the risk associated with maintaining an inventory can be approached from three perspectives. 1. Replacement cost if total inventory was lost. In this case use the highest inventory value for the year. 2. The cost of food losses during the previous year. If this is the choice, disregard the potential of total inventory loss and deal only with the routine cost of food spoilage. Routine food spoilage in the warehouse must be recognized as a cost of operation. A just-in-time product movement policy would lower food spoilage rate because you would own the product for a shorter period of time. 3. The cost of insurance on the average monthly inventory value is the most practical approach. Most product insurance will have a deductible, so add the cost of routine spoilage to the insurance premium.	
Formula: $_____ (your choice of costing options) =	$
Total cost of inventory investment	$
Summary of Warehouse Cost	
1. Warehouse Occupancy	
2. Delivery Equipment	
3. Salaries and Fringe Benefits	
4. Inventory Investment	
Total Warehouse Cost	$

continues

Self-Assessment of Warehouse
Delivery Volume

The second step in determining the cost of operating a warehouse: Convert the total cost to a per-case cost. Use a per-case cost to determine if you can save enough on the purchase price of an item to cover the cost of warehouse operations.

Determining the total cases of product delivered to or from the warehouse during the year. This assumes that you are not building inventory but maintaining it at a pre-established level; therefore, the number delivered *to* will be about equal to the number delivered *from* the warehouse. Use the number that is the easiest to find from your inventory records. If you are building inventory you should use the number of cases shipped from the warehouse. This calculation is called warehouse "throughput."

Total cases: Purchased food   _____
              Donated food   _____
              Paper and supply items _____
              Other   _____
Total cases received/delivered   _____

Don't get too detailed with this calculation. Questions such as "do I count one mop as a case?" make the calculation more difficult than necessary. The normal delivery unit is the best guide. All you want is a realistic estimate of throughput.

Divide the total cases received/delivered (throughput) by the total cost from the summary above.

Formula: $_____ (warehouse cost) divided by
_____ (throughput) = $_____ per-case cost of warehouse operation.
Example: $258,756 ÷ 164,652 = $1.57

When you know the per-case cost, compare product cost to determine if warehousing will become part of your product movement policy. When making product comparisons avoid the tendency to "cherry pick" the items which you compare. A true comparison must deal with 100 percent of the items. If you compare only the high-volume items, you might find that there is a cost savings; however, often the price paid for low-volume items will offset any savings on high-volume items.

If you are currently operating a warehouse, take the current cost of items plus the cost per case for warehousing and compare it to the price paid by a similar school district with direct-to-site delivery.

Example: Your district   Applesauce 6/#10 invoice cost = ... $20
                          Warehouse cost = ... $1.57
                          Actual food cost...................................... $21.57
                          Comparison district—Applesauce 6/#10 = ... $20.98
                          Cost savings with site delivery =.................... $.59 per case

Probably you will see a trend early in the comparison and you won't need to complete comparison of 100 percent of the items. Be certain before you stop the comparison that you have compared low- and high-volume, frozen, dry, and refrigerated items. Compare some items in all product categories before you reach a conclusion.

continues

If you are in a state with commercial distributors delivering donated food, the cost per case paid for direct-to-site delivery is also a good comparison. Except for the cost of financing the inventory, a distributor's cost for donated or purchased food is about the same. If the school district cost per case for warehouse operation is more than the donated food delivery fee, then you have an indication that direct-to-site delivery may save money. The professional distributor should be more efficient than the school district. Remember that a food service distributor devotes 100 percent of his time to product movement, which is only one of hundreds of tasks you must accomplish in school food service.

If you are in a district without a warehouse and are considering the capital investment to create a school district–operated warehouse, then you can make the reverse comparison presented above. Compare the purchase cost of an item in your district to a similar-sized district that operates a warehouse, adding the cost of operating a warehouse to the purchase cost the other district pays.

Source: Reprinted with permission from M. Gunn, *First Choice, A Purchasing Systems Manual for School Food Service,* © 1995, National Food Service Management Institute.

Sample Protocol for Screening New Products or Brands of Existing Products

A four-part process to screen new products:

1. Paper screen
2. Product committee screen
3. Appearance screen
4. Student taste screen

A three-part process to screen new brands of existing products:

1. Paper screen
2. Appearance screen
3. Student taste screen

Paper Screen

- Design a product comparison sheet with the following basic information:
  - a. Brand of product
  - b. Manufacturer's code number
  - c. Establishment number of the manufacturer if a meat product
  - d. If applicable, the CN label number and the meal pattern contribution
  - e. Meal pattern contribution
  - f. Portion size and case size
  - g. The first five ingredients on the label ingredient statement
  - h. Nutrient analysis showing total calories, total fat, saturated fat, carbohydrate, protein, and sodium and whether values are from laboratory analysis or calculated from a standard database.

- Get a copy of the product label and nutrient analysis from the company.
- For a new product, create a new product comparison sheet, list product as the first brand, and add the product to the agenda list for the next product committee meeting.
- For an existing product list, add to the product comparison sheet and determine if the product meets the description.
- Notify manufacturer's representative of results of the paper screening.

Product Committee Screen

- Appoint a product committee. Possible members are the CN purchasing specialist, specialists who have routine contact with schools, building level manager, and the director of food service.
- Maintain an agenda of products for consideration at each regularly scheduled meeting.
- Report appearance and taste screen results to the committee.
- Allow any staff member to add items to the agenda list. Member who submits the item will present the following information to the committee:
  - a. How the product will be used
  - b. Whether the product will replace an existing item or will expand the product list

c. How product will impact cost
d. Availability of the product from other manufacturers and, if sole-source item, impact on cost.
e. Copy of product label and nutrient analysis.
- Committee may take one of three actions:
    1. Refer to appearance testing
    2. Reject as not appropriate for food service system
    3. Table for future review with additional information
- Report product committee screening to the appropriate sales personnel.

Appearance Screen

- Appoint a committee of those involved daily in hands-on food preparation.
- Get a full-case sample from a production line—not a specially made sample. Obtain the sample from a stocking food service distributor. Get samples directly from a manufacturer or broker if there is no other way to obtain them.
- Record the results of the appearance screen in narrative form, signed by all present.
- Include the following:
    a. Compare the label to that provided during the paper screening. If the label is not identical, suspend appearance screening.
    b. Record the date/shift coding on the packaging for the record if product is rejected.
    c. Screen the packaging for acceptability to your food service operation. Record the style and condition of the packaging.
    d. Evaluate the appearance of the product in the raw and cooked state for acceptability—shape, texture, color, smell, plate coverage and availability

of recommended preparation equipment.
    e. Committee takes one of two actions;
        1. Reject the product based on appearance.
        2. Refer the product for student taste screen.
- Provide sales personnel with the results of the appearance screen. See product tracking sheet.

Student Taste Screen

- Serve the product as part of a regular meal service. Do not use a special group of students.
- Test the product in three schools on the same day with the identical other foods.
- Rate food product as acceptable or unacceptable. Do not rate food products on a competitive basis.
- Place the rating scale by the cashier's stand for the students to pick voluntarily. Encourage all students who choose the item being tested to complete a rating scale. Use a hedonic scale (smiley faces or frowny faces) for lower grades or the words *acceptable/unacceptable* with older students.
- Test only one product per day.
- Approve product with a simple majority of acceptable ratings unless school district Food and Nutrition administrators prefer a higher acceptance rating. If the product is unacceptable in two schools and acceptable in the third school, test the product again in two different schools.
- Prepare a summary of the test results and report to the product committee and the sales personnel representing the product. Retain the summary of all test results for documentation related to expenditure of federal funds.

Special Considerations

Do not allow sales personnel or company representatives at the product committee meeting or the appearance or taste testing.

Source: Reprinted with permission from M. Gunn, *First Choice, A Purchasing Systems Manual for School Food Service,* pp. 186–187, © 1995, National Food Service Management Institute.

CHAPTER 14

Food Production Systems for the Future

Mary B. Gregoire and Betty Bender

OUTLINE

INTRODUCTION

The food production system for the future must be capable of delivering acceptable meals consistent with education, health, and nutrition goals to all children within the school district. The production system defines the parameters of all food offerings in the school's nutrition program. Menu development must recognize the adequacy of the facility design yet maximize the use of equipment and labor. More than 90 percent of the nation's elementary and secondary schools participate in the federally funded child nutrition programs that define national nutritional standards for meals served. The emphasis of the programs is to reach all students with nutritional meals and establish eating habits that will benefit them for life. In planning for the future it is imperative that school decision makers design a production system that will meet the goals of the district and the child nutrition program.

Many production systems currently in use were designed 25 or more years ago to meet the need of producing a school lunch that generally consisted of a single nonselective menu. Since that time student expectations have changed, research has identified the role of nutrition in physical and intellectual health, and more is known about how food behaviors are influenced. Publication of the *Dietary Guidelines for Americans* and subsequent federal and state legislation prompted schools to expand meal services and menu offerings to provide students regular access to healthful meals from a variety of foods. The school menu has grown from a single nonselective menu to one of multiple choices. Menus offer a variety of hot and cold foods, including multicultural menus that encourage students to eat a variety of foods and establish positive eating habits.

School nutrition programs in 94,000 schools have the potential of producing breakfast, lunch, after-school snacks, and supplemental food offerings, meals for young children in child care, children with disabilities, and those with special diet needs; and often provide catering services and a variety of other food offerings to more than 51 million children daily. The production system and the available labor force are major determinants of how well the school district can achieve its goal. Both have a major impact on financial and nutritional accountability as well as customer acceptance of the school meal offerings. The food production systems sets the parameters for variety, quantity, and quality of foods that are prepared and served. The production system must accommodate the range of services needed to meet the school and community needs.

Program goals, demographic considerations, financial parameters, and personnel factors combine to form the framework for determining the most appropriate food production system for a school district. The school food and nutrition director and designated school business official are challenged to identify program goals based on student and community needs and envision a production system to meet them. The production system is a long-term investment and should reflect the district's goals and plans for the future. There is no single best production system. The design of new or renovated production systems begins with clearly identified goals for the school food and nutrition program and the development of a strategy to meet them.

The purpose of this chapter is to provide information for consideration in designing and implementing a cost-effective food production and delivery system that will offer all children healthful and acceptable meals. This information will help identify factors to consider in selecting a food production system that will meet the needs today and in the future.

The specific objectives for this chapter are as follows:

- Identify the role of the food production system in meeting program goals and customer expectations.
- Identify competencies needed by the food service director/manager in designing and managing a food production system.

- Provide a conceptual framework for a food production system.
- Present an overview of different food production systems, including advantages and disadvantages of each.
- Discuss issues and strategies for designing and equipping food production systems for the future
- Identify design considerations, including ingredient control, storage, production, delivery service, and transportation

FOOD PRODUCTION SYSTEMS

The food production system is a vital component in the comprehensive performance plan of a school or school district in implementing its school food and nutrition program.[1] The food production system should be a reflection of the school board's philosophy for nutrition services in the district. The menu, food offerings, and services should determine the specific design of the system. High costs in the production area result from the following:

- Poor or no planning
- Overstaffing
- Poor employee training and instruction
- Poor or no written procedures
- Waiting for materials
- No internal monitoring or reviews

Requirements of the Food Production System

The food production system is the core function of food service operations. It should be designed to enhance the nutrition quality and customer acceptance of food.[2] Without the production and delivery of food, all other functions become meaningless. It is through the food production system that the school food and nutrition department meets the goals of providing healthful, acceptable meals for students. The food production system is a unique process of manufacturing a product to specifications in the desired quantity that controls costs and provides high-quality food.

In order to achieve these goals the production system

- must be efficiently designed and appropriately equipped
- should have dry, refrigerated, and freezer storage located appropriately with adequate space
- must include a storage and delivery system that is easily managed and capable of maintaining all products at the correct temperature and managed easily.

Competencies of the School Food and Nutrition Director/Manager

Effective management of the food production operation is one of the major responsibilities of school food and nutrition director/manager. Results[3-9] of several research studies indicate the importance of food and nutrition directors and managers being competent and knowledgeable in the areas of facility layout and equipment selection, food production, food safety, and financial management. School food and nutrition directors and managers should be skilled in these competencies to manage and direct school food and nutrition programs effectively. These competencies comprise the major portion of the workday of the school food and nutrition professional. Being proficient in the listed competencies indicates that the food service professional is capable of implementing a food production system that meets or exceeds the district goals.

Researchers at the National Food Service Management Institute[3-6,9] reported that the most important competencies performed by school food and nutrition program managers were monitoring food production, setting up and maintaining standards of control for food production, and monitoring and improving productivity. Competencies most important for directors included evaluating food quality, operating the department within budget, and assessing compliance with federal regulations.

The constant challenge faced by the school food and nutrition manager or director is to precost effectively and to produce acceptable, high-quality, nutritious, and appealing meals in a safe and sanitary manner. The importance of these efforts is clear in standards that are suggested for program success. The American School Food Service Association (ASFSA) published the Standards of Excellence in 1989. Many states also developed standards manuals. Reports of the development of some of these manuals have been published.[10–12] The National Food Service Management Institute (NFSMI) developed standards[13] to facilitate the implementation of the ASFSA nutrition integrity core concepts. These standards placed emphasis on the importance of menu planning, purchasing, production, and service. The ASFSA incorporated these nutrition integrity standards into a comprehensive document, *Keys to Excellence*,[14] which details specific quality goals for food and nutrition operations and includes a focus on the importance of production activities.

The production of food for students, staff, and visitors is a major responsibility of school food and nutrition managers and directors. This task is challenging because of the great variety of production systems that currently exist in school food and nutrition operations.

FUNCTIONS OF FOOD PRODUCTION SYSTEMS

Overview

Bobeng[15] published a model that identified processes in conventional, cook-chill, and cook-freeze food service systems that occurred between the initial procurement of food and supplies and service of meals. Bobeng's model was the first to illustrate processes common and unique to each system. Matthews[16] illustrated product flow in five types of food production systems: cook/serve, cook/chill, cook/freeze, thaw/heat/serve, and heat/serve. Product flow in each started with procurement and ended with service to the customer. The

number of steps varied from four in the heat/serve system to nine in the cook/freeze system.

Another approach to describing how food service systems differ was proposed by Escueta et al.[17] They classified activities into various stages and developed unique flowcharts depending on the particular activities that occurred in a given operation. Their classification scheme consisted of six components (purchasing, manipulation, processing, preservation, reheating, and distribution) which, when combined in various ways, explain the processes of any food service operation. Jones and Heulin[18] expanded this classification concept in their proposed flowchart, which included 10 stages (storage, preparation, production, holding, transportation, regeneration, service, dining, catering, and dishwashing). They combined these stages in various ways to characterize 10 generic food service systems.

The application of systems theory to a food and nutrition program operation was first introduced by Spears and Vaden[19]; a continued refinement of this model was detailed by Spears.[20] The food service systems model detailed input, transformation, and output components specific to a food service operation. This model did not characterize how operations using various production systems differed but rather provided a conceptual framework for components of a food service operation.

Gregoire and Nettles[21] and Greathouse and Gregoire[22] built on these previous models and developed a food and nutrition operations diagram to illustrate the major processes that can occur in food service operations preparing and serving food to hospital patients. This food service operations diagram has been modified for use in detailing the flow of product through school food service operations (Figure 14–1). The diagram includes all possible steps; the arrows designate the potential flow between each step. Every step does not occur in every school food service operation. The three key steps in every school food service operation are receiving–storage, production, and service. What oc-

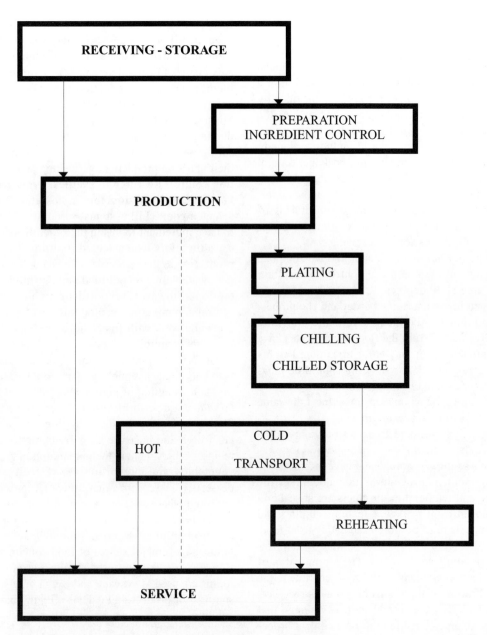

Figure 14–1 Flow of Food Products through School Food and Nutrition Operations from Receiving through Service. *Source:* Adapted from M.B. Gregoire and M.F. Nettles, Alternate Food Production Systems, in *Nutrition and Food Services for Integrated Health Care*, R. Jackson, ed., pp. 330–354, © 1997, Aspen Publishers, Inc.

curs between these three key steps differs depending on the specific operation at a particular school and/or district. This diagram will be used throughout this chapter to illustrate particular flow patterns for different types of operations.

Receiving and Storage

The production kitchen should have written procedures and forms for receiving products. The person receiving products should have a specific description of the product, the quantity ordered, and specific instructions such as the type of packaging or temperature requirements. The receiving form should include a place to verify quantity, temperature, package, time of delivery, and initials of the receiving personnel. The receiving process is one of the most important parts of food service management as it affects product quality and costs. Refer to Chapter 13 for discussion on receiving.

The dry storage area should have adequate airflow and temperature control to maintain the area at 70 degrees. Products should be arranged in predetermined order and should be a minimum of six inches from the wall and twelve inches from the floor. Some states have identified requirements for maximum heights for stacks. Racks or shelving should be movable for ease in cleaning. Central commissaries that store product on skids must meet the same air and sanitation requirements.

Refrigeration and freezer storage areas require the same airflow and sanitation requirements as for dry storage and have the added requirement of procedures that document the time and temperature products are stored and removed from storage. Cleaning supplies and chemicals must be stored separately from food, but the same airflow and sanitation requirements apply in this area. The storage area of production kitchens is highly susceptible to the infiltration of insects from products received, particularly paper products. It is essential that storage areas have regular pest control procedures in place.

Preparation and Ingredient Control

Once food has been received into a food service operation, ingredient control becomes an issue that is important regardless of the type of food production system. Effective utilization of a centralized ingredient room has been identified as a cost-effective measure for food and nutrition directors to implement.[23] Advantages to central assembly of ingredients include increased production control, quality control, and improved security.[23] According to Spears,[24] employing less costly employees to do simple tasks such as assembling and measuring ingredients allows cooks to concentrate their skills on production, garnishing, and portion control. Research by Nettles,[25] however, has indicated that directors in hospitals who selected cook-chill systems were more likely to have ingredient rooms in their facilities than were directors who selected traditional food production systems. Similar published data are not available for school food and nutrition operations; however, school districts utilizing central commissaries, central kitchens, or bakeries and cook-chill/freeze have implemented ingredient control.

The primary function of the ingredient room is to coordinate assembly, preparation, measuring, and weighing of ingredients.[26] The actual tasks that are performed in this area vary from facility to facility. In some facilities, employees weigh and measure all ingredients for all recipes; others include the preparation of fresh vegetables and preportioning of fruit and desserts.[27–30] Facilities that utilize an ingredient room where staff prepare and portion fresh products are able to reduce contamination in the production area. Fresh products, such as lettuce, are a major source of food contamination in a production area. Some ingredient rooms are used to measure and weigh only seasonings for production kitchens utilizing batch cooking.

Food Production

Definitions first proposed by Unklesby et al. in 1977[31] are commonly used as a means of grouping food production systems. A conceptual framework of the food and nutrition industry was developed that categorized food and nutrition systems as conventional, commissary, ready food, and assembly-serve. The way food production was conducted in schools across the country was fairly consistent until research in the 1960s [32-35] introduced ideas that dramatically changed the process.

Food Service Systems

Conventional: Often referred to as traditional or on-site preparation. Food is prepared and served at the same site.

Commissary: A central facility that prepares food for a number of schools and other outlets and transports it to a number of sites. The receiving schools are referred to as satellites or receiving schools. Food may be transported in bulk, preplated or partially prepared. The receiving school may have either a finishing kitchen or a receiving kitchen.

Ready food: Includes cook-chill, cook-freeze, and *sous vide*. In these, menu items are always stored and ready for final assembly and/or reheating.

Assembly-serve: Sometimes called convenience food. Food arrives in the facility ready to serve. May be used in both on-site and commissary systems. When used in a contral production facility, food is packaged for delivery to sites.

Base: A base food production systems is housed in a school where food is prepared and served on-site and also transported for service to one or more sites. The receiving sites are referred to as satellites.

Traditional food production remains the most prevalent in school food and nutrition programs. It was reported in 1993[36] that 45 percent of major city directors were using traditional food production, 49 percent used a combination of traditional and convenience, and less than 5 percent used cook-chill. The central production preplated meal facility was not reported. The traditional or conventional food service system has three major steps, as shown in Figure 14–2. Food is prepared and held until serving.[37] Making an appropriate selection of a food production system requires an understanding of the advantages and disadvantages of each type (Exhibit 14–1).

The traditional on-site production kitchen offers greater flexibility in food preparation. The emphasis can be on batch cooking rather than cook-and-hold procedures. The holding time for cooked and prepared products is less than that of other food production systems, thereby increasing the freshness of the product for the customer. The on-site production kitchen has the capability of customizing service if needed. The conventional production kitchen, when equipped properly, can produce all food products without the quality and temperature constraints of holding foods. The disadvantages of the conventional production kitchen are increased labor hours, the cost of space and equipment, and increased amount of supervision required.

Research of the 1960s led to modifications in this traditional process by introducing cook-chill and cook-freeze technology as a way to prepare and chill or freeze food at one location or one point in time and then reheat foods closer to the point of service, thus reducing hot holding time (see Figure 14–3).

Commissary systems are defined as those with a centralized food procurement and production function with distribution of prepared menu items to several remote locations for final preparation and service. Most menu items are processed completely in the central facility and then are transported in a heated or chilled state to satellite units. Commissary systems are used by some school food and nutrition program directors as an opportunity to expand their services and to become a revenue-generating center providing food for other school districts, day-care centers, and other facilities.[38-40] Operating a commissary kitchen requires attention to three subsystems—production, distribution, and service at a remote site.

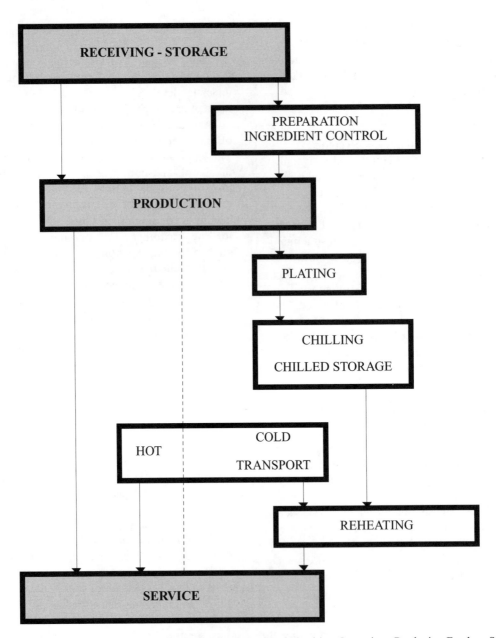

Figure 14–2 Flow of Food Products through School Food and Nutrition Operations Producing Food on Site for Immediate Service. *Source:* Adapted from M.B. Gregoire and M.F. Nettles, Alternate Food Production Systems, in *Nutrition and Food Services for Integrated Health Care*, R. Jackson, ed., pp. 330–354, © 1997, Aspen Publishers, Inc.

In commissary systems such as the ones operated in Dayton and Olatha public schools,[41] the production and service of food are con- ducted in separate facilities. A modification of this concept is the "central or base kitchen." This production unit, which is located in a

Exhibit 14–1 The Conventional Food Service System

ADVANTAGES	DISADVANTAGES
• Schools are not dependent on other sites for food.	• Requires more skilled employees.
• The system is more responsive to school preferences and customer wants.	• Cost of labor may be higher and meals per labor hour less.
• The system provides for more flexibility in offering choices.	• Requires space and fully equipped kitchen.
• Food is prepared nearer time of service and appears fresher; holding time for food is less.	• Quality varies from school to school.
• Preparation facilities are available for community use.	
• The kitchen facility provides a laboratory for food experiences for students.	

Source: Reprinted with permission from D.V. Pannell-Martin, *School Foodservice Management*, 5th Ed., p. 150, © 1999, InTEAM Associates, Inc.

school with facilities, produces food for on-site service as well as for transporting to other schools. In some school districts, food is prepared at a central commissary and then shipped in bulk to individual schools. At other schools the food is plated at the central commissary prior to shipping individual schools (Figure 14–4).

The advantages and disadvantages of central commissaries vary with each system. The central commissary that produces preplated meals similar to commercial TV dinners is equipped with automated equipment and is less labor intensive than the conventional production facility. Depending on the packaging equipment available, products must be one specific size to be placed in the packaging container. The types of food and the consistency of food limit the food combinations placed in the same container. The central production kitchen producing preplated meals is structured to maximize production and packaging equipment. This limits the flexibility of the types of products produced and may require the purchase of convenience food products, which increase food costs. The menu is limited as a result of cost and availability of product. The advantage to the central food production system is reduced labor cost, reduced waste, and reduced cost of cleaning and sanitation.

Schools receiving food from a commissary or central kitchen often are termed *satellite schools* or *receiving schools*. A satellite school is defined as one in which foods are prepared at a central kitchen and transported, either hot or cold, to another kitchen.[42] Variations of the satellite concept include the satellite finishing kitchen. The finishing kitchen has limited equipment, usually only refrigeration, storage, and an oven and steamer for reheating foods or cooking foods that do not transport well such as vegetables.[43] Due to the inability to maintain food quality of some products when shipped hot, the finishing kitchen may include fryers, ventilating, and a ventilating hood. A dishmachine, triple and double sinks, and disposals also are available on site for warewashing. This type of finishing kitchen must also be stocked with pans and cooking utensils.

A distinct feature of ready-food systems, which include cook-chill, cook-freeze, and *sous vide*, is that menu items are always stored and ready for final assembly and/or heating. Foods are produced in quantities needed to meet inventory levels rather than daily customer counts. In ready-food systems hot food items go through a second heat processing before being served. In cook-chill operations, foods are partially heat processed, chilled either in serving pans in a blast chiller or in bags

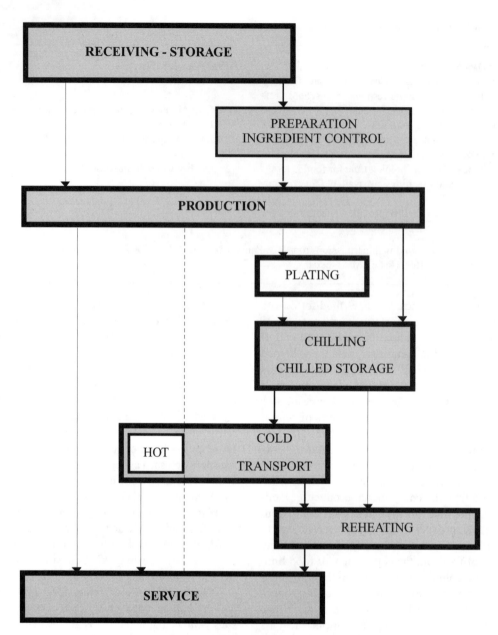

Figure 14–3 Flow of Food Products through School Food and Nutrition Operations Using an Ingredient Room, Cook-Chill Production, Bulk Transport, and Reheating prior to Service. *Source:* Adapted from M.B. Gregoire and M.F. Nettles, Alternate Food Production Systems, in *Nutrition and Food Services for Integrated Health Care*, R. Jackson, ed., pp. 330–354, © 1997, Aspen Publishers, Inc.

in a tumble chiller, and then stored in refrigerators for 5 (panned and blast chilled) to 40 (bagged and tumble chilled) days. Two examples of the flow in cook-chill systems are shown in Figures 14–3 and 14–4. In Figure 14–3, food is produced, chilled in bulk, trans-

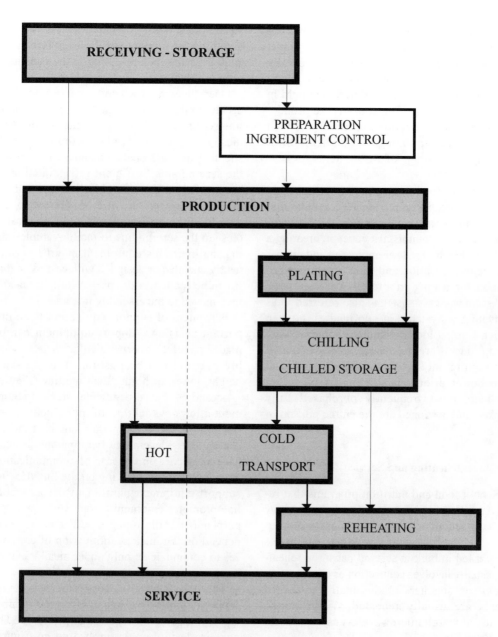

Figure 14–4 Flow of Food Products through School Food and Nutrition Operations Producing Products and Portioning and Distributing Products in a Central Facility. *Source:* Adapted from M.B. Gregoire and M.F. Nettles, Alternate Food Production Systems, in *Nutrition and Food Services for Integrated Health Care*, R. Jackson, ed., pp. 330–354, © 1997, Aspen Publishers, Inc.

ported, and then reheated prior to service. Figure 14–4 illustrates the production, plating, chilling, distribution, and reheating of food at the service site.

Sous vide differs somewhat from cook-chill in that raw foods are placed in special bags that are vacuum sealed. The foods then are partially or fully cooked in low-temperature circulating water and rapidly cooled before being held in refrigerated storage. The cook-freeze production system involves partial processing of food items, panning or plating of food items, blast freezing, and storage of frozen items for several weeks.[44–47]

Cook-chill food production systems are becoming more prevalent in large school districts. This type of production usually is combined with the commissary concept, creating a system whereby foods are prepared and chilled at a central location and then transported to schools for heating prior to service.

Assembly-serve systems, also referred to as convenience systems, are defined as those in which limited food production occurs. Many food products are purchased already prepared and require only portioning, packaging, and distribution prior to heating and service.[46,47] Products most frequently purchased fully cooked and portioned are the entree portion of the meal.

Product Reheating and Service

School food and nutrition programs that receive chilled food from a central commissary or base school will need appropriate equipment to reheat food on site. When food items are chilled in bulk in serving pans, the reheating usually involves convection or combination ovens or steamers. Individually packaged meals are usually reheated in convection ovens, although microwave ovens sometimes are used.

Products that were bagged and chilled can be reheated in several ways. The bags of product can be placed in steam-jacketed kettles of boiling water for heating; once heated, the product can be transferred to a steam table for service. The contents of the bags can be emptied directly into steam-jacketed kettles or tilting fry pans, reheated, and then transferred to steam table pans. A final method involves emptying the contents of the bags into steam table pans and then reheating in the pans in an oven or steamer.

Operations that use central packaging of individual meals usually have a meal assembly line set up for packaging the meals. Because these meals are nearly always transported off site, they are packaged cold and are reheated at the serving site. Sufficient refrigerated units are needed on the assembly line to maintain the proper temperature of food. Most food service facilities will have refrigerators located close to the serving line to facilitate replenishing the line. This equipment may be permanently installed or designed with casters so that it can be loaded in the preparation areas and then moved to the assembly line area.

Placement of support equipment is an important decision. Support equipment can be placed parallel or perpendicular to the assembly line and can be positioned at the same height, lower, or higher than the line (Figures 14–5 and 14–6). Perpendicular support equipment allows availability of more menu items without adding to the overall length of the assembly line. Placement of equipment also can have an impact on the ease of communication among employees working on the line. Having support equipment parallel to the assembly line promotes communication, while having it perpendicular discourages it. The choice may depend on the internal motivation of employees to communicate only about meal assembly issues as they arise.

The use of parallel versus perpendicular support equipment also can affect the number and type of motions required of personnel. The goal in designing assembly-line configurations, the layout of the support equipment, and the placement of the dishes and supplies should be to minimize the number of turns and reaches the employees will need to make while assembling meals.

Several types of conveyor belts are available for use. Some are mechanized, others are not. Powered conveyors move trays by means of a

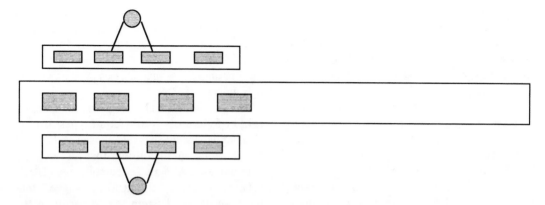

Figure 14–5 Example of a Parallel Placement of Support Equipment

mechanized belt. The belt may be a solid fabric or made of slats or chains. Slat-and-chain belts have the advantage of being able to negotiate corners so that different configurations can be accomplished. Bandveyor belts are four continuous bands that run vertically the length of the assembly line. They are the least expensive to purchase and have lower maintenance costs. However, they work only with full-sized trays; they are not appropriate for use with small individual food containers.

The multienergy cooking tunnel is a new concept in bulk reheating.[48] The tunnel uses four different forms of energy transfer (microwave, low-pressure steam, forced-air convection, infrared), separately or in combination depending on the product being processed. The rationale for each form of energy use is that the microwaves will ensure rapid cooking to the center of the product, low-pressure steam will provide moisture to preserve the color and nutrient content while reducing weight loss,

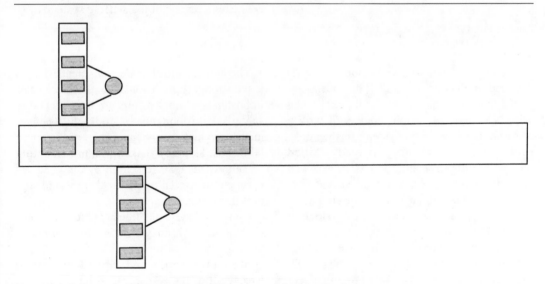

Figure 14–6 Example of a Perpendicular Placement of Support Equipment

forced-air convection provides crispness and deep browning, and infrared allows rapid surface cooking and browning. The oven can be preprogrammed for a particular food item to ensure the appropriate amount of energy from each source.

School food and nutrition directors are faced with many issues when deciding how best to prepare food for service to the students. Key factors that should be considered in this decision are menu and food offerings; customer preferences and acceptance; cost of food, labor, and supplies; distribution of product; availability of skilled labor; flexibility of production scheduling; service temperature of food; microbiological safety; sensory quality; nutrient retention; equipment required; and energy use.

FOOD SERVICE PRODUCTION ISSUES

A comparison of the impact of the four production systems on production issues will be useful in selecting a new or renovated production system. Among issues to be discussed include cost of food, cost of labor, cost of supplies, skill level of available labor, and production scheduling.

Cost of Food

Authors vary in their beliefs as to whether differences in food cost exist among the various food production systems. It has been suggested that food cost savings will occur when using a cook-chill system compared with a conventional production system. In the cook-chill system, an inventory of ready-chilled food is maintained and food is used when needed; therefore less food is wasted.[49–51] Durocher[51] also suggests that cooking food products such as meats in bags, as is done in some cook-chill operations, reduces the shrinkage in those products. However, cooking and then bagging food products can negatively affect yield. Average losses of 10 to 20 percent

are found in food products that are cooked in large steam-jacketed kettles, pumped into bags, reheated in bulk, transferred to steam table pans, and held hot on steam table lines; the amount of loss increases as product viscosity increases.

Most of the research addressing the comparison of food costs for different types of food production systems has been based on hospital food service, and results of this research are contradictory. Although predictive models[52–54] have been developed that would suggest that the cook-freeze system would result in the lowest hospital meal cost, research[55-58] has failed to support food cost savings for either cook-freeze or cook-chill systems when compared with conventional production systems.

School food and nutrition directors and managers operating base kitchens with satellite receiving kitchens have been able to maintain the low food cost reflected in the traditional food service operation. The highest food costs are found in convenience systems, where all food products are purchased ready to serve. This higher cost results from having the production labor, packaging, and other costs incorporated into the selling price of the food products. The use of ready-to-serve foods necessitates a review of the staffing system.

Cost of Labor

The number of full-time equivalents (FTEs) is the strongest predictor of food service costs in hospitals; similar results are likely found in schools.[59] Proponents of cook-chill convenience production systems report reduction in labor cost as a key reason for implementing these systems.[60–66] Research by the U.S. Department of Agriculture and others would support this claim.[67,68]

Cook-chill systems often are able to run production as a Monday through Friday, eight-hour-a-day operation because food is being cooked in quantity and chilled or frozen. Nearly all of the research that has addressed the cost of labor has focused on hospital food service operations, which usually operate a kitchen 12 or more hours a day, seven days a week. Because schools currently operate kitchens for fewer hours each day and for only five days a week, the expected labor savings by implementing a cook-chill operation may not be as substantial as that reported in hospitals. Another difference betweeen hospital food service and school food service is the length of time the customer is served by the system. There is less likelihood that the hospital patient will become bored with the food than the school customer, who is in school for 180 days each year and in the building for several years.

Most school districts using a cook-chill systems have one large production facility in which food is prepared and then shipped to numerous schools. Directors considering implementation of a central production facility should evaluate carefully total labor needs, including the finishing kitchen requirements, to determine whether labor savings will occur.

Time spent cleaning cook-chill equipment is another issue that can affect labor cost.[69] Hospital food service directors have indicated that more labor hours are spent on sanitation activities such as cleaning additional equipment used in cook-chill production. One director indicated that sanitation represented 20 percent to 25 percent of the labor hours in the cook-chill area, because staff had to pay more attention to the cleanliness of production equipment. The University of Iowa Hospitals and Clinics[70] provided guidelines for cleaning the kettles, food hoses, and bag filler outlets in their cook-chill operation. Their guidelines indicated that cleaning kettles between products can take 5 to 35 minutes depending on the product, and cleaning at the end of the day takes at least two hours.

Cook-chill and convenience systems maintain an inventory of prepared food items. Monitoring, rotating, and managing this inventory can require additional labor. Colleges and universities using convenience products, when compared with conventional, cook-chill, and cook-freeze systems, were unable to demonstrate a total labor cost saving.[71] A study by the Department of Veterans Affairs[72] in 1993 indicated that there appeared to be no guarantee of labor savings when using a cook-chill rather than conventional system.

The central commissary using convenience preportioned entree is able to demonstrate increased productivity to offset the higher food cost of convenience foods. Cleaning of the facility, sanitizing of equipment, and trash removal are less than 10 percent of the cost of operation and the work hours assigned to the central facility. A facility using a combination of convenience foods and traditional preparation methods is able to produce as many as 90 to 100 meals per work hour when all production, warehouse, janitorial, and supervisory labor hours are included in the calculation. When this labor productivity is blended with the labor in the finishing kitchen at the serving site, it is possible to achieve 30 to 35 meals per work hour productivity. The use of automated equipment in production and packaging functions is a major factor in reducing labor cost.

Cost of Supplies

Very little has been written about the cost of supplies in the various production systems. Supplies that are unique to particular systems include disposable bags/casing and tipper ties for some forms of cook-chill systems, and disposable serving dishes and covers or plastic wrap for individually plated items in cook-chill or cook-freeze systems. It has been suggested that the cost of packaging supplies can be 20 to 25 percent higher in cook-chill operations compared with conventional production systems using permanent serving trays, dishes, and utensils.

When the cost of water, dishwashing chemicals, and replacement equipment is included in the calculation, the cost of an all disposable system does not exceed the traditional food service operation by more than 10 percent.

Skill Level of Available Labor

Another positive outcome cited for use of convenience and cook-chill systems compared to conventional systems is the reduction in number of skilled employees[73–75] needed because food services using these systems typically operate a production unit for fewer hours in a week than do conventional operations. Research is limited, however, comparing the actual number of skilled employees needed for each type of production system. Results of a research study conducted in the United Kingdom[76] indicated that the cook-chill operations that were most successful actually had an increase in skill level of employees because of recipe development, temperature, and microbiological controls.

Operating a cook-chill or preplate system does not mean that there is no need for skilled employees. Development of recipes that will produce a quality product, monitoring of microbiological issues, and rotation of items in chilled storage are but a few of the specialized skills needed in addition to the traditional preparation skills. The need for skilled production employees is probably least in operations using total convenience systems. Such systems require limited preparation, usually only reheating of product at the school site. School production facilities using a combination convenience and traditional system require skilled employees, standardized recipes, and menu development that combines foods correctly. The combination foods from the two systems present special problems when packaging food components in the same package for delivery off site. Exceptional menu development skills are needed to achieve quality at time of service when the combination systems are used, as packaging and delivery present unique challenges. The labor market for attaining and maintaining employees is a major consideration when planning either renovation of existing food service facilities or designing new ones.

Production Scheduling

In *conventional systems*, all food items needed for a meal are generally prepared or finished on the day of service. Production is geared to having food ready for service once or twice a day with peak periods of activity. Daily adjustments in recipes and forecast quantities are common, based on student census. Batch-cooking, used to have food prepared just in time for each serving period, reduces the amount of holding time for each food item and control leftovers.

Production scheduling is another often cited advantage for use of cook-chill and convenience systems.[77–81] Production scheduling for *cook-chill systems* is quite different. Production is not linked to the service process, thus the peaks and valleys of activity are reduced or eliminated. Not all food items on a menu are prepared each day; rather production is planned to meet inventory levels. Large quantities of fewer items are produced each day. Cook-chill technology cannot be used for all items on the menu. A discussion of the items that can be appropriately prepared using cook-chill technology is included under the section on menu development.

Total *convenience systems* usually require limited production scheduling. Since convenience items need only to be heated, production scheduling focuses on the utilization of labor for packaging and production. Convenience systems with limited production require carefully planned or engineered menus in order to control labor cost. Menus that require production must be automated when packaging. Menus that require employees on the packaging line cannot require production employees. Labor cost control cannot be achieved without carefully engineered menus. Quality meals cannot be produced unless careful attention to food combinations is in place. There cannot be transfer of odor, moisture, or taste in any sealed package if the meal is to be of high quality and acceptable to students.

Central commissaries using a mixture of convenience foods require careful scheduling of production. In a large central kitchen facility a simple production process such as opening and disposing of cans is a major operation. If more than one item on the menu is a canned product, the workload in the preparation area cannot be achieved with the normal number of personnel and work hours. For example, if the facility normally averages 200 cases of product to be opened each day, a major increase of personnel time for opening of cans and trash disposal is required when two canned items, such as baked beans and applesauce are scheduled. Menus must be carefully engineered to maximize the use of labor and equipment while producing highly acceptable nutritious meals.

Food Service Equipment

Food service equipment needs will differ based on the type of food production system used. A food service consultant can guide the school food and nutrition director in determining the specific equipment requirements for the proposed food production system. Equipment should be selected and sized based on an analysis of the menus to be offered and the number of servings to be prepared in each facility. Several textbooks contain information that can assist food service managers with equipment selection decisions. [182-87]

In conventional kitchens, the equipment should be selected based on the menu, method of preparation, and production of food items. Many school food and nutrition operations use batch-cooking concepts where smaller quantities of food products are prepared closer to the time of service. Use of such batch-cooking techniques can decrease the size of equipment needed and thus the capital expenditure required. Space requirements for this equipment also may be reduced. The types of equipment needed could include walk-in refrigerators and

freezers, ovens (convection, combination convection oven/steamer, deck revolving, roll-in, conveyor, microwave), steam-jacketed kettles, steamers (pressure, convection, combination convection oven/steamer), tilting fry pans, ranges, griddles/grills, fryers, and/or food warmers. Innovations in production equipment include the development of hot air impingement/jet sweep ovens, infrared light ovens, combination ovens/steamers, microwave hotair convection ovens, multienergy cooking tunnels, and direct steam-heating kettles.[88-90]

A cook-chill system has many of the same pieces of cooking equipment that are found in conventional kitchens. Since food is not served the same day it is prepared, specialized chilling equipment is needed. Systems using blast chilling will need to have a large supply of steam table pans because products are prepared and stored for several days. Facilities utilizing the tumble-chill type of cook-chill will have some special production equipment. Steam-jacketed kettles in sizes ranging from 50 to 200 gallons are equipped with automatic temperature controls that ensure uniform cooking of the entire batch of food. Recording temperature gauges maintains a time-temperature record for every batch. To further ensure even cooking, the kettle is equipped with a mechanical agitator arm that is activated during cooking yet will not damage delicate items. An airoperated three-inch draw-off valve works with a pump-fill station to rapidly transfer preset amounts of product from the kettle into plastic casings. Filled casings are immediately loaded into a tumble chiller to allow for rapid chilling of the product.

Water-filled cook tanks often are used to cook meat and poultry products in cook-chill operations. Using this technique, pieces of meat are placed in multilayered bags and vacuum sealed prior to cooking. Cook tanks use direct steam as a heat source and can be set to cook overnight during off-peak utility hours to effect energy savings. During cooking, the water temperature is maintained between 150 and 175 degrees Fahrenheit. At the end of the cook cycle, the hot water is drained and re-placed with chilled water, which stops the cooking process and rapidly drops the temper-ature of meat before it is refrigerated.

The costs of production equipment and re-frigeration for cook-chill operations are usu-ally 15 percent to 20 percent more than those required for a conventional production opera-tion.[91] The cost of energy in a cook-chill oper-ation usually is higher when compared with conventional systems.

Total convenience systems using prepared products usually require limited production equipment. Often the only production equip-ment needed at the receiving site are refrigera-tors for storage, automatic can openers, ovens for reheating products prior to service, and steamers for cooking vegetables.

The large central kitchen using both pre-pared and nonprepared foods requires auto-matic can openers, mixers, kettles that will both cook and cool, transfer pumps and tubes for moving product, special equipment for use when packaging food, ovens for baking, dish-machines, disposals, packaging equipment, special pumps and fillers, and refrigeration for storage before shipping and reheating the product at the satellite operation. All equip-ment should be portable, if possible, and easily cleaned and sanitized. Containers such as bas-kets that are used to deliver food to the satellite location must be washed and sanitized daily. Regular testing for bacteria is a standard pro-cedure in central production facilities.

Energy

Energy use is another consideration in the selection of a food service system. Energy has been categorized in food service operations into direct and indirect energy expenditures. Direct energy includes the energy used to store, heat, cook, package, reheat, distribute, and serve food. Indirect energy is used to sup-port other functions and includes waste dis-posal, sanitation, and maintenance of optimal work environment. Many school food service

operations are now expected to pay for indirect energy cost in both central facilities and satel-lite locations.

The importance of conserving energy use was widely discussed during the 1970s and early 1980s. Research during that time focused on energy use for cooking and holding equip-ment. Food service equipment was redesigned to minimize energy usage. Features added in-cluded solid-state controls to allow for pro-grammed cooking times; reduced equipment size to minimize energy use; and use of multi-ple-energy sources such as hot air jets, mi-crowave, and electromagnetic induction to de-crease cooking times and energy use.[92-94] It has been suggested that eliminating the pre-heating of ovens could result in 10 percent to 15 percent energy savings for the operation without negatively impacting on food qual-ity.[93,94] Energy consumption increases as the oven load increases. A fully loaded oven re-sults in higher energy savings per serving than a partially loaded oven.[95,96] Energy consump-tion during the holding of hot products was not affected by the quantity of food being held.

Several studies have been conducted to ex-amine energy use of the various food produc-tions.[97,98] Energy consumption is influenced by the thermostat setting, the quantity and den-sity of product prepared at one time, the length of the heat-processing period, and the type of equipment used. The cost of electricity is mini-mal for chilling, freezing, holding under re-frigeration, and reheating foods in ready pro-duction systems.

Contradictory findings have been reported from studies examining whether energy use differed in conventional and ready food sys-tems.[99-101] Studies indicate that cook-chill and cook-freeze systems require more energy use. There appears to be little difference in energy use between cook-chill and conventional sys-tems. The differences are the results of the menus produced and the scheduled production.

Conservation of energy is an important con-sideration for the environment and for the food service budget. The cost of energy is considered minor compared to food and labor costs within an organization. However energy costs are important and should be monitored regularly. Energy conservation should be one of the primary goals of a food service operation. There are publications which assist school food service directors monitor and conserve energy.[100–106]

Menu Development

The menu should drive the food production system. However, the type of food production system must be considered when determining foods offered on a menu. Many food products that can be prepared and served on site in a conventional system are not suitable for preparation in cook-chill, convenience, or central production systems for transport to other sites. This fact should be considered in planning a new or renovated food production system.

The development of the menu as discussed in Chapter 10 is the key to cost-effective, high-quality, nutritious food production. Menus should be engineered to maximize the use of personnel and equipment. Although many of the same ingredients and products can be used in different menu items, it is the correct combination of these products that maintains cost control and maximum efficiency. Each menu should be evaluated for labor intensity. It is not practical to have all foods on any one day have the same preparation procedures regardless of food production system. The goal should be to maximize both personnel and equipment by developing a menu that provides an even flow of work with effective use of equipment.

When developing a menu for cook-chill or convenience systems, each will have to include items in the menu that can best be prepared in that system. Products such as soups, sauces, casseroles, gravies, and meats can be prepared using cook-chill technology, and the majority of hospital food service directors who have cook-chill operations indicate using it for these products.[107,108] In facilities that use cook-tumble chill technology, menu items must be

"pumpable" to move from the kettle into the plastic casings or from the filler into the packaging pan. This limits the food items that can be processed. Foods that usually are not prepared using cook-chill technology include fried foods, vegetables, sandwiches, bakery items, egg dishes such as omelets, and breakfast items such as waffles or French toast. Convenience systems can package successfully precooked meats, vegetables, sandwiches, bakery items, and breakfast items such as waffles and French toast.

In developing the menu in food service systems that preplate foods, it is important to consider the transfer of odor and moisture of products when packaging two or more items in one container. An example would be the packaging of an unwrapped bread product with an unwrapped cookie. The moisture transfer will make the bread stale and cookie soggy; therefore, it is necessary that one of the products be wrapped or that a barrier be placed between the two products.

Facilities transporting foods have menu considerations as well. Food items that are transported hot need to be able to withstand being held at 165 degrees Fahrenheit without a reduction in food quality. Products that do not maintain quality well during hot transport include selected cooked vegetables, grilled sandwiches, and the like. All vehicles used for transporting either hot or cold food must be properly constructed to maintain appropriate/safe temperatures and meet sanitation standards.

Food Quality

Food quality is probably the most highly debated issue in comparing food production systems. Some authors[109,110] support the use of cook-chill technology because standardized recipes are used. Food is produced in uniformly controlled batches, and small amounts of food can be reheated closer to the point of service that prevents long holding times.

Assessment of food quality is not only a system selection question but a continuous quality improvement issue. Food quality is affected by the recipes used and the quality of the ingredients. Evaluation of food quality requires standards for each product served and a systematic process for evaluating food items to see that standards were met. Teaching food production personnel to use a scorecard regularly for each product will promote consistency of product regardless of the food production system used. Standards for food items have been published that can be used or adapted for use in school food and nutrition operations.[111–113]

Having food quality standards eliminates managers' and employees' judging food products acceptable one day and unacceptable the next. Food standards are an objective measure of what a school food and nutrition team believes is desirable for service to its clientele. Use of cook-chill or convenience systems may require two standards for a food product, one for the quality as it leaves the production process, another reflecting quality after reheating at the service site.

Although a test kitchen is desirable for any production system, it is more frequently used in districts utilizing a central production system because considerable time must be spent in recipe modifications to achieve quality food products. Seasoning levels, percentages of liquid versus solid ingredients, shapes, thickness, and product consistency can be affected by the chilling and reheating processes. The dietary department of the University of Iowa Hospitals and Clinics[114] published information on problem solving in cook-chill recipe production and included several recipes that had been developed for their cook-chill operation.

The acceptance of food by the customer is the ultimate measure of quality. *The customer is interested in the quality of the product not the type of food production system.* The school food and nutrition director/manager must consider the variety of products to be offered and the customer acceptance of food offered when

making the decision about the food production system.

Food Safety

Food safety is an issue for all school food and nutrition operations regardless of the type of food production system being used. The importance of thoroughly cooking and cooling food and preventing food contamination cannot be emphasized too much.[115–117] Food safety concerns are particularly important in cook-chill systems because of the additional critical control points introduced by the chilling and reheating of food items. Conventional food production systems typically have six major stages that require risk evaluation; ready-prepared systems may have as many as eleven stages.

Some of the studies conducted in actual operations or in simulated operations indicate that microbial quality appears to be dependent on issues such as type of food, quality of raw ingredients, batch size, type of equipment used for cooking, type of food-handling procedures established, and the position of the food item in cooking equipment.[118–120] Management of time-temperature relationships throughout all processes is critical. Improper cooling has been identified as the most frequent cause of outbreaks of foodborne diseases.[121,122] The 1997 Food Code requires that cooked, potentially hazardous food be cooled from 140 degrees Fahrenheit to 70 degrees Fahrenheit within two hours and from 70 degrees Fahrenheit to 41 degrees Fahrenheit or below within four hours.

Research in hospitals indicates that the appropriate safe temperature in cook-chill systems is not always maintained. After tracking the internal items of 93 food items, only a few were found to be in the recommended temperature range at meal assembly.[123]

A food safety program incorporating concepts such as hazard analysis critical control points (HACCP) as presented in Chapter 18 should be established in each school food and nutrition program operation to assure food safety. Critical control points in food service systems are storage and ingredient control; equipment sanitation; personnel sanitation; and time and temperature.[124] The 1997 Food Code, issued by the U.S. Public Health Service, defines several HACCP principles and describes how to implement these principles.

School food and nutrition operations using convenience or cook-chill technology need to consider microbiological testing of product samples. There are increased safety concerns for food items prepared in cook-chill operations that pass through the temperature danger zone several times and often are held for extended periods of time.[125–127] Microbiological testing can be expensive. A report by the Department of Veterans Affairs indicates costs could be $100 or more per sample if testing includes total plate count anaerobic organisms, *Clostridium perfringens, Escherichia coli,* and *Listeria monocytogenes.* Certified local laboratories will usually test for *E. coli, Salmonella*, total plate count, and *Staphylococcus* coagulase positive for $30.00 or less.

Transportation

The transportation of food whether hot or cold must be handled carefully. Equipment selected should allow easy movement of food products, exact temperature control, and ease in cleaning and sanitizing. The traditional production kitchen moves product short distances and usually requires hot carts and refrigeration for short periods of holding product. The production kitchen that produces either hot or cold food products for finishing kitchens should select equipment with the capability of retaining food temperatures with less than 10 degrees variation for a minimum of two hours or a maximum of six hours. The equipment selected should be easily cleaned and sanitized, and should transport with minimum difficulty. All baskets and containers must fit the trans-

port cart. The transport cart should fit the truck or van carrying the products to an off-site location, and refrigeration units and ovens should be made to fit the transport dollies. The less movement of individual product, the least spillage, the minimum labor hours, and the fewer pieces of equipment to clean.

Factors that must be considered by central commissaries and central kitchens utilizing trucks for delivery include the following:

- Carts or dollies of product sized to fit the inside bed of the truck
- Inside measurements of the truck that allow stacking of product in such a manner that product will not spill and will allow easy rotation of product and empty containers
- Refrigerated truck with thermometers built into the interior front, rear, and near each opening. The driver should be able to read the temperature of each thermometer from the outside of the truck
- Tailgates that both lift and lower
- Depending upon the difficulty of the delivery entrance, special ramps may be needed

Measures of Operational Efficiency

Efficiency of school food and nutrition program operations can be measured in several ways. All measurements, however, involve some comparison of input to output. Efficiency measures of the meal preparation or assembly process reflect use of resources (employee work hours or number) to produce an output (meals). The food and nutrition program should establish a standard for these efficiency measures so that a comparison of actual performance to this standard can be made. School food and nutrition directors, managers, and employees need to know methods of measuring and monitoring factors that have an impact on productivity and methods to enhance productivity if they are to increase efficiency and productivity.[128]

Efficiency of the meal preparation or assembly often is measured by calculating a ratio of the amount of time spent preparing or assembling meals to the number of meals produced or assembled. Common calculations include meals per minute or minutes per meal. Labor time to produce a reimbursable meal ranges from 2.69 to 16.52 minutes with a mean of 7.16 minutes.[129] It is recommended that the mean time plus or minus one standard deviation be used as a standard for school food and nutrition program operations. The most common method used by schools for calculating efficiency of meal preparation is meals produced per labor hour. This calculation is derived from the number of full meals and the number of meal equivalents[130] divided by the number of hours assigned. (A meal equivalent is defined as two reimbursable breakfasts and/or $2.00 in supplemental food sales.) Since implementation of "offer versus serve" a more equitable method to allocate labor in schools is based on the number of food servings produced.[131] The range of servings of food per labor hour ranges from 56 to 90 with a mean of 71 (see Table 14–1, Sample Staffing Guidelines).

FACILITY DESIGN AND EQUIPMENT SELECTION

The impact of facility design and equipment selection is an ongoing cost to the food service operation.[132] When designing a kitchen facility and selecting equipment, it is critical to have clearly stated production goals and proposed menus available. School food and nutrition directors and managers need to consider the child nutrition and food service programs in which the district currently participates as well as future programs. In addition to operating the current programs, which include NSLP, SBP, after-school snacks, and à la carte programs, the food service operation may be expanded to include summer food service programs, supplmenetal feeding programs, day care for children and adults, catering, special diets, and year-round school programs—all factors that will make a major impact on the space required for storage, production and service, as well as equipment selection and layout. Traditionally most school food and nutrition programs have operated only eight hours per day, 180 days per year. In the future there is the possibility that schools will be year round and other community services may use the facility when it is not in use for school meal purposes.

With back-to-work programs of the federal government, some secondary schools are offering culinary training using the school meal facility after school hours.

In designing a new facility or updating an existing facility, the food service director/manager must be aware of available utilities and the cost of increasing or changing the existing utilities. The layout of the kitchen facility should reflect supervisory controls, work simplification, low-maintenance equipment, and efficient product movement.

Supervisory controls should allow the manager to view receiving, storage, product issues, production, packaging, and distribution. In large central commissaries or central kitchens, receiving, storage, and issue of product may be under the supervision of a warehouse manager, allowing the central kitchen manager to devote time to efficient production of high-quality food products.

Work simplification should include equipment placement that maximizes personnel performance without placing undue physical strain upon the employee. This requires equipment well placed that is not labor intensive. Labor costs are ongoing, whereas the cost of good facility design and proper equipment selection is a one-time expenditure.

The traditional food service operation that delivers food to off site-locations requires additional equipment for shipping and transporting. The transportating equipment required is determined by the method used to distribute

Table 14–1   Sample Staffing Guidelines for On-Site Production

Meals per Labor Hour (MPLH)/Total Hours

Number of Meal Equivalents[a]	Conventional System[a]		Convenience System[b]	
	Low	High	Low	High
Up to 100	8	10	10	12
101–150	9	11	11	13
151–200	10–11	12	12	14
251–300	13	15	15	16
301–400	14	16	16	18
401–500	14	17	18	19
501–600	15	17	18	19
601–700	16	18	19	20
701–800	17	19	20	22
801–900	18	20	21	23
901+	19	21	22	23

[a]Meal equivalents include breakfast and à la carte sales.
[b]Conventional system is preparation of some foods from raw ingredients on premises (using some bakery breads and prepared pizza, and washing dishes).
[c]Convenience system is using the maximum amount of processed foods (for example, using all bakery breads, prefried chicken, and preportioned condiments and washing only trays or using disposable dinnerware).
Source: Reprinted with permission from D.V. Pannell-Martin, *School Foodservice Management*, 5th Ed., p. 150, © 1999, InTEAM Associates.

food to the receiving site, whether preplated or in bulk. Depending on the delivery and pickup schedule, it is possible that these central facilities may require either a two- or three-day inventory of packaging containers and delivery equipment.

The chilling/chilled storage process occurs only in cook-chill systems. Special equipment is needed in these operations to chill food items quickly. Blast-chill units are used to chill pans of cooked food items rapidly. A blast chiller is a quick-chill cabinet that usually holds roll-in racks of food pans. Blast chillers direct frigid air at 1,000 feet per minute over the steam table pans. The smallest blast chiller is capable of dropping the temperature of up to 44 pounds of foods to 37 degrees Fahrenheit within 90 minutes. For large-scale operations, blast chillers capable of chilling 360 pounds or more per batch are common.

Tumble chillers are other pieces of equipment used to chill food rapidly. In tumble-chill operations, hot food is bagged into plastic casings. These casings are loaded immediately into a tumble chiller, which is filled with ice water. The bags are then agitated in the ice water. Depending on product viscosity and casing size, product emperatures are reduced to 40 degrees Fahrenheit in 20 to 60 minutes. Once the bags of food are chilled, they are transferred to holding crates and stored in refrigerated units until needed.

Operations using tumble chillers and cook tank/chillers will need an ice builder to supply the ice water for the chiller units. The amount of water used in these systems can be of concern, especially in drought areas. Additional refrigerated space is needed for cook-chill operations for storage of the inventory of chilled food products. The amount of refrigeration will depend on the length of time food products will be stored. Convenience systems also require additional refrigeration and freezer space. Large freezers are required to store the inventory of frozen food products, and refrigerated space is needed to temper the frozen items.

SYSTEM SELECTION PROCESS

Planning for a school food and nutrition production system involves many important decisions. Food service staff need to be very much involved in the planning and selection process. Planning for the remodeling of current or construction of new facilities can take several years. Research has not been done to examine the food service system selection process by school food and nutrition directors. Research on this decision process by hospital food and nutrition directors suggested that directors spend differing amounts of time in the decision process to select a food service system, varying from a few months to several years.[133–136] Issues that must be considered in selecting a food production system include production operation, support and information, and construction and quality. A list of system selection issues is shown in Exhibit 14–2.

Directors should be involved in the planning process from the beginning. The first step in the planning process should be writing a program paper that explains the major goals of the new design.[137] Directors need to be assertive in working with architects and should be involved in the hiring of a food and nutrition consultant. The selection of the appropriate food service consultant can be critical to the success of the project. The food service director should remain an active participant in the selection process after a food and nutrition consultant has been hired. Research[138] indicated that although food and nutrition directors in Mississippi had been very much involved in school food and nutrition renovation or construction projects, many indicated the need for continuing education to improve their skills in this process.

Directors involved in the system selection decision should gather information from a variety of sources, such as users of the system(s) under consideration; information from food service equipment manufacturers, manufacturers' representatives, food service consultants, seminars and conferences, industry journals, and professional journals; and visits to other facilities.[139–141]

Issues to consider when selecting a food production system should be categorized as operational, including cost, and financial data; support and information; construction; and food quality concerns (Exhibit 14–2).[142,143] The importance of these issues should be determined by the planning committees. Each facility has different goals and expectations that should be considered in the selection decision. The food service director/manager cannot think only of the current operation, but must look to the future for possible additional programs or use of the facility and equipment. One indicator in ASFSA's *Keys to Excellence* states that "a long-range facility and equipment service and replacement plan should be in place to improve the production and delivery system."[144]

Food and nutrition directors should evaluate the costs associated with recipe development in test kitchens and microbiological testing of food products. Directors selecting convenience or cook-chill systems should explore the issues of chilled/frozen storage of food products and reheating. In order to make an intelligent decision it is necessary to be aware of the current and future labor market, the strategic plan of the school district and how it will affect students, future expansion projects of the district and the community, and, when possible, future regulations and funding from the state and federal governments. All food and nutrition directors should build in time and money for training and employee jobs redesign when planning for a new system. When changing services to students, it is important to create a public relations plan for the educational community, employees, unions, and parents and students.

Exhibit 14–2 Food Service System Selection Issues

Issues Related to Production Operation
- Actual and projected food cost
- Actual and projected production labor cost
- Actual and projected service labor cost
- Actual and projected total departmental cost
- Actual and projected meals per labor hour
- Employee training
- Operation of an ingredient room
- Payback period and return on investment
- Break-even point
- Computerization
- Plate waste
- Ability to provide food to other facilities
- Availability and skill level of labor
- Centralization of production
- Cost of distribution
- Actual and projected overhead costs

Issues Related to Support and Information
- Dollars available for new food and nutrition system
- Viewing actual operation of other facilities/discussion with other system users
- Food and nutrition consultant advice
- Manufacturer technical assistance and training
- Journal articles/seminars/conferences
- Administration support
- Staff acceptance/staff involvement in decision process
- Community acceptance
- Perception that food and nutrition operation is innovative

Issues Related to Construction
- Additional or new production, delivery/transportation, refrigeration and/or rethermalization equipment
- Installation costs
- Production area and/or satellite facilities construction or renovation

Issues Related to Food Quality
- Temperature and holding time of prepared foods
- Food texture
- Standardized recipes

Source: Adapted from M.B. Gregoire and M.F. Nettles, Alternate Food Production Systems, in *Nutrition and Food Services for Integrated Health Care*, R. Jackson, ed., p. 350, © 1997, Aspen Publishers, Inc.

SUMMARY

The production system is a major determinant in the level of effectiveness, including customer satisfaction and efficiency of a school food and nutrition program. It must be capable of producing quality products, flexible enough to accommodate expanded services, allow for growth, and be cost effective. When selecting the production system for a new or renovated facility, some factors to be considered are as follows:

- Menu
- Equipment required
- Layout and design of the facility
- Available labor market and costs
- School district demographics
- Food services offered

Both internal and external concerns will have an impact on production systems of the future. Internally, the menu, food availability, service system, safety issues, labor availability, and cost constraints will affect the system; externally, technological changes that affect food and equipment, energy cost and availability, safety requirements, recycling, union contracts, transportation cost, and the labor market will influence the decision when implementing a new facility or renovating an existing facility. The major decision to be made regarding the food production system is to select a system that will provide the most cost-effective educational/health services to the students in the school district. The goal of the cost-effective production system is to produce a variety of healthful foods of consistent quality, acceptable to the customers of the district.

CASE STUDY
THE CHALLENGE OF EXPANDING FOOD SERVICE

Betty Bender

Prior to 1970 the structure of the Dayton, Ohio, school system was kindergarten through grade eight as elementary; grades nine through twelve were secondary. The district was designed as neighborhood schools. All elementary students and the majority of secondary students walked to school. Lunch was offered at all secondary schools and two special schools; a limited number of elementary schools received a cold box lunch. The majority of students were required to go home for lunch, and the school building was closed for one hour and fifteen minutes during the lunch period. Because of the changing economy of the city, increased numbers of working mothers, and a federal court order that mandated that all schools should be integrated, with each school reflecting the racial composition of the city, it became necessary to offer a school lunch program in each building.

When the board of education voted to provide school lunch in every building, there were many obstacles to overcome. The two most difficult were funding and the mind-set of the administrative and teaching staff. The board of education had closed schools because an operating levy did not pass. It appeared foolish to spend monies to implement a new program that required purchasing and equipping a new building when the district had just closed its doors to students due to lack of operating funds. Teachers and administrators viewed the lunch program as an infringement on their personal time. Negotiations with each union had to be reopened. In order to avoid a strike, the board of education accepted an article in the teachers' contract that stated that no teacher shall be required to supervise a child feeding program. Supervision of the school lunch program became the responsibility of the building administrator.

Challenge

The challenge was to provide food service in 60 elementary schools. The superintendent assigned the business manager to oversee the project and to provide a recommendation on how to proceed.

Following the process that was put into place:

- The district engineer was asked to assess each elementary building for space, electrical power, and plumbing.
- The estimated cost of establishing a production kitchen and cafeteria in each building was projected. The new facility had to meet the requirement of feeding all students in no more than three lunch periods, to be consistent with the negotiated teacher agreement.
- The director of food service was asked to provide an estimate of the cost of equipping each facility including tables and chairs for the cafeterias.

After totaling the anticipated costs and submitting them to the superintendent, we were instructed to find a different method of feeding children because the total dollar package to construct on-site production facilities plus cafeteria space was not within the financial constraints of the budget. It was at this point that the real challenge began.

Action

A core committee consisting of the business manager, engineer, and director of food service was appointed and charged with submitting a complete plan to implement school lunch in all elementary schools. The final plan could not spend more than the budgeted amount of dollars. The committee met and assigned the following tasks:

- The business manager would request information from the state department of education concerning other successful methods of providing food service in schools, possible sources of additional funding, and the future of school food service legislation at both the state and the federal level.
- The superintendent and board of education were asked to develop a policy that stated the district philosophy about the child nutrition program.
- The food service director researched other types of feeding operations and presented the core committee with the following options:
  1. Establish a central kitchen/central commissary that produces and distributes preplated meals to schools either
     a. Frozen
     b. Chilled
     c. Hot and/or cold
  2. Purchase frozen preplated meals—distribution to be handled by the district or commercially.
  3. Establish small reconstituting kitchens in each elementary building. Kitchens shall contain an oven, refrigerator, milk cooler, storage cabinet, and desk.
  4. Purchase meals in bulk either frozen or chilled—distribution to be handled by the district or commercially.
  5. Establish a small reconstituting kitchen and portable serving lines.
  6. Employ a company to operate the food service program.

A cost estimate was prepared, and it was determined that the funds available restricted the district to either establishing a central kitchen/central commissary facility that produced preplated meals or utilizing a company to provide the service. The philosophy of the board of ed-

ucation and the wording of the current union contract prohibited contracting this service to a company. It was agreed to establish a pilot program in five elementary schools and evaluate its success or failure after six months. The district received federal non–food assistance (NFA) dollars to establish the pilot program. [Editor's note: Non-Food Assistance Funds were eliminated by the 1981 Budget Reconciliation Act].

The district designed and implemented a small production kitchen that produced baked goods, salads, and fruit for packaging and distribution. The district entered into a contract with a manufacturer to produce the entrees and vegetables. Distribution was handled by refrigerated trucks owned by the district. Equipment needed at the receiving school was selected. The production and packaging equipment were chosen and carefully evaluated for speed, automation, ease of cleaning and sanitizing, and mechanical difficulties and maintenance. Although the production and packaging equipment selected were successful when preparing 5,000 meals, it was determined that this equipment would not produce 20,000 meals on a daily basis at a reasonable cost or in a reasonable time period.

The business manager, engineer, and food service director then visited other major cities that were preparing preplated meals. We asked each district to provide us with a list of equipment, the name of the architect who designed the facility, and an evaluation of the facility. If they had to build a central facility again, what would they change? In addition, we visited three companies that manufactured and packaged meals and other products.

At the end of six months, the committee conducted an evaluation of the pilot program with students, parents, administrators, and teachers. The evaluation was positive, and the original program had expanded from five pilot schools to twelve schools. This gave a clear indication of success within the community.

The core committee then assembled the data and presented a recommendation to the superintendent and board of education to establish a central kitchen/central commissary facility. The facility was to produce, package, and distribute school lunches to 60 elementary schools. Upon receiving approval and a firm commitment of dollars the project began.

The project timetable was as follows:

February
1. Building was selected and purchased.
2. Architect was selected.

March
1. Kitchen design company was selected.
2. Kitchen design was begun.

April
1. Kitchen design completed.
2. Equipment specifications completed.
3. Building design approved.
4. Equipment advertised for legal bid.

May
1. Building construction began.

June
1. Equipment bids were awarded.

July/August
1. Building completed.

Like all new construction, Dayton had a number of delays and problems that had to be overcome. Training personnel in new procedures and on new equipment was difficult. Because of the school calendar and delays in installation of some equipment there was insufficient time for training.

Outcome

The Dayton central kitchen/commissary has been an excellent operation. It has produced quality meals and has been cost effective. If we had to undertake this project again, we would take more time and plan carefully. The worst mistake made was lack of vision. The Dayton schools planned to produce school lunch for all elementary schools from the facility. Consideration was not given to future programs such as the school breakfast program, catering, day-care services, centralized bulk food services for secondary schools, the summer feeding program, and contracted services for other school districts. The second mistake made was an unrealistic timetable. There was insufficient time for training of personnel, and some equipment was delayed and not available for the opening of school. The other mistake was developing the menu. We quickly learned that menu development had to be engineered to meet available labor and equipment constraints. The most successful characteristic of the facility is the flexibility of the layout and equipment selected. This flexibility has allowed the district to meet other demands successfully with minimal changes.

REFERENCES

1. American School Food Service Association (ASFSA), *Keys to Excellence* (Alexandria, VA: 1995), 17.
2. California Department of Education, *School Nutrition Facility Planning Guide* (Sacramento, CA: 1992), 9–10.
3. J. Sneed and K.T. White, "Development and Validation of Competency Statements for Managers in School Food and Nutrition," *School Food and Nutrition Research Review* 17 (1993): 50–61.
4. M.T. Conklin, "Job Functions and Tasks of School Nutrition Managers and District Directors/Supervisors," *NFSMI Insight* 2 (1995).
5. M.T. Conklin et al., "Preparing Child Nutrition Professionals for the 21st Century," *School Food and Nutrition Research Review*, 19 (1995): 6–13.
6. M.B. Gregoire and J. Sneed, "Competencies for District School Nutrition Directors/Supervisors," *School Food and Nutrition Research Review*, 18 (1994): 89–99.
7. J. Martin, "Validating Competencies," *School Food and Nutrition Journal* 38 (1984): 129–134.
8. "Recommended Functions and Tasks for School Nutrition Program Personnel," *School Food and Nutrition Journal* 7 (1984): a–p. American School Food and Nutrition Association, Denver, CO.
9. Sneed and White, "Development and Validation of Competency Statements."
10. S. Borden and E. Matthews, "Taking Steps toward Program Excellence: Development and Implementation in Wisconsin of Program Standards of Excel-

lence, *School Food and Nutrition Research Review* 17 (1993): 98–102.

11. E.W. Cross et al., "Texas School Food and Nutrition Associations Standards of Excellence Program Part 1: Development of Standards and Manual," *School Food and Nutrition Research Review* 13 (1989): 114–118.

12. E.W. Cross et al., "Texas School Food and Nutrition Association Standards of Excellence Program Part 2: Program Evaluation," *School Food and Nutrition Research Review* 13 (1989): 119–129.

13. M.B. Gregoire and J. Sneed, *Nutrition Integrity Standards* (University, MS: National Foodservice Management Institute, 1993).

14. ASFSA, *Keys to Excellence.*

15. B.J. Bobeng, "Alternative for Menu Item Flow in Hospital Patient Feeding Systems," in *Hospital Patient Feeding Systems* (Washington, DC: National Academy Press, 1982), 113–117.

16. M.E. Matthews, "Foodservice in health care facilities," *Journal of Food Technology* no. 7 (1982): 53–71.

17. E.S. Escueta et al., "A New Hospital Foodservice Classification System," *Journal of Foodservice Systems* 4 (1986): 107–116.

18. P. Jones and A. Heulin, "Foodservice Systems—Generic Types, Alternative Technologies and Infinite Variation," *Journal of Foodservice Systems* 5 (1990): 299–311.

19. M.C. Spears and A.G. Vaden, *Foodservice Organizations: A Managerial and Systems Approach* (Englewood Cliffs, NJ: Merrill, 1985).

20. M.C. Spears, *Foodservice Organizations: A Managerial and Systems Approach*, 3rd ed. (Englewood Cliffs, NJ: Merrill, 1995).

21. M.B. Gregoire and M.F. Nettles, "Alternate Food Production Systems," in *Nutrition and Food Services for Integrated Health Care,* A.R. Jackson (Gaithersburg, MD: Aspen Publishers, Inc., 1997), 330–354.

22. K.R. Greathouse and M.B. Gregoire, "Options in Meal Assembly, Delivery and Service," in *Nutrition and Food Services for Integrated Health Care,* ed. R. Jackson (Gaithersburg, MD: Aspen Publishers, Inc., 1997), 354–384.

23. J. Payne-Palacio et al., *West's and Wood's Introduction to Foodservice*, 7th ed. (New York: Macmillan, 1994).

24. Spears, *Foodservice Organizations.*

25. M.F. Nettles, *Analysis of the Decision to Select a Conventional or Cook-Chill System for Hospital Foodservice.* Unpublished Doctoral Dissertation, Kansas State University, Manhattan, KS, 1993.

26. Spears, *Foodservice Organizations.*

27. P. King, "A Gamble Pays Off," *Food Management* 24, no. 9 (1989): 80, 86.

28. P. King, "A Vision Comes to Life," *Food Management* 24, no. 12 (1989): 66, 68.

29. P. King, "Something Old, Something New," *Food Management* 26, no. 7 (1991): 56, 58.

30. P. King, "The Beginning of a Dream," *Food Management* 29, no. 12 (1994): 35.

31. N. Unklesbay et al., *Foodservice Systems: Product Flow and Microbial Quality and Safety of Foods* (Columbia, MO: University of Missouri—Columbia Agriculture Experiment Station, 1977).

32. H.A. MacLennan, "Ready Foods: The Application of Mass Production to a la Carte Food Service Using Prepared-to-Order Food," *Cornell Hotel and Restaurant Administration Quarterly* 6, no. 2 (1965): 21–63.

33. H.A. MacLennan, "Ready Foods for Hotels," *Cornell Hotel and Restaurant Administration Quarterly* 10, no. 2 (1969): 21–31.

34. A. Bjorkman and K.A. Delphin, "Sweden's Nacka Hospital Food System Centralizes Preparation and Distribution," *Cornell Hotel Restaurant Administration Quarterly* 7, no. 3 (1966): 84-87.

35. A.T. McGuckian, "The A.G.S. Food System—Chilled Pasteurized Food," *Cornell Hotel Restaurant Administration Quarterly* 10, no. 1 (1969): 87–92, 99.

36. N.L. Mann et al., "An Assessment of Solid Waste Management Practices Used in School Food Service Operations," *School Food and Nutrition Research Review* 17 (1993): 109-114.

37. California Department of Education, *School Nutrition.*

38. P. King, "Expanding a Foodservice System," *Food Management* 22, no. 10 (1987): 64, 68.

39. P. King, "Production for Profit," *Food Management* 22, no. 3 (1987): 68, 76.

40. King, "A Gamble Pays Off."

41. "Surveying the Scene," *School Food and Nutrition Journal* 48, no. 2 (1994): 40–45.

42. B.P. Klein et al., *Foodservice Systems: Time and Temperature Effects on Food Quality* (North Central Regional Research Publication No. 293) (Urbana-Champaign: University of Illinois, 1984).

43. D.M. Rieley et al., "Evaluation of Three School Food Service Systems," *School Food and Nutrition Research Review* 10 (1986): 109–115.

44. J. Durocher, "Cook-Chill Systems," *Restaurant Business* (1992): 154,156.

45. B.A. Byers, et al., *Food Service Manual for Health Care Institutions* (Chicago: American Hospital Association. 1994).

46. Spears, *Foodservice Organizations.*

47. Unklesbay et al., "Foodservice Systems."

48. Y. Lambre, "The Multi-Energy Cooking Tunnel," *The Consultant* 26, no. 1 (1993): 32–33.

49. R.M. Corsi, "The Ready Foods System," *The Consultant,* Winter 1984: 23–25.

50. R. Pizzuto and E. Winslow, "Why Cook/Chill Systems Don't Work When They Should," *The Consultant* 22, no. 1 (1989): 32–34.

51. Durocher, "Cook-Chill Systems."

52. P. Hysen, "Ready Foods May Provide Ready Savings," *Modern Hospital* 116, no. 6 (1971): 95–98, 117.

53. M.L. Herz and J.J. Souder, "Preparation Systems Have Significant Effect on Costs," *Hospitals* 53, no. 1 (1979): 89–92.

54. J.F. Freshwater, *Least-Cost Hospital Food Service Systems.* Marketing Research Report No. 1116. (Washington, DC: Department of Agriculture, Agricultural Marketing Service, 1980).

55. A.L. Moorshead, *An Empirical Investigation of the Reliability and Validity of the USDA Model To Determine Least-Cost Hospital Food Service Systems.* Unpublished Master's Thesis, Virginia Polytechnic Institute and State University, Blacksburg, VA, 1982.

56. K.R. Greathouse et al., "Comparison of Conventional, Cook-Chill, and Cook-Freeze Systems," *Journal of the American Dietetic Association* 89 (1989): 1606–1611.

57. Department of Veterans Affairs, *Advanced Food Preparation Systems.* Final Report. (Milwaukee, WI: 1993).

58. Nettles, *Analysis of the Decision to Select.*

59. Greathouse et al., "Comparison of Systems."

60. G. Glew and J.F. Armstrong, "Cost Optimization through Cook-Freeze Systems," *Journal of Foodservice Systems* 1 (1981): 235–254.

61. C.M. Goldberg and M. Kohligian, "Conventional, Convenience, or Ready Foodservice," *Hospitals* 48 (1974): 80–83.

62. J.F. Halling and B.M. Frakes, "Product-Oriented Production in a Cook Freeze System," *Journal of Foodservice Systems* 4 (1981): 355–361.

63. Durocher, "Cook-Chill Systems."

64. Byers et al., *Food Service Manual.*

65. Corsi, "The Ready Foods System."

66. Pizzuto and Winslow, "Why Cook/Chill Systems Don't Work."

67. Freshwater, *Least-Cost Hospital Food.*

68. Greathouse et al., "Comparison of Systems."

69. K. Schuster, "Is Your Future in Cook-Chill?," *Food Management* 28, no. 7 (1993): 90, 94, 96, 98, 123–124.

70. University of Iowa Hospitals and Clinics, *Cook Chill Cookbook* (Iowa City, IA: 1994).

71. C.L. Rappole, "Institutional Use of Frozen Entrees," *Cornell Hotel and Restaurant Administration Quarterly* 14, no. 1 (1973): 72–89 99.

72. Department of Veterans Affairs, *Advanced Food Preparation System.*

73. J. Maahs, "Cook/Chill from Preparation through Service," *The Consultant* 26, no. 2 (1993): 16–18.

74. Byers et al., *Food Service Manual.*

75. Glen and Armstrong, "Cost Optimization."

76. A. E. Walker, *The Transfer of Technology: A Study of KU Cook Chill Catering Operations.* Unpublished Doctoral Dissertation, Dorset Institute of Higher Education, Dorset, England, 1988.

77. M.S. Pinkert, "Basic Planning Concepts for Ready Foods Systems," *Canadian Hospital* (1972): 32–34.

78. Durocher, "Cook-Chill Systems."

79. Byers et al., *Food Service Manual.*

80. Glen and Armstrong, "Cost Optimization."

81. Halling and Frakes, "Product-Oriented Production."

82. A.K. Jernigan and L. N. Ross, *Food Service Equipment,* 3rd. ed. (Ames, IA: Iowa State University Press. 1989).

83. Spears, *Foodservice Organizations.*

84. Payne-Palacio et al., *West's and Wood's Introduction.*

85. Byers et al., *Food Service Manual.*

86. C.R. Scriven and J. W. Stevens, *Equipment Facts, Revised* (New York: Van Nostrand Reinhold, 1989).

87. C.R. Scriven and J. W. Stevens, *Manual of Equipment and Design for the Foodservice Industry* (New York: Van Nostrand Reinhold, 1989).

88. R. Kent, "Turbo-Charged 'EasyBake' Oven Speeds Cooking with Light," *Hospital Food Service Management* 1, no. 5 (1993): 73–75.

89. R.A. Lampi et al., "Perspective and Thoughts on Foodservice Equipment," *Journal of Food Technology* 44, no. 7 (1990): 61–69.

90. Lambre, "The Multi-Energy Cooking Tunnel."

91. USECO. CATR, *Chilled Food System* (Murfreesboro, TN: 1994).

92. R. Lampi, "New Developments in Energy Saving Equipment," *Journal of Foodservice Systems* 1 (1980): 27–38.

93. L. McProud, "Reducing Energy Loss in Foodservice Operations," *Journal of Food Technology* 37, no. 7 (1982): 67–71.

94. D. Odland and C. Davis, "Products Cooked in Preheated versus Non-Preheated Ovens," *Journal of the American Dietetic Association* 81 (1982): 135–144.

95. J. Hsieh and M. Matthews, "Energy Use, Time, and Product Yield of Turkey Rolls at Three Oven Loads

and Cooking Temperatures in a Convection Oven," *Journal of Foodservice Systems* 4 (1986): 97–106.

96. M. Tutt et al., "Comparison of Energy Consumption in Fully and Partially Loaded Institutional Forced-Air Convection Ovens: Preheated and Nonpreheated," *School Food and Nutrition Research Review* 13 (1989): 146–149.

97. M.J. Barclay and M.J. Hitchcock, "Energy Consumption Assessment in a Conventional Foodservice System," *Journal of Foodservice Systems* 3 (1984): 33–47.

98. C.J. Thomas and N.E. Brown, "Use and Cost of Electricity for Selected Processes Specific to a Hospital Cook-Chill/Freeze Food-Production System," *Journal of Foodservice Systems* 4, no. 3 (1987): 159–169.

99. L. McProud and B. David, "Energy Use and Management in Production of Entrees in Hospital Foodservice Systems," *Journal of the American Dietetic Association* 81 (1981): 45–151.

100. A.M. Messeersmith et al., "Energy Used to Produce Meals in School Food and Nutrition," *School Food and Nutrition Research Review* 18 (1994): 29–36.

101. A.M. Messersmith et al., "School Food Service Energy," *School Food and Nutrition Research Review* 18 (1994): 38–44.

102. National Restaurant Association, *Facilities Operations Manual* (Chicago: 1986).

103. A. Thumann, *Handbook of Energy Audits*, 3rd. ed. (Lilburn, GA: Fairmont Press, Inc., 1992).

104. N. Unklesbay and K. Unklesbay, *Energy Management in Foodservice* (Westport, CT: AVI Publishing, Inc., 1982).

105. Jernigan and Ross, *Food Service Equipment.*

106. McProud, "Reducing Energy Loss."

107. Nettles, *Analysis of the Decision to Select.*

108. Department of Veterans Affairs, *Advanced Food Preparation Systems.*

109. Byers et al., *Food Service Manual.*

110. Pizzuto and Winslow, "Why Cook/Chill Systems Don't Work."

111. Spears, *Foodservice Organizations.*

112. Payne-Palacio et al., *West's and Woods Introduction.*

113. K. Ruf, *Manual for Food and Nutrition Services: Quality Control, Quality Assurance* (Gaithersburg, MD: Aspen Publishing, Inc., 1989).

114. University of Iowa Hospitals and Clinics, *Cook-Chill Cookbook.*

115. J.R. Chipley and M.L. Cremer, "Microbiological Problems in the Food Service Industry," *Journal of Food Technology* 34, no. 10 (1980): 59–68.

116. K.P. Penner, "Food Safety," *School Food and Nutrition Research Review* 15 (1991): 123–126.

117. Klein et al., *Foodservice Systems.*

118. C.A. Dahl et al., "Fate of *Staphylococcus aureus* in Beef Loaf, Potatoes and Frozen Green Beans after Microwave-Heating in a Simulated Cook/Chill Hospital Foodservice System," *Journal of Food Protection* 43 (1980): 916–923.

119. S.J. Ridly and M.E. Matthews, "Temperature Histories of Menu Items during Meal Assembly, Distribution and Service in a Hospital Foodservice," *Journal of Food Protection* 46 (1983): 100–104.

120. P.G. Williams and J.C.B. Miller, "Warm-Holding of Vegetables I, Hospitals: Cook/Chill versus Cook/Hot-Hold Foodservice Systems," *Journal of Foodservice Systems* (1993): 117–128.

121. P.O. Snyder and M.E. Matthews, "Microbiological Quality of Foodservice Menu Items Produced and Stored by Cook/Chill, Cook/Freeze, Cook/Hot-Hold and Heat/Serve Methods," *Journal of Food Protection* 47, no. 11 (1984): 876–885.

122. F.L. Bryan, "Application of HACCP to Ready-to-Eat Chilled Foods," *Journal of Food Technology* 44, no. 7 (1990): 70–77.

123. Ridley and Matthews, "Temperature Histories of Menu Items."

124. B.L. Bobeng and B.D. David, "HACCP Models for Quality Control of Entree Production in Hospital Foodservice Systems. I. Development of Hazard Analysis Critical Control Point models. II. Quality Assessment of Beef Loaves Utilizing HACCP Models," *Journal of the American Dietetic Association* 73 (1978): 524–535.

125. M.A. Beasley, "Implementing HACCP Standards," *Food Management* 30, no. 1 (1995): 38, 40.

126. D.A. Corlett, "Refrigerated Foods and Use of Hazard Analysis and Critical Control Point Principles," *Journal of Food Technology* 43, no. 2 (1989): 91–94.

127. Bryan, "Application of HACCP."

128. California Department of Education, *School Nutrition Facility Planning Guide.*

129. M.D. Olsen and M.K. Meyer, "Current Perspectives on Productivity in Food Service and Suggestions for the Future," *School Food Service Research Review* 11 (1987): 87–93.

130. D. Pannell, *School Foodservice Management* (New York: Van Nostrand Reinhold, 1990).

131. C.R. Mayo and M.D. Olsen, "Food Servings per Labor Hour: An Alternate Productivity Measure," *School Food and Nutrition Research Review* 11 (1987): 48–51.

132. R. Jackson, "Equipment Can Sabotage Your Budget," *Hospital Food and Nutrition Focus* 11, no. 5 (1995): 1, 3–5.

133. G.G. Green, *Decision Making Strategy in the Selection of Cook-Chill Production in Hospital Foodservice*. Unpublished Doctoral Dissertation, Virginia Polytechnic Institute and State University, Blacksburg, VA, 1992.

134. P. King and D. Boss, "The Politics of a Renovation," *Food Management* 26, no. 7 (1991): 104–117, 166.

135. Nettles, *Analysis of the Decision To Select.*

136. Walker, *The Transfer of Technology.*

137. H.D. Van Brunt and M.S. Joynt, "Renovating on a Tight Budget," *School Food and Nutrition Journal* 48, no. 2 (1994): 19.

138. M.E. Richardson et al., "School Food Service Supervisor's Involvement in Layout and Design of Facilities," *School Food and Nutrition Research Review* 14 (1990): 118–123.

139. Nettles, *Analysis of the Decision To Select.*

140. Walker, *The Transfer of Technology.*

141. Green, *Decision Making Strategy.*

142. M.F. Nettles and M.B. Gregoire, "Satisfaction of Foodservice Directors after Implementation of a Conventional or Cook/Chill Foodservice System," *Journal of Foodservice Systems*, 9 (1997): 107–115.

143. Pannell, *School Foodservice Management.*

144. ASFSA, *Keys to Excellence.*

CHAPTER 15

Preparation of Nutritious Food That Students Accept and Choose

Charlotte B. Oakley

OUTLINE

INTRODUCTION

Meal production is one operational function of the school food and nutrition program that is driven by the menu. The concept that the availability of a healthful, student-acceptable school meal depends on the application of proper cooking and serving techniques is supported by the key achievements outlined in the *Keys to Excellence*.[1] As students select school meals from an array of healthful food choices at breakfast and lunch each day, they learn to make good nutrition choices that lead to the development of lifelong healthy eating behaviors. Healthful meals begin with a well-planned menu (refer to Chapter 10 for details on menu planning)—a menu that takes into consideration the principles of nutrition; federal, state, and local requirements; available resources; customer preferences; and all other restraints to the operation of the school food and nutrition program. The school food and nutrition program director/manager and the food service production staff must follow the standardized recipes and food preparation techniques indicated on the menu and production schedule to ensure that the nutrient content of the meal (as prepared and served) is the same as when the menu was analyzed during the planning process. The purposes of this chapter are to explore the various managerial aspects of food production and to look at both the art and science of food preparation. Specific objectives are as follows:

1. Discuss the various elements of production of the menu that support the delivery of healthful school meals to the student customer.
2. Discuss the importance of developing production standards and quality standards for foods that meet the nutrition goals of the program and that meet the taste preferences of the student customer.
3. Review the various cooking, flavor enhancement, presentation techniques, and recipe development and modification processes necessary to the production of healthful, student-acceptable school meals.
4. Promote the importance of training the food service staff in the techniques described to produce school meals that meet the nutrition recommendations in the *Dietary Guidelines for Americans*.

Thinking of food preparation simply as cooking can be a limiting factor in the preparation of meals that students find acceptable. The application of the culinary arts to the preparation of school meals is an essential component in the success of programs that offer healthful school meals. Bringing the art of cooking to the school kitchen ensures more than student satisfaction. Well-prepared foods that look and smell good and taste delicious are important goals for the school food and nutrition program. The availability of high-quality foods that meet the taste preferences of students will help make eating in the school cafeteria an exciting and fun experience. Students will look forward to breakfast and lunch in the cafeteria because they can count on having a meal that they will really enjoy eating.

PRODUCING THE MENU

The nutrition integrity of the menu (as served) depends on the proper application of the principles of various aspects of food preparation. These include selecting high-quality ingredients for items cooked from scratch and for preprepared food products, using standardized recipes, weighing and measuring ingredients properly, following the production schedule, and selecting the proper cooking methods. In *On Cooking: A Textbook of Culinary Fundamentals*,[2] professional cooking is defined as "a system of cooking based upon a knowledge of and appreciation for ingredients and procedures." Spears[3] defines production as "the managerial function of converting food items purchased in various states into menu items that are served to a customer." As in all other types of food service operations, producing the menu in school food and nutrition programs involves the integrated management functions of planning, organizing, and controlling. As a first step to production, planning involves analyzing the work to be done and making the necessary assignments. The production schedule serves as a written plan for accomplishing all tasks necessary to produce the menu.[3]

High-Quality Ingredients

The finished product can only be as good as the ingredients that go into it. The selection criteria for high-quality ingredients vary with the type of food product under consideration. For example, fresh produce should look fresh. Plump, crisp, succulent-looking produce is really fresh and indicates quality. Frozen products are delivered completely frozen without any signs of previous thawing and refreezing. All foods are held and delivered at the correct temperatures and levels of humidity. Telltale signs of improper holding temperatures include water marks on packaging and other damage to the containers of ingredients or preprepared food products. Quality is also indicated by the grade standards for many agricultural products. Purchase the highest grade financially feasible that is appropriate for the menu item to be prepared. For example, it is desirable to purchase the best quality of fresh produce available for a menu item that will be served with minimal preparation, such as a fresh apple or peach, while a lower grade of canned fruit would be acceptable for a fruit cobbler.

Standardized Recipes

Standardized recipes are the basis for consistent quality and quantity of foods prepared in the school food and nutrition program operation. Standardized recipes will produce the same quality and the same quantity of a food

each time it is used when the food and nutrition program assistant follows the recipe exactly. To standardize a recipe it is tested several times until the results are consistent. When recipes are used for the first time, the recipe is tested in the facility, since the equipment in various kitchens will vary and perform differently. For example, ovens do not always cook the same, even though the temperatures are carefully set. Also, individuals preparing the recipe may use slightly different techniques in measuring, and so forth, that result in variations to the characteristics of the final product.

Once all recipes are standardized for the local school, copies must be on file in all food and nutrition programs in the school district, and a master standardized recipe file maintained in the central office. All production staff understand the concept of using standardized recipes and are trained in the use of the standardized recipes needed to produce the menu. Training emphasizes following the cooking procedures outlined in the recipe. A well-trained food production staff understands that following the recipe—avoiding adding extra fat, sodium, and/or sugars or altering the cooking method—ensures the nutritional integrity of the menu, quality of product, and consistency.

Following a standardized recipe exactly will result in a good-quality product in flavor, texture, and appearance. Standardized recipes have been tested several times under the same conditions that normally exist in a particular school setting, which includes

- using correct procedures for weighing and measuring;
- selecting the right-sized containers, preparation, and cooking equipment; using correct cooking and holding temperatures;
- and considering any other aspect of preparation unique to the recipe being standardized.

Following the recipe exactly each time it is prepared will produce a good-quality product and a specific number of servings.

Standardized recipes are also part of the cost controls in the day-to-day operation of the school food and nutrition program. The cost of a recipe is affected by several factors: adding the correct amount of an ingredient, serving the correct portion size specified in the recipe, using the size pan specified in the recipe, using appropriate cooking procedures and temperatures that result in an acceptable product, and scraping the bowl or pan to get the last few servings. Correct yield is a critical factor in successful food production. Too little of a product will result in not enough portions to meet the demands of customers, and too much means unnecessary additional cost to the program. Running out of menu selections can also mean disappointed customers who may lose confidence in the program's ability to meet their personal food preferences.

Repeated experience with standardized recipes allows the food and nutrition program assistant to become familiar with the recipes, thus saving time in preparation that can be used for other tasks. Time saved in preparation translates into dollar savings to the program. The recipes produced by the United States Department of Agriculture (USDA) contain clear step-by-step directions for combining ingredients and cooking. Ingredients are listed as either a weight or measure (or both) and in the order that they are used in the recipe. Times and temperatures for cooking and holding, optional ingredients, recipe variations, serving suggestions, portion size, and other yield information are included on the USDA standardized recipes. When recipe sources other than USDA are used in school food and nutrition programs, the recipes should be selected from other reliable sources and standardized. For those programs that do not participate in the National School Lunch/Breakfast Programs, the same standards for recipe selection also apply.

The *Tool Kit for Healthy School Meals*[4] and the *USDA Recipe File*[5] recipes have been analyzed for key nutrients, including protein, fat, saturated fat, cholesterol, sodium, iron, cal-cium, vitamin A, vitamin C, and calories per serving. This same information is included in the USDA nutrient database, which serves as the foundation database for all USDA-approved software for the nutrient analysis of school meals. Use of the USDA standardized recipes limits the number of recipes that the school food authority or state agency must enter during the nutrient analysis process.

Some state agencies have developed menus using the nutrient standard planning system that is available to the local school districts. Readers may contact the state agency responsible for the school food and nutrition program in their state on the availability of menus and recipes developed under the Assisted Nutrient Standard Menu Planning (Assisted NSMP) menu-planning system. State agencies that have developed Assisted NSMP are also generous in sharing these (and other school food and nutrition program-related materials) across state lines. Recipes standardized for Nutrient Standard Menu Planning (NSMP) and Assisted NSMP may not meet meal component requirements of food-based menu systems. Recipes should conform to the menu system chosen and may need adjusting to meet this requirement. For additional information on this topic, contact the National Food Service Management Institute (NFSMI).

Weighing and Measuring

Weighing and measuring are critical steps in the correct application and use of standardized recipes. Using the correct measuring equipment most appropriate to the ingredient being measured and using the correct procedures are critical to accurate yield and product quality. Small volumes of ingredients may be measured, but all other ingredients are weighed when possible. When the standardized recipe lists both the weight and volume measurement for ingredients, weighing is more efficient and accurate than measuring. Weighing is generally more accurate than measuring, especially for ingredients such as flour, which may pack down in the container. To be accurate, the scales used must be of good quality and properly maintained. Refer to Table 15–1 for examples of food weight and approximate equivalents in measures.[6]

Portion Control

Portion control is essential to ensure that the nutrient content of each meal as served is accurate and that the meal pattern requirements are met. Good portion control requires the production of the expected number of servings from a recipe and includes serving the right amount of food to each customer. Inconsistency in portion sizes of a food item may lead to unhappy customers. When some customers receive larger or smaller servings, dissatisfaction with the service offered may occur. Serving the planned portion size will also help control costs, minimize waste, serve as a guide to ordering and preparing food, and ensure customer satisfaction in getting the amount of food expected.

Portion control begins with establishing specifications or product descriptions for the purchase of food products and ingredients. The school food and nutrition program production and serving staff work closely with the food buyer when determining the amount of each serving to be sure that the planned portion size is served. Serving a larger portion than was planned when the food was ordered or prepared results in inadequate food to serve all customers. Accurate forecasting to determine the amounts of food products and ingredients is dependent on portion control at the serving line.

It is critical for schools participating in federally assisted school food and nutrition programs to use consistently and accurately portioning equipment that ensures that each student receives the required amount of food, thus ensuring the service of the appropriate amount of nutrients to each customer. Various sizes of scoops are available for portioning and serving foods to achieve accurate portion control. The recipe will specify the size disher needed to yield the specified number of servings. When products are cut and served by the piece, the standardized recipe will indicate the proper cut to make to yield the correct number of servings (i.e., size of pan used to yield 48 portions cut 6 × 8). Employees must be skilled in proper use of appropriate equipment, which may require training. Bun dividers, spoodles, biscuit cutters, expandable cake cutters, pie markers, and food slicing machines are examples of other equipment used to portion foods for service.

Weighing and measuring sample portions and serving them in the appropriate container prior to meal service allows the server an opportunity to visualize the correct portion of a food item and how it is placed on the dish or tray. (When spoons are used to serve food, this becomes an important step toward proper portion control.) Preparing the sample plate or tray not only helps the server visualize the correct serving, but when placed on the line, helps market the menu. Students can see what they are going to be served as they make their selections from the line.

Serving level measures from scoops, spoons, spoodles, and ladles will also ensure that adequate food is available for the projected number of servings. Knowing the size and yield of all pans, dishers, and ladles is important. The scoop or disher number indicates the number of servings of a specified size that are in one quart; therefore, it takes eight portions served from a No. 8 scoop to yield one quart. Larger numbers indicate smaller size servings, for example, a No. 60 scoop holds one tablespoon[7] (Table 15–2).

Dishers are used on the serving line and during meal preparation to portion products such as muffin batter, cookie dough, and meatballs. Prepared items may be purchased in individual servings, such as breakfast cereals, hamburger patties, fruit juices, and condiments. These and other products purchased by count (i.e., apples, potatoes, oranges) make portion control easier and more predictable.

Table 15–1 Food Weights and Approximate Equivalents in Measures

Food	Weight	Approximate Measure
Allspice	1 ounce	4½ tablespoons
Apples, A.P.	1 pound	3–4 medium
Applesauce	1 pound	2 cups
Apples, canned pie pack	1½ pounds	1 quart
Baking powder	1 ounce	2 tablespoons
Bananas, A.P.	1 pound	3 medium
Bran, All Bran	8 ounces	1 quart
Bread crumbs, dry	1 pound	4 cups
Bread crumbs, soft	1 pound	2 quarts
Butter	1 pound	2 cups
Celery, diced (depends on size)	1–2 bunches	1 quart
Cheese, cottage	1 pound	2 cups
Cheese, grated or ground	1 pound	1 quart
Chili powder	1 ounce	4 tablespoons
Cinnamon, ground	1 ounce	4 tablespoons
Cloves, ground	1 ounce	5 tablespoons
Cocoa	1 pound	4 cups
Coconut, shredded	1 pound	6–7 cups
Corn flakes	1 pound	4 quarts
Cornmeal	1 pound	3 cups
Cornstarch	1 pound	3½ cups
Cream of tartar	1 ounce	3 tablespoons
Flour, all-purpose	1 pound	4 cups
Gelatin, flavored	1 pound	2⅓ cups
Ginger, ground	1 ounce	5 tablespoons
Lettuce, average head	9 ounces	1 head
Macaroni, A.P.	1 pound	4 cups
Margarine	1 pound	2 cups
Milk, fluid whole	1 pound + 1 ounce	2 cups
Milk, nonfat dry	1 pound	4 cups
Mustard, ground dry	1 pound	4½ cups
Noodles, dry A.P.	1 pound	6 cups
Nutmeg, ground	1 ounce	3½ tablespoons
Oats, rolled, A.P.	1 pound	6 cups
Oil, vegetable	1 pound	2–2⅛ cups
Onions, A.P.	1 pound	4–5 medium
Paprika	1 ounce	4 tablespoons
Peanut butter	1 pound	1¾ cups
Peanuts, E.P.	1 pound	3¼ cups
Pepper, ground	1 ounce	4 tablespoons
Rice, A.P.	1 pound	2 cups
Salt	1 ounce	1½ tablespoons
Shortening	1 pound	2¼ cups
Soda,	1 ounce	2⅓ tablespoons
Spaghetti, A.P. (2-inch pieces)	1 pound	5 cups
Sugar, brown, light pack	1 pound	3 cups

continues

Table 15–1 continued

Food	Weight	Approximate Measure
Sugar, brown, solid pack	1 pound	2 cups
Sugar, granulated	1 pound	2 cups
Sugar, powdered	1 pound	3 cups
Vanilla	½ ounce	1 tablespoon

Source: Adapted with permission from the National Food Service Management Institute, *On the Road to Professional Food Preparation,* © 1993, National Food Service Management Institute.

Foods are often portioned in the kitchen (back of the house or line) into individual servings for self-service by the customer. As with serving on the line, it is necessary to use the proper portioning equipment to ensure uniformity of serving sizes. Preportioning menu items in the kitchen can be more accurate than portioning on the line when the server is likely to be hurried by the need to move students quickly through the line, allowing little time for accurate portioning of food onto plates or trays. The attractive arrangement of an assortment of carefully portioned items on the serving line attracts customers to the cafeteria. Students enjoy the speed and autonomy that self-serve offers. Also, if the food is there ready for quick pickup, students may choose items that they would have refused if they had to wait to be served.

Whether food is portioned on the line, in the back of the house, or purchased preportioned, good portion control is ensured when the food and nutrition program staff use established specifications or descriptions for purchasing, standardized recipes, proper portioning equipment and techniques during production and service to promote customer satisfaction, meet the nutrient needs of each student, and manage resources to control cost.

Production Records and Production Schedules

Production records and schedules are organized plans for the accomplishment of all the tasks necessary to produce the menu. Production schedules are detailed plans that list each menu item and related tasks, the food and nutrition program assistant responsible for each task or menu item, and a time schedule for each task. The amount of each menu item to be prepared is recorded on the production record. Production of all food items is based on the historical data available to the school food and nutrition program director/manager. Each time the menu is produced, the amount of each menu item prepared and the amount of leftovers are recorded. These data become the basis for the production record for the menu when prepared again. Additional information may be recorded on the production record, but effective production records list the menu item, amount to produce, size of each portion, person responsible, date of service, and the number actually served.

The importance of production records to the forecasting process cannot be overemphasized. Accurately recorded data on number of servings produced and selected by customers are studied by the director/manager. What trends are seen in the data recorded on the production record? Are there days that are consistently lower or higher in participation? What factors are related to these variances in participation (i.e., certain menu items, school events, flu season, etc.)? Are some menu items consistently more popular than others? When students consistently refuse components of the school meal as reflected by data recorded on the production record, the director/manager

Table 15–2 Portion Control

The recipes are standardized to yield a certain number of servings of the size specified in the recipe. To obtain that number of servings, follow the specified serving size as closely as possible. Scoops, ladles, or spoons of standard sizes help in serving equal-size portions.

Ladles	Scoop (or Disher) Number	Serving Spoons
The following sizes of ladles will help in obtaining equal-size servings of soups, sauces, creamed foods, and other similar foods. Perforated ladles are available for accurate portioning of foods that need draining.	The number of the scoop or disher indicates the number of level scoopfuls it takes to make 1 quart. The following gives an approximate measure for each scoop:	A serving spoon (solid or slotted) may be used instead of a scoop. Since these spoons are not identified by number, it is necessary to measure or weigh the quantity of food from the spoons used. This will help ensure that the proper portion size is served.

Ladle Size	Approximate Measure	Scoop or Disher Number	Approximate Measure
1 oz	⅛ cup	6	⅔ cup
2 oz	¼ cup	8	½ cup
4 oz	½ cup	10	⅜ cup
6 oz	¾ cup	12	⅓ cup
8 oz	1 cup	16	¼ cup
		20	3⅕ Tbsp
		24	2⅔ Tbsp
		30	2 Tbsp
		40	1⅗ Tbsp
		50	3¾ tsp
		60	3¼ tsp
		70	2¾ tsp
		100	2 tsp

Source: Adapted from U.S. Department of Agriculture, Food and Nutrition Service, *Recipe File*, p. 95, 1988, U.S. Government Printing Office.

can develop strategies to market those menu items. Nutrition education activities can be planned to target the appropriate customers with the information they need to encourage the selection of all menu items.

Offering choices will enhance the probability that students will select a wider variety of foods from the different food groups. It has been well documented that when student customers can select from a choice of menu items within the different food groups and meal components, they are more likely to take foods from each of the categories. This is especially important and effective with foods in the vegetable group—often children's least favorite food group. As the menu becomes more complex, there is a greater need for accurate and consistent use of the production record. Offering choices makes forecasting quantities of foods to prepare more challenging for the director/manager. Maintaining accurate records of servings produced and served is especially critical when choices are offered. Regardless of the complexity of the menu, forecasting is critical to ensure that adequate amounts of foods are prepared for each meal and, equally important, to ensure that too much food is not prepared. Leftover food means higher cost to the program, since leftovers may become waste. Establishing cycle menus helps with forecasting the amounts of foods to prepare. (Refer to Chapter 10 for a discussion on forecasting and cycle menus.)

Production records and schedules are essential for quality control as well as cost control. Schools participating in the National School Lunch Program are required by USDA Food and Nutrition Service (FNS) to use production records (see Table 15–3 for an example of a production record appropriate for school use).[8] The production record is therefore a guide to follow to produce the meal and a record of what is produced and to whom it is served. Computer software programs are available that will prepare the basic production record and schedule from a selection of the recipes included in the program database. These reports or schedules can be customized to include any additional information the operator wishes to include.

The school food and nutrition program director/manager calculates the nutrient analysis of the menus based on the numbers of servings available to students as recorded on the production record. In a similar manner, the production record is a tool used by the state agency to verify the school food and nutrition program's compliance with the nutrition standards for the school meal.

Using production schedules ensures that foods reach the customer at the peak of freshness. The production schedule is organized to include the preparation and cooking times for each menu item. Beginning preparation times and serving times for each item set the time parameters for the food and nutrition program assistant responsible for the food product. Schedule production so that freshly prepared food products are placed on the serving line as they are needed to meet the demands of the customers. According to the *Keys to Excellence*,[9] all phases of production are planned in advance with the following points being considered:

- Work schedules are developed, posted, and reviewed periodically.
- Kitchen production is organized into preparation areas and assigned storage space.
- School food service delivery systems ensure maximum product quality and freshness.
- A long-range facility and equipment service and replacement plan is in place to improve production and delivery systems.

Batch cooking has long been a standard for production in school food service operations. Batch cooking refers to cooking in small quantities that can be served while the quality of the product is at its best. Batch cooking generally applies to preparing foods that require only short cooking times and do not hold well on the serving line, such as steamed broccoli and other vegetables and pasta products. Not only does batch cooking ensure higher-quality food products on the serving line, but batch cooking balances the use of equipment and allows the food and nutrition program staff to spread the workload over a longer period of time. This leads to less downtime and a more efficient work pattern.

Today, the school food and nutrition program production staff is encouraged to cook-to-the-line and use just-in-time food preparation.[10] Just-in-time food preparation or cooking-to-the-line takes the concept of batch cooking a step further. While the techniques are the same, food and nutrition program operations committed to just-in-time food preparation extend the batch cooking concept to most menu items. For example, freshly baked breads are baked off throughout the meal service time, as they are needed to ensure that each serving period has fresh-from-the-oven bread throughout the serving period and not just at the beginning. Enough pizza—a favorite among student customers—to meet the demands of an entire school meal is too often

Table 15–3 Sample Format #1 Food-Based Production Record (Traditional or Enhanced)

Site _____   Meal Date _____

Menu

Food Item Used and Form	Recipe or Product (name or #)	Person Responsible	Grade Group	Portion Size* (#/wt/qty)	Student Projected Servings	Total Projected Servings	Amount of Food Used** (lb or qty)	Student Servings	À la carte Servings	Adult Servings	Leftovers

(Actual)

*Portion size: Must be same as planned. Use separate line if adjusted for age.
**Amount of food used: Based on USDA Food Buying Guide or USDA recipe.
Source: Adapted from U.S. Department of Agriculture, Food and Nutrition Service, *Healthy School Meals Training,* Menu Planner, FNS-303, p. 195, 1998, U.S. Government Printing Office.

baked and held for service. It is just as easy, and far more desirable, to bake the pizza as needed. Some foods hold better than others, but most (except products requiring chilling) are best served as they come from the oven, fryer, or steamer.

Prepreparation of foods on the day before they are to served may assist the school food and nutrition program to shift to a just-in-time production schedule. Preprepared products, such as meat patties, breakfast sandwiches, and pizza, have excellent application with just-in-time food preparation. Cooking-to-the-line will also save cost, since only the amount of food needed is prepared. Carefully watching the line will prevent the overproduction of menu items that are not needed. Producing all the expected number of servings at one time may result in unnecessary food cost in leftovers.

Just-in-time service in the satellite facility requires different considerations due to the general lack of cooking equipment in these facilities. Satellite kitchens may receive food products that are fully prepared and ready for service or foods that require further preparation or finishing. Foods are prepared at a central or base kitchen and transported to the satellite kitchen, which may only have the equipment capability to hold foods warm or chilled until needed on the line. In such operations, proper holding and serving temperatures help ensure that foods are served at the peak of freshness, quality, and safety. Properly held foods maintain a fresh appearance and flavors.

The satellite food and nutrition program operator and the central kitchen manager should work closely to ensure that foods do not arrive overcooked or at temperatures inappropriate for serving. When equipment is available for finishing foods in the satellite kitchen, such as steaming frozen vegetables, preparing salad ingredients, and baking preprepared pizzas, just-in-time preparation and service will be easier to implement. Regardless of the type of operation, every effort should be made to serve all foods at the peak of freshness to meet the established quality standards for food production.

Just-in-time food and nutrition program preparation may require training the food and nutrition program staff to think differently about the way they work. Changing the pace and spreading the workload over a longer period of time may take some getting used to, but the freshness and improved flavor of the foods served to students are worth the efforts.

The heart of the production schedule is the hand-and-foot work or tasks needed to prepare the meal. The organization of each of these tasks has three parts: the get ready, the do, and the clean up. *Mise en place* is the French term used to mean to put in place and refers to the parts of the "get ready" part of the task. *Mise en place* is the organization of the task and begins with a careful study of all the recipes to be prepared. All ingredients are collected, weighed and measured, and prepared according to the recipe. All equipment is available, and the food and nutrition program assistants understand the correct operating procedures. According to *The New Professional Chef* written by chef instructors at the Culinary Institute of America,[11] *mise en place* means being able to keep many tasks in mind and establishing priorities to each task. Organizing each recipe that appears on the menu and prioritizing tasks in the kitchen will increase efficiency. The various cooking techniques have their own unique *mise en place*. Food and nutrition program assistants who plan ahead and adopt *mise en place* as a routine approach to food preparation are thinking and working like true food and nutrition program professionals.

Quality Standards

Each school food and nutrition program must establish quality standards for the various menu items offered. Quality standards set food preparation goals the food and nutrition program assistants work to achieve. Preparing and serving high-quality foods can be a source of pride for the food service staff and the school food and nutrition program. Certainly, programs striving for excellence only serve foods of which they are proud—foods that meet the high-quality standards established by the program. When food and nutrition program assistants are proud to acknowledge that they prepared certain foods, the school food and nutrition program is likely to be held in high regard by the customers and enjoy a high participation in the program.

Food quality is evaluated by various methods—sensory, chemical, and physical. Generally, the quality standards for foods can be grouped into those that evaluate appearance, texture or consistency, flavor, and temperature of the food when served (Table 15–4).[12] The study of food preparation has always included the characteristics of high-quality products. For example, all basic food preparation textbooks include a description of standard products that are produced when the recipes are followed correctly. Experienced cooks know that the standards for muffins are rounded top, no tunnel in the interior, slightly coarse crumb, medium cell wall, and tender texture. The food preparation steps to achieving the characteristics of the standard product for muffins are carefully followed to achieve the desired quality. [13]

While there are established standards of quality for many foods prepared in the school food and nutrition program, the staff will need to evaluate each menu item to ensure that an acceptable standard is in place. The quality standards become part of the standardized recipe, and all food service staff are familiar with each standard. Foods that do not meet the quality standard for that product should not be served to customers. How is the quality standard established in school nutrition programs?

- Begin with any established standards that are available and work to produce the standard product.
- Involve students and other customers in tasting and evaluating the standard product. Regional and individual preferences

are important aspects of establishing quality standards. For example, the preferred amount of chili powder added to a meat topping for tacos in southwestern states may be unacceptable to students in the northeast. The age of the students will also be a factor in establishing quality standards, as will the experience of the students with various foods.

- Acknowledge the lack of food experiences that many students have had and build on what they know about flavor, texture, and appearance. It is possible to start with a high-quality boxed pasta and cheese product that the students really like and move them along with more complex flavors and combinations of foods through experiences with new foods introduced at tasting parties or along with familiar foods on the serving line.
- Work with the food and nutrition program production staff to adjust the recipe and/or preparation techniques to improve the acceptability of foods when needed. Record the changes in writing to ensure that future use of the recipe reflects the changes.
- Use quality scorecards for each menu item. The quality scorecards list the desirable characteristics of the various foods. The cook responsible for preparing each food scores it before placing the food on the line. Foods that do not meet the quality standard are not served to customers. Some items may be recycled, while others become waste.

Quality standards and product evaluation are important aspects of any food and nutrition quality control program. The school food and nutrition program director/manager will develop a systematic approach to quality assurance. Formal and informal evaluations are planned as part of a comprehensive quality assurance program. Formal evaluations require more forethought and preparation, but are worth the effort. Set up a tasting session or test products directly on the serving line and fol-

Table 15–4 Quality ScoreCard for Baked Fruits and Fruit Desserts

Date _____ Name of Menu Item _____ Proudly Prepared by _____
Quality Scored By _____

Directions: When the food is ready to serve, use this quality scorecard to evaluate the quality. Mark Yes when the food meets the standard and No when it does not. Mark NA (not applicable) when a specific quality standard does not apply to the food being evaluated. Use the Comments section to explain why a food does not meet a standard.

Remember, if a food does not meet the quality standards, it should not be placed on the service line.

Quality Standard	Yes	No	NA	Comments
Appearance				
▲ Fruit pieces are similar in size	☐	☐	☐	
▲ Fruit pieces are intact	☐	☐	☐	
▲ Garnish is edible and appropriate for the dish	☐	☐	☐	
▲ Pastry or topping has a golden brown color	☐	☐	☐	
▲ Pastry has a blistery surface	☐	☐	☐	
Texture or consistency				
▲ All pieces of the fruit have the same texture	☐	☐	☐	
▲ Pastry has a flaky or mealy texture	☐	☐	☐	
▲ Pastry cuts easily	☐	☐	☐	
Flavor and seasonings				
▲ Fruits have a pleasing, slightly sweet, ripe flavor	☐	☐	☐	
▲ If seasonings have been used, they are detectable but not overpowering	☐	☐	☐	
▲ Seasonings enhance the fruit flavor	☐	☐	☐	
▲ Pastry has a pleasant, bland flavor	☐	☐	☐	
Service temperature				
▲ Pastry desserts −60° to −70°F	☐	☐	☐	
▲ Hot baked fruit −160° to −180°F	☐	☐	☐	

Source: Adapted with permission from National Food Service Management Institute, Culinary Techniques for Healthy School News, *Proud Times Lesson Booklets,* © 1996, National Food Service Management Institute.

low up with a questionnaire about the product. Informal evaluations include the casual observation of how well a food product is accepted by the students and other customers. For example, a walk through the cafeteria to visit with students who have selected the food being evaluated will reveal much about its acceptability, as will a stop by the dish return window to see how much is left on students' plates or trays. Student customers are the best source of information on the quality of the foods offered in the school cafeteria, and all standards reflect the taste preferences of these customers.

Training in proper food preparation techniques and the relationship of time and temperature of holding foods is key to the success of any quality assurance program. A well-trained food production staff prepares foods of high quality to meet the established standards; it understands the relationship of time and temperature to the maintenance of quality of foods held for service or on the line; and it takes appropriate measures to ensure that the quality meets the expectations of the customer and the program. The application of just-in-time food preparation is part of the quality assurance measures employed to achieve a quality program.

A well-trained staff applies the same quality assurance measures to the preparation and service of preprepared products. Many manufacturers include storage, preparation, and holding directions with their products. Some directions are better than others, so food and nutrition program assistants will need to apply their knowledge and expertise in cooking to these products in much the same way they do with from-scratch foods. When directions are given, they are followed for best results. Additional information on the handling of preprepared products may be available from the manufacturer. Requesting preparation and handling information from the manufacturer will stimulate the development of more precise directions for the use of various products.

The *Keys to Excellence*[14] quality standards state, "Management procedures assure the delivery of high quality food to all students." The *Keys* recommend that production be evaluated for efficiency and improvement measures implemented based on the following points:

- Staffing is adjusted for changes in participation.
- Productivity is measured monthly using meals per labor hour or other calculated indicators of productivity.
- An ongoing training program for food production is implemented.
- Daily food production records are accurate and complete.

Cooking Methods

Food cooks when it is heated. The heat may be transferred to the food from some source or created within the food. Heat energy is transferred from its source to the food by means of conduction, convection currents, or radiation. Induction cooking and microwave cooking are examples of cooking taking place without a heat source. Induction cooking relies on the generation of heat within the food being cooked by creating a magnetic field between the induction unit and the metal cooking utensil. Only the food gets hot. The cooking surface and the metal handles of pots and pans maintain a comfortable skin temperature. Induction cooking is becoming increasingly more affordable for commercial food service use.[15] Cooking occurs when food is exposed to electromagnetic waves in a microwave oven. Commercial microwave ovens are available and have application in the school food and nutrition program operation.

Selecting the correct cooking method is essential to the production of high-quality foods. The correct preparation techniques and the right equipment are needed to implement the method of choice. When certain equipment is not available, acceptable alternate methods must be selected. For example, it is possible to steam frozen or fresh vegetables in an oven if the school kitchen does not have a steamer. Flexibility and versatility are desirable characteristics for all food service equipment. For example, the tilting skillet or braising pan has many uses—braising meats, boiling pasta, stir-frying, and many others.

A complete analysis of the menu for the cooking methods most appropriate for each menu item and the equipment to be used is a critical step in the operation of an excellent school food and nutrition program. Training in the use of existing equipment and an understanding of the principles of cookery will give the food and nutrition program assistant the skills needed to produce the menu efficiently and make adjustments in equipment selection and cooking techniques when necessary.

All cooking methods are classified as either moist heat or dry heat. Moist heat cooking methods transfer heat to the food through either water or steam. Dry heat cooking methods transfer heat to the foods through dry air, contact with the hot metal of the cooking equipment, radiation (heat rays), or hot fat. New equipment technology combines moist and dry heat during the cooking process (i.e., convection streamers), while other new equipment technology allows for more than one dry heat application, such as the quartz grill that simultaneously grills and broils to cook foods from the top and bottom. Dry heat methods of cooking are usually used for tender meats, fish, poultry, and batters and doughs. Dry heat cooking methods include roasting, baking, oven frying, broiling, grilling, barbecuing, and frying.

Moist heat cooking methods include boiling, simmering, stewing, poaching, blanching, braising, and steaming. All of these methods are variations on the same theme, with the temperature of the water or other liquid used being the distinguishing factor.

Deep-fried foods are some of the favorite items on school menus, and students demand that they be served often. The amount of fat absorbed by the product being fried can be decreased to some degree, if proper frying techniques are followed: use the proper temperature; time the frying process; keep frozen products solidly frozen until ready to cook; and remember that products with a high percentage of eggs, fat, and/or sugar absorb more fat than other products. Select the frying oil that is most appropriate for the fryer being used. Fats that have less saturated fatty acids may be a better nutrition choice, but following the manufacturer's recommendations on the selection of the cooking oil will generally give better performance and the highest-quality product with less fat absorption.

Keeping the cooking oil free of food particles and using the correct frying temperatures for the product being cooked will prolong the life of the frying oil and prevent off-flavors that result when the oil starts to deteriorate. Modern deep-fat fryers have solid-state electronics that monitor the cooking cycle and control cooking temperatures. A built-in filter system is a necessary feature to consider when selecting a gas or electric fryer. Pressurized fryers that cook food faster are also available. In addition to keeping the oil clean, it is important to add new oil to the fryer and to store the cooking oil properly between uses to prevent a rancid flavor or smell to the oil, which transfers easily to the food being cooked.

When selecting oils for cooking methods, such as sautéing, and food preparation techniques, such as preparing salad dressings, choose cooking oils that are less saturated. Recent research indicates that both poly- and monounsaturated fats can be included in a healthy diet. Flavorful oils such as olive oil, a good source of monounsaturated fatty acids, not only serve as a cooking medium but add a desirable characteristic favor. A good rule of thumb might be that when adding fat during cooking or to prepared foods such as salads in the form of a dressing, be sure flavor is added and not just fat and calories.

MENU PRODUCTION TECHNIQUES FOR HEALTHY SCHOOL MEALS

School food and nutrition personnel are trained in food preparation techniques that preserve food quality and nutrient content. Value-added products, such as preprepared salad ingredients; precooked meat patties; bakery products; prepared pasta, vegetable, and meat salads; and many other convenience products, are widely used in school food and nutrition programs. The food industry is constantly presenting new value-added food items that require little or no preparation. These foods are priced with the labor required to prepare them built into the cost of the product. When selecting value-added products in preference to preparing the foods in the school kitchen, follow the manufacturer's directions for proper storage and finishing to ensure food quality and food safety. Although more and more school food and nutrition programs rely on preprepared food products, from-scratch cooking is still very much a part of their operations.

The correct application of cooking and holding techniques to all foods prepared in the school food and nutrition program are critical to quality standards established for the program. This chapter includes a brief discussion of the major points to consider when preparing the various food products.

Vegetables, Fruits, and Salads

The nutritional contribution of fruits and vegetables to the school meal is well documented, as is the increasing evidence of the health benefits derived from eating a wide variety of fruits and vegetables, especially fresh fruits and fresh vegetables. Vegetables and fruits are good sources of many vitamins and minerals, incomplete protein, and carbohydrates, while they are low in fat and sodium. Processing, including drying, canning, and preparation for freezing, may alter the vitamin content of vegetables and fruits. Careful handling to prevent bruising, proper storage temperature, and proper preparation techniques that control time and temperature of cooking and holding enhance the retention of the vitamin content of vegetable and fruits. The *Dietary Guidelines for Americans* recommends a diet that includes plenty of vegetables and fruits each day. The Food Guide Pyramid recommendation for vegetables is three to five servings a day and two to three servings of fruit each day.

Vegetable items are consistently the least-often selected foods served in the school cafeteria. New and fun ways to prepare and serve vegetables are needed if children and teenagers are going to choose them. Serving fresh, raw vegetables with a low-fat dip, salad bars, and preplated salads are ways to increase vegetable selection by the students. Offering a variety of vegetable choices each day or all-you-can eat vegetable bars will also improve vegetable selection. Proper cooking and holding of cooked vegetables and vegetable dishes is also essential to their acceptance.

When cooking vegetables it is important to remember that the chlorophyll, the green pigment in vegetables, turns a dark olive green color when overheated or overcooked. The addition of strong acid to cooked green vegetables will also turn the color an unappealing olive green. Overcooking and prolonged holding on the serving line can also ruin the flavors of vegetables—strong flavors get stronger and mild flavors fade. Following the preparation techniques on the standardized recipe and preparing vegetables for just-in-time service will ensure that vegetables are served at the peak of freshness.

Salad preparation will incorporate the principles of fruit and vegetable preparation discussed here, as well as the following considerations. Salads offer a wonderful opportunity for encouraging students to eat more vegetables and fruits. Salad ingredients may include fresh, canned, dried, and frozen ingredients. Preprepared salads of all kinds, including pasta, potato, bean, tuna, chicken, ham, and many others, may be purchased and served in the school food and nutrition program. Select the highest-quality preprepared salads available and purchase those products that contribute positively to the nutrition goals established for the program. Many preprepared salads contain mayonnaise and oils as principal ingredients and should be served in moderation and/or in combination with lower-fat selections for proper nutrient balance. Value-added salad greens are available washed, chopped, and bagged in combination with other salad vegetables, such as grated carrots and red cabbage. Although preprepared fresh salad ingredients such as these are prewashed, it is a good practice to rinse all fresh produce with cool water as part of the preparation. Look for signs of freshness when receiving value-added produce, and use all of these products within the freshness date recorded on the packaging to ensure highest quality and food safety.

When preparing fresh tossed green salads, consider the following: store fresh produce at the right temperature; use a variety of ingredients for contrast in color, flavor, texture, and shape; prepare all ingredients so that they are clean, drained, chilled, and crisp; and offer a variety of low-fat or fat-free salad dressings for students to add to the salad. Add salad dressings close to the time of service.

Preplated salads are salads that are placed on a separate plate or small bowl. Preplated salads have a base or underliner to hold or frame the salad, a body or main ingredients of the salad, a dressing that is either part of the salad ingredients or served on the side to be added by the customer, and an edible garnish. Fresh vegetable ingredients in salads, such as carrots, broccoli, and cauliflower, may be blanched to improve and retain their color and make them easier to eat.

Serve salads often and offer a variety of salads to increase selection of vegetables and fruits by the student customers. As with fruit and vegetable menu items, establish quality standards for all salads offered as part of the school menu and serve only those products that meet these quality standards.

Entrees: Meats and Meat Alternates

Meats

Entrees or the center-of-the-plate items are generally meat, fish, or poultry item. Meat items include beef, pork, lamb, and veal. Poultry and fish have similar preparation principles as meats. When meat and poultry are cooked, the texture, flavor, appearance, and safety of the food is affected. While cooking destroys harmful microorganisms that may cause illness in humans, it also improves the flavor of meats and poultry. Proper cooking is essential to ensure optimum texture, appearance, and yield of meat and poultry products. Cooking times and temperature affect the finished product. You

---

For further food safety information call the USDA's nationwide, toll-free meat and poultry hotline at 1-800-535-4555; TTY: 1-800-256-7072.
Source: Reprinted from U.S. Department of Agriculture, *Kitchen Thermometers*, Food Safety and Inspection Service, p. 8, 1997.

---

should follow the guidelines for the safe cooking and handling of meat and poultry discussed under Processed Meat Products.

Moisture and fat are lost during most methods of cooking, particularly dry heat methods such as roasting and baking. This "cooking loss" is evidenced by the shrinkage of the product during cooking and the amount of drippings in the pan. Prolonged holding will contribute further to the cooking loss. Just-in-time cooking is applied whenever possible to decrease cooking loss and maintain product quality.

Select cooking methods for meat and poultry that use a minimal amount of fat and sodium. Since many meats are potentially high in fat, especially ground meats, selecting grilling, baking, or similar methods of preparation allow for some of the fat to drain and be discarded. Rinsing cooked ground meats results in flavor loss and may create a food safety hazard. Over the last few decades there has been a discussion among food professionals on the need for and the desirability of rinsing cooked ground beef to remove fat that has liquefied during the cooking process. Generally when cooked ground beef is rinsed, rinsing under warm tap water follows thorough draining. Numerous studies have explored the benefits of rinsing cooked ground beef to remove fat. It is generally agreed that rinsing cooked ground beef does lower the fat content of the beef, but it also lowers the content of water-soluble nutrients, and flavor is lost along with the fat and meat juices. The safe handling of cooked ground beef before, during, and after rinsing and how to properly dispose of the rinse water have created much debate. In September 1997 USDA, FNS issued the following statement (posted on Meal Talk, an internet discussion group), "Rinsing Beef—USDA recognizes rinsing beef is one of several techniques available to lower the fat content of meat. USDA does not encourage nor discourage the use of rinsing beef. If a school chooses to use this technique, food and nutrition program managers should be sure local food safety and sanitation practices are followed." School food authorities are recommended to consult with their state agencies for policies regarding the rinsing of cooked ground meat products.

Moist heat methods such as braising and stewing are recommended for meats from less tender cuts—those parts of the animal that get the most exercise. Grinding, cubing, and cutting meat into strips will also help to tenderize less tender cuts of meat. Browning of meats and poultry pieces to be braised and stewed allows excess fat to be drained away. The residue or *fond* left on the pan where the meat juices evaporate can add flavor to the dish being prepared. The liquid for moist heat cooking can be a stock or broth made from meat bases, cooked or canned vegetables, or water. If purchasing commercial stock products, select low-sodium varieties.

Processed Meat Products. Processed meat products are sometimes referred to as value-added products. Processing has removed some of the preparation steps needed and time is saved in the preparation and service of value-added food products. Examples of processed meat products include canned meats; breaded chicken and meat items; skinless, boneless chicken breasts; uncooked and precooked meat patties; burritos; casseroles; and egg rolls. Processed meat products should be selected carefully, with attention to the sodium and fat content of the product being considered as part of the quality standard for these products. The culinary techniques used to finish these products should add little or no fat or sodium.

Processed meat products have the cost of labor built into the cost of the product; therefore, school food service operations need fewer labor hours when using processed products than when cooking from scratch.

Finishing processed meats requires careful attention to the directions recommended by the product manufacturer. When adequate directions are not given on the packaging for the storage, finishing, and holding of processed foods, contact the manufacturer for more detailed instructions. Most processed products must be cooked for just-in-time service and held for only a short time during service in order to maintain product quality. Processed meats (as well as all meat items) are always cooked to the *internal* temperature recommended by the manufacturer to ensure food safety. Color change in cooked meats and meat products is no longer recognized as a reliable indicator of doneness. Foodborne bacteria and other illness-causing microorganisms may survive cooking beyond the temperature that causes the meat to lose its pink color. An internal temperature of at least 165° F is required to kill bacteria.[16] Products should be checked with a calibrated thermometer (see Figure 15–1).

If the meat or poultry product is not served immediately, it is covered and kept in a warmer at the correct temperature or chilled in the refrigerator until needed. Meat and poultry products are never held at room temperature. (Refer to Chapter 18 for a detailed discussion of food safety and proper procedures to follow when determining the internal temperature of various food products.)

Follow these additional suggestions when preparing and serving processed meat products in the school food and nutrition program

- keep frozen products frozen until time for cooking;
- do not refreeze extra portions that have been removed from the freezer if they have thawed;
- always follow the recommended cooking techniques, times, and temperatures;
- follow the steps for just-in-time cooking; and
- deep-fat fry only those products that cannot be successfully prepared using an alternate method such as baking or grilling.[17]

Meat Alternates

Meat alternate main dishes rely on eggs, cheese, and grain-legume (dried beans and peas) combinations to provide protein and

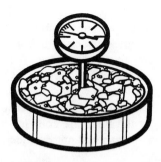

Calibrating a Thermometer

There are two ways to check the accuracy of a food thermometer. One method uses ice water; the other uses boiling water. Many thermometers have a calibration nut under the dial that can be adjusted. Check the package for instructions.

ICE WATER

To use the ice water method, fill a large glass with finely crushed ice, add clean tap water to the top of the ice, and stir well. Immerse the thermometer stem a minimum of 2 inches into the mixture, touching neither the sides nor the bottom of the glass. (For ease in handling, the stem of the thermometer can be placed through the clip section of the stem sheath and, holding the sheath horizontally, lowered into the water.) Without removing the stem from the ice, hold the adjusting nut under the head of the thermometer with a suitable tool and turn head so pointer reads 32°F. Allow a minimum of 30 seconds before adjusting.

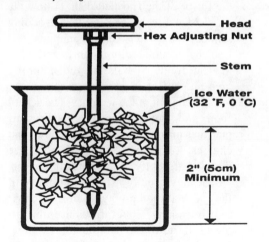

BOILING WATER

To use the boiling water method, bring a deep pan of clean tap water to a full rolling boil. Immerse the stem of a thermometer in boiling water a minimum of 2 inches and wait at least 30 seconds. (For ease in handling, the stem of the thermometer can be placed through the clip section of the steam sheath and, holding the sheath horizontally, lowered into the boilding water.) Without removing the stem from the pan, hold the adjusting nut under the head of the thermometer with a suitable tool and turn head so the thermometer reads 212°F.

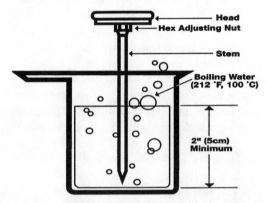

For true accuracy, distilled water must be used and the atmospheric pressure must be one atmosphere (29.921 inches of mercury). A consumer using tap water in unknown atmospheric conditions would probably not measure water boiling at 212°F. Most likely it would boil at least 2°F and perhaps as much as 5°F lower. And remember that water boils at a lower temperature in a high-altitude area.

Check with your local Cooperative Extension Service or Health Department for the exact temperature of boiling water in your area.

Even if the thermometer cannot be calibrated, it should still be checked for accuracy using either method. Any inaccuracies can be taken into consideration when using, or the thermometer can be replaced. For example, if the thermometer reads 214°F in boiling water, subtract 2 degrees from the temperature registered when taking a reading in food.

Figure 15–1 Calibrating a thermometer. *Source:* Reprinted from U.S. Department of Agriculture, *Kitchen Thermometers*, Food Safety and Inspection Service, p. 7, 1997.

other nutrients supplied by meat-based entrees. Additionally, grain and legumes provide carbohydrates, starch and fiber, and are naturally lower in fat than other protein foods, such as meats and cheese. Special attention is given to the preparation of eggs and cheese for just-in-time cooking, since these food products lose quality quickly during holding.

Meat alternate main dishes are some of the most versatile foods on the menu. Many ethnic and culturally diverse food items fall into this category. Bean burritos, couscous, bean and rice dishes, bean and corn salads, vegetable lasagna and pizza, and omelets are some examples of meat alternate main dishes that students choose. Many students in the 1990s have begun to adopt various degrees of vegetarianism. Explore the various cultures and nationalities represented in the student population serviced by the school food and nutrition program for ideas in food selection and preparation methods to liven up the school menu.

Challenge students' taste preferences by offering a wide variety of entrees that break with the hamburger/pizza tradition prevalent in some programs. Meatless main dishes fit well into any menu-planning option. Because the cost is generally less per serving, the portion size can often be increased to help keep the calories and nutrient content of the meal high without adding extra cost. Similarly, since the fat content of many meat alternate dishes is low or moderately low (menu items with greater proportions of some types of cheese may be an exception), meat alternates are a good nutrition buy as well.

Follow these suggestions when preparing meat alternate entrees.

- Sort dry beans and peas to remove any foreign material that may be present. Soaking dry beans and peas shortens the cooking time. Cook the soaked beans in fresh water if desired. (The soaking water will contain soluble carbohydrates and oligosaccharides, which may cause gas to develop in the lower gastrointestinal tract.

Starting with fresh water may help relieve this distress for some individuals.) Alkaline ingredients such as baking soda are often used to speed cooking of dried beans and peas due to the softening effect on the structural carbohydrates in the legumes. But since alkaline ingredients also destroy some of the thiamine content in the legumes, they should not be added for any reason.

- Select canned beans and peas rather than dry ones when either preparation time and/or availability of cooking equipment are limited. Canned legumes are ready to heat and serve and save time and effort during preparation.

- Chill cooked beans and peas in shallow pans in the refrigerator if they are not prepared for just-in-time service. Overheating during cooking or holding on the steam table will cause legumes to have a floury or pasty taste and texture. Use just-in-time service or batch heating of prepared dishes.

- Season legume-based menu items with spices and herbs and a minimal amount of salt. Some salt added during the cooking process of dry beans and peas enhances the flavor of the finished dish. Follow the standardized recipe carefully when adding salt to avoid using excessive amounts.

- Use cheese along with legumes and other low-fat foods to balance the naturally high-fat content of many cheeses with the low-fat content of the legumes. The school food and nutrition program director/manager may also choose to use lower-fat cheeses. Remember that lower-fat cheese melts differently than natural cheese, which may greatly affect the quality of the finished food product if correct cooking times and temperatures are not followed. Refer to the manufacturer's directions for details on how to handle low-fat cheese during cooking.

- Heating and holding will cause cheese to become tough and rubbery over time. Use just-in-time cooking when preparing pizza and other cheese-based food products. Adding the cheese topping for casseroles, such as lasagna, at the end of the cooking period will help to maintain the quality of the finished menu item.

- Use eggs by themselves or in combination with other ingredients for great low-cost, nutritious main dish menu items. In addition to their high nutritive value, eggs are used in various food products to add color, flavor, texture, thickness, and moisture, and to act as an emulsifier. Eggs are added to baked products, puddings and custards, and cooked dressings. They may be hard-cooked and used in salads and casseroles. Eggs are a good nutrition buy, providing protein of high biological value and various vitamins and minerals, including iron. They are also good buys related to their cost. Eggs are less expensive than meats and cheese per portion.

- Prepare egg dishes such as scrambled eggs and quiche as needed, using just-in-time preparation techniques. Cooked egg products do not maintain their quality long during holding. Egg dishes are an excellent place for foodborne illness–causing microorganisms to grow. Cook all eggs and egg-containing food products to 165°F to ensure that all possible salmonella bacteria common to egg and poultry products are destroyed. All cracked or whole eggs are cooked until the white is completely set and the internal temperature has reached 165°F.

- Substitute pasteurized egg products for whole eggs in cooked egg dishes that require long cooking times; however, it is still necessary to cook to the recommended 165°F internal temperature, since any product is subject to contamination during food preparation. When using frozen egg products, thaw in the refrigerator only the amount needed within a 24-hour period. Do not refreeze unused thawed egg products.

- Egg substitutes made from egg whites or soy or milk protein cannot be credited toward meeting the meat alternate requirement in reimbursed school meals.

- Use grains such as rice and barley in entree items to extend meats and other meat alternates. Try the many pasta products and other grain products available to add interest and eating enjoyment to the school menu at breakfast and lunch.

- Refer to the *USDA Recipe File* and the *Tool Kit Recipes*[18–20] for recipe suggestions using grain, legumes, eggs, and cheese as meat alternates or in combination with meat and poultry as a meat extender.

Breads

Breads have been referred to as "the staff of life." They have an important role in providing proper nutrition as evidenced by their prominent position at the base of the Food Guide Pyramid. Therefore, school food and nutrition programs are recommended to serve a wide variety and plentiful amounts of breads. High-quality bread products require a thorough understanding of the principles of preparing batters and doughs.

Breads may be classified in several ways; for example, breads are either made from batters, flour mixtures that pour; or doughs, flour mixtures that are shaped. Breads are also classified according to the source of leavening gases responsible for the increase in volume of the bread during baking. Carbon dioxide is the principal leavening gas in baked products, while air and steam also contribute to the leavening, in varying amounts, in all baked products, including breads. When carbon dioxide is produced by a chemical leavening agents such as baking powder or baking soda, the bread is referred to as a quick bread because the reaction takes place quickly.

Carbon dioxide is also produced biologically during the process of yeast fermentation. Breads that rely on yeast fermentation to produce the carbon dioxide needed to leaven the product are referred to as yeast breads. Yeast fermentation takes time. The fermentation period is referred to as proofing. Generally, the soft dough or sponge is proofed and the bread is proofed again after shaping and panning.

All breads rise in the heat of the oven, as the reaction of the baking powder and fermentation are enhanced during the early part of baking. This increase in volume during baking is known as oven spring. All breads, including quick breads and yeast breads, are evaluated for consistency and texture largely based on the correct amount of leavening of the product. If the rise is not adequate, the finished product will be heavy and compact. If the batter or dough has increased in volume too much, the texture may be open and airy or the bread my collapse during baking.

In addition to the importance of the proper amount of leavening in breads are other basic ingredients, which play a functional role in the baked product. All breads contain some type of flour. Generally, wheat flour is used as the principal flour in breads due to the high protein content of the wheat grain. When rye bread is made, some wheat flour is required to provide the protein needed to develop the gluten—protein matrix—of the dough. Without gluten, the bread will rise during proofing and baking and collapse due to a poor structure. Some commercial low-protein flours are enhanced with gluten extracts to improve their protein content without having to add wheat flour.

The ratio of flour to liquid in the mixture determines whether or not it is classified as a batter or dough. Quick breads made from batters include muffins, waffles, pancakes, cornbread, and fruit breads, such as banana bread. Biscuits and cream puffs are examples of quick breads that are made from doughs. Yeast breads such as rolls, loaf breads, and cinnamon rolls are all made from doughs. Yeast breads may be batters as well, but most yeast breads are stiff enough to knead (work with the hands)

and roll or shape into rolls or loaves. Milk and water are the most commonly used liquid ingredients in breads. Milk adds extra nutrients to the bread and enhances crust formation and browning. Lean (low in fat) breads such as pizza dough and French bread are made with water and little fat.

Breads also contain a fat, salt, and a liquid, usually milk; batters and doughs may also contain eggs and sugars, as well as other flavoring ingredients. The fat in breads contributes to the texture of the bread. Fat interferes with the formation of gluten in the batter and dough and thus tenderizes the product. Fat also improves the flavor and keeping quality of the finished bread. Solid fats are generally used in quick breads and pastry crust because as the fat melts during baking the space left in the dough creates the characteristic layers or flakes desirable in these products. Oils also tenderize baked products in the same way as solid fats do, but oils do not produce layers in biscuits or flaky pastries.

Eggs are added to breads to improve their flavor, color, and texture. Eggs also contribute to the overall nutritional value of breads. Breads that are more delicate in texture, such as muffins, rely on the protein in the egg for structure. Egg protein provides structure to the baked product without adding toughness, as would using a higher ratio of flour or overmixing the batter. Eggs contribute moisture for steam formation during baking, which helps to leaven the product. Cream puffs rely primarily on the egg protein for structure development, and steam and air beaten into the dough are the only leavening gases in this easy-to-prepare product. Eggs also improve the overall quality of yeast breads.

Sugar is added to batters and doughs to improve the texture. Sugar, like fat, shortens the gluten strands to cause a more tender product. Flour mixtures with high percentages of sugar withstand greater mechanical manipulation than those with little or no sugar. Sugar contributes to the browning of the bread and the development of the crust. Sugar is the food that feeds the yeast during fermentation. The addition of sugar also improves the flavor, of course. Salt is a functional ingredient in yeast breads, since salt helps control the fermentation process. Salt also adds flavor to batters and doughs. With the exception of yeast breads, salt could be eliminated from the batter or dough of baked products without adverse effects.

Breads are popular foods for all students. Take advantage of the wide variety of grains and other ingredients available today to create wholesome, interesting breads for the school menu. The aroma of freshly baked breads is an irresistible calling card for the school food and nutrition program. If the program elects not to prepare breads from scratch, then fresh-baked breads from mixes or frozen products are a good substitute. All breads, whether served warm or hot, are prepared for just-in-time service. The power of the aroma drifting down the classroom halls is equally effective in bringing customers to the cafeteria for breakfast as lunch.

Desserts

Healthful desserts made from grain products and fruits may be offered to ensure that adequate calories are in the meals when fats are reduced as recommended in the *Dietary Guidelines for Americans*. Desserts are typically popular menu items and add much to the overall enjoyment of eating. Many techniques and ingredients can be used to create flavorful, lower-fat, lower-sugar desserts that fit into a well-balanced school meal.

What are healthful desserts? Healthful desserts are those food products that are consistent in composition to the recommendations in the Food Guide Pyramid. Desserts provide the menu planner with another opportunity to use fruits and grains in school meals. When developing dessert recipes, consider the taste and feel of the food. Some desserts are delicate in flavor, such as baked custard, while others

have a robust flavor, such as cherry crisp. Desserts may also be served warm or cold, which affects the flavor and consistency of many dessert products. For example, fruit pies, cobblers, and crisps have more pungent flavors and flakier topping when served warm. Frozen desserts are served while completely frozen to maintain texture, consistency, and flavor.

Fresh, canned, and frozen fruits always make an appropriate and simple dessert. These fruits may be served plain or cooked in some way. Poaching and stewing are examples of cooking fruits for service. A simple sauce or topping completes the dessert. Fruits also make excellent toppings for plain cakes or served along with cookies or brownies. Fruit salads also may serve as a dessert. Fresh fruits slices served with a dip made from yogurt or honey or peanut butter is another idea for a sweet finishing touch for lunch.

Baked desserts may include sweet breads made with fruit, such as banana bread, applesauce muffins, or pound cake. Fruit purées make a very good fat substitute in many baked desserts. Consult with the state agency to determine the crediting of any baked dessert offered under the USDA food-based menu-planning option. Follow the quality scorecard example given in Table 15–4 to evaluate the quality of a baked fruit dessert.

Recipe Development and Modification

Healthful school meals are planned and prepared to meet the nutrition recommendations of the *Dietary Guidelines for Americans*. The use of only a moderate amount of fat, salt, and sugars is recommended in food preparation to meet the nutrition goals of the program. When necessary, recipes are modified to achieve appropriate levels of fat, sodium, and sugar in considering student acceptability.

Recipe modification begins with a nutrient analysis of the standardized recipe. The director/manager decides which recipes are to be modified to lower the fat, saturated fat, salt, or sugar based on the analysis, keeping in mind that not all recipes are required to meet the nutrient standards established by USDA for the school food and nutrition program. It is the combination of menu items in the meal and the average of the nutrient contents of the school meals over time that is evaluated for meeting the nutrient standards. Ideally schools that do not participate in the National School Lunch or Breakfast Programs also use the same nutrition standards established for the federally funded programs.

The successful school food and nutrition program director/manager works to accomplish the most student-acceptable blend of recipes. Many school food and nutrition programs offer foods on a regular basis that food and nutrition program personnel are most proud to serve to the students. Very often those foods are dessert items or other special comfort foods that may be higher in fat, salt, sugar, or some combination of these than other menu choices. This may lead the director/manager to decide to either eliminate the item from the menu, serve it less often, serve it along with lower fat or salt or sugar menu choices, or modify the recipe to improve the nutrient profile. It is probably wise to resist modification of these signature items—those foods on the menu that the school food and nutrition program is famous for and that students really enjoy and look forward to eating—in order to avoid disappointed customers.

All foods can fit into a healthy diet, and most have a place on the school menu. The menu teaches students to select healthful foods by offering a wide variety of healthful foods from which to choose, and offering foods that need to be selected in moderation and/or balanced with healthier choices. Properly prepared and attractively served, nutrient-dense foods, such as fresh-baked whole-grain breads, can become students' favorites also and can become the signature items of the school food and nutrition program.

Successful recipe modification that helps the program achieve the goal of healthful school meals incorporates the suggestions outlined in the *Keys to Excellence*.[21]

1. The school food and nutrition program staff tests and evaluates modified recipes before serving them to the students.
2. Recipe modifications are tested by student panels or committees before they are added to the menu.
3. Information about recipe modifications is communicated to parents and students.
4. Modified menu items are served to the students, and the acceptability is assessed by using meal counts and other measures.
5. New or modified menu items are promoted through planned promotions, tasting parties, and point-of-sale marketing (some directors/managers have reported that nutrient disclosure increases acceptance of lower fat and sodium items, while others say that just the opposite is true in their schools).
6. Nutrition education activities in the classroom and the cafeteria are coordinated with the menu changes.

When modifying existing standardized recipes or developing new ones, it is important to follow the basic rules of recipe development, which include the following:

- Complete the nutrient analysis and make a decision on what modifications are to be made; remember that in addition to adding flavor, fat, sugar, and salt may serve as functional ingredients in the recipe.
- Modify only one kind of ingredient in a recipe at a time—once the fat is adjusted to an acceptable level, for example, the salt content might be adjusted.
- Make small changes and evaluate the results; continue adjusting the recipe until the desired results are achieved and the product meets the quality standards of the program.
- Record all modifications and evaluation results so that the recipe can be reproduced successfully.

- Work in small batches of 25 servings, and repeat successful modifications to 50 servings.
- Use substitute ingredients that will serve the same function in the recipe, such as puréed fruit in the place of fat in many baked products.
- Taste-test all modified items before offering them on the menu.

When recipes undergo major modifications and no longer taste or look like the original item, but are tasty and meet the nutrition and quality standards of the program, introducing them as new menu items and giving them a new name may enhance student acceptance. Recipe modification and development to lower fat, salt, and sugar are only part of the efforts that can be made to serve healthier school meals.

Purchasing ingredients and prepared foods that are lower in fat, salt, and sugars should be the first step when menu modifications are needed. For example, lowfat dairy products and reduced sodium condiments are available, as are lean cuts of meats and higher lean to fat ratios in ground beef. Cooking methods that require little or no additional fat can be used by the school food and nutrition staff. A well-trained production staff knows the techniques of dry *sauté*, grilling, baking, steaming, microwaving, and other lower fat cooking methods. Not only do these cooking techniques lower the fat in the school meal, they produce foods that are flavorful and well accepted by the student customer. The *Culinary Techniques for Healthy School Meals* is one example of an excellent training package for teaching food service assistants healthy cooking techniques.

CULINARY SKILLS ATTRACT STUDENT CUSTOMERS

Flavor Enhancement Techniques

The concept of flavor and the individual's perception of flavors is complex. The old saying, "if it doesn't taste good, they won't eat it," is still true. When recipes and meals are modified for fat, salt, and sugar content, flavor is lost. If students are accustomed to high-fat, high-sodium, or high-sugar foods and meals, participation may decrease as the school food and nutrition program implements the nutrition recommendations in the *Dietary Guidelines for Americans*. Flavor enhancement is an essential component of the process of producing student-acceptable healthful school meals. Flavor enhancement techniques including the addition of spice, herbs, and other flavoring ingredients, and the cooking techniques that build flavors of foods are discussed here.

Spices

Spices[22] are aromatic ingredients produced primarily from the bark and seeds of plants. The flavor of most spices is intense and powerful. Spices are nearly always sold in the dried form and may be available whole or ground. In addition there are a number of spice blends, such as curry powder, chili powder, and pickling spice. Various other spice blends are possible and may be purchased as a commercial product or prepared on site to the specific taste preferences of the students in the school.

Herbs

Herbs[22] are the leaves of aromatic plants used primarily to add flavor to food. Most herbs are available both fresh and dried, although some dry more successfully than others. Aroma is a good indicator of quality in both fresh and dried herbs. The scent of the herb can be tested by crumbling a few leaves between the fingers and then smelling the leaves. The aroma should resemble the fresh herb and not dry grass.

Herbs can be used to flavor numerous preparations. They should be used to enhance and balance, not overpower, the flavors in the food products. Overuse or the inappropriate use of herbs can result in food product that tastes of nothing but herbs. Certain herbs have special affinity for certain foods, such as basil and tomato dishes. Refer to the seasoning chart, Table 15–5, for additional suggested uses of spices and herbs.[23]

Dried herbs are often stored too close to the top of the range, are kept too long, and are purchased in overly large quantities. Purchase only the amount of dried herbs that can be used within two or three months and store away from any sources of heat. Discard herbs that a have a musty or flat aroma.

Other flavoring ingredients include vinegars, fruit juices, citrus zest, lily family vegetables (i.e., onion and garlic), peppers, stocks, horseradish, and ginger root. Commercial ingredients also include low-sodium soy sauce, Worcestershire sauce, smoke flavor concentrate, meat bases, vegetable stock, flavorful oils and butter, hot sauce, prepared mustard, and flavoring extracts such as vanilla and almond. Select commercially prepared products carefully to avoid increasing the sodium content of the food product unnecessarily. Use oils and other flavorful fats in moderation. For chocolate-flavored recipes, use cocoa as a low-fat replacement.

Cooking Techniques That Add Flavor[24]

Deglazing of pans and equipment where meats and vegetables have browned adds great flavors to cooking liquids. Little or no fat is needed to accomplish this technique. Roasting vegetables also enhances flavors through caramelization of the sugars in the vegetables. Grilling and marinating are also preparation techniques that add delicious flavors to foods. Heating brings out the natural volatile component of spices. Remember the wonderful aroma of cinnamon rolls as they bake? To further enhance the flavor, try heating ground spices before adding them to other ingredients. A word of caution: watch the temperature closely to avoid burning the spice during heating.

Vegetables and Fruits

Use spices and herbs to enhance the flavor of vegetables and fruits. Refer to Table 15–5 for suggestions of seasoning appropriate for these foods. Be careful not to overpower the natural flavors of vegetables and fruits, especially delicately flavored ones. Remember that no herb or spice will make up for improper cooking that has ruined the natural flavor of a vegetable. If strong-flavored vegetables, such as broccoli or cauliflower are overcooked, they should not be served. No amount of seasoning will repair the damage caused by overcooking strong flavored vegetables.

Meat and Meat Alternates

The fat in meat and poultry releases flavors when heated. Take advantage of this principle by applying dry heat to meat and poultry when possible. After any excess fat is drained from pans, incorporate the *fond* (dry residue of the meat juices that collects on the pan when meats are cooked) that is left on the pan into the liquid or sauce that becomes part of the food product.

Make a *mirepoix* of flavorful vegetables such as onions, celery, and carrots to season these products.

Dry rubs of spices and ground or chopped herbs also add flavors to roasted and baked meat and poultry. Placing fresh or dried herbs just under the skin of poultry gives a real boost to the flavor and the appearance of baked chicken breasts. Meat and poultry may also be marinated in a flavorful oil and acid mixture to add a distinct flavor as well as enhance the tenderness of the product.

Spices and other flavorful ingredients are added during cooking and final preparation to add distinctive flavor to meat alternate food products. For example, try the addition of ground cinnamon and cloves to cooked beans and chopped fresh cilantro to a black bean salad. Add cooked beans or peas to caramalized chopped onions, prepared by the dry sauté method, for great flavor and color. Chopped peppers—select from a wide variety of colors and flavors—add great color and flavor to egg and cheese dishes, such as omelets. Use small amounts of lean meats as a seasoning for meat alternate dishes; for example, small dices of

Table 15–5 More about Spices and Herbs

More about Spices

Spices are prepared from the roots, buds, flowers, fruits, bark, or seeds of plants. Table 15–5 shows some of the basic information about spices.

Name	Forms	Taste	Uses
Allspice	Whole berries, ground	The aroma suggests a blend of cloves, cinnamon, and nutmeg; sweet flavor	Fruit cakes, pies, relishes, preserves, sweet yellow vegetables (e.g., sweet potatoes), and tomatoes
Cardamom seed	Whole, ground	Mild, pleasant, sweet ginger-like flavor	Baked goods, apple and pumpkin pies; an important ingredient in curry
Cinnamon	Whole sticks, ground	Warm, spicy, sweet flavor	Cakes, buns, breads, cookies, and pies
Cloves	Whole, ground	Hot, spicy, sweet penetrating flavor	Whole cloves for baking hams and other pork, in pickling fruits, and in stews and meat gravies; ground cloves in baked goods and desserts and to enhance the flavor of sweet vegetables—beets, sweet potatoes, and winter squash
Ginger	Fresh, whole, cracked, ground	Aromatic, sweet, spicy, penetrating flavor	Baked goods and rubbed on meat, poultry, and fish; in stir-fry dishes
Mace	Ground	Strong nutmeg flavor	The thin red network surrounding the nutmeg fruit; used in baked goods where a color lighter than nutmeg is desirable
Mustard	Whole seeds, prepared, ground	Sharp, hot, very pungent	Meats, poultry, fish, sauces, salad dressings, cheese and egg dishes; whole seeds in pickling and boiled with beets, cabbage, or sauerkraut
Nutmeg	Whole, ground	Spicy, pleasant flavor	Seed of the nutmeg fruit for baked goods, puddings, sauces, vegetables; in spice blends for processed meats; mixed with butter for corn on cob, spinach, and candied sweet potatoes
Paprika	Ground	Sweet, mild pungent flavor	A garnish spice, gives an appealing appearance to a wide variety of dishes; used in the production of processed meats such as sausage, salad dressings, and other prepared foods
Peppercorns: black, white, red, and pink	Whole, course ground, ground	Hot, biting, very pungent	Many uses in a wide variety of foods; white pepper ideal in light-colored foods where dark specks might not be attractive
Red pepper (cayenne)	Crushed, ground	Hot, pungent flavor	Meats and sauces

continues

Table 15–5 continued

More about Herbs

Herbs come from the leaf or soft portions of plants.

Name	Forms	Taste	Uses
Anise seed	Seeds	Sweet licorice flavor	Cookies, cakes, fruit mixtures, chicken
Basil	Fresh, dried chopped leaves	Mint licorice-like flavor	Pizza, spaghetti sauce, tomato dishes, vegetable soups, meat pies, peas, zucchini, green beans
Bay leaves	Whole	Sweet balsamic aroma, peppery flavor	Fish, soups, stews, stocks, sauces, grain dishes
Caraway seed	Whole	Sharp and pungent	Rye bread, other baked goods, cheeses, sauerkraut dishes, soups, meats, stews
Celery seed	Whole, ground	Flavor distinctly different from celery	Fish, soups, tomato juice, potato salad dressing
Chives	Fresh, freeze-dried	In the onion family; delicate flavor	Baked potato topping, all cooked green vegetables, green salads, cream sauce, cheese dishes
Coriander seed	Whole, ground	Pleasant lemon-orange flavor	Ingredient in curry; ground form used in pastries, buns, cookies, and cakes; in processed foods such as frankfurters
Cilantro (Coriander leaves)	Fresh, dried	Sweet aroma, mildly peppery	Ingredient in Mexican foods
Cumin	Whole seeds, ground	Warm, distinctive, salty-sweet, resembles caraway	Ingredient in chili powder and curry powder; German cooks add to pork and sauerkraut, and Dutch add to cheese
Dill	Fresh, whole as seeds or weed	Aromatic, like caraway but milder and sweeter	Dill pickles; seeds in meats, sauces, salads, coleslaw, potato salad, and cooked macaroni; dill weed in salads, sandwiches, and uncooked mixtures
Fennel seed	Whole	Flavor similar to anise, pleasant sweet licorice flavor	Breads, rolls, apple pies, seafood, pork and poultry dishes; provides the distinctive flavor to Italian sausage
Marjoram	Fresh, dried whole or ground	Faintly like sage, slight mint aftertaste, delicate	Vegetables, one of the ingredients in poultry and Italian seasoning; processed foods such as bologna
Mint	Fresh, dried flakes or leaves	Strong and sweet with a cool aftertaste	Peppermint is the most common variety; popular flavor for candies and frozen desserts; many fruits, peas and carrots

continues

Table 15–5 continued

Name	Forms	Taste	Uses
Oregano	Fresh, dried leaves, ground	More pungent than marjoram, reminiscent of thyme	Pizza, other meat dishes, cheese and egg dishes; vegetables such as tomatoes, zucchini or green beans; an ingredient in chili powder
Parsley	Fresh, dried flakes	Sweet, mildly spicy, refreshing	A wide variety of cooked foods, salad dressings, and sandwich spreads
Poppy seed	Whole, crushed	Nut flavor	Whole as a topping for rolls, breads, cakes, cookies, and pastries; crushed in fillings for pastries; over noodles and pasta, or rice; in vegetables such as green beans
Rosemary	Fresh, whole leaves	Refreshing, pine, resinous, pungent	Chicken dishes and vegetables such as eggplant, turnips, cauliflower, green beans, beets, and summer squash; enhances the flavor of citrus fruits

Source: Adapted with permission from the National Food Service Management Institute, Culinary Techniques for Healthy School Meals, *Proud Times Lesson Booklets*, © 1996, National Food Service Management Institute

ham add just a touch of flavor to dishes without adding much fat and no fat when fat-free varieties are used.

Presentation Techniques

Foods that look good help student customers want to eat.[25] Nice-looking and appealing foods perk up the appetite of most people, especially children. Serving appealing foods gives the food service staff a feeling of satisfaction and pride in the meal service offered to customers. Meals are served with the intent to stimulate all of the student customer's senses. Maintaining a clean, neat serving line, salad bar, and other food service areas by food service assistants who are neatly dressed is also part of the presentation of foods. The carefully planned placement of foods on the serving line, whether in steam table pans or preplated, makes a statement that every effort is made to create a pleasing arrangement to meet the customer's needs.

An attractive and appealing appearance stimulates the desire to taste food. Prepare show plates or trays to guide students in selecting a variety of visually appealing, nutritious foods. Food should look natural. Main colors should be soft, natural, and compatible. The execution of basic culinary principles is important to avoid complicating the food through unnecessary ingredients and combinations.

Compatible cooking methods enhance the experience of basic tastes, textures, and appearance of food. Basic presentation concepts include consideration of the color, texture, shape, form, height, and movement created by the placement of food items on the plate or tray. Foods served at their peak of freshness are visually more appealing than foods that are served after being held too long or after improper reheating; and cold and frozen foods are served at the proper temperature for better flavor and to prevent loss of consistency and texture.

Garnishes are used only when the plate or pan of food needs an extra touch. Garnishes are always part of the overall plan and are always edible. The color and flavor of the garnish are compatible with the food product. Because garnishing can be time consuming, consider the use of only those garnishes that can be executed quickly and efficiently. Simple garnishes such as an orange wedge with a pre-plated chicken salad sandwich is easy to prepare and adds to the overall eating quality of the menu item. Do not overgarnish. Just a sprinkle of fresh chopped parsley in the cooked carrots works better than a larger amount.

TRAINING BASICS

Qualified employees are the keys to effective school food and nutrition programs. The National Food Service Management Institute recognized the importance of training to develop professionals by conducting a multiphased research project to determine the competencies, knowledge, and skills required of effective district school food and nutrition directors/managers. The results of this study are reported in two documents, *Competencies, Knowledge, and Skills of Effective District School Nutrition Directors/Supervisors* and *Competencies, Knowledge, and Skills of Effective School Nutrition Managers.*[26,27] Refer to Table 15–6 for a summary of the competencies, knowledge, and skills outlined for directors.

The food service staff responsible for transforming the menu into meals that appeal to the taste preferences of students should be well trained in the art of food preparation. Training the food production staff is a major management function and should not be left to chance. A well-trained staff is equipped with the knowledge and skills necessary to produce the menu as planned to meet the goals of the school food and nutrition program. Not only is the staff trained in the proper procedures of various cooking methods that deliver high-quality products, they are trained in work simplification and resource management related to the production aspects of operating the program.

A well-trained staff feels personally responsible for the quality of the school food and nutrition program and works to ensure that the program is successful. Providing appropriate

and timely training programs for the staff is evidence that the program is managed for excellence and that a commitment to the professional development of the staff is important to top management. Any investments of time or money made in training the staff will come back to the program many times over in greater productivity and higher-quality meals prepared and served to the student customers.

Training increases job satisfaction and builds employee loyalty to the program, which may lead to less turnover and lower absenteeism among employees. The provision of training sends a clear message to the staff that they are valuable members of the school food and nutrition team and empowers individuals to make a commitment to the quality of the program.

Training opportunities may take various forms in the school setting. (See Chapter 5 for more information or training.) Food preparation skills are best learned when hands-on training is provided. Educators tell us that adults learn best when they know why they are learning a new task, when they know how to do the new task, when they are given an opportunity to see the task performed, when they are given an opportunity to practice the new task, and when the trainer provides feedback on their progress. Training may take various forms and incorporates these principles of adult learning.[28]

Both formal and informal training sessions are needed in the food and nutrition program environment. A training plan should be based on assessed needs. Formal training sessions are scheduled outside the regular workday and allow the trainer and the learner to focus on the training being offered. After-work hours and special staff development days generally provide opportunities for formal training sessions in food production skills.

Materials should be selected for the training that reflect the training needs of the audience. Since formal training requires an investment in time and material resources of the program, topics, and materials for training must focus on the assessed needs of the food and nutrition

Table 15–6 Competencies, Knowledge, and Skills of Effective District School Nutrition Directors

Competency 4.1
Develop procedures to ensure the food production system provides nutritious food of maximum quality.

Entry-Level	*Beyond Entry-Level*
KNOWLEDGE STATEMENTS	**KNOWLEDGE STATEMENTS**
Knows standards for control of quality and quantity food production and distribution, reflecting nutrition objectives.	
Knows principles of food science and fundamentals of flavor enrichment related to quantity food production, holding, and serving.	
Knows fundamentals for developing a continuous quality improvement system for food production.	
SKILL STATEMENTS	**SKILL STATEMENTS**
Establishes procedures of food processing, storing, preparation, and serving that conserve the nutritive value and enhance flavor and attractiveness of final product.	Ensures staff receive proper training and instructions on food preparation techniques, scheduling food preparation, and procedures for making adjustments when necessary.
Evaluates menus for cost, customer acceptability, equipment demands, time requirements, and personnel availability.	Implements procedures that are flexible and allows adaptability to a conventional/non-conventional system of production.
Establishes procedures for high-quality production.	Establishes guidelines for work station design to achieve high production standards.
Implements production planning procedures to include work schedules, standardized recipes, prepreparation plans, and portion control instructions.	Develops effective work methods to complete tasks, based on time and motion principles.
Implements procedures for evaluating food quality on a regular basis.	

Competency 4.2
Ensures that operational procedures for food production and distribution adhere to district, state, and federal guidelines and regulations.

Entry-Level	*Beyond Entry-Level*
KNOWLEDGE STATEMENTS	**KNOWLEDGE STATEMENTS**
Knows procedures for documenting and evaluating meal amounts planned, prepared, and served.	
Knows portion-control guidelines as appropriate.	
Knows relationship of menu planning to purchasing, food preparation, and productivity.	
Knows methods to determine productivity ratios.	

continues

Table 15–6 continued

Competency 4.2
Ensures that operational procedures for food production and distribution adhere to district, state, and federal guidelines and regulations.

Entry-Level	Beyond Entry-Level
SKILL STATEMENTS	SKILL STATEMENTS
Implements a procedure for portion control.	
Develops a system of consistent and accurate documentation for food production and nutrient analysis.	
Directs the use of standardized recipes in controlling food quality, recipe yield, and portion size.	
Develops and monitors child nutrition	
Program food production methods to ensure the yield of high-quality foods that meet nutrition objectives.	
Establishes and applies work standards for productivity of meal (i.e., meals per labor hour/meal equivalents).	

Competency 4.3
Monitors food production procedures for effectively implementing changes and improvement within program requirements.

Entry-Level	Beyond Entry-Level
KNOWLEDGE STATEMENTS	KNOWLEDGE STATEMENTS
	Knows impact of operational influences and resources on food production.
	Knows how to effectively implement change.
SKILL STATEMENTS	SKILL STATEMENTS
Works with staff to evaluate the food production system and food quality and revise the system as needed.	Employs forecasting procedures for maximum operational efficiency of current and future outputs.
Develops a system to effectively train child nutrition program personnel in the preparation of meals.	Trains staff in production and forecasting procedures.
	Implements procedures to involve the customer in testing new recipes and food products.
	Evaluates and responds to change as needed.

Source: Adapted with permission from the National Food Service Management Institute, *Competencies Knowledge, and Skills of Effective District School Nutrition Directors/Supervisors,* © 1996, National Food Service Management Institute.

program assistants. Implementing new methods of preparing foods to meet the nutrition goals of the school food and nutrition program, operation of new equipment, and the addition of new menu items are examples of situations that may require training for the entire staff; and new school food and nutrition employees must always be trained on the procedures used in the operation. Many resources are available for training materials and programs, as are food service consultants who specialize in training who will deliver the training for the school food and nutrition program.

Training may also take place on a continuous basis during the day-to-day operation of the program. Informal training allows the food and nutrition program assistant to learn on the job with the help of the experienced staff, who show and guide the food service assistant through each task. Establishing a mentoring program for training is a positive approach to training and benefits the new employee and the experienced food and nutrition program assistant as well. Mentoring has long been recognized as an important aspect of training. A mentor is one who teaches, advises, or counsels someone else.

In the school food and nutrition program operation, the manager or an effective food service assistant can be the mentor for the new food assistants. Mentoring generally is more effective when the mentor is paired with one person for the purpose of training. The mentor becomes the adviser or source of help to the food service assistant as new skills are learned during the daily production of the menu. Mentoring works well as a means of training new food and nutrition program assistants when formal job or skills training is not available. As a follow-up to formal training, mentoring assures that the food and nutrition program assistant has someone who can continue the training during the regular workday as new food preparation skills are put into practice. Mentoring should always be viewed as a positive interaction between staff members who are willing to work closely together to achieve the goals of the program.

Coaching[29] is a technique that can be applied to training in both formal and informal settings. Coaching is the technique of training that encourages the food and nutrition program assistant to learn a new task, to practice the task correctly, and to continue to perform the task the correct way every time it is performed. The four steps in the coaching process are understanding the task, showing the task, experiencing the task, and doing the task. Following the steps in the process each time a new task is taught will allow the trainer to follow the progress of the food and nutrition program assistant until the correct execution of the task becomes part of standard operational procedures. Very simply stated, coaching is the trainer interacting with the food and nutrition program assistant in just the same helpful and respectful way the trainer would also expect to be treated. Coaching is a positive approach to training and retraining and requires a consistent message of support from the manager/coach. For additional information on coaching employees, refer to Chapter 16.

APPLICATION

The application of correct food preparation techniques to the production of the school menu is necessary to accomplish the goals of healthier school meals that meet the taste and personal preference of the student customers. Training and a consistent message of management's commitment to the operation of a quality program are essential to the success of the school food and nutrition program in meeting these goals. It is the responsibility of the school food and nutrition program director/manager to lead the food and nutrition program staff in thinking creatively about the menu and the way it is prepared, presented, and served to continue to excite and interest the customers.

The development of the menu must be a continual process that reflects the needs and wishes of the students who are actively involved in the menu-planning process. A quality program also requires the individual commitment of the school food and nutrition program assistants who are responsible for the day-to-day operation of the program and the preparation and service of the meals to the students. Leadership for excellence in the twenty-first century involves a total commitment to preparing and serving the highest-quality food products possible to ensure that all the goals of the school food and nutrition program are met.

SUMMARY

Production is the end of the line for ensuring quality in the school food and nutrition program. Once the food is prepared the quality is established. In the final analysis it is the students' perception of the quality of the foods offered on the line that defines the overall quality of the program. Although school food and nutrition program directors cannot be present every day to personally supervise the production of the menu, they are the persons most responsible for the integrity of the program. Various tools such as the production record and the quality score cards discussed in this chapter are alternate methods of supervising the production of the menu by the director. Both the completed production record and the scorecards are reviewed daily by the director and/or manager to ensure consistent quantity and quality of all foods prepared.

Results of recent surveys conducted by the NFSMI[30] support the notion that the quality of the foods served to the student customer is the single most important aspect of the operation of the program. Whether or not students participate in the program on a regular basis is highly correlated to their perception of the flavor and appearance of the meal. To provide leadership for excellence in food production, the school food and nutrition program director must know quantity food production and have some practical experience in the production techniques and quality standards for foods produced by the staff. It is not reasonable to assume or propose that directors can direct or manage processes such as food preparation if they have little or no knowledge of or experiences with production. Training is also more effective and purposeful. Being able to actually work in the production area to prepare the foods on the menu is a powerful skill for the director/manager who expects the food service assistants to perform at a highly skilled level.

The interpretation of the menu into a production record that is carefully and consistently followed requires the director to direct the process. Excellent school food and nutrition programs are led by directors/managers who practice a hands-on approach to directing the program. Successful directors are those that step away from the desk and move outside the office to observe and participate in the day-to-day operation of the program as often as possible. Successful directors know what happens in the school production areas and in the cafeteria; they influence the quality of the program through their knowledge and expertise, and their presence demonstrates the value they place on the preparation of the meal and the professionals who labor every day to make it all happen.

CASE STUDY
FOOD PYRAMID CHOICE MENUS:
OREGON'S STRATEGY FOR PROVIDING SCHOOL LUNCHES THAT
MEET THE RECOMMENDATIONS OF THE *DIETARY GUIDELINES*
FOR AMERICANS AND REDUCING FOOD WASTE

Jennifer Parenteau and Jane Gullett

INTRODUCTION AND CHALLENGE

Food Pyramid Choice Menus

Since 1993, the Oregon Department of Education Child Nutrition Programs has promoted Food Pyramid Choice Menus (FPCM), a type of school lunch service that offers students a wide variety of food choices. Students in FPCM schools are given the daily opportunity to self-select lunches from a minimum of three entrees, six or more fruits and vegetables choices, three bread/grain items (preferably one whole grain) and two types of low-fat milk. Variety bars (better known as salad bars) are key to offering the fruit, vegetable and bread/grain choices which are the FPCM hallmark. It has received praise from all students, parents, food service staff, teachers and administrators. FPCM evolved from a project initiated to reduce food waste.

Prior to implementing Food Pyramid Choice Menus, students in one elementary school in Portland, Oregon, threw away about 70 pounds of food waste daily at lunch. This amounted to about one-third pound of food waste per lunch served. "Some students went directly from the serving line to the garbage can, throwing away what they wouldn't eat," noted a waste reduction education specialist with the Oregon Department of Environmental Quality.

Two months after Food Pyramid Choice Menus was started at the school, the students weighed and measured the lunch food waste for five days. Cafeteria generated food waste had dropped to a daily average of 23 pounds, a whopping 68% reduction in food waste.

History

In 1993 a private environmental eingineering firm in Portland, Oregon was granted funding to help develop innovative methods, other than recycling, to reduce solid waste in schools. Three elementary school cafeterias were recruited for this pilot project. These schools, like most in Oregon, offered the traditional one entree lunch, one bread/grain, one vegetable, one fruit and one milk choice at lunch. During the project, each school implemented a lunch service that offered students a wide variety of food choices.

All schools weighed their cafeteria food waste before and after implementation of the choice system. Food waste decreased significantly in all three schools. At one school the average daily lunch participation increased from 61% to 73% while food waste per lunch served dropped 47%. (See Figure 15–2)

Other changes were encouraging as well. Customer satisfaction increased for both students and adults. Polled students indicated that they enjoyed making their own food choices and teachers were impressed with the fruits and vegetables students were selecting and eating from the variety bar.

Action

Results from this pilot program were so promising that the Oregon Department of Education (ODE) Child Nutrition Programs' staff decided to develop the choices program into a comprehensive menu planning system. After much deliberation the program was named Food Pyramid Choice Menus. A complete

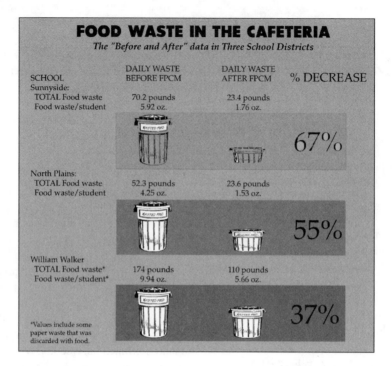

Figure 15–2 Food Waste in the Cafeteria. *Source:* Reprinted with permission from Child Nutrition Staff and NETPRO Trainers, Child Nutrition Programs, *Food Pyramid Choice Menus Tabloid*, p. 4, © 1996, Oregon Department of Education.

training program was constructed which included videos, menus, production sheets, training manuals, and more. ODE even funded independent nutrition consultants to go into the schools to assist them in the correct implementation of Food Pyramid Choice Menus.

Offering students choices in the school lunch program is not a new concept. In the 1920s a Philadelphia Home and School League report stated: *Children preferred making food choices instead of taking the 3-cent combination plate, which was preplated.*

Benefits of Food Pyramid Choice Menus

First and foremost, students are offered a wide variety of fruits, vegetables, and grain foods daily at lunch. This corresponds to the Dietary Guidelines for Americans to eat a wide variety of foods; and to eat more grains, vegetables and fruits. FPCM does not advocate desserts

School Meals Initiative (SMI) is a comprehensive, integrated plan for promoting the health of our nation's school children by updating nutrition standards for the National School Lunch and School Breakfast Programs. SMI is based on the recommendations of the Dietary Guidelines for Americans. Children are 21% of the nation's population and they are 100% of our future and 58% who have school meal programs available participate. The vision of SMI is to improve the health and education of children through better nutrition.

Five Guiding Principles provide the framework making this vision a reality.

1. **Healthy Children**—to provide our Nation's children with access to

school meal programs that promote their health, prevent disease and meet the Dietary Guidelines for Americans.

2. **Customer Appeal**—to provide nutritious food which children will eat.

3. **Flexibility**—to reduce paperwork and offer schools different menu planning options to meet the required Nutrient Standards: Calories, Total Fat, Protein, Calcium, Iron, Vitamin A and C.

4. **Investing in People**—to provide schools with the training and technical assistance necessary to bring about nutrition changes in the school meals program by building the nutrition skills of our nation's children and improve their health.

5. **Building Partnerships**—to meet our nation's health responsibility for children and to increase cost effectiveness; we must forge partnerships in the public and private sectors.

but instead relies on a variety of fruits, both fresh, canned and frozen, to bring a satisfying end to lunch. This harmonizes with the Dietary Guideline to choose a diet moderate in sugars.

Food Pyramid Choice Menus

- Allow children to self-select the foods they intend to eat giving them the autonomy to make healthful food choices. This has the added benefit of decreasing food waste, as children are encouraged to take only those foods they intend to consume. This intriguing feature of FPCM—entrusting children with a say in the foods they select to eat— fits solidly into Ellyn Satter's "division of responsibility" in regard to the child/adult

feeding relationship. Ms. Satter, MSW, RD, one of the nation's leading authorities on feeding children, basically states that adults are only responsible for what, when and where children eat, and that children are responsible for how much and even whether they eat.

- Enriches the adult and child feeding relationship. Research shows children will eat when they are hungry and children are able to regulate their food intake. The key here is to offer healthy choices like those available in FPCM.

- Can accommodate vegetarian and ethnically diverse food preferences by offering a daily variety of entrées, including at least one vegetarian entrée every day. Children with specific medical conditions, like diabetes, food allergies or lactose intolerance, are also more easily served with FPCM than with the traditional meal service.

- Has motivated Oregon schools to prioritize nutrition education, linking food choices to the food guide pyramid and transforming the cafeteria into a learning laboratory for students.

- Supports the United States Department of Agriculture's School Meals Initiative (SMI) which emphasizes food choices and nutrition education.

In one elementary school where 11 different languages are spoken, the garbage decreased by half the first day of FPCM service. Teachers were amazed at the change in their students and the foods eaten. Even the food service director stated: "This is the first school lunch where I have had my choice. What a difference!

As of 1998, 30% of Oregon schools offer Food Pyramid Choice Menus. The adoption of Food Pyramid Choice Menus in schools is strictly voluntary.

Food Pyramid Choice Menus: A Successful Formula

FPCM fit comfortably into all four of the National School Lunch Program's menus planning options. The recommended daily food pyramid choices for FPCM are as follows:

- Three or more entrée choices (one vegetarian)

  Common daily entrées include pizza, burgers, South of the Border (nachos, burritos, tacos), deli sandwiches, and a rotating entrée such as chicken nuggets, spaghetti, or casseroles. One vegetarian entrée is recommended and might include cheese pizza, bean burritos, cheese nachos or garden burgers. For holidays or other special occasions some schools prefer to revert back to a single entree meal. For example, for a Thanksgiving celebration, a school may choose to serve turkey with all the trimmings and not follow the FPCM recommendations.

- Six or more fruit and vegetable choices (a variety of fresh, frozen, canned, or dried)

  A typical variety bar may offer carrot sticks, rounds or baby-size, celery, broccoli, cauliflower florets, cucumbers, tomatoes, plus salad mix. Other vegetables like canned corn or green beans or mixed vegetables (either served warm or cold) and/or frozen peas round out the selections. Fruits offered include apples, bananas, oranges, melons, kiwi, dates, figs, prunes and raisins and all varieties of canned fruits. Oregon children love canned pineapple.

- Three or more bread/grain food choices (preferably one whole grain)

  Other items offered on variety bars include whole-wheat rolls, bread sticks, biscuits, steamed rice (either brown or white), oriental rice and refried beans.

- Two or more milk choices (such as lowfat white and nonfat chocolate)

Variety bars are key to offering the fruit, vegetable and bread/grain choices which are FPCM hallmark. Different textures, colors, shapes, sizes and tastes provide eye appealing choices for students. The variety bar is School Meals Initiative in living reality. Flexibility in offerings is one of the most useful features of the variety bar. Recipes from *USDA's Tool Kit for Healthy School Meals, NFSMI Culinary Techniques for Healthy School Meals* and *Healthy Cuisine Workshop for Kids* are excellent resources to expand students' choices.

Food Safety

Safe food handling is critical for food service staff, students and school staff to reduce the risk of food-borne illness. Variety bars have the most potential for food borne-illness. To reduce this risk ODE staff developed protocol for schools to use when implementing Food Pyramid Choice Menus. The protocol calls for intensive training for students and school staff concerning handwashing and variety bar etiquette.

ODE developed food safety resources to accompany FPCM training, including two handwashing videos: *Hands Down on Germs* for grades K–5, and *War on Germs* for grades 5–12. Also developed were handwashing sequence pictures, in both English and Spanish, using the Mayer-Johnson Boardmaker program. Schools laminate and post over sinks in student restrooms to remind students how to successfully wash their hands. These are available upon request from the Oregon Department of Education Child Nutrition Programs. (www.ode.state.or.us/stusvc/Nutrition)

Meeting National School Lunch Program (NSLP) Requirements

As mentioned. Food Pyramid Choice Menus fit comfortably in all four of the National School Lunch Program's menu planning options. Yet, ODE staff was curious if Food Pyramid Choice Menus met USDA's NSLP nutrient standards for elementary student lunches. To answer this question, ODE contracted with Oregon's land grant university, Oregon State University, to conduct research on Food Pyramid Choice Menus. Dr. Constance Georgiou,

Ph.D., Associate Professor, Department of Nutriton and Food Management headed the study. The study was conducted during the 1996–97 school year. The primary focus of the research was to answer the following question: Do Food Pyramid Choice Menus meet the energy and nutrient requirements specified by USDA for third graders?

Careful research protocol was designed to determine whether Food Pyramid Choice Menus, planned for one week for elementary students, complied with USDA standards for energy and nutrient content of lunches as offered (energy, total fat and saturated fat as a percentage of energy, protein, calcium, iron, vitamins A and C). Cholesterol, sodium and the dietary fiber content of the lunches were also measured. The research was also designed to detect differences, if they existed, between the energy and nutrient content of the meals planned by schools which use onsite, satellited and centrally-planned/site prepared methods of menu planning and preparation of meals.

Research results showed that elementary school lunches planned under Food Pyramid Choice Menus succeeded in, or closely approached, meeting all the nutrient standards for energy and nutrient content for third graders. The schools in the study, on average, generously met the standards for energy, protein, vitamin and mineral content. Over 50% of the 23 schools selected for the study met the nutrient standards for fat and saturated fat. Food Pyramid Choice Menus also provided more vitamin A and less cholesterol than elementary school lunches nationwide.

The average energy content was 709 calories, which exceeds the nutrient standard of 664 calories/day. The mean protein was 30 grams, about three times the nutrient standard. The mean calcium, iron, vitamin A and C content exceeded the nutrient standards generously. Although there are no current nutrient standards for fiber, cholesterol and sodium, it is required that these nutrients be monitored. Food Pyramid Choice Menus school lunches averaged 5.8 grams of dietary fiber, 62 milligrams of cholesterol, and 1461 milligrams of sodium per lunch.

What is Next? "Any Reasonable Approach"

Congress has authorized schools to use any reasonable means for planning menus with a requirement that the approach would neet the Dietary Guidelines for Americans. USDA's proposed rule for implementing the any reasonable means legislation states that "the State Agency may establish a general policy allowing school food authorities to adopt such approaches without prior USDA approval." Oregon Department of Education Child Nutriton Programs will investigate the potential writing of criteria to establish FPCM as "any reasonable approach." Under the proposed rule "This is one alternative consisting of relatively minor modifications of one of the four existing menu planning options. Menus continue to be required to meet the Dietary Guidelines. FPCM has the potential to meet "any reasonable means."

Conclusions

Oregon's children, teachers, administrators, parents and food service personnel are pleased with Food Pyramid Choice Menus. Waste is reduced and children tend to consume more fruits, vegetables, and bread/grains. This delivery system allows students to make healthy choices and thus meets the intent of SMI.

CASE STUDY
REACHING HIGH SCHOOL STUDENTS IN A NEW CONSOLIDATED SCHOOL

Harriet Deel and Julia Sanders

The Challenge

"How can school food service reach high school students with appealing, nutritious meals?" was the challenge for the newly consolidated Huntington High School. Consolidation of the Huntington Central High School and the East High School was generally viewed by many with a negative attitude. Those who opposed consolidation believed that neighborhood schools would be superior to the new school in spite of improved, modern facilities, expanded curriculum, and enhanced programs. More particularly, participation in school lunch at the two schools to be consolidated had been much less than desirable, with average daily participation at 125 and 150 from combined enrollments of 2,200. School breakfast participation was minimal, with fewer than 100 meals served per day at Huntington East. Even students eligible for free meals participated at a low rate. The action plan developed for attacking the challenge consisted of nine strategic steps.

Action Plan Involved Partnerships and Training

Step one of the action plan called for bringing together representatives of each school community to determine what they wanted in the new school food and nutrition program. This step was designed to help each community group share ownership in the new program. It was necessary that each community group view the new school as its own.

Step two provided for the District Food and Nutrition Director and the newly appointed school food and nutrition manager to visit both schools and speak to various groups, including the student body. This phase of communicating with students yielded not only suggestions for types and quality of foods the student wanted, but also provided vital admministrative ideas for a successful program. Among these were the necessity of speed of service, since students' social time is much too important to them to stand in lines, and the unequivocal need to protect student esteem. Students also clearly stated that they wanted food choices, and their french fries, hot and crisp.

Step three involved developing and implementing training for personnel in the new school. Useful training initiatives included the following:

1. The food and nutrition manager trained the school food service staff, using prepared work schedules.
2. With the help of the District Food and Nutrition Director, the manager also trained a pool of 20 computer operators for point-of-service meal counting.
3. State Department of Education coordinators provided training in effective use of production records.
4. State department personnel worked with school faculty, administrators, secretaries, counselors, and nurses to ensure that the school met state policy provisions. For example, it was important that the school plan to meet the needs of pregnant students.

Step four involved the development of core customer service strategies, which included planning for four serving periods. Five serving lines were utilized, each with different, complete nutritious meals. Service equipment and procedures facilitated speed of service. Food preparation catered to student appeal. Food items were customized for ease of service.

Step 5 involved preparing a detailed implementation plan for scheduling meals. The meal schedule provided four serving periods. With five serving lines, 500 students could be served in 10 to 13 minutes. All point-of-service counting was computerized.

Step 6 provided for a variety of menu choices on the five service lines, including

- a sandwich service (both hot and cold)
- country cooking
- pizza (three choices)
- soup and salad bar with a taco bar added periodically
- a modified sandwich line that was served from a truck in the student center.

Additionally, on each line a variety of fresh, seasonal fruit, fresh-baked desserts, gelatin dessert, puddings, yogurt, assorted fruit juices, and assorted milk choices were offered. Second servings were given as desired; however, full second meals were available only if purchased. The purchase prices were $1.75 and $1.25 for lunch and breakfast, respectively.

Step six focused on strategies for speed of service. These included menu boards located at the beginning of each line, tableware designed for ease of self-service, and food items customized for ease of service. For example, baskets were available at the pizza line; single-service containers were routinely used; and bowls, plates, and trays were available at the salad bar.

Step seven focused on preparation of quality food to insure that the freshest possible food be served to the students. Preparation was characterized by batch cooking. Student appeal is high when pizza is just out of the oven, fries are just out of the cooker, fresh or frozen vegetables are steamed in small batches and are green, crisp, bright, and nutritious. Mashed potatoes are prepared as students go through the line, with pans freshly filled. With batch cooking, foods on the serving lines were fresh, and the fourth lunch period student had the same high-quality food as did those in the first lunch period.

Step eight gave focus to the importance of the food service staff to customer satisfaction. Customer service elements of speed and qual-

lity were matched by an emphasis on a pleasant demeanor of the food and nutrition program staff. The important words were "smile" and "listen."

Step nine combined high-quality service with vital nutrition education initiatives. Parent involvement and community partnerships were essential for effective nutrition education. Nutrition education initiatives included "Body-by-Choice," designation as a Team Nutrition School, establishment of a Nutrition Advisory Council, and participation of the school food and nutrition department in health fairs. Additionally, the food and nutrition manager served on the Healthy Schools committee, and parents were encouraged to informally discuss their concerns with the communications-conscious manager.

Outcomes Verified Value of Focused Efforts

Important outcomes resulted from implementing the vigorous and visionary action plan. Among these results were the following:

1. Student participation improved significantly, and is considered excellent. School lunch participation averaged 1,400 daily out of a school population of 2,200. Daily school breakfast participation increased to 465.
2. Students benefit from nutritious choices. All meals served meet the *Dietary Guidelines for Americans*. À la carte sales, limited by state policy, are neither available nor needed.
3. New food and nutrition program personnel were employed to meet the needs of increased participation. The two original schools had employed three persons and the new school employs 16. Program expansion resulted in an employment boost for the community.
4. Student, faculty, and community satisfaction is high. Any discipline problem in the cafeteria is extremely rare. Students show respect for the food and nu-

trition program employees, reflecting the respect the workers consistently show for the students.

Highlander Café, named for the school mascot, is the place for students to be at lunchtime at Huntington High. Is there more that needs to be done? Certainly, improvement goals have been established. Breakfast participation of at least 500 daily is desired. Keeping up to date on changing student tastes is an important goal, also. Use of computer skills to chart trends is vital in the demanding student environment.

Any evaluation of the Huntington High school food and nutrition program would rate it a big success in reaching students, as evidenced by the increased participation. This success can be attributed to a number of important factors that begin with a strong, professional on-site manager, skillful in communica-

tions, scheduling, and organizing; a manager who understood the strengths and motivation of each of the staff and earned their confidence. A strong commitment to nutrition integrity and to the demonstration of respect and kindness to students also contributed to the success of the program. Much credit goes to the students and the community for their involvement, to the faculty for their cooperation, to the school administration for its support, and to the use of computer technology.

The importance of a supportive state policy related to limiting à la carte food sales must be recognized. And, perhaps most importantly, success of the new school food and nutrition program is attributable to the appealing presentation of an excellent variety of foods that were fresh and prepared for just-in-time service and that met the needs and tastes preferences of individual customers.

REFERENCES

1. American School Food Service Association (ASFSA), *Keys to Excellence: Standards of Practice for Nutrition Integrity* (Alexandria, VA: 1995).

2. S.R. Labensky and A.M. Hause, *On Cooking: A Textbook of Culinary Fundamentals.* (Englewood Cliffs, NJ: Merrill/Prentice Hall, 1995).

3. M.C. Spears, *Foodservice Organizations: A Managerial and Systems Approach*, 3rd ed. (Englewood Cliffs, NJ: Merrill/Prentice Hall, 1995).

4. US Department of Agriculture (USDA) Food and Consumer Service, *A Tool Kit for Healthy School Meals* (Washington, DC: U.S. Government Printing Office, 1996).

5. USDA Food and Consumer Service. *USDA Recipe File* (Washington, DC: U.S. Government Printing Office, 1988), 95.

6. National Food Service Management Institute, *On the Road to Professional Food Preparation* (University, MS: 1993).

7. USDA, *Recipe File.*

8. USDA Food and Consumer Service, *Healthy School Meals Training* (Washington, DC: U.S. Government Printing Office, 1996).

9. ASFSA, *Keys to Excellence.*

10. National Food Service Management Institute (NFSMI), *Culinary Techniques for Healthy School Meals.* (University, MS: 1996).

11. Culinary Institute of America, *The New Professional Chef*, 6th ed., ed. M.D. Donovan (New York: Van Nostrand Reinhold, 1996).

12. NFSMI, *Culinary Techniques for Healthy School Meals.*

13. M. Bennion, *Introductory Foods*, 10th ed. (Englewood Cliffs, NJ: Merrill/Prentice Hall, 1995).

14. ASFSA, *Keys to Excellence.*

15. Foodservice Equipment Report, *Demystifying Induction Cooking*, 1997.

16. US Department of Agriculture, Food and Consumer Service. *Serving It Safe: A Manager's Tool Kit.* FCA-295 (Washington, DC: 1996).

17. USDA, *Healthy School Meals Training.*

18. USDA, *USDA Recipe File.*

19. USDA, *A Tool Kit for Healthy School Meals.*

20. USDA, *Serving It Safe: A Manager's Tool Kit.*

21. ASFSA, *Keys to Excellence.*

22. C.B. Oakley and C. Powers, *Healthy Cuisine for Kids Workshop Trainer's Manual* (University, MS: National Food Service Management Institute, 1995).

23. NFSMI, *Culinary Techniques for Healthy School Meals.*

24. Culinary Institute of America, *The Professional Chef's Techniques for Healthy Cooking*, ed. M.D. Donovan (New York: Van Nostrand Reinhold, 1993).

25. Oakley and Powers, *Healthy Cuisine for Kids*.

26. National Food Service Management Institute, *Competencies, Knowledge, and Skills of Effective District School Nutrition Directors/Supervisors* (University, MS: 1995).

27. National Food Service Management Institute, *Competencies, Knowledge, and Skills of Effective District School Nutrition Managers* (University, MS: 1996).

28. M. Knowles, *The Adult Learner: A Neglected Species*, 3rd ed. (Houston, TX: Gulf Publishing Co., Book Division, 1984).

29. A. Robinson, *Instructor Manual for a Coaching Guide for School Nutrition Managers* (University, MS: National Food Service Management Institute, 1995).

30. National Food Service Management Institute, *The High School Foodservice Survey* (R-28-97) (University, MS: 1996).

CHAPTER 16

Managing Employees for Outstanding Customer Service

Mary Kay Meyer

OUTLINE

INTRODUCTION

School food and nutrition programs are much different from those of 1946, when the National School Lunch Act was passed. Although the program's purpose, "to safeguard the health and well-being of the nation's children by serving nutritious meals," has not changed, our primary customers—students—have.[1] If school food and nutrition programs are to close the participation gap, decision makers at all functioning levels must give more attention to managing employees for outstanding customer service.

Students are more sophisticated and are exposed at an earlier age to a variety of types of food and services. They grew up in an environment of fast-food restaurants and food courts, where quick service with a smile is the norm. Student customers will continue to demand a higher level of service than ever before. The school food and nutrition program no longer has a captive audience. Child nutrition programs are competing with fast foods, vending machines, brown-bag lunches, not eating, and competitive food sales for school lunch participation. One key to school food and nutrition programs maintaining a competitive advantage in school meal participation is to maintain a sound customer base. A strong customer base results from a school food and nutrition program's being managed with a service orientation that flows from its vision of being customer focused.

Incorporating service into the vision of the organization requires managers to think strategically about service. They must also understand the dynamics of the dual technical core service delivery system and the role the food service staff play in this technical core.[2] In the traditional manufacturing model of human resources, employees were involved only in production of products for sale. School food and nutrition programs not only prepare meals, but serve the students. This involves two technical cores: food production and customer service. Food service operations are unique. They must deal with both production and customer service simultaneously to be successful. It is not economically feasible to have a production staff and a service staff in most schools. However, in larger schools, with multiple meal offerings and districts with centralized food production, regular part-time service delivery staff are employed.

Traditionally the focus in food service management emphasized the technical core of production in training dietitians, food service directors, and managers. It was the strategy of the school food and nutrition program to prepare healthful meals and serve the students in the allotted time. Minimal attention was given to training or practice of the service delivery system beyond getting the students through the line as rapidly as possible. The service orientation of student customers demands that we shift part of the focus to the service delivery component or service technical core of the food and nutrition program.[3]

The service technical core of the operation is essential in maintaining a sound customer base and financial stability in school food and nutrition programs and other food service programs. This need has been recognized and is reflected in the American Dietetic Association's *Standards of Professional Practice*; *Competencies, Knowledge, and Skills of Effective District School Nutrition Directors/Supervisors*; and the *Nutrition Integrity Standards* developed by the National Food Service Management Institute; and the American School Food Service Association's *Keys to Excellence*.[4–7]

Watchwords for the Service Revolution in the Twenty-First Century

If you're not serving the customer, your job is to serve someone who is.
Everyone has a customer.
Quality service starts *inside* the organization.

These service watchwords clearly focus on the role of the employee. Employees will play a prominent role in service delivery in the twenty-first century. Service literature in the late 1970s and 1980s focused on the intangibility of service and how service could be operationalized.[8,9] However, as the concept of service technology evolved into a technical core, the concept of internal service (the idea that the whole organization must serve those who serve) has emerged as an important principle.[10,11] The principle of the internal customer has become the focus and will play a more prominent role in the twenty-first century as school food and nutrition program directors face changing demographics and higher customer demands for service. It is impossible to become a customer-focused company without being truly people oriented and recognizing the internal customer.[11,12] The question must be asked by the school food and nutrition program director and manager, "How can we create a staff that cares about all customers?" Employees who believe that they contribute to the organizational goals and are valued want satisfied customers. Satisfied customers generally become repeat customers, thus maintaining a sound customer base.

Leading for excellence in the twenty-first century requires managing for outstanding customer service. Customer service will be the differentiating factor for a successful school food and nutrition program. The purpose of this chapter is to provide information to assist the food and nutrition program director and manager in managing employees to achieve an emotional environment where both internal and external customers believe that they are valued. Strategies to create and maintain a customer-focused staff will be discussed. To achieve this goal, the food service decision maker must recruit people with the right skill sets, train them effectively in the technical cores of production and service, coach them for effectiveness, and reward desired outcomes. The specific objectives of the chapter are the following:

- Help the reader understand the dual-core nature of the service delivery system in school food and nutrition programs.
- Help the reader understand the role employees play in the service delivery system of school food and nutrition programs.
- Provide strategies for the school food service decision maker to use in creating and maintaining a customer-focused staff.

EMPLOYEES AS A CORE COMPONENT OF THE SERVICE DELIVERY SYSTEM

Service delivery in school food and nutrition programs involves constant interaction with our primary external customer, the student. The employees listen to the students' views, talk with them daily, ask about their wants and needs, and create part of the atmosphere in the food service. Just imagine an average day in a school food and nutrition program.

A Day in School Food Service

It is 6:45 A.M. when the manager and a food service assistant arrive at school to begin the preparation for serving breakfast at 7:30 A.M. to approximately 200 students. The food service assistant begins the preparation of ham and biscuits. When the oven is preheated, she places both the biscuits and ham in it and sets the timer. While the biscuits and ham are cooking, the food service assistant fills the dish machine and prepares the dish room to receive the trays used at breakfast. When the biscuits are cooked, the food service assistant places them in the warmer. The manager has placed the utensils, condiments, fruit, milk, and juice on the serving line. She has also prepared the computer for line service.

Serving begins at 7:30 A.M. The food service assistant serves breakfast to 198 students, most of whom she knows by name. When Johnny comes through the line, she asks about his grandmother, one of her neighbors. He says, "She will be home from the hospital tomorrow." While the food service assistant is serving the meal, the manager works at the cashier station. She smiles and speaks to each student as she records their meal. One girl asks for jelly for her biscuit. The manager politely with a smile directs her to the bowl sitting on the serving line.

A second food service assistant begins work at 7:45 A.M. She goes directly to the dish room where she bumps and racks the trays returned as the students finish eating breakfast. She talks with the students and asks them how they enjoyed their breakfast. When breakfast is finished all of the trays are washed and placed in the tray carts. The cashier counts the money and compares it to the total on the computer.

Two additional food service assistants begin work at 8:15 A.M. One begins the preparation of the garlic rolls and tossed salad while the other begins the spaghetti and meatballs. While the ground beef browns, she cleans her work area according to the daily cleaning tasks. Sanitation is important not only to be sure the food is safe for the students but for other customers who frequently come to the department. While gathering the ingredients from the refrigerator for the tossed salad, the food service assistant notices that there are only two pounds of bell pepper. The recipe requires four pounds of bell pepper. She substitutes two pounds of spinach for two pounds of the bell pepper needed. Preparation for tomorrow's breakfast and lunch is done as time permits during the lunch preparation.

The fifth food service assistant begins work at 9:30 A.M. She opens the chilled peaches and places them in the refrigerated pass-through. She is careful to be sure the serving dishes are not too full or sloppy. She knows students "eat with their eyes as well as their taste." She also prepares the serving line, the condiment stand, and the milk box for serving lunch. She then sets up the computer and cash drawer for customer service.

As the meal preparation nears an end, the staff focus their attention on the serving and dining area. All tables in the dining room are sanitized, any trash from breakfast is removed, and final touches are put on the service area. A clean, cheery dining area is important to the students. The staff pride themselves on how the dining area looks. The manager and staff then eat lunch in shifts as the final preparation is completed. A final check of the serving line from the customer's view is done by the manager. A garnish is added to the spaghetti and peaches. A food service assistant then prepares a sample tray. Students like to see the meal as they enter the line. The staff have found this helps the students make their choices more quickly. Just before serving begins, the staff check their appearance and put on their clean aprons over their blue golf shirts.

As the cashier sets up her register, she notices a lady entering the dining area. She stops and introduces herself, "Hi, I am Sarah, one of the food and nutrition staff. May I help you?" "Yes," the stranger answers, "I am Jane Smith and we have just moved here. I wanted to see where my little Mary will be eating because she is a picky eater." Sarah asks her to be seated and tells her she will get the manager. The manager greets the new student's mother, and assures her she will take special care of her daughter. She invites the mother to eat with her daughter any time she can. She tells her several parents eat breakfast at the school with their children. It is a quiet time for them to spend with their child as they start the busy day.

The food service assistants are preparing to serve. They love to see the bright eyes of the students as they parade through the line. One young man named Tommy asks for parmesan cheese for his spaghetti. The food service assistant serving the spaghetti smiles and directs him to the condiment stand. The food service assistants smile and make eye contact with the students as they move through the line. This takes a focused effort by the food service assistants since they are very concerned about serving the students in the allotted time. After serving, the food service assistants scrape and rack the trays and silverware. All clean dishes are put away, leftovers are properly stored, and the floors are swept and mopped before the staff leave for the day. The cashier counts the money and the manager verifies her count.

The manager posts the production schedule for the next day.

During an average day food service assistants need several skills. Not only must employees be knowledgeable in equipment operation, food preparation, sanitation, managing their time and making decisions, but also must know how to create and maintain a customer service atmosphere in the school food service operation.

The service delivery system in a school food and nutrition program is composed of three parts: staff, physical environment, and food production (Figure 16–1).[13] School food and nutrition employees are considered high-customer-contact employees and influence the customer's perception of service and food quality.[14–16] Think for a moment about what goes with the students as they leave the food service department. The physical product, the food, was consumed. The experience of staff contact and dining area atmosphere are removed. The only thing the students take with them is a feeling, which is the residual of the interface of the three parts of the service delivery system (the staff, physical environment, and food production).[17–19] This feeling determines their satisfaction with the school food and nutrition program and future participation.

The Service Profit Chain, developed by a group of Harvard professors, says that satisfied employees lead to satisfied customers. When employees are happy, they exhibit enthusiasm to the customer. Customers are influenced positively by the employees' attitude. In a research study Schneider showed that courtesy, competency, adequate staffing, and employee morale were strongly related to customers' evaluation of the service received.[20] The service customers received strongly influenced their intentions to continue using the service.[21] In a study of 1,217 high school students, the National Food Service Management Institute (NFSMI) of Applied Research Division found that the staff was one of the top three factors influencing students' satisfaction with school food services.[22]

Employees set the mood, part of the atmosphere, in every food service operation. If the employees smile and greet students by name, a positive impression is left in the mind of the student. If they plop the food on the plate and snarl at them, a negative impression is left. Students are less likely to remember that the chicken nuggets were too brown or the potatoes were dry if there is a positive impression left by the staff. The mood created by the staff is part of some feeling students have when they leave the food service. Students perceive this as important, and the mood the food and nutrition staff create greatly affects the satisfaction and participation of the students in school food and nutrition programs.

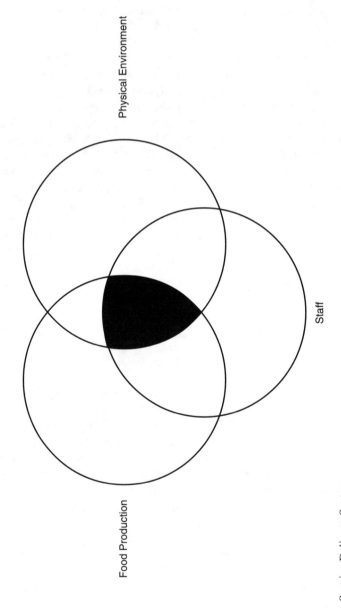

Figure 16–1 Service Delivery System

Customers perceive atmosphere as part of the mood of the dining experience. Appearance of the staff is an ingredient of the atmosphere along with layout, cleanliness, and furniture placement that relates to the mood.[23] The perception of the customer is that the service person and the service encounter cannot be distinguished. They are one in the mind of the customer.[24] If the service person is wearing a dirty shirt or uniform and has unkempt hair hanging from under a hairnet or cap, the perception in the minds of customers is that of poor service. They question, "Was the kitchen clean?" "Were proper hygiene practices used by the staff?" "Were the dishes clean?" If customers convince themselves that these problems exist, whether true or not, it will affect their willingness to continue to be a repeat customer. This will affect participation in the school food and nutrition program. If the scenario was positive and they cannot convince themselves these questions are correct, then a positive residue was created in the service delivery. When a positive residue is created, students are more likely to become regular customers.

ESSENTIAL SKILLS FOR SCHOOL FOOD SERVICE EMPLOYEES

During the workday employees must use technical skills in food production, equipment use, and sanitation; managerial skills to manage their time and coordinate all the tasks that need to be done; and interpersonal skills to be the service "ambassadors" to every person who walks in the school food and nutrition program door. This requires a unique set of skills.

Interpersonal Skills

Interpersonal skills relate to the communication process involved in the service transaction. These skills are a large component in the staff function of the service delivery system.[25] All functional levels of personnel, from director to food service assistant, need these skills to create and maintain a customer-focused organization. SCANS identifies interpersonal skills as a foundation skill needed for competency in the workplace.[26] More is discussed about this topic in Chapter 5.

Interpersonal skills may be perceived by some as common sense. However, employees use these daily as they interact with a variety of internal and external customers, including students, teachers, administrators, fellow workers and parents. The communication techniques and styles used in the information exchange can affect the mood created in the operation.[27] Communication skills are essential in a customer-focused organization. The next few paragraphs on communication, appearance, and patience are not intended to be new information for the reader, but to serve as a reminder of the importance of these interpersonal skill components. Of growing concern is

Skills Needed during an Average Day for a Food Service Assistant		
Technical Skills	*Managerial Skills*	*Interpersonal Skills*
Food preparation	Time management	Verbal and nonverbal communication
Equipment use	Decision making	Dealing with cultural diversity
Sanitation		Patience
Standardized recipe use		Self-management
Substitution procedures		Being a customer service ambassador
		Maintaining a customer-focused culture

the skill of dealing with cultural diversity. This skill is briefly addressed. The concept of self-management may provide new information for the reader. Self-management is thought by the author to be the most important interpersonal skill component.

Communication

The communication process involves verbal and nonverbal techniques. The verbal techniques encompass language and inflection, that, is what is said and the way it is said. Do an experiment for a moment. Say the word "yes" in two different tones of voice. Listen to the two different meanings. Just in how a word is said, a message is sent to the listener. If the listener is a customer, it is important that the meaning intended is the message the listener heard. Part of the mood that employees create in the food service is determined by the tone of their voice. They can create an inviting mood that leads to the customer's satisfaction or a tense mood that creates apprehension and avoidance. When a tense mood or unfriendly environment is created, student customers decrease their participation. No matter how good the food or how meaningful the mission, if the customer is not comfortable in the environment, the operation will not be successful.

Nonverbal communication is another part of the communication process. Making eye contact, standing tall, and appropriate use of gestures are all part of nonverbal communication. Try carrying on a conversation with someone who will not make eye contact. What emotion was aroused? Probably that of being ignored or discounted. Students feel this way when servers fail to make eye contact or frown as they serve the food. A pleasant employee can inadvertently create an uncomfortable mood by gestures used. The nonverbal communication of plopping food on the plate is very evident to our customers. To the customers it may say, "I don't care or I don't want to be here." How does this make customers feel? They do not want to be there either. Nonverbal communication, no matter how small, is remembered

by customers. It influences their decision to become a repeat customer.

Dealing with Cultural Diversity

Growing cultural diversity will greatly affect communications with both internal and external customers in the twenty-first century. Prior to the 1970s, the major growth in population in the United States consisted of white men and women. By 2000, 85 percent of the population growth will consist of African Americans, Asian Americans, and Hispanic Americans.[28] Additionally one of every five students will be nonwhite and many will have English as a second language.[29] Staff must be able to communicate effectively and maintain a customer-focused atmosphere with each student. Nonverbal communications will be extremely important in serving non–English-speaking customers. Alternative methods of communication will become more widespread. For example, it is common in Japan to see wax models of menu items in restaurant windows with the Japanese name and menu number. This reduces the fear of the language barrier for foreign visitors when ordering food from a Japanese menu. They can point to the food model or use the number when ordering. This increases the customer base for the restaurant by encouraging non–Japanese-speaking customers to frequent their restaurant. Other alternative communication techniques such as tasting parties, picture menu boards, and display plates can assist with creating a customer-focused school food and nutrition program.

Economists report that the labor pool for service employees is shrinking. By the year 2000 the labor force will be composed of more immigrants than since the turn of the century, be older, and have more women and people of color than ever before.[30] Managers must be willing to accept differences in cultures and languages in staffing programs. In the past it was the responsibility of the employee to learn to communicate with the staff and management. In the future, it will be the manager's responsibility to communicate with employees. This does not mean that the manager must learn two or three languages; it does mean that the manager must find creative ways to accomplish this task. Some school food and nutrition programs and many contract food service companies, restaurant chains, and hotels have created the following:

- Recipes in Spanish and French
- Production sheets using pictures of the food
- Color codes for amounts to produce
- Serving line diagrams with pictures
- Bilingual training and training aids
- Contracts with interpreters to be available by phone for emergencies

By adopting some of these or other creative solutions, school food and nutrition programs can plan strategically to meet the challenge of cultural diversity and become customer focused.

Patience

Another component of interpersonal skills needed by the food and nutrition staff is patience. This may be a common-sense skill, but it is vital in school food service. Customers do not always know what they want when they enter the service area. Food service employees frequently need to explain the foods, ingredients used, and how it tastes before students will select an item. The other extreme may happen when 20 students all want the same thing at the same time. Either situation requires patience and understanding by food and nutrition staff. If the server is impatient, the customer perceives this as part of the mood of the dining experience and a negative residue is left in the mind of the customer. This negative impression if repeated, even periodically, will negatively influence customer satisfaction of the customer and participation.

Self-Management

Self-management is a form of self-leadership, self-control, or self-influence.[31-33] Self-managed individuals are self-starters. It is the influence members of an organization exert over themselves.[34] Leadership has been replaced with the self-induced actions of the employee.[35] Self-managed persons do not depend on someone telling them to do certain tasks; they know what to do, how to do it, and do it without direction. The motivation of these individuals is the consequence directly involved in the self-controlling process or those resulting from the outcomes of the behavior. The reward is a result of the behavior, generally a sense of self-satisfaction. In order for self-management to evolve the individual must have: requisite abilities, skills, training, an understanding of what the job entails, and understand what is expected.[36]

In a school food and nutrition program, it is impossible for a manager to be present at all service points at all times during the service period. Therefore, employees must take the leadership responsibility for meeting customer needs without being told by the manager what to do or how to do it. If a customer has a request the employees should know what to do and how to meet the customer needs. In school food service this happens often during a meal period. It is common for a student customer to ask for ketchup on a sausage biscuit. But how does the food service worker handle the situation? Do they get the ketchup,? Tell the student they cannot have it,? Tell them they do not need it for breakfast or do they have the ketchup available for all students who ask? The self-managed employee would anticipate the request and have ketchup available for the student who asks, or, get the ketchup for the student when first requested and have it available for others who may asks.

Manager-led employees would wait until they were told by the manager to get the ketchup for the student before acting. It's possible that many dissatisfied customers would go through the line before the manager took action. The customer may be lost before the manager recognizes the situation. Hours of time can be saved in a manager's schedule when a staff of ten or twelve or even three or four practice self-management. Many unhappy customers could be converted to satisfied customers. When students are satisfied, participation is positively impacted. The self-management skill is inherent in many people, latent in others, and nonexistent in some. It can be cultivated and trained with special techniques and modeling. In order for the training to be effective, an organization culture of customer service must be present. Employees must feel comfortable in the environment and lack fear of repercussions resulting from initiating actions.

Empowerment should not be confused with self-management. Empowerment is classically defined as giving official authority.[37] It was one of many human resource buzz words of the 90s and thought to be the fix-all in the workplace for involvement, support, and commitment of employees. It, however, backfired on many managers.

Organizations empowered employees to make suggestions and changes without providing the training, materials, or support to allow this to occur. They often did not assess whether the employee was willing to make these decisions. Empowerment is a process that happens in the relationship between people. Empowerment is not a set of techniques, but a way of constructing an inner understanding of the relationship between oneself and the people with whom one works. Empowerment is different from the traditional concept of control. It is finding the right balance between personal freedom on the job and the freedom to take action. Some aspects of running a food service operation require controls, while others can be improved with suggestions and changes made by creative employees. Empowerment is that balance. Many employees resisted the process of being empowered and withdrew from these well-intentioned efforts. These individuals frequently lacked the self-management skill. Managers cannot just wave a magic wand and empower employees.[38] To empower employees the following must occur:

- Employees must be willing to accept the power.
- Managers must provide the resources necessary for the employee to make decisions that will satisfy a customer want or need.
- An open, constructive environment must be present before the concept of empowerment is introduced. This implies that employees are comfortable discussing opportunities for improvement with the manager.
- Employees must be trained in any boundaries established for meeting the wants and needs of the customers. It is important that employees know to what extent they can go to satisfy a customer.

How does empowerment differ from self-management? Self-management is an inner drive within a person that allows him or her to accept empowerment and use it for the good of the organization.[39] Give self-managed individuals the resources to satisfy the customers and they will work endlessly to meet that goal. Their motivation will be the self-satisfaction of meeting this goal. Self-managed individuals do not wait to be empowered by a manager to initiate change and make suggestions. They often find ways around the system when the work environment is not conducive to changes they

---

Case of the Self-Managed Food Service Assistant

A food service assistant had been working in the high school food service for about six months. She noticed several ways the serving line could be reorganized to make it easier and faster to serve students. Students were always complaining they never had enough time to eat after they got through the line. One day the food service assistant approached the manager with her ideas. The manager said, "You may have something there. Try your idea tomorrow." The food service assistant was excited about the opportunity to try to make the serving line more efficient. That night she made a detailed diagram of the line. The day of the trial she spent extra time setting up the line, and the manager came out to check the line. She turned to the food service assistant and said, "You may experience some problems with this setup, but we will see what happens today." The food service assistant watched eagerly as students filed through the line. Her idea did not slow the line nor did it increase efficiency. After lunch, the food service assistant asked the manager about another idea. Her reply was similar to the one she had given the day before. The food service assistant asked the manager to review her idea before she tried it the next day. The manager was happy to discuss her ideas. The food service assistant eagerly planned her next trial. When the manager came out the next day to check the lunch, she told the food service assistant she thought her setup was good. That day the line did move more smoothly and the students seemed to like the new setup. The food service assistant was proud of her accomplishment. After the lunch was over, the manager approached the food service assistant and congratulated her on a job well done. The manager truly empowered the food service assistant to try new ideas. She supported her ideas, offered suggestions, and rewarded her accomplishments.

RECRUITING AND HIRING HIGH-CUSTOMER-CONTACT EMPLOYEES

A major personnel issue for the twenty-first century is how to equip school food and nutrition programs with staff possessing these customer service and self-management skills in this dynamic environment. It is not easy to find employees in some areas of the country. Many restaurants and hotels are experiencing similar problems, and bus employees over an hour each away. The literature suggests that present employees are the best source of recruiting future employees.[40] The concept of "internal customers" follows this line of thinking. If employees are satisfied with a job, they are the best marketing tools a business can have. If they are dissatisfied, they will not positively market the work opportunities, and turnover rates will be high.

The selection process is a challenge in the food service industry because both technical and interpersonal skills are necessary. Traditionally in the food service industry during the interview process the focus was on assessing the technical skills of the interviewee. Could they use a slicer or had they ever made a meat loaf from scratch? The philosophy is changing.[40] Customer service and communications are major skills for the school food and nutrition program staff. Employees create the mood to satisfy customers and support repeat participation. The interpersonal skills needed in food service are much more difficult, and some say impossible to train. Therefore, the interpersonal skills should be the focus of the selection process. *Look for these skills during the selec-*

see as helpful. Food service employees can become frustrated when managers and directors do not create the proper environment for self-management and provide the resources to allow empowerment to be effective. The best situation is to provide an open environment and one in which empowerment flourishes to allow the self-managed individual to be successful.

The Selection Process for High-Customer-Contact Employees

Step one. The first step in the selection process is to decide what specific skills are important for an employee in a certain position. One of the main points emphasized in this chapter is the value of interpersonal skills in meeting program goals. But what specifically are the interpersonal skills for specific employees in specific roles? This will vary from food service to food service depending on the service delivery system and how the technical core is configured. Earlier in the chapter some interpersonal skills were discussed in general.

One easy way of deciding the interpersonal skills needed in a specific food service operation is to identify the most successful customer service "ambassadors" from the customer's point of view. Next, interview the customers to decide what characteristics they most value in these employees. After completing this step, interview the employees to determine from their perspective what characteristics have made them successful.

The most challenging part of this exercise is how to translate these characteristics into measurable skills. For example, if an employee says, "My pleasant attitude makes me popular with the kids," what skills are involved? Attitude may include communication, appearance, and tone of voice. Which of these is most important? All skills are not equal in value. Each job category will have a skill set especially important for that job based on the configuration of the service delivery system. Although all customer-contact employees should possess interpersonal skills, within each job category and facility the ranking of these skills will be different. This ranking is different because customer wants and needs are different depending on the general and specific environment of the food service operation. What may rank high in importance in one school

may not rank as high in another. Many of the top 500 service companies have adopted this strategy and credit it for their success in customer service.

Step two. Once the essential step of identifying the skills has been completed, interview questions must be developed for each job category. A useful technique patented by Behavioral Technology Inc. of Memphis, Tennessee, is behavioral interviewing. Behavioral interviewing is based on the premise that past performance predicts future behavior. If past behavior can be determined during the interview, then future performance can be predicted. The key is to zsk questions that make the person explain how he or she handled a situation or experience of the past. This will help predict the future.

Traditional Interview Questions To Assess Interpersonal Skills

How do you feel about listening and following directions?
Do you like talking with people?
How do you deal with an angry customer?

Questions Using the Behavioral Interviewing Technique To Assess Interpersonal Skills

Tell me about a specific time when your ability to listen helped you perform your job more efficiently.
In your past job when you had to spend a large amount of time talking to people, how did it affect you?
Tell me about a specific time when you had to calm an angry customer and how you turned the situation around.

Step three. After the interview questions have been composed, they need to be structured for a smooth-flowing interview. Asking each candidate interviewing for a specific job category the same questions will ensure a fair and equitable decision. There are "people" people and there are "technical" people. The recruiting techniques just discussed will help identify those "people" people during the selection process and give insight into their future performance.

tion process and train for the technical skills once hired is the new philosophy and one the food service industry has found very successful. The concept of training site-based employees in technical skills on the job is not new in school food and nutrition programs. The emphasis here is assessing the potential employees interpersonal skills during the interview process.

TRAINING AND DEVELOPING HIGH-CUSTOMER-CONTACT EMPLOYEES

Training and development begin weeks before new personnel walk through the door of the operation and continue throughout their career. Following the hiring process, a training plan should be developed for each employee. The training plan should be based on the technical and customer service skills needed for the job and the skills possessed by the person hired. Although the most wonderful "people" person has been hired, he or she must be trained in the service techniques specific to an operation. Assumptions cannot be made that a newly hired individual knows how to do the job. Even when the right person is hired, that person must be trained in the specific procedures unique to the organization in order to maintain quality standards. It cannot be taken for granted that when a "people" person is hired to work in a school food and nutrition program, that person will do the job to organizational specifications. All employees must be taught to perform tasks according to established procedures of a particular program.

Phase one of training begins with a well-orchestrated orientation. There is no worse feeling to a new staff member than to be told, "You must wait until I am finished before I can show you around" or "Sally, show Susan around and get her started on her job." Should a customer, whether internal or external, be treated this way? Employees, internal customers, are our most valuable marketing tools. New staff members should be treated as valued customers beginning the moment they walk through the door. The ideal first day for new employees would begin with the manager waiting for them to arrive. Then the manager should take as much time as needed to show new employees the preparation areas, dining areas, where to hang their coats, how to record their time, where and when to take breaks, and any other policies specific to their operation. In some organizations, orientation lasts two days. In small operations, orientation may last only a few hours. The length of the orientation is not as important as comprehensiveness.

Phase two of training and development is training in specific customer techniques to meet the organizational quality standards.

Phase three of the training plan is technical skill training. A job plan or master task list with times is essential for employees. This gives them a framework for the workday. Specific technical training must accompany the job plan or master task list. Training can be enjoyable for employees if presented in accordance with sound principles of adult education or boring and dreaded if the staff is not engaged in the process. A variety of training resources are available through the National Food Service Management Institute and the Education Foundation of National Restaurant Association.

Training does not stop when a new employee knows how to do the specified job tasks. Training and development should continue as long as an employee is in the operation. "Never stop learning" is a good motto. School food and nutrition programs operate in a dynamic environment that necessitates con-

rning to stay up to date. Even without changes in the environment, there are always new and easier ways to do the job. A continuing challenge of management is to find these ways and present them to the staff in a manner that motivates them. All ideas do not have to be original. Employees are good sources of training materials. Frequently the staff will discover an easier way to do many tasks, and they should be encouraged to share them with their fellow internal customers.

Effective Customer Service Training Techniques

Effective customer service training involves active participation and practice by the employee. Limiting training to the use of passive training techniques such as lectures or videos will not achieve the desired result of outstanding customer interaction. Neither will providing training at only one setting. Some research indicates that a person must have 50 hours of training prior to a modification in behavior.

Scripting is an effective technique frequently used in the service industry for teaching service techniques. "Good morning, may I help you?" is a simple example of a script. Scripting involves training the employees in the verbalizations appropriate for the customer and situation. Scripts include how to address a customer, how to ask what you may serve the customer, and how to move a customer through the serving line more quickly, as well as how to handle the dissatisfied customer. Hotels, restaurants, banks, and quick-service operations such as car washes use this technique for training. These scripts must be developed prior to the actual training. All employees must have a uniform plan of action and receive consistent training. If the employees are told to use their judgment and no examples are given, quality of service may be sacrificed. If Jane, a food service assistant, is asked to teach Sally, a newly hired employee, how to serve the customers, consistent training may not occur.

Training by using scripts will provide consistency in serving customers.

Another technique used in training customer service techniques is role playing. Role playing is an effective method to use for some in-service meetings or monthly staff training on topics such as dealing with upset customers or how to answer the phone with a customer-friendly tone. Each member of the group must be comfortable with others, however, and be willing to perform in front of one another. It is important that group members be comfortable with the group before this type of training will be successful.

Self-management is one skill that may require development in some individuals. No simple training program can teach an employee this skill. It requires a desire by the employee, a conducive environment, and an active role model.[41] Modeling is an effective technique for the development of self-management. Continuous encouragement and reinforcement of desired behavior can enhance the self-management skill. Managers must use self-management for employees to role model. Employees must see it being practiced on a daily basis and encouraged to practice self-management themselves.

To enhance the development of self-management in employees, the physical surroundings need to be conducive and nonthreatening. If an employee is meeting the needs of the customer who wanted ketchup with a sausage biscuit, the employee must have space to put the ketchup on or near the serving line and be encouraged to use the space available creatively. When an employee is being encouraged to practice self-management, a small roadblock such as lack of space or lack of management encouragement can become a large roadblock in the mind of the employee. Employees can quickly revert to old habits if the physical and organizational environments are not conducive for self-management.

Behavioral programming can also be helpful in developing self-management skills. Behavioral programming involves consequences administered contingent upon the performance of targeted behaviors. In everyday life we frequently practice this technique. We might reward ourselves with a new dress for saving $200 that month by not ordering out fast food and staying home rather than going to the movies. This technique can also be applied to the work setting. To encourage self-management, managers should set goals with their staff to give them a performance target and reward them for performance.

COACHING FOR EFFECTIVENESS

Coaching is a directive process to train and orient an employee to the realities of the workplace and help remove barriers to optimum work performance.[42,43] When the word *coach* is mentioned, the vision of sports teams such as football, basketball, and soccer are often recalled. Managers, directors, and supervisors of school food and nutrition programs are also coaches. Coaching involves realizing the potential in employees, setting realistic goals for performance, and helping employees excel. Frequently managers must remove the roadblocks for employees or help them see the roadblocks. Coaches are cheerleaders, motivators, role models, trainers, and counselors.

Training is an important coaching function. In school food and nutrition programs managers are key trainers. A helpful tool for coaches, when functioning in the training role, is the USED model.[44] Another name frequently used for this model is the Four-Step Method of Training. The USED model first assesses the *understanding* of the task assigned and explains the task to the worker. The task is then demonstrated, *showing* the worker each step. The worker then practices what was demonstrated while the coach observes. The worker *experiences* performing the task. The workers then allowed to *do* the task while the coach encourages and praises their good work. This model incorporates several valuable concepts: (1) The coach is the trainer. The workers see the manager doing tasks they will be perform-

ing daily. This creates a positive image in the mind of the workers, an image that portrays a competent manager with skills necessary to perform many tasks. (2) The workers see the task demonstrated the correct way. (3) The workers are allowed to practice with the coach alongside to ensure that they understand the proper procedure for doing the task. (4) The coach encourages the workers and gives immediate positive reinforcement. The model is appropriate for training a variety of skills, from using a piece of equipment safely to the proper way of moving a customer through the line.

Counseling is another important function performed by a coach. Counseling is helping employees deal with a personal problem. The personal problem may involve being late, losing a loved one, or other personal matters. One aspect often overlooked in counseling an employee is getting to the root cause of the problem. The behavior exhibited may be a result of a deeper problem and usually is. Active listening is one skill that will assist with getting to the root problem. Active listening is doing more than hearing words. It is understanding expressions and feelings of the person talking. Active listening does not come naturally. It is a skill developed over time, as are many coaching skills. Getting to a root problem experienced by a worker takes patience, skill, and a conducive environment.

Being a coach requires creating an environment of safety in which employees are comfortable talking and letting you help them. It requires confidentiality, knowing the staff, and dealing with one person's concern at a time. If this is the first discussion between a manager and an employee, the employee will more than likely resist assistance. One key is to become knowledgeable about employees. Get to know what they are like as people and something about their families. Coaching requires managers to understand and appreciate cultural differences. Not everyone thinks or acts the same. Each person is different partly because of background and heritage. For example, in the traditional Native American culture public praise is embarrassing. They consider public praise selfish and shameful. They will resent such actions, but may never say this for fear of causing more shame. All cultures have specific values.[45] If several cultures are represented in the workplace, getting to know the individuals, their customs, and beliefs is important. This may require checking out a book from the public library or talking to teachers who may be familiar with a specific culture. One way to find out about a specific culture and customs is to talk to the employees and ask about their heritage. Encourage them to share and help the staff learn about their ways. One suggestion would be to have an International Festival Day in the cafeteria and prepare various ethnic dishes. Have the employees develop the menu. Or organize an employee pot luck for a holiday celebration.

Division of values also exists along generation lines. The younger generation of today is more inner directed and seeks more self-fulfillment. They do not "live to work," like their grandparents, but "work to live." To them work must be fun or they will seek other employment. Personal development, leisure time, and quality family time have become more important than company goals or loyalty. Challenging work, job satisfaction, a sense of achievement, and recognition have become the main elements of today's generation's desire from their jobs.[45] The coach must understand the differences in the generations represented in the staff. The coaching role is the most important role a school food and nutrition professional plays. It is important to remember that to make personnel feel valued they must be known and understood.

REWARDING VALUED EMPLOYEES

Rewards classically have been thought of as a way to encourage personnel to exhibit desired behaviors. However, the system often fails to recognize what is truly important. Traditionally the employee was rewarded for being to work on time, preparing quality food products, and keeping work areas clean. These are not all of the tasks that are important in a service-related job. Customer satisfaction, repeat business, and profitability are important aspects in today's environment.[46] It is difficult to measure these aspects; therefore, employees may not be rewarded for assisting with these tasks. These outcomes are a result of the skills for which the person was interviewed and the criteria used for hiring. Then shouldn't they be the skills rewarded? Management will get the behaviors from employees it rewards. This basic idea was proven by Pavlov and his experiments with rats and dogs. If employees are not rewarded for good customer service, they will not continue to provide good customer service. The difficulty in rewarding desired behavior is twofold: (1) how are these behaviors measured? and (2) what can be used to reward employees given limited budgets? Measuring customer service can easily be done, but it takes planning and thought. Customer service surveys are very useful in school food and nutrition programs for gathering these data. They measure how the students perceive the food, service, and dining atmosphere. As we have discussed, employees directly affect these aspects of the operation, not just the food. Students are more than willing to assist by voicing their views. Surveys are covered thoroughly in Chapter 20. No more time will be devoted to them here, except to emphasize the importance of asking the students how the food service and employees are satisfying their wants and needs.

The other area of concern is rewarding employees for good customer service on a limited budget. We have previously discussed that employees today are different and have different values. The key is to know what motivates each employee. Employees can be internally motivated by self-satisfaction and knowing they have done a good job. This does not require a monetary gift, just recognition from management and customers for the job well done. A smile and "thank you" are valued rewards for a self-managed individual. Other individuals are externally motivated and require material rewards. Herzberg theorized that individuals are not motivated by praise until the basic life-sustaining needs have been met.[47] If employees do not have the money to support their family, then they may not be motivated by praise alone. These individuals will not be motivated until their basic needs have been met. Coaching skills should be used to determine how these employees can be motivated. There may an underlying reason why the motivational techniques available are not working. Getting to know and understand an individual is the key to motivating her or him. This takes time and a comfortable open environment. When an internal customer service attitude is created, employees are more likely to be motivated. Motivation is giving them something they value. This is very often as simple as praise, whether a private "job well done and thank you" or recognition in front of the work group.

ROLE OF THE MANAGER IN DEVELOPING A CUSTOMER SERVICE–FOCUSED STAFF

Providing superior customer service begins with developing a customer-focused vision, mission, and strategic plan for the organization. Creating customer service and a customer-focused organization does not begin with the staff. They are an extension of the strategies initiated at the top. School food service decision makers set the tone for customer service. A customer service environment must be created to allow a school to focus on the customer.[48] The staff cannot be expected to create the customer-focused atmosphere without leadership from the top. This involves leaders: living the strategy, communicating the vision, believing in and investing in people, being students for life, putting the customer first, being part of and encouraging teamwork, and being dedicated to the process. Without leaders who exhibit these components, employees cannot successfully focus on the customer.

SUMMARY

A major challenge of managers and directors in the twenty-first century is managing the food service environment for superior customer service. Competition in the school meal arena is increasing. Students have more alternatives to school lunch than ever before. School food and nutrition programs must provide levels of services offered in other food service establishments. This means developing a vision, mission, and strategic plan with the customer as the focus. A customer service–focused staff is a critical part of the strategic plan. To have a customer-focused staff, child nutrition professionals must hire the right persons, treat employees as customers, support their desire to service the customers, and motivate them to become the best possible. A customer-oriented environment of self-management, pleasing the customer, and setting quality standards that meet the needs of all customers is essential. When these things happen, the school food and nutrition program will be recognized for outstanding customer service. A strong customer base and financial stability are natural byproducts of adopting a customer service focus in school food and nutrition programs.

CASE STUDY
THE PROBLEM AT SUNSHINE SCHOOL

Mary Nix

The Challenge

To produce and serve quality food every day requires each school food and nutrition staff person to be productive at his or her workstation during normal work hours. At Sunshine School, Betty Jo had been at least 20 minutes late four times within the last two weeks. When she was at work, she was quiet and sullen. Jessie, the manager, was concerned about Betty Jo as a person and as an employee. She observed the resentment of the other staff members when they had to help Betty Jo finish her jobs.

On the fourth day that Betty Jo was late, the following scenario happened: Betty Jo walked in the back door at 8:20, 20 minutes late. Edna looked at Josie. Josie looked at Evelyn. Then they all looked at Jessie, the manager. But she barely glanced up from stirring the chili in the steam kettle. Betty Jo said nothing to anyone as she pulled off her sweater, tied on her apron, and went to the walk-in for the salad vegetables. As she came out, Evelyn nudged Josie. Betty Jo had put down the vegetables and was wiping reddened eyes. A half hour later, meal preparation was in full swing. Nobody paid any attention to Jessie when she motioned Betty Jo to follow her out onto the loading dock. Betty Jo wasn't herself. Normally, she was quiet-spoken and cool as a cucumber. She would share laughter, but she never started it. If she had a sense of humor, she kept it to herself. In the last month, however, she had not even shared laughter. Betty Jo was withdrawn and her work was haphazard. Where before there had been pride, there was now only a vacuum. Jessie had worked with her for three years, yet she still felt that she didn't know Betty Jo. At lunch she had sat with Betty Jo most times and tried to draw her out without

much luck. Of her three children, only one was still at home, and he had finished school and was working. Her husband was a carpenter and was home much of the time. Betty Jo needed to work. As she stepped out the back door onto the loading dock, Betty Jo was sullen. "Betty Jo, this is the fourth time. . . ." That was as far as Jessie got. Betty Jo lashed out angrily with words that were too loud. "I knew you were laying for me. Edie and Josie have been late before, and you've never called them out. But then, they're your pets, aren't they?" Jessie didn't answer. The silence lengthened. "Well, aren't they?" Betty Jo demanded. "Betty Jo, as I started to say, you've been late four times in the last two weeks. Now, if something is wrong at home, and you need . . ." Too quickly, Betty Jo retorted, "What happens in my home is none of your business as long as I do my . . ." "Your work?" Jessie said firmly, completing her sentence. Betty Jo's mouth became a straight white line. She turned her head away from Jessie and stared at nothing. "It's not just your being late, Betty Jo." Jessie spoke quietly and then waited. She waited until their eyes met. "Are you satisfied that you've been doing the best job that you could have done these past few months?" "What's been wrong with my work? If you mean that mess with the cookies . . ." Jessie shook her head slowly. "No, not that." "Then what?" Betty Jo asked. Some of the anger was gone, but the belligerence was still there. "Have you been treated fairly here, Betty Jo?" Jessie asked "Well, sometimes you. . ." Jessie quietly interrupted. "Have you been treated fairly? Your work schedule, your kitchen assignments, your cleanup jobs?" The reply came slowly. The belligerence was gone. The voice was dead. "Yes," she answered. "I won't be late again." She turned to go. Jessie gently laid a hand on her shoulder and spoke

"Just a minute, Betty Jo. It's more than being late. We both know that. Something is happening that is affecting your work. Several times you have snapped at the students and not created a good atmosphere in the cafeteria. We pride ourselves in being friendly and courteous to the students. Your work has been affected and it is affecting the team. Whatever it is, perhaps we can make some changes here to help you out." For the briefest moment, the stirring of anger was there. Then it died. Betty Jo sighed again, and then she smiled warmly. "Jessie, I'm really sorry. For what I said and for being late." Her voice was quiet. The eyes were no longer hostile. They glistened as she said, "Jessie, I need some help, but I've just been too proud to ask for it. My husband has been out of work for two months and one of our cars was repossessed. I was afraid we were going to lose our house until he found a job two weeks ago, but we are still hurting for money.

"The reason I have been late is that I drop off Melinda at kindergarten as soon as the doors open and then take my husband to work. Sometimes the traffic is so bad, I just can't get here from Bill's workplace on time. It makes me a nervous wreck. I know it's affecting my work and I'm really sorry. I just have to have this job." Jessie smiled and said, "If you can stay ten minutes after work this afternoon, we will work something out."

After all of the employees had left for the day, Betty Jo timidly came into Jessie's office and sat down. Jessie said, "Betty Jo, I've been reviewing the production schedule and thinking about your need to have a few more minutes in the morning to get through the traffic. Would you be willing to change your work schedule and come in at 8:30 A.M. and stay 30 minutes later in the afternoon to prepare the after-school snack?" "Oh yes," Betty Jo said without hesitation. "I can be on time with this schedule."

The next day, Jessie explained to the staff that she had asked Betty Jo to come in to work 30 minutes later and stay 30 minutes later to prepare the after-school snacks. They were delighted because none of them wanted to do it. Betty Jo was on time the next day and every day thereafter. She was back to being the quiet, cooperative person that all of the staff admired.

The Outcome

Strategies that Jessie, the manager, used are as follows:

- She recognized that open and honest communication is essential for a good work environment. She knew that a conducive work environment was essential for a well-functioning, customer-focused school food and nutrition program.
- She observed the tardiness, performance, and attitude shift of Betty Jo and its effect on the other staff members.
- She used appropriate counseling skills and waited for the best time and place to discuss the situation with Betty Jo.
- She listened with concern and worked out a mutually beneficial solution.
- She kept open communications, and all staff knew about the change in the schedule.

Principles exhibited in the case include the following:

- Jessie knew her staff. She recognized something had been wrong during the last month.
- She waited until the lunch preparation was underway before finding a quiet place to talk to Betty Jo.
- She actively listened. She listened to words and actions.
- Jessie addressed only Betty Jo's situation. She did not talk about other employees' problems.
- Jessie offered to work with Betty Jo in solving her problems.

REFERENCES

1. United States Department of Agriculture, Child Nutrition Act, 1966: Public Law 89-642.

2. W. Sasser et al., *Management of Service Operations* (Newton, MA: Allyn & Bacon, 1978).

3. L. Daniel, "Overcome the Barriers to Superior Customer Service." *Journal of Business Strategy*, January/February 1992, 18–24.

4. American Dietetic Association. *Standards of Professional Practice* 98(1) (1998): 83–87.

5. D. Carr et al. *Competencies, Knowledge, and Skills of Effective District School Nutrition Director/Supervisors* (Oxford, MS: University of Mississippi, National Food Service Management Institute, 1996).

6. M.B. Gregoire and J. Sneed, *Report on Indicators and Evidences of Achievement of Nutrition Integrity Standards*. R-13-94 (Oxford, MS: University of Mississippi, National Food Service Management Institute, 1993).

7. American School Food Service Association, *Keys to Excellence: Standards of Practice for Nutrition Integrity* (Alexandra, VA: American School Food Service Association, 1995).

8. K. Albrecht and R. Zemke, *Service America* (Homewood, IL: Don Jones-Irwin, 1985).

9. Sasser et al., *Management of Service Operations*.

10. K. Albrecht, *Service Within: Solving the Middle Management Leadership Crisis* (Homewood, IL: Business One Irwin, 1990).

11. W. Sherden, "Gaining the Service Quality Advantage," *Journal of Business Strategy,* March/April, 1998, 45–48.

12. D. Bowen and E. Lawler, "Total Quality Human Resource Management," *Organization Dynamics* 20 (1992): 29–41.

13. Sasser et al., *Management of Service Operations*.

14. B. Losyk, *Managing a Changing Workforce* (Davie, FL: Workplace Trends Publishing, 1996).

15. J. Heskett et al., "Putting the Service Profit Chain to Work," *Harvard Business Review*, March–April, 1994, 165–174.

16. W. Samenfink, "A Qualitative Analysis of Certain Interpersonal Skills Required in the Service Encounter." *The Council on Hotel, Restaurant, and Institutional Education,* 17 (1994): 3–15.

17. Sasser et al., *Management of Service Operations*.

18. M.K. Meyer, "Service in the Hospitality Industry" in *Hospitality Management: An Introduction to the Industry*, ed. R. Brymer (Dubuque, IA: Kendall Hunt Publications, 1991).

19. M.K. Meyer, "Enhancing the Client Acceptance of Nutrition Counseling: Understanding the Service Concept and Developing a Positive Residual, *Journal of the American Dietetic Association* 11 (1989): 1655–1656.

20. B. Schneider, "The Perception of Organizational Climate: The Customer's View," *Journal of Applied Psychology* 37 (1973): 248–256.

21. Sherden, "Gaining the Service Quality Advantage."

22. M.K. Meyer et al., *Report on High School Foodservice Survey*. R-29-97 (Oxford, MS: University of Mississippi, National Food Service Management Institute, 1997).

23. Schneider, "The Perception of Organizational Climate."

24. W.R. George and L.L. Berry, "Guidelines for the Advertising of Services," *Business Horizon*, July/August, 1981, 407–410.

25. B. Sparks, "Communicative Aspects of the Service Encounter," *Council on Hotel, Restaurant, and Institutional Education,* 17 (1994): 39–50.

26. United States Department of Labor, *Skills and Tasks for Jobs: A SCANS Report for America 2000* (Washington, DC: U.S. Government Printing Office, 1992).

27. Sparks, "Communicative Aspects of the Service Encounter."

28. Losyk, *Managing a Changing Workforce.*

29. United States Department of Education, *Projection Statistics to 2006: Highlights* [on line]. Available: http://www.ed.gov/NCES/pubs/proj2006/projhil.html.

30. Losyk, *Managing a Changing Workforce.*

31. C. Manz, "Self-Leadership: Toward an Expanded Theory of Self Influence Process in Organizations," *Academy of Management Research* 11 (1986): 585–600.

32. C. Manz and H. Sims, "Self-Management as a Substitute for Leadership: A Social Learning Theory Perspective," *Academy of Management Research* 5 (1980): 361–367.

33. F. Luthans and T. Davis, "Behavioral Self-Management: The Missing Link in Managerial Effectiveness," *American Management Association*, Summer 1979, 42–60.

34. Manz, "Self-Leadership."

35. Luthans and Davis, "Behavioral Self-Management."

36. P. Mills et al., "Motivating the Client/Employee System as a Service Production Strategy," *Academy of Management Research* 18 (1983): 301–308.

37. C. Scott and D. Jaffe, *Empowerment* (Los Altos, CA: Crisp Publishing, 1991).

38. K. Blanchard et al., *Empowerment Takes More Than a Minute* (San Francisco, CA: Berrett-Koehler Publishers, 1995).

39. Manz and Sims, "Self-Management as a Substitute for Leadership."

40. Losyk, *Managing a Changing Workforce*.

41. Manz and Sims, *Self-Management as a Substitute for Leadership*.

42. M. Minor, *Coaching and Counseling: A Practical Guide for Managers* (Los Altos, CA: Crisp Publishing, 1989).

43. D. Kinlaw, *Coaching for Commitment: Managerial Strategies for Obtaining Superior Performance* (San Diego, CA: Pfeiffer & Co., 1989).

44. A. Robinson and B. Hankin, *Coaching for Improved Performance in Child Nutrition Programs* (Oxford, MS: University of Mississippi, National Food Service Management Institute, 1994).

45. Losyk, *Managing a Changing Workforce*.

46. D.E. Bowen, "Managing the Customer as Human Resource in Service Organizations," *Human Resource Management* 25 (1986): 371–383.

47. F. Herzberg, "One More Time: How Do We Motivate Employees?," in *Manage People Not Personnel* (Boston: Harvard Business Review, Harvard Business School Publishing, 1990).

48. J. Brager, "The Customer Focused Quality Leader," *Quality Progress*, May 1992, 51–53.

CHAPTER 17

Customer Service Design and Implementation

Nena P. Bratianu and Sheila G. Terry

OUTLINE

Source: "Customer Service Design and Implementation." Portions of this chapter including tables, figures, and exhibits have been reprinted with permission from the *School Food and Nutrition Service Design Manual,* pp. 7–38, © 1996, Maryland State Department of Education.

INTRODUCTION

Leading for excellence in child nutrition programs demands a new way of looking at how students are served in the school food and nutrition programs as noted in Chapter 16. The service and dining available in a school food and nutrition program may be the most critical factor in attracting customers and in causing them to want to return. Ambiance encompasses everything from the appearance of the food items and the manner in which they are marketed in the service area to the décor of the dining area and the attitudes of the school food and nutrition staff in interacting with the customers. *Keys to Excellence* identifies standards for customer service design and implementation in school food and nutrition programs. These are some of the standards that must be covered in the educational specifications for both new and remodeling projects. These standards provide a benchmark for results that can be used to assess the impact of each decision made in the planning process.[1]

Challenges

The school food and nutrition programs of the present face more challenges than ever before since their inception. They face challenges from competing external forces such as widely appealing commercial food services and from internal forces such as design, operation, and education concerns. The external challenges stem from a prolific and sophisticated restaurant and food service industry that spends millions of dollars vying for the attention and business of the student consumer. Commercial fast-food enterprises and shopping mall food courts compete with school food and nutrition programs, even if the schools have closed campuses, by affecting students' expectations. Students' expectation of food services have been defined mostly by dining-out experiences in fast-food chains and mall food courts. These expectations have risen greatly in the last twenty years due to the ever-increasing variety of commercial food types and services.

Higher expectations of students place a real demand on school food and nutrition programs to provide a wider variety of foods. Traditional school meals cannot compete with the variety of commercially available foods. Commercially available ethnic foods and specialty foods have dramatically increased choices. Commercially available health foods such as lower-fat and high-fiber vegetarian foods have increased consumer awareness of nutrition and affected eating habits. Higher expectations of students also place real demand on school food and nutrition programs for enhanced dining environments. The physical presentation of commercial food products and the dining environment in which they are offered are perceived to be dynamic, exciting, and inviting when compared with traditional institutional school cafeterias. The variety of activities that occur in school dining spaces will benefit from a higher level of design energy that responds to these external forces.

In order to gain the competitive edge, the school food and nutrition program must respond to these forces that are shaping students' expectations. The program must embrace the future education landscape and food service marketplace and address these challenges by creating opportunities for education, design, and operation viability.

The challenge is to design inviting dining and service environments that keep student customers by providing high-quality, nutritious foods in a cost-effective and informative manner. Many school food and nutrition programs must be financially self-sufficient. The initial step in designing the customer service area is to determine the most appropriate meal services to be offered. This decision will profoundly affect design concepts, construction costs, staffing, and operating expenses of the facility.

The design challenge is first to identify the appropriate type of food service and nutrition education program that will best meet the school's and students' needs. Second, incorporate into the program the appropriate design guidelines. This will require the collective understanding, effort, and agreement of the design committee for the particular project. The aspirations for the design must mesh the program with the allowable construction budget, as well as with the future operating and maintenance budget of the project.

Value is added by

- Creating an efficient food service operation, which ensures financial viability
- Improving the quality and variety of foods and therefore increasing student participation in the school food and nutrition programs
- Enhancing the dining environment, thereby increasing student participation in the school food and nutrition programs
- Designing for the multiple uses of the dining space, thereby increasing its effectiveness as a program area
- Increasing student knowledge of nutrition

Nutrition Considerations

The National School Lunch and School Breakfast Programs are designed to promote the health and well-being of the nation's children by offering nutritious meals and nutrition education. In June 1995, the United States Department of Agriculture (USDA) published new regulations as part of an integrated plan for promoting the health of the nation's children. The nutritional requirements of the programs incorporate the 1995 Dietary Guidelines for Americans. In accordance with the USDA regulations, the school lunch and breakfast programs will, over a week

- Limit total fat to 30 percent of total calories
- Limit saturated fat to less than 10 percent of total calories

- Reduce the levels of sodium and cholesterol
- Increase the levels of dietary fiber

Schools are encouraged to publish the nutritional content of menus. Display and signage in customer service areas are needed to convey nutritional information.

The proper selection of food service equipment can promote compliance with USDA meal requirements by enabling the operation to use preparation methods that can reduce fat, such as steaming. Schools are encouraged to limit the use of other pieces of equipment that may increase fat consumption, such as fryers.

Purpose and Objectives

The purpose of this chapter is to provide a strategy for meeting the challenges facing school food and nutrition leaders seeking excellence in their service to students. This chapter will do the following:

- Identify components to be addressed in order to create and develop a successful customer service design that supports the mission of the programs.
- Provide guidelines for identifying these components during programming and design phases to ensure that they will be included in the final design for construction. It identifies certain education, operation, and design concerns that should be augmented with specific requirements of the local food and nutrition program. Applying these strategies to the design process will result in increased value.

Specific objectives of the chapter include the following:

- Present the critical importance of the design and implementation of the customer service area in school food and nutrition programs
- Describe the planning process for the customer service area, including formation of the planning committee, development of educational specifications, and the scope

of decisions to be made during the planning process

- Identify the design considerations for the customer service area
- Enumerate the factors affecting the decisions to be made for the dining area
- Discuss the design impact on customer service regarding food flow, customer relationships, and staffing
- Highlight general considerations that have an impact on the design and implementation process
- Present case studies that highlight the successful application of the processes and procedures presented in this chapter.

THE PLANNING PROCESS

The Process

In planning a facility, a school system must translate an educational philosophy into a three-dimensional place. In order to ensure that the facility is appropriate and well-designed, many points of view and areas of expertise must be tapped. A planning committee is assembled to bring together individuals with the diverse experience that is required. Sometimes the committee is charged with planning a new facility; other times the task at hand may be to renovate an existing facility. The committee will see the project progress through a number of distinct phases, from inception to occupancy. Although the process will vary from place to place and project to project, the basic sequence is consistent.

The following steps outline a planning process:

Planning the Project

- Project approval and site identification
- Planning committee and planning subgroup formation
- Committee discussions and decisions on program philosophy, content, staffing, organization, and so forth

- Educational specifications preparation
- Selection of an architect
- Selection of a food service consultant (if required)

Design

- Predesign meeting with the architect and food service consultant
- Schematic design
- Design development
- Preparation of construction documents

Construction

- Bidding and contract award
- Construction
- Acceptance of project and occupancy of facility

Occupancy

- Installation of moveable equipment and furnishings
- Occupancy
- Postoccupancy evaluation

The Planning Committee

The planning phase encompasses the identification of a need for a project, the definition of a solution involving construction of a new facility or renovation of an existing one, and a preliminary budget and funding source. Decisions are made within the framework of a master plan. Once a project is approved to proceed, a planning committee is formed to define the parameters of the project. The resulting document, the educational specifications, serves as the basis for the design phases that follow.

Most food service projects take place within larger frameworks, such as new school construction or major renovation projects. Some projects, however, are specifically for the modernization of a food and nutrition facility. In either case, there will be a planning committee that has a key role in the decision-making process for the overall project. The planning committee is a collection of people with diverse interests and expertise. Although the planning process takes longer with many persons involved, divergent frames of reference and points of view provide a broad basis for valid decision. These decisions will guide the planning and design processes, creating a functional facility.

Planning committees vary in size and composition, but all planning committees should include at minimum the following:

- Principal
- Local school facilities planner
- Project architect
- School food and nutrition program manager/director
- School district office representative

Other members may include

- Support services staff
- Parents
- Teachers
- Students
- Food service consultant
- Nutrition consultant
- Representative from state food and nutrition service department

The local administration ensures that educational programs, budget constraints, and facilities standards are incorporated into the project. The facilities planner is usually responsible for coordinating the process. Even while the project is being developed as a whole entity, each of its programmatic components is studied and developed individually. The food service facility will be one of these components. As such, it will be developed and reviewed by appropriate members of the planning committee.[2] The future users of the facility are represented by the principal, teachers, students, and support staff. For a new facility that has yet to be assigned staff, personnel and students from other facilities can assist. The participation of the future users will achieve an ownership of and relevance to the decisions to be made during the planning stages.

For major renovation projects or new school construction, the architect may join the project at its inception or after the development of the educational specifications. It is the architect's responsibility to transform the text of the educational specifications into a design and then produce two-dimensional drawings and technical specifications. These will form the contract documents for construction.

Decisions and the Educational Specification

Developing an educational specification provides insurance to the future owner that the facility will meet the needs of the student body for which it is planned. Decisions made regarding the following areas will become part of the educational specification the architect will use in developing the design. The school administrators and school food and nutrition personnel, with involvement of each representative customer group, will need to make some initial decisions on such areas as

- Meal services to be provided
- Scheduling options
- Philosophy that will guide decisions about nutrition, nutrition education, and educational specifications
- Additional services to be included (Some of the additional services may include catering, serving a community facility for the elderly or preschool ages, sales of items for take-out dining such as school-made pizza, breads, etc.)
- Methods to secure customer input
- Funding options
- Open versus closed campus
- Initial time frames

Analyzing School Needs

Customer preferences are critical in this stage of developing the service-oriented plan. The first steps to secure these data will be to announce the intention of making changes, and conduct focus groups and surveys to gather the information. The results from the focus groups and surveys will provide the framework for all future discussions and plans. If the designing or retrofitting project is for an elementary school, a survey should be administered to parents as well as the students and faculty. A positive approval rating of the food service by parents in the early years can make a difference in the children's acceptance. One may also learn how willing the parents are to reinforce the nutrition education messages that are provided at school and what the children's eating habits are away from school. The surveys and focus groups for middle and high school students will be the first step in letting them know that this project is for them. An open approach to getting their opinions will give information on their opinions about what they like and dislike about the current school food and nutrition program and their preferences for all areas of the service and dining environment from food items to temperature and sanitation.

The faculty survey is very important to the reputation of the school food and nutrition program. The faculty may indicate a desire for types of foods different from those chosen by the students or for a more private dining area. A serving line or even the main menu on one day a week might be the responsive solution to the faculty preference. It may be that they would be pleased to see ice tea, coffee, or some other à la carte item offered. Securing their input and having the committee consider it along with the student preferences is important.

Identifying Funding Sources

New plant construction funds from local, state, or federal sources are usually available for new schools, which may include funds for the food service area. Federal regulations prohibit the use of school food service funds for capital expenditures such as expanding or building a new facility. Identifying funding sources for remodeling projects may require more effort on the part of the planners. The primary funding source for retrofitting or redesigning the service area may be funds that will result from increased student participation. Student participation will generate revenue from both student payments and federal reim-

bursement and, in some cases, state reimbursement. Often the improved environment and student-influenced menu selections will generate ample revenue to fund the improvements. As this is not guaranteed at the initiation of the project and some funds will be necessary in advance, other sources should be considered.

The district food service account may be adequate to fund the improvements in advance. If this would mean using funds generated by other schools in the district, it will be important for those school food and nutrition program directors and school principals to have an understanding of the project objectives and plans for recovering the funds once the project is completed. A long-range plan and policy should be developed based on an analysis of all of the districts schools that will identify the following:

- Priority of schools to be selected for similar redecorating efforts
- Equipment that other schools don't currently have that will be tested in this project for possible inclusion in other schools

If the school is sponsored by a local business an inquiry about the availability of employees to donate labor or benefits from their artistic talents such as assisting students and faculty in painting murals, making screens to partition senior or faculty dining areas, or making a donation to offset the cost of supplies may be useful. If there is not a school sponsor and it isn't in conflict with school board policy, students might solicit local businesses for similar contributions. Receiving recognition for their support in a school newsletter or a sign displayed at the grand opening of the project may be adequate incentive to those businesses that rely on the students and parents from the school community.

Health promotion organizations, state departments of education, and federal agencies sometimes have grant funds available to assist in projects that would promote or enhance special initiatives that they have targeted. Inquiries made with local and state organizations will help determine whether grant possibilities exist.

The school district custodial/engineering staff is a valuable resource as a member of the planning group. Often they can provide a service in doing such things as modifying service counters, arranging special lighting, disguising unsightly areas, or remodeling spaces not previously considered a part of the food service area. These first steps are necessary to make the project successful and responsive to customer needs.[3]

In their book, *Service America!* Karl Albrecht and Ron Zemke make the case for service being paramount to success.[4] They state that service is the competitive edge. Organizations must be committed to service from the top levels of management and throughout the organization. Effectively and efficiently managing the design development and delivery of service will make the difference in the survival of both nonprofit and for-profit organizations in the future. Albrecht and Zemke define service management as a philosophy, a thought process, a set of values and attitudes, and a set of methods. Transforming the organization to a customer-driven one takes time, resources, planning, imagination, and commitment. Boorstin says that the challenge facing the entire food service industry is not so much food as it is service. Service, like quality, is a perception, and each individual holds the power to choose to be (or not to be) a customer of the school food and nutrition programs.[5]

What is the source of the student's first impression of the school food and nutrition program? It's the way the facility looks, feels, the aromas—in other words it's the ambiance of the program. Knowing this, as school food and nutrition programs move into the next decade, they face many challenges both internally and externally. The internal forces include education concerns, both time and money; external forces include the rapidly expanding commercial food services. The question that school food and nutrition program directors must address is, "How do we maintain the competitive edge amid the internal and external challenges?" Many challenges are beyond the scope of the food and nutrition program director; however, the design of the customer service area and service management are within the boundary of opportunity.

Decisions on the design and décor of the menu offerings and service areas lead to positive results when all customers are involved in making the decisions. Representatives from the students, faculty, employees of the school, administration, parents, and community should all be involved in the decision process. Focus groups and surveys are two of the most popular and successful methods for securing input.[6] These procedures not only secure valuable guidance in the decision-making process, they also begin the educational process for all customer groups about the requirements for an effective school food and nutrition program. The guidance from these activities should include menu preferences; perceptions of customers about present employee attitudes, sanitation, and physical comfort of existing facilities; and ideas for future decorating themes, color preferences, and seating arrangements. Several resources are available to assist in conducting focus groups and surveys. Initially ideas and opinions should be gathered in the most creative and constraint-free environment. Details regarding cost, space, and labor constraints will follow once the ideal service and dining environment has been defined.

DESIGNING THE CUSTOMER SERVICE AREAS

It is the responsibility of the planning committee to identify the functional and area requirements for the dining and serving areas for the school food and nutrition program. The educational specifications for the facility will need to address the considerations and ideas resulting from the planning committee.

Location of the Customer Service Area

The location of the food service program and dining area within the school is of primary importance, as it controls the type of programmed activities that can occur there. The relationship between the food service program and adjacent programs can have a dramatic impact on the potential uses of the dining area and adjacent spaces.

Adjacency considerations for dining areas are as follows:

- Near active student circulation areas
- Accessible to the public for after-hours use
- Near other major student activity spaces
- Near gymnasium and/or auditorium for after hours use
- Near outdoor dining/activity area
- Near student government space (high schools)
- Near toilet facilities
- Near guidance and career center (high schools)
- Near stage (elementary and middle schools)
- Readily supervisable from nearby administration
- Acoustically separated from quiet program areas (such as media centers and teaching spaces)

Consideration for Other Uses

A dining area in a school can be used for many activities other than dining. A dining area, which is designed to function well as a multiuse space both during school and after-hours, is a wise investment. The key is integrating the necessary and diverse components of different use groups with the necessary components of dining use.

Many activities other than student dining may occur in dining areas, including student assemblies, ceremonies, banquets, testing, public meetings, faculty dining, community dining, dramatic events, athletic events, social events, instructional activities, gymnastic events, musical events, and after-school programs.

The diverse activities to be accommodated in the dining area must be anticipated in order for the design to meet anticipated need. The educational specifications should clearly define the area requirements and the kind of relationship desired between the food service program and surrounding program areas. They should also define the various activities/uses envisioned for the dining area. Certain functional activities require specialized equipment, such as sound systems and dimmable light systems, which must be programmed into the specifications, designed into the construction documents, and provided for in the project's construction budget and future operation budget.

Further, many diverse activities that will occur in a dining area require different, often conflicting, material finishes. For instance, a dining area in an elementary school frequently serves as a recreation or physical education space for activities such as basketball and volleyball. This same cafeteria space may also serve as an auditorium for drama and music. The preferred floor surfaces for these individual activities are different: wood (physical education), carpeting (auditorium) and vinyl composition tile (cafeteria). Thus, design/planning committee members must be aware of the inherent conflicts associated with multiuse spaces and prepare to make decisions that may involve some level of compromise for either functional uses or material finishes.

Careful consideration should be given to the following items, which are frequently sources of material selection conflicts and compromises in the development of multiuse dining spaces:

- Floor, wall, and ceiling finishes
- Daylighting and artificial lighting
- Spatial quality and ceiling heights
- Maintenance
- Access to outdoors
- Signage and displays
- Degree of closure

Dining Environment Design Considerations

- Provide natural daylight whenever possible. School food service is primarily a daytime activity. Maximize opportunities for introducing natural daylight through windows or skylights. Control direct sunlight with sunscreening elements, blinds, or shade cloths.
- Provide views and access to outdoor dining areas for students and staff whenever possible.
- Provide a colorful, well-lighted environment. Supplement natural light with appropriate levels of artificial light. Plan for evening uses of the space. Provide separate switching of light fixtures to maximize energy efficiencies and minimize operating costs. Coordinate color schemes with artificial light source, color, and temperature.
- Locate the long side of the kitchen adjacent to the dining room to maximize the length of the serving area. Multiple serving lines need to be accommodated in almost every school type. Considerable frontage along the kitchen is required in order to create an efficient and effective serving area. High school food courts require the greatest length of serving area (see Figure 17–1 and Figure 17–2).
- Provide visual connection between serving area and dining room by utilizing transparent materials such as glass doors, windows, and glass blocks.
- Provide interesting and comfortable furniture arrangements. Furniture can enhance attractiveness, create intimacy, and provide visual relief. Furniture can break down the scale of a large room. It can be movable and provide for a variety of arrangements for dining, instruction, and assembly.
- Provide for efficient waste management and recycling with integrated collection stations.
- Break down large-scale spaces into more intimate smaller spaces through the use of ceiling treatments, planters, furniture, floor patterns, and lighting. Fixed items such as booth seating and planters should occur near the perimeter of the space and not interfere with or limit other nondining uses of the space.
- Create an attractive environment that suggests a comfortable and pleasant dining experience.
- Maximize sight lines throughout space and design for easy supervision of space. Avoid deeply recessed areas that are difficult to supervise.
- Provide for future flexibility by designing a space that can be subdivided with operable walls or curtains. These items and their structural framing requirements may be specified as "add alternatives" to the project if not in the original program or budget.

Over the past several years, many high schools have experienced a decline in on-campus dining. This has resulted in lost revenue opportunities for the schools. Recently, numerous high schools have been designed with food courts to compete with off-campus food services such as mall food courts and fast food establishments. These on-campus food courts have been designed to attract back the off-campus dining population. They are also intended to increase school revenues by creating an attractive and profitable school food and nutrition program. Accordingly, these schools have increased the number of seats required by their program. Then they have either increased the area for seating in their dining rooms or they have designated areas outside of the dining room (such as a major lobby space or commons area) for overflow dining (whether sitting or standing). Limit other nondining uses of the space. Floor level changes can also break down the scale of the space; however, they should be carefully considered and reviewed by the planning committee to ensure that they do not limit nondining uses of the space.

Consider specific design elements required by specific program uses:

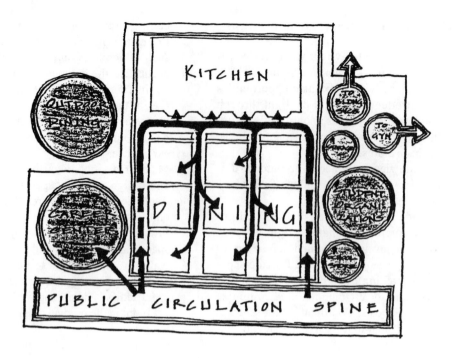

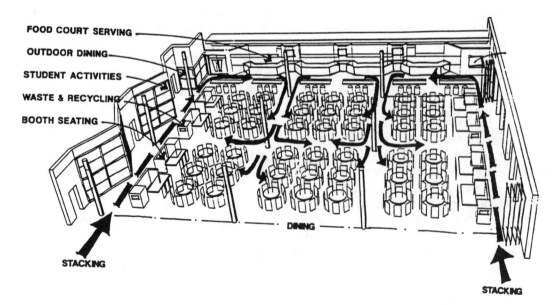

Figure 17–1 High School Food Court Concept Plan. *Source:* Reprinted with permission from the *School Food and Nutrition Service Design Manual,* p. 30, © 1996, Maryland State Department of Education.

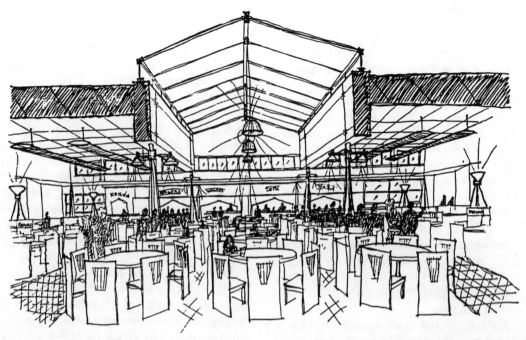

Figure 17–2 High School Dining Space. *Source:* Reprinted with permission from the *School Food and Nutrition Service Design Manual,* p. 10, © 1996, Maryland State Department of Education.

- Recreational activities and physical education: Provide game lines on floor, resilient flooring for physical activities, wall pads, retractable game boards, climbing ropes, and so forth.
- Theatrical activities: Provide dimmable house lighting, stage curtains, public address system, projection screen, blackout curtains, and other items as needed.
- Instructional activities: Provide tackboards; markerboards; chalkboards; display cases; access to power, voice, video, and data cabling.
- Dining activities: Provide floor and wall finishes that are stain resistant, durable, easy to maintain, and attractive. Flooring must be nonslip and compatible with programmed activities and furniture supports (i.e., metal, plastic, or nylon rollers, casters, etc.).

- Miscellaneous activities: Some activities may require specific design elements such as booth seating, specialty lighting, planters, mirrors, supergraphics, multimedia display systems, music, white noise, video displays, and signage.

FACTORS AFFECTING THE DINING AREA

The following factors affect the area needed and the seating capacity required for a dining area:

- Room use requirements
- Meal periods and schedules
- Student population and seating arrangements
- Storage requirements
- Circulation/aisle space requirements

Room Use Requirements

As previously discussed, the dining room may be designed for various activities. The size of the room will depend on the most demanding use of the space. Elementary school dining spaces frequently combine auditorium or gymnasium (or both) functions with the dining functions. For example, if a dining area is to function as a gym and an auditorium, the program that requires the greatest area should govern the size of the space. In addition to the room size, the area should be provided for the ancillary spaces that support the programmed functions of the room. For example, additional storage space should be provided for cafeteria tables with attached seats and auditorium seats (loose/stackable/interlockable chairs) when the space is functioning as a gym.

The educational specifications should provide net dining area parameters or requirements. However, the final gross area will be affected by the following:

- Aisles and circulation zones within the space
- Clearance requirements between program components
- Efficiency characteristics of selected seating styles
- Number of meal periods—which proportionally affects number of seats required

Meal Periods

The educational specifications may state the number and types of meal periods that are to be designed for. However, it may also require comparative consideration of more than one approach and may call for a recommendation of one type. If so, there are several ways to schedule meal periods: single meal periods, multiple meal periods, and staggered meal periods. Each has advantages and disadvantages depending on the evaluation criteria.

Single Meal Periods

The dining room is designed to seat the entire school population at one time for one meal period. The serving area must house enough serving equipment to accommodate those who participate in meal programs. The food and nutrition program must also provide a staff large enough to serve (or supply in self-serve operations) the needed quantities in the time period provided. Because the method can be capital intensive, it is used predominantly in small schools (population less than 300). Although this method provides students with the most social interaction, it has numerous disadvantages. In larger schools, it requires a very large dining area, large operating staff, large supervising staff, and a lot of serving equipment, any of which may be economically prohibitive. Some of the capital expense can be offset if the large dining area serves double duty as the school's gymnasium during the time when it is not functioning as a dining room.

Multiple Meal Periods

The dining room is designed to seat a fraction of the entire school population at one time, for two or more distinct meal periods. The greater the number of meal periods, the smaller the dining area and serving area that is needed. With multiple meal periods, economies may be achieved through repetitive use of a smaller dining area, fewer tables and seats, fewer serving lines, less serving equipment, and fewer serving or supply staff. The greater number of meal periods also reduces staff required for supervision during a meal period. The major disadvantage, depending on the number of meal periods, is that some students may eat lunch very early or very late in the day. A smaller dining area also reduces the potential of the area for other educational purposes.

Staggered Meal Periods

The dining room is designed to seat a certain percentage of the entire school population at any given moment, for the duration of the meal periods. Students are released for lunch on set intervals, a few minutes apart, so that there is a constant flow of students at the serving areas. This method can be developed to minimize the required dining area and seating capacity. However, there is considerably more administrative effort required to stagger the class releases effectively. Supervision and student body control is more complex and difficult due to overlap of dining periods. This method is used primarily in elementary schools.

Seating Plans: Requirements and Consideration

The number of seats that must be provided during a lunch period depends on the overall student dining population divided by the number of meal periods. Elementary and middle schools can anticipate a dining population equal to that of the entire school. High schools, however, are more site- and lunch program-sensitive. The student dining population for a high school is affected by the school policy relating to open or closed campus. This number can vary dramatically depending on the quality of the on-campus school food and nutrition program and the quality of off-campus food service. Urban and suburban high school locations with open campuses can expect a certain percentage of students to go off-campus for lunch. Rural school locations with open campuses should consider the distance to the nearest off-campus food establishments when determining their student dining population. Program committee members should carefully consider how the high school dining program will respond to off-campus dining forces. A basic decision to be made by school authorities relates to the issue of open versus closed campus.

Establish the number of seats needed, as required by the education specifications, and then determine the quality, efficiency, and type of seating for the appropriate school type.

Quality Considerations for Seating

- Durable construction and components
- Easy to move, portable lightweight
- Compact, stores easily, foldable, stackable
- Lockable rollers, casters, or wheels
- Rollers/wheels compatible with specified flooring material
- Easy to clean, maintain, repair
- Nontrendy colors that will endure and not appear dated
- Styles and colors that will coordinate easily with other finishes

Efficiency Considerations for Seating in Dining Area

- Maximize efficiency of seating capacity and safety of furniture arrangement and coordinate these with all applicable codes.
- Utilize double-loaded aisleways, six feet four inches width minimum, for two-way flow with food trays.
- Maximize efficiency of circulation flow into and out of seating areas.
- Utilize table types, shapes, and sizes that optimize seating capacity and are appropriate for the education level of the student population.
- Balance efficiency considerations with inviting, friendly layout and program requirements.
- Refer to Building Officials and Code Administrators (BOCA) International, Inc., and the National Fire Protection Association's (NFPA) Life Safety Code 101 for additional assembly seating requirements, such as required clearances between seatbacks and aisles and/or aisleways, number of required exits from space, clear egress width minimums depending on furniture arrangement and room occupancy load.

Seating and Table Type Considerations (Figure 17–3)

- The shape and capacity of the dining room will influence seating and table type selection.

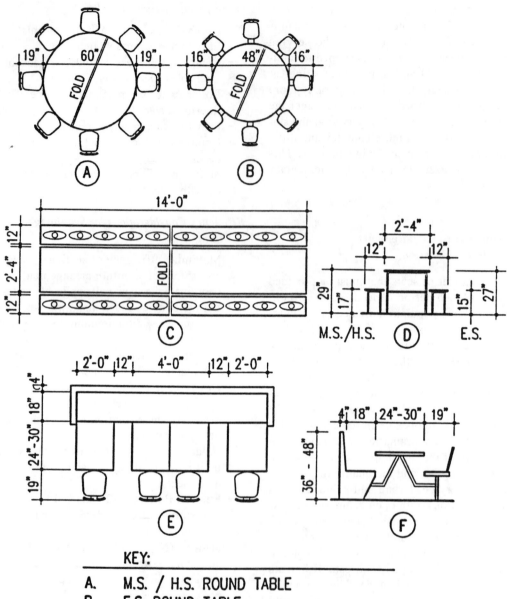

KEY:

A.　M.S. / H.S. ROUND TABLE
B.　E.S. ROUND TABLE
C.　FOLDING TABLE WITH ATTACHED BENCH
D.　SECTION THROUGH FOLDING TABLE
E.　H.S. BOOTH STYLE SEATING
F.　SECTION THROUGH BOOTH STYLE SEATING

Figure 17–3 Seating Types. *Source:* Reprinted with permission from the *School Food and Nutrition Service Design Manual,* p. 26, © 1996, Maryland State Department of Education.

- The maturity level of the student population will influence seating and table type selection: tables with attached seats require fewer social decisions by students and are appropriate for elementary schools and some middle schools. Tables with detached seats require more maturity and are appropriate for some middle schools and high schools.
- Long, rectangular tables with eight or more seats are very efficient, but are less social and awkward to be seated.
- Round, 60-inch-diameter tables with eight seats are very social while moderately efficient.
- Small rectangular tables with two or four seats are not very efficient when used individually, but they can be combined to create longer, more efficient seating arrangements when needed.
- Long, rectangular tables with bench style seating can allow for temporary occupancy increases for special events such as assemblies.

Seating Selection Guidelines for an Elementary School (Figure 17–4)

- Provide tables with attached seats or benches—this simplifies social decisions.
- Provide colorful tables and chair heights economically proportioned for two sizes: prekindergarten, kindergarten, and first grade (first size) and grades two through six (second size)
- Provide 12 to 14 net square feet per person.

Seating Selection Guidelines for a Middle School (Figure 17–5)

- Provide mostly tables with attached seats or benches, some with detached seats.
- Provide a variety of table shapes and capacities.
- Provide tables and chair heights proportioned for ages 12 to 14 years.

- Provide 12 to 14 net square feet per person.

Seating Selection Guidelines for a High School

- Provide mostly tables with detached chairs.
- Provide some fixed booth type seating (10 to 20 percent when possible).
- Provide numerous (10 to 20 percent) small tables (two to four seats).
- Provide a variety of table shapes and capacities.
- Create interesting arrangements.
- Allow for students to arrange furniture themselves.
- Provide tables and chair heights proportioned for ages 15 and up.
- Provide 14 to 16 net square feet per person.

Service Areas and Traffic Flow

Stacking Considerations

Stacking refers to students lining up at serving areas during lunch periods. Stacking preferences will vary with the physical dining environment as well as with the school staff members responsible for supervising the lunch period. Key stacking considerations are the following:

- Avoid conflicts between those standing in line waiting to be served and those already served and looking for seating.
- Provide adequate clearances for one-way and two-way traffic flow as needed by the food service program and the design of the dining space.
- Utilize dining room features (such as columns, condiment counters, and booth seating) to establish natural edges along stacking areas.
- Provide three feet two inches minimum (four feet preferred) aisleways for one-way traffic with trays.

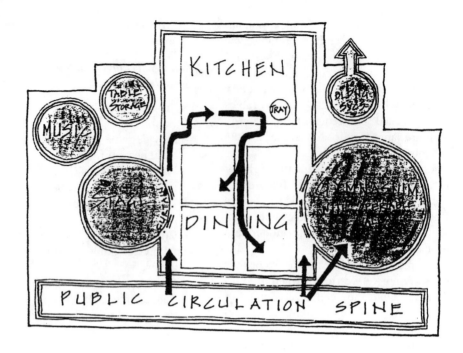

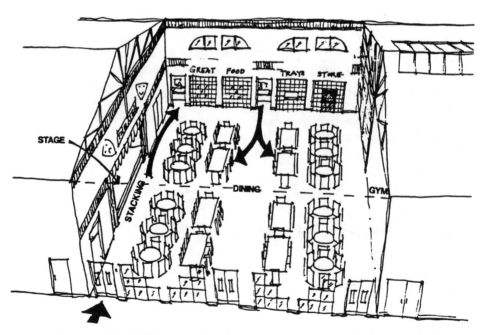

Figure 17–4 Elementary School Dining Concept Plan. *Source:* Reprinted with permission from the *School Food and Nutrition Service Design Manual,* p. 28, © 1996, Maryland State Department of Education.

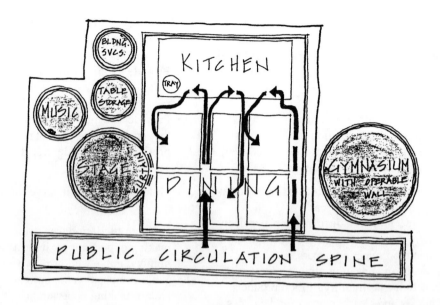

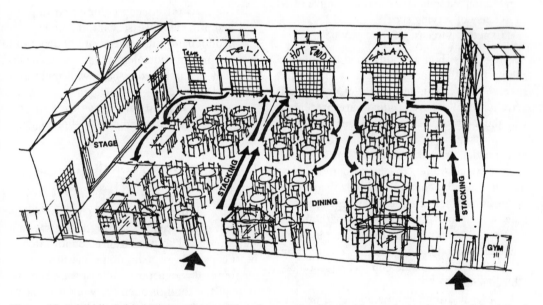

Figure 17–5 Middle School Dining Concept Plan. *Source:* Reprinted with permission from the *School Food and Nutrition Service Design Manual,* p. 29, © 1996, Maryland State Department of Education.

- Provide six feet four inches minimum (eight feet preferred) aisleways for two-way traffic with trays.
- Align entrances to serving lines with stacking aisles in dining area.

- Refer to requirements of the American with Disabilities Act (ADA).
- Refer to BOCA and Life Safety Code (NFPA–101) for minimum requirements in assembly seating areas.

- Refer to the dining room flow diagrams in Figure 17–6, which illustrate stacking areas, aisle areas, food service areas, and seating areas.

Serving Areas

Serving areas are critical to the success of the school food and nutrition program for several reasons. When they are designed well, serving areas do the following:

- Facilitate the flow of students from stacking areas to seating areas.
- Provide nutrition information precisely when and where needed—at the time when food selection occurs.
- Provide an appealing atmosphere that enhances the desirability of food products.
- Quickly and clearly convey food choices.
- Minimize redundancy and maximize efficiency of serving staff.
- Expedite purchase of food products.

Serving areas should be designed to a higher energy level than the remainder of the dining space. This area can be thought of as a "retail activity zone" where students are presented with the food service product (Figure 17–7).

The serving area is where the school food and nutrition program displays its product and entices its customer. In closed-campus elementary, middle, and high schools there is an opportunity to attract more students to participate in the food service program with an appealing presentation. In open-campus high schools, the food serving area is essentially in competition with outside commercial food establishments.

In order to attract more students to participate in the food service program, this "retail activity zone" should be exciting and appealing.

- Provide lighting levels appropriate to commercial food product display with lamp types (which adhere to code-regulated energy guidelines) that are easy and affordable to maintain and replace.
- Provide colorful, durable, and easily cleanable finishes appropriate to commercial food product display.
- Provide clear, colorful signage that is suited to the educational level of the reader.
- Provide a bright, attractive atmosphere that enhances the presentation of the food product. Clearly identify degree of self-service available.

Utilize materials that serve multiple functions:

- Ceramic tile introduces color and pattern-making opportunities; it is an economical, highly durable wall or floor finish.
- Vinyl composition tile introduces color and pattern-making opportunities; it is durable, easily maintained, and economical.
- Signage introduces color opportunities and provides necessary information.
- Wood trim and veneer provide natural warmth and complement man-made materials as durable edge, base, wall, and wainscot treatment.
- Mirrors expand spatial qualities and increase sightlines and ease of supervision.

IMPACT OF DESIGN ON CUSTOMER SERVICE

A school food and nutrition program can be thought of as a manufacturing facility with a retail outlet. The design of a school kitchen must consider two main flows: the flow of the customer through the public spaces and the flow of the food through the working spaces. This flow as it relates to the serving and dining areas must be maintained to promote an efficient operation.

Food Flow Relationships

- Serving adjacent to production—to provide the freshest food to the serving area and ease replenishment

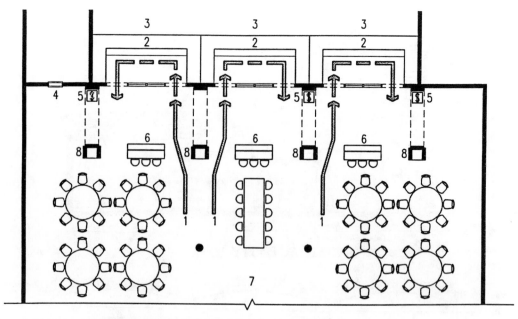

1. STACKING AREAS AND AISLEWAYS
2. SERVING AREAS
3. KITCHEN PREPARATION AREA
4. TRAY RETURN AT DISHWASH/ RECYCLE
5. CASHIER
6. SEATING / COUNTER
7. DINING AREA
8. TRASH / RECYCLE

Figure 17–6 Functional Flow Diagram Between Dining and Serving. *Source:* Reprinted with permission from the *School Food and Nutrition Service Design Manual,* p. 32, © 1996, Maryland State Department of Education.

- Serving and production adjacent to warewashing—to maintain an efficient cleaning and sanitation program
- Internal trash collection adjacent to or part of the warewashing—to maintain an efficient cleaning and sanitation program and avoid cross-contamination
- Recycling area near trash to encourage participation in recycling programs

Service Area Layout/Scheduling Considerations

There are four factors to consider in determining service area layout/scheduling:

1. Number and length of meal periods, which is usually determined by the school principal or board policy

2. The *Keys to Excellence* standard that no student should stand in line more than 10 minutes
3. The school district standard regarding the number to be served per minute
4. Style of service—self-serve, served by personnel

The following examples illustrate the need for the planner to consider the need to base decisions on the four factors and the expectations of the service area.

Example: An elementary school serves 500 lunches daily. The lunch period begins at 11:30 A.M. and all children must be served by 1:00 P.M. Students are released on 10-minute intervals. In order to meet the standard for standing in line when there is only one serving line, it would be necessary to serve 6.6 meals every

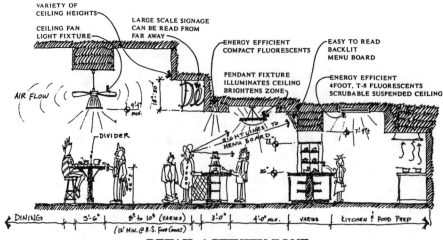

RETAIL ACTIVITY ZONE

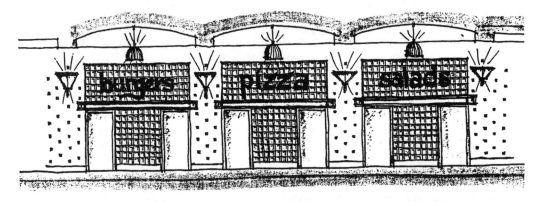

ELEVATION STUDY FROM DINING AT SERVING ENTRY

Figure 17–7 Retail Activity Zone. *Source:* Reprinted with permission from the *School Food and Nutrition Service Design Manual,* p. 33, © 1996, Maryland State Department of Education.

minute. If the meal-per-minute standard was set at 10, children could be served in 50 minutes. This would allow food service 5 minutes in between groups to replenish the serving line.

Example: A high school serves 500 meals and the lunch period is from 12:00 to 1:00 P.M. All students have an hour for lunch. To meet the standard for standing in line in this situation requires a different configuration. Even with two service counters, 250 students would be in line for each counter. If the meal standard is 10 meals served per minute, the last students

would be standing in line 25 minutes. Increasing the number of serving stations to four would allow all students to be served with the longest standing-in-line time being 12 minutes.

Example: The school district policy provides for self-service in elementary schools and provides a standard that three students per minute are served on each serving line. The district also strives to achieve the goal that no student stands in line more than 10 minutes. The architect has proposed that four serving lines be provided in each school. To assess the adequacy of four lines to meet the standards, the school food and nutrition program director/ manager must calculate the number of students that can be scheduled for the cafeteria for any 10-minute interval.

Calculation: Each serving line can serve 30 customers in 10 minutes; therefore, four serving lines would accommodate 120 customers. To keep the line flowing the school policy would be to schedule 120 customers into the cafeteria on 10-minute intervals.

The school administrator and the school food and nutrition program director must determine if this is a feasible schedule. If not, either the serving schedule must be changed or the designer must devise another serving center alternative. Decisions of this type should be a part of the planning process.

Customer Flow Relationships

- Serving area easily accessible to entrance to expedite and simplify the customers' access to the serving area
- Serving adjacent to the dining area for ease and convenience of the customers
- Warewashing adjacent to the dining area to encourage the students to remove their dishes easily to the warewashing area
- Exit near warewashing to facilitate orderly departure from space for crowd control

Staffing

Design is a critical factor for efficiency and effectiveness in staffing. The following staffing principles should be considered in the development of the food service programs:

- The principle of critical period staffing is used. Critical period staffing provides the largest number of staff members at the time most needed. The critical period for school food service is during the serving time for lunch.
- Nutrition integrity standards recommend that customers should not stand in line for more than 10 minutes and that meal peri-

ods should allow a minimum of 20 minutes to eat lunch and 10 minutes to eat breakfast.
- Staff levels are reduced for satellite schools since the preparation labor takes place at the preparation site. Part-time staff can be utilized for satellite schools.

GENERAL CONSIDERATIONS

Acoustics

Sound transmission and absorption can be controlled through design decisions such as physical adjacencies, volumetric shapes, and material selections.

- Acoustic control begins with initial schematic design concepts. Sound transmission can best be controlled by room adjacency relationships. The dining area will be a noise source at times and because of this it requires sound isolation from adjacent quiet areas. This may be achieved by requiring physical separation at the basic programming level.
- Key views into and out of the dining area should be maintained as required for security and observation purposes, but the remainder of perimeter interior wall areas should be acoustically isolated from adjacent program areas.
- Place program buffer areas such as storage rooms, toilet rooms, school stores, utility closets, janitor's closets, and ticket booths between the dining area and adjacent programs.
- Where programmatic isolation is not feasible, refer to Architectural Graphic Standards for Sound Transmission Coefficient (STC)–rated partitions, which are recommended for isolating different room types.
- Room shapes are also important factors in acoustic design. Acoustic analysis of various volumetric shapes will reveal reverberation times and whether sound is being focused at any particular location. Non-

parallel walls can reduce reverberation problems.

- Certain shapes can focus sound and amplify decibel levels dramatically in particular areas. This can be very disruptive in an educational environment, even a cafeteria. The use of sound baffles or acoustic dampers can control this phenomenon. Acoustic analysis and design is very important in dining areas, especially those that also serve as auditoriums.

- Noise reduction works best when noise is eliminated or controlled at its source. Employ high-performing noise reduction, sound-absorbing material as close to the sound source as possible in order to control it. Floors and low wall areas are the closest surfaces to noise sources, however, and they tend to be made of hard, durable, easy-to-maintain materials that offer little opportunity for sound absorption. Therefore, maximize use of available upper wall areas and ceiling surfaces for placement of acoustic wall panels and acoustic ceiling tiles. Noise reduction coefficients (NRC rating) of 0.50 to 0.75 are economically available in these products.

Lighting

Lighting levels, aesthetics, energy consumption, and the ease of relamping are primary design issues that can be addressed in the lighting design and fixture selection.

- Illumination levels in a dining area will depend on the specific uses of the space. For instance, dining uses require a 30-foot-candle illumination level, while testing uses require a 50-foot-candle illumination level (compared to a typical classroom's 70-foot-candle level). Theatrical uses require a wide range of illumination levels (from completely darkened at 5 foot-candles to 50 foot-candles), which is usually accomplished through dimming controls.

- Illumination levels should be designed in accordance with current Illumination Engineer's Society Lighting Handbook standards, American Society of Heating, Refrigeration and Air Conditioning Engineers (ASHRAE), Illumination Engineer's Society of North America (IES) standard 90.1, 1989, *Energy Efficient Design of New Buildings Except Low-Rise*, state energy conservation guidelines of state buildings, and any applicable local code requirements.

- Pendant-mounted fluorescent light fixtures can provide direct down-lighting for dining and some up-lighting for ceiling plane illumination. These energy-efficient fixtures can be specified with dimmable electronic ballast and can provide a multitude of lighting levels.

- Recessed, dimmable, compact fluorescent fixtures can be employed to create different "scenes" or provide "mood" lighting for special activities. These energy-efficient fixtures must be specified with dimmable electronic ballast.

- Separate switching of different fixtures can increase flexibility of lighting scenarios, maximize energy efficiency, and minimize operating costs.

- Color and temperature of the lamp light source should be appropriate for dining, food displays, and assembly functions. Lamp life, availability and cost of relamping should be considered when selecting color and temperature of light source.

- A variety of light fixture housings can enliven the design; however, the number of different lamp types should be minimized to facilitate maintenance and relamping.

- Care should be taken to select energy-efficient and long life span lamp types, such as T-8 fluorescent with electronic ballast and dimmers, compact fluorescent, and color-corrected metal halides. Incandescent light sources should be used sparingly, if at all.

Mechanical, Electrical, and Fire Protection Considerations

The dining area may also serve as a multimedia instruction and assembly space. It should be well ventilated, pleasant, and free of odors. The space should provide for the use of computers in several locations. Outlets for voice data, video, and power will allow for future multimedia use in providing nutrition education music and other activities.

Mechanical, electrical, smoke control, fire detection, and alarm systems should be designed in consultation with the owner, the mechanical/electrical/plumbing (MEP) engineer, the food services designer, and the architect. The design team for these systems should consider the following:

- Heating, ventilating, and air conditioning (HVAC) systems should be designed and installed in accordance with ASHRAE 62, *Ventilation for Acceptable Indoor Air Quality*, and NFPA 90A, *Installation of Air Conditioning and Ventilating Systems* or NFPA 90B, *Installation of Warm Air Heating and Air Conditioning Systems,* as applicable.
- Electrical systems should be designed and installed in accordance with NFPA 70, *National Electrical Code.*
- Equipment utilizing gas and related gas piping should be designed and installed in accordance with NFPA 54, *National Fuel Gas Code,* or NFPA 58, *Standard for Storage and Handling of Liquefied Petroleum Gases.*
- Ventilating or heat-producing equipment should be designed and installed in accordance with NFPA 91, *Standard for Exhaust Systems for Air Conveying of Materials*; NFPA 211, *Standard for Chimneys, Fireplace Vents, and Solid Fuel-burning Appliances*; NFPA 31, *Standard for Installation of Oil-burning Equipment;* NFPA 54, *National Fuel Gas Code*; or NFPA 70, *National Electrical Code,* as applicable.

- Commercial cooking equipment should be designed and installed in accordance with NFPA 96, *Standard on Ventilation Control and Fire Protection of Commercial Cooking Operations.*
- Smoke control systems should be designed and installed in accordance with NFPA 92 A, *Recommended Practice for Smoke-Control Systems*; NFPA 92B, *Guide for Smoke Management Systems in Malls, Atria, and Large Areas*; NFPA SPP-53, *Smoke Control in Fire Safety Design*; and *ASHRAE Handbook and Product Directory—Fundamentals.*
- Rubbish chutes and incinerators should be designed and installed in accordance with NFPA 82, *Standards on Incinerators and Waste and Linen Handling Systems and Equipment.*
- Fire detection, alarm, and communication systems should be designed in accordance with the requirements of Life Safety Code/NFPA 101, BOCA, and all applicable local building codes and regulations.

Security

Security includes the protection of people, cash, merchandise, equipment, and supplies. Theft in any form represents a loss of revenue and is of concern. Theft tends to occur in three areas in the food service industry: money thefts, food pilferage, and collusion between employees and purveyors. Good school food service design can help prevent theft of money and food, but cannot prevent collusion. Some design considerations are the following:

- Design serving areas to prevent student pilferage. Consider the use of low railings or glass partitions to separate students in serving areas from students in seating areas. Most student theft takes place in between the serving lines and the seating areas of the dining room.

- Provide storage areas separately keyed from the rest of the school to prevent any unauthorized access by school personnel.
- Provide adequate room for a safe in the manager's office or plan to remove the cash every day to a secure location.

Equipment for the Serving Area

Food service equipment manufacturers and designers are continually making improvements in the products available to provide maximum flexibility and quality for food service operations. When selecting serving equipment keep in mind that it needs to be flexible, mobile, versatile, and adjustable to future needs. Some of the items essential to a successful service area are the following[7]:

- Pass-through heated cabinets
- Pass-through refrigerators
- Heated serving counters
- Refrigerated serving counters
- Milk cooler
- Ice cream freezer
- Cashier counters
- Point-of-sale computer
- Ice machine
- Chilled water dispenser
- Tray dispensers
- Dish dispensers
- Utility carts
- Hand sink

Numbers of serving counters, coolers, and tray and dish dispensers to be placed will be determined by the decisions made about menus, service styles, and expected participation.

SUMMARY

The prevalence of fast-food and specialty restaurants, buffets, and take-out services have had an impact on the customer expectations and sophistication of even our youngest school food and nutrition program customers. Kindergarten and first-grade students have been successfully taught to select a reimbursable lunch and breakfast from a self-service counter. In addition to self-service, which has labor-saving advantages, some of the service trends include the following:

- Kiosks with specialty or combo meals offered at popular student gathering areas on the school campus.
- Specialty bars, including favorites such as taco or Mexican bar, potato bar
- All-American bar (hamburgers, hot dogs, barbecue)
- Pasta bar
- Salad bar
- Soup bar
- Deli bar

As space and labor are a premium in most schools, the input from a student survey is essential to making wise decisions about the most popular foods for an individual school's population. This is best done with the realization that food popularity changes, and capital investment should be made with future flexibility possible.

The adoption of a computer system that will allow point-of-service counts and collections is a necessity to maximize the potential for alternative service areas and the variety of offerings necessary to satisfy today's customers (see Chapter 6). Decisions on specialty bars should be reviewed periodically, and acceptance of the individual products should be a part of an ongoing assessment. The school food and nutrition program manager must constantly be ready to make a switch in line offerings should there be a swing in customer preferences.

The use of a variety of seating or dining accommodations should be considered. It is generally recognized that the use of long tables with attached benches or stools is perhaps the least popular but most economical option available. Because of space constraints, elementary schools often determine that these are still the best option. Early in the planning stages it is important to have the planning committee consider many options. Desire and ingenuity have been known to devise methods of achieving what might seem initially to be impossible. Some of the dining potentials that may be considered include the following:

- Conversational groupings with tables for four, six, and eight
- Variously shaped tables
- Counters or pedestal tables for stand-up eating
- Booths
- Special areas for seniors, honor students, athletes, band
- Faculty dining/service area
- Outdoor seating in climates that permit
- Dining in popular student areas (gym, lobby, covered courtyards, student lounge)
- Special seating needs of children with disabilities.

It is important to approach the brainstorming portion of this planning with an open mind and a belief that the majority of your customers would respect having such options.[8]

Involvement of students, faculty, and community supporters in the planning process is a great way to get creative solutions to service area issues. Such solutions as the custodial/engineering staff volunteering to modify existing service counters, parent/teacher groups offering to contribute to the cost of decorating, and school sponsors offering their time and talents to do some of the work needed have often been the result of such involvement. Creating a feeling of joint ownership with other members of the school team will pay great dividends in your quest for excellence in child nutrition programs.

CASE STUDY
DEVELOPING AND IMPLEMENTING A PLAN TO IMPROVE PARTICIPATION

Barbara Gilbert

The Challenge

How to increase student participation in Cedar Grove High School in DeKalb County, Georgia.

Action

The Dekalb County School Food and Nutrition Department was awarded a small Nutrition Education and Training Program (NET) grant by the Georgia Department of Education. The purpose of the grant was to develop and implement a plan to improve the lower than average participation of Cedar Grove High School. The district school food and nutrition staff, school administration, Cedar Grove food and nutrition manager, student representatives, and custodial staff were brought together to form the planning committee. Student input was secured on the following

- Menu preferences
- Name and decorating theme for cafeteria
- Colors for decorating
- Special seating areas

The student survey revealed the following:

- Students wanted to have access to food court–style food choices every day.
- The cafeteria should be named "Café des Saints" with school colors of Columbia blue and navy blue for decorating.
- Seniors, athletes, and faculty should have a separate dining area.
- There should be special meals on game days for the athletes.
- Music should be provided in the dining area.
- The cafeteria should lose its traditional institutional appearance in favor of a café atmosphere.

- Service should be speeded up to allow sufficient time for eating and socializing.

The custodial staff said that they could do the following:

- Convert the area adjacent to dining area, used for storage, into a serving area.
- Provide the labor necessary to paint serving lines and dining and service areas, and provide support to the food and nutrition staff for other retrofitting projects such as electrical access for signage, installation of additional serving line, and cashier station.

The Cedar Grove and Dekalb County School food and nutrition staffs agreed that they could

- Provide three serving stations (two that already existed and the new one to be set up in a previous storage space):
  1. Pizza express with alternate options of Mexican bar/potato bar/training table bar
  2. Traditional type entrées—two main entrée choices
  3. Deli express/ready-to-go salads
- Provide color-coordinated awnings over each serving station, window curtains, table clothes for all tables, and umbrellas for senior/faculty dining area.
- Provide a jukebox in the dining area.
- Provide equipment necessary for the new service area, including a glass-door reach-in refrigerator for ready-to-go salads and alternate beverages.
- Provide employee uniforms in school colors.
- Provide clear plastic fast-food trays and colored baskets to replace institutional trays.

- Provide neon signage over serving stations and menu boards.
- Provide funds to pay for school food and nutrition program employee training on quality food production and food court–style service with emphasis on batch cooking, dietary guidelines, and merchandising.
- Provide nutrition training for coaches; special high-carbohydrate meals on game days; nutrition education displays in the cafeteria emphasizing the Food Pyramid

The school administrators gave full and continuing support to the project:

- Scheduled and participated in the grand-opening ceremony
- Assured that school scheduling would allow adequate time for lunch.

The retrofitting work and action planning occurred during the summer of 1995, with the grand opening ceremony held at the beginning of the 1996 school year.

Outcome

Student participation in reimbursable meals increased 100 percent in school year 1996 from the low 49 percent in school year 1995. Adult participation increased 110 percent. Cedar Grove has been able to maintain a higher level of participation. Dekalb County School Food and Nutrition staff expanded this approach for increasing high school participation through improved customer service design to other district high schools.

CASE STUDY
DESIGNING SMALL TOWN SUCCESS

Deborah H. Carr

The Problem

In 1993, the Quitman School District, Quitman, Mississippi, was faced with growing pains brought about by increased student participation at the high school. The 1960-model school cafeteria did not adequately meet the customers' needs. A Band-Aid approach would no longer suffice when addressing the issues of an inadequate serving area, limited production space, and an overcrowded dining area.

Background

The high school population of 700 had outgrown the 160-seat child nutrition program (CNP) facility. The dining facility was very traditional in style and function. Food service assistants served food behind a traditional T-line. Employees were trained in customer relations and suggestive selling for both hot and cold items. Menu choices were available to encourage healthy eating of all meal components. To meet the changing needs and desires of customers, however, additional serving and dining space were badly needed. The CNP director and school administration thought that the situation provided an opportunity to evaluate immediate and long-range needs. With the modernization of the commercial food service industry, the students were more sophisticated customers than those of the early 1960s. Customer satisfaction was important to the decision makers and now was the time to make a difference.

Solution

Planning

The CNP director thought that assured success would be better achieved if customers were involved in the reimaging project. A student advisory group was formed to determine the needs and wants of the customers. A student satisfaction survey was developed and pilot-tested by the student advisory groups. The survey was designed to measure customer satisfaction and desired changes for the CNP facility.

A random sample of 110 high school students used the student satisfaction survey to rate the CNP during the planning stages of the project.

Data from the student satisfaction survey were analyzed with interesting results. The following factors were identified as most important to the customers:

- Colors or visual perception of the dining area
- Facility logo
- Meal service style
- Table groupings and length of time allowed to eat
- Meal scheduling

Administrators used the information from the survey to develop and implement renovation plans. The design of the project centered on a practical approach to meeting customers' needs and expectations while providing a futuristic atmosphere that attracted customers. Specific objectives of the project were as follows:

- Develop a plan for renovation of the high school cafeteria serving/dining area based on cafeteria ambiance factors students value as determined by the student satisfaction survey.
- Determine student satisfaction levels with menu choices, food quality, meal schedules, and overall association with CNP staff before renovations.

- Compare participation rates before and after implementing renovations.
- Compare levels of student satisfaction before and after renovations.

Reimaging

The serving and dining areas of the Quitman High School cafeteria were transformed within the constraints of space and money. The former dining area was transformed into the serving area, and new construction of approximately 4,000 square feet of dining space was funded by the school district. The CNP director paid all other allowable costs for improving the existing facility and operation from school food service funds. The total costs were approximately $300,000.

New lighting was installed in the dining room that increased foot-candles over what had been available in the previous dining area. Windows were replaced with modern glass blocks. Bright, designer colors were used that incorporated a more intense version of the school colors of blue and gold with gray as a neutral and fuchsia as an accent color. The CNP director conducted a survey to name the new dining area. The name "Hot Spot" won, and a neon sign spelling out the name of the facility was installed above the serving area. Seating was changed from traditional long tables to a variety of seating styles. Booths, cluster seating, and regular tables for four, in coordinating colors, were used to provide mixed seating options.

The serving line was changed to allow more self-service. Space was a consideration, so a modular line was chosen with one cashier. Customized modular serving lines were installed with special features to allow self-service of prewrapped sandwiches, soup, fruit, salads, and breads. Students were able to serve themselves beverages from a chilled water dispenser and reach-in refrigeration units. Pass-through warmers and refrigerators were added to the back counter areas. The CNP director and school administration joined with teachers to release students for lunch on a continuous schedule to minimize waiting time in line. Throughout the renovation process and afterwards, the menu did not change. Only a few signature items were renamed to reflect the school mascot, the panther.

Evaluation

Measurable steps were incorporated into the two-year planning and renovation commitment. The philosophy was to operate the CNP with flexibility, adaptability, and customer orientation. The student satisfaction survey was given again to 110 randomly chosen high school students when the renovation project was complete and CNP operations had returned to "normal." The pre- and postsurvey results indicated that the customers were more satisfied with the changes related to the dining furniture, general appearance of the facility, decrease in noise, and total environment/ambiance (Figure 17–8). The pre- and postsurvey comparisons indicated an increase in participation in all meal classification categories, with the greatest increase in participation occurring with the paying student. The participation rate with the latter category went from 22 percent to 29 percent (Figure 17–9).

An interesting finding was that the perception of the food improved even though there had been no changes in the menu or food items. This would suggest that the service method and dining surroundings impact customer perceptions in a positive way. It also was surprising to learn that the customers viewed the CNP staff as less friendly at the end of the project. We thought these results could be attributed to the diminished contact with CNP staff due to the new self-service system. Because of this finding, CNP cashiers made a special effort to be more attentive and customer-focused. To paraphrase the service guru, Peter Glen, "food service is just finding out what customers want, determining how they want it . . . and giving it to customers just that way." We did this in Quitman, and the high school became an "in" place for students to eat.

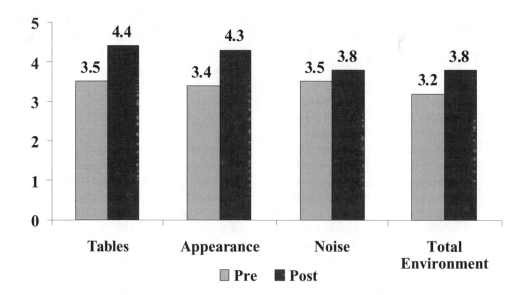

Scale: Strongly Disagree (1) to Strongly Agree (5)

Figure 17–8 Significant Improvements in Dining Ambiance: Pre- and Postsurvey Comparisons. *Source:* Reprinted with permission from the National Food Service Management Institute, *Child Nutrition Program Director/Supervisor Survey Guide,* © 1997, National Food Service Management Institute.

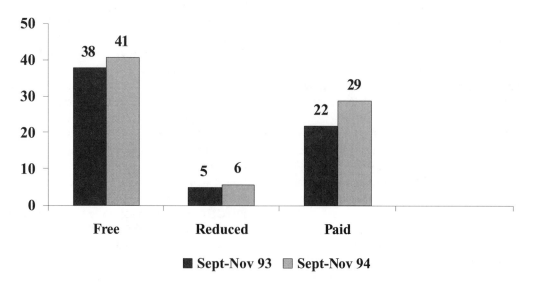

Figure 17–9 Percentage Participation in CNP: Pre- and Postsurvey Comparisons, September–November. *Source:* Reprinted with permission from the National Food Service Management Institute, *Child Nutrition Program Director/Supervisor Survey Guide,* © 1997, National Food Service Management Institute.

This project provided immediate improvement in the area of student satisfaction. We found that involving the customer in changes at the high school level has the potential for increasing participation and customer satisfaction, particularly with the paying students. The following are implications of this project:

- Student involvement at the planning stage should be considered as a strategy for CNP changes, particularly in designing service and dining areas.
- Changing the menu is not the only way to increase customer satisfaction and participation.

- Changing the dining ambiance in a high school CNP has the potential for increasing customer participation by improving customer satisfaction.
- When making high tech changes, don't forget high touch. There may be an inverse relationship between converting to more self-service and the students' perceptions of the CNP staff. Actively planning to promote more staff involvement with students when contemplating a similar change in service style should be considered.

REFERENCES

1. American School Food Service Association, *Keys to Excellence: Standards of Practice for Nutrition Integrity* (Alexandria, VA: 1995).

2. Maryland State Department of Education, School Food and Nutrition Service Design Manual (Baltimore: Maryland State Department of Education, 1996).

3. American School Food Service Association, *Keys to Excellence.*

4. K. Albrecht and R. Zemke, *Service America!* (New York: Warner Books, 1985).

5. D.J. Boorstin, *Restaurants and Institutions* 10, no. 11 (1992): 102.

6. National Food Service Management Institute, *Child Nutrition Program Director/Supervisor's Survey Guide* (Oxford, MS: University of Mississippi, July 1997).

7. M.F. Nettles and D.H. Carr, *Guidelines for Equipment to Prepare Healthy Meals* (University, MS: National Food Service Management Institute, 1996).

8. Maryland State Department of Education.

CHAPTER 18

Sanitation, Safety, Energy Conservation, and Waste Management

Nadine L. Mann and Evelina W. Cross

OUTLINE

INTRODUCTION

Two of the most basic concerns and requirements that food and nutrition program directors face are those of preparing and serving meals under safe and sanitary conditions and effectively managing resources to protect the environment. This chapter provides the reader with a comprehensive plan for implementing a preventive approach to safe food handling, called the Hazard Analysis Critical Control Point program (HACCP), and practical methods of controlling energy and waste-generating/hauling expenses.

The most basic requirement and concern of the food and nutrition program director is that of serving meals under safe and sanitary conditions. With more processed and ready-to-serve foods utilized in school kitchens, as well as the work force's becoming more ethnically diverse, a dynamic process to ensure that our goal of healthful, safe food is essential. The environment presents new hazards and risks that create public concern about the dangers of unsafe food and food-borne illness. While food safety principles rarely change, new issues emerge and school food service operators no longer can be complacent.[1] The rapid and far-reaching evolution of technology and American society is precipitating change at unprecedented speed. In the next decade, many familiar concepts and paradigms will be altered.[1] Successful school food and nutrition professionals must be prepared to anticipate and facilitate these changes. HACCP centers on examining the processes or steps necessary to achieve the desired outcome of serving safe food to school food and nutrition program customers.

The second basic concern is the management of cost-effective programs that protect the environment. Visionary food service directors leading school food and nutrition programs into the twenty-first century must be vigilant in the control of financial and human resources and continually monitor the hidden, operational costs that do not provide direct customer service.[2–5] Energy usage and waste generation/removal are operational costs incurred by all school sites and district-level administrative offices, including school food service departments located in school sites, central kitchens and warehouses, and other administrative offices. School preparation kitchens are extremely energy intensive and, along with the cafeteria service area, can contribute a significant amount of waste generated at the school. Since both energy and waste-generation/hauling expenses are common financial and environmental concerns shared by the entire school district, a team approach is essential to control the variable expenses of energy and solid waste management most effectively.

The ultimate responsibility for implementing effective safety and sanitation measures, and energy utilization and waste-management practices at the site of food storage, preparation, and service begins as an administrative decision. Effectiveness depends on a team effort with leadership stemming from the school board and superintendent, with a flow down to departments, schools, and administrative sites. The school food and nutrition program director and other members of the district-level team determine procedures, establish guidelines, plan training sessions, and establish a time frame for implementing and monitoring the energy-management and solid waste–management programs. In order for district success to occur, participation must be required of all school, department, administrative, and warehouse personnel. With a move toward site-based management and more decision making occurring at the school level, it is equally important to have a collaborative school team that includes students, parents, and school business partners. The school food and nutrition program director, working closely with each school's food service team, has the ultimate responsibility for making the program work.

The purpose of this chapter is to prepare the child nutrition professional to lead for excellence in the twenty-first century by becoming more process oriented to achieve expected outcomes, to focus on controlling hidden operational costs, and to become a more powerful and credible school team player. This chapter explores three standards of school food service management practice enumerated in the American School Food Service Association's *Keys to Excellence*: to follow food safety and environmental health regulations, to establish procedures to ensure a safe working environment, and to participate in a coordinated waste management effort that is part of the total school program.[6] Specific chapter objectives are (1) to provide the steps to implement a preventive approach to a safe and sanitary food preparation program—the HACCP; (2) to outline of an effective energy-conservation program; and (3) to define systematically a cost-effective, practical plan to implement a districtwide solid waste–management program.

HAZARD ANALYSIS CRITICAL CONTROL POINT: A PREVENTIVE APPROACH

Definition and Rationale

The Hazard Analysis Critical Control Point (HACCP) is a food safety and self-inspection system that focuses on potentially hazardous foods (PHF) and how they are handled in the food service environment. The goal is to eliminate hazards from biological, chemical, and physical sources before the product is contaminated. It is a systematic process to ensure food safety through the identification and control of any point or procedure in a food system that may result in an unacceptable health risk. HACCP focuses on the flow of food through the operation, beginning with the decision as to which foods to include on the menu and continuing with recipe development, food procurement, delivery and storage, preparation, holding or displaying, serving, and reheating. Success relies on identification of critical control points.[7]

A basic requirement of school food and nutrition programs is the provision of safe and wholesome foods. The safety of the American food supply has been questioned because of a rise in outbreaks of food-borne illness, the occurrence of natural contaminants, and the use of pesticides in farming.[8] The Food and Drug Administration (FDA) estimates that as many as 81 million cases of food poisoning occur in the United States yearly, with associated costs estimated to be between $10 and $23 billion.[9] School food and nutrition program directors can be proactive by implementing an HACCP program to ensure that the food prepared and served by child nutrition personnel is safe and free from contamination.

Prevention of food-borne illness has become the guiding philosophy of the FDA, and this new direction is reflected in the model Food Code 1993.[10] The Food Code provides the most recent scientifically based guidelines for safe food handling and contains a framework for the development of HACCP plans.[11] The increased focus on the mechanisms of disease and related preventive factors have led state and federal regulatory agencies to incorporate the HACCP concept in the food inspection process and recommend its use by the food service industry.[12]

Background

HACCP is not a new concept. It was developed in the early 1960s by the Pillsbury Company for the National Aeronautics and Space Administration to ensure that the foods consumed by the astronauts would not cause illness during space missions.[13] Although HACCP did not gain immediate acceptance, it now is considered the benchmark of food safety programs. The FDA approved HACCP as the mandatory inspection system for the seafood industry, and the United States Department of Agriculture (USDA) has recommended that the meat and poultry industry adopt HACCP procedures. In addition, the FDA and the National Academy of Sciences have recommended HACCP as the mandatory inspection system for all food service operations.

This recommendation includes school food and nutrition programs. While not a formal mandate, HACCP concepts strongly influence regulatory agencies that oversee food safety and sanitation in school food and nutrition programs. Many state health departments have revised their inspections to incorporate HACCP principles, and the definite and distinct recommendation by federal agencies for use of HACCP in all food service operations provides the impetus for comprehensive implementation of HACCP concepts. Concern for ensuring the nutritional integrity of food and the well-being of schoolchildren requires a safety and sanitation system that consistently provides the certainty that foods are prepared and served under safe and sanitary conditions. A more ethnically diverse work force, increased use of processed and ready-to-serve goods, sophisticated technology, and rapidly changing consumer needs and expectations are reasons to demand a food safety and sanitation system that prevents problems before they occur. HACCP offers a flexible, scientific tool that can be integrated into existing school food and nutrition programs to assist in meeting the need for excellence in practice in the twenty-first century.

Benefits

HACCP provides a preventive direction for food safety and sanitation that is more effective than conventional quality assurance procedures. Quality assurance tends to rely on finished product testing as evidence of safety. HACCP does not rely solely on visual inspection of facilities, laboratory examination of food, and correction of problems after the fact but focuses on verifying that well-designed systems for preventive controls are in place and functioning properly.[14] HACCP is a sophisticated and powerful tool for meeting food safety responsibility.[15] Table 18–1 illustrates the change in focus.[15,16]

The HACCP Process

The HACCP system consists of seven steps (see Figure 18–1).

Step 1: Identify and assess hazards in the flow of food throughout the operation and develop procedures that reduce or eliminate the identified risks. A hazard analysis should be conducted to identify potential biological, chemical, and physical hazards. Biological hazards include harmful bacteria, viruses, or other microorganisms. This category accounts for approximately 93 percent of food-borne illnesses. Chemical hazards include toxins, heavy metals, pesticides, cleaning compounds, and food additives. Physical hazards are foreign objects, such as metal, glass, plastic, and wood, that may cause injury or illness.[17] The procedures for implementing the first step follow.

Table 18–1 Comparison of HACCP Focus and Quality Assurance Focus

HACCP Focus	Quality Assurance Focus
• Food safety	• Sanitation
• Disease prevention	• Final product inspection
• Rapid cool, refrigerate	• Cover, refrigerate
• Handwashing	• Hair restraints
• Food-handling processes	• Physical environment
• Total time in danger zone	• Temperatures, hot/cold

Source: Reprinted with permission from A.M. Messersmith et al., Energy Monitoring: Organization and Procedures, *Energy Conservation Manual for School Food Service Managers*, pp. 7, © 1994, National Food Service Management Institute.

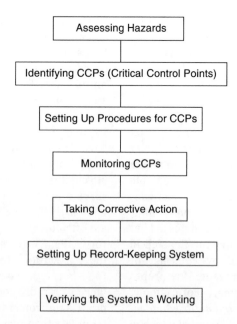

Figure 18–1 The Seven Steps in the Hazard Analysis Critical Control Point Process. *Source: The HAACP Food Safety Manual*, J.K. Loken, Copyright © 1995, p. xvi. Reprinted with permission of John Wiley & Sons, Inc.

Menus and recipes should be reviewed and PHF items and ingredients identified. Potentially hazardous foods include cooked or raw products of animal origin, cooked vegetables and starches, and raw seed sprouts. Fish and shellfish present unique risks, as do refrigerated foods and those processed utilizing the *sous vide* method. *Sous vide* is a method of food processing in which freshly prepared foods are processed with low-temperature cooking and vacuum-sealed in individual pouches. Other sources of potential contamination are food handlers, temperature of refrigerated and frozen storage areas, and food contact surfaces, including equipment and utensils.[18]

Develop a flowchart describing the path that food travels in the school food service operation. The flow diagram describes the steps in the process that are directly under the control of the school food service operation. It should be a simple, clear description of steps that can be used by others to understand the process.[19]

Assess hazards at each step of the food flow and develop procedures to lower risks. This may involve deciding to include an item on the menu, developing recipes, purchasing ingredients and supplies, delivering ingredients and supplies, receiving and storing ingredients and supplies, preparing (thawing, processing, cooking), holding or displaying foods, serving food, cooling and storing food, and reheating food for service.[20]

Determine situations where the probability of unacceptable contamination, microbial growth or survival, or persistence of toxins exists. This can be accomplished by asking questions about the menu and recipes, observing employees, seeking additional facts about the operation, measuring temperatures, testing foods, and reviewing records. When a large number of PHFs are served or complicated recipes used, the opportunities for food-borne illness increase.[21] Equipment capacity and ability to produce or maintain proper temperatures also should be monitored. Vendors and suppliers who have a verifiable HACCP program may be given preferential treatment in the procurement process.

After completing the analysis, the significant hazards associated with each step in the flow diagram should be listed along with any preventive measures to control the hazards.[22] Exhibit 18–1 presents factors to be considered when assessing potential hazards in the flow of food through a school food service.

Step 2: Determine critical control points (CCPs). The USDA defines CCPs as any point or procedure in a specific food system where loss of control may result in an unacceptable health risk.[24] It is the step in the product handling process where control will reduce, eliminate, or prevent hazards that procedures at later stages will not correct. It may be the step in which bacteria are killed by cooking, or growth is controlled or prevented by proper chilled storage or hot holding.[25] For example, raw poultry may carry *Salmonella* when received. Receiving is a control point at which to monitor temperatures and time in the food safety danger zone. Later in the food flow, the *Salmonella* is eliminated by the cooking process. Thus, cooking is the CCP.[26] CCPs differ for each type of food and method of preparation. The most critical items in food service are personal hygiene; time/temperature; cooking, cooling, reheating, and holding; advance preparation; and cross-contamination. Answers to the following questions will help identify CCPs:

- Can the food become contaminated at this step of preparation or can contaminants increase or survive?
- Can the hazard be prevented through corrective action?
- Can the hazard be prevented, eliminated, or reduced by actions taken later in the preparation process?
- Can the critical control point be monitored, measured, and corrective actions documented?

Once the CCPs are identified critical limits or standards can be established to reduce or eliminate potential hazards.[27]

Step 3: Establish control procedures and standards for CCPs. Determine the critical limits or criteria that must be met at each identified CCP. Every critical limit or standard must be specific and capable of being immediately monitored by measurement or observation.[27] Once CCPs are identified, critical limits that will reduce or eliminate potential hazards can be formulated. School food and nutrition program personnel must monitor closely the food items transported to satellite service centers and document temperatures upon arrival. Time and temperature measures are often identified as critical limits or criteria for CCPs. Since improper cooling of potentially hazardous foods is a leading cause of food-borne disease transmission, the importance of rapidly cooling foods following heat processing from 140° F (60° C) to 70° F (21° C) in less than two hours and from 70° F (21° C) to 40° F (4.4° C) in four hours or less is essential.[28] Establish standard operating procedures that delineate employee hygiene, cleaning and sanitizing utensils and equipment, waste disposal, purchasing, receiving and storage, handwashing, and temperature maintenance.[29,30]

CCPs and critical limits should be incorporated into recipes. Instructions would include required temperatures, times, and container sizes. The instructions must be capable of being measured and documented. For example, employees might be instructed to refrigerate an item in a covered, two-inch deep pan for 10 hours or overnight and to check the temperature to ensure that it drops to 40° F (4.4° C) within 4 hours. A place to note the process completion time and initials of the individual completing the procedure should be included. When this information is included on recipes, food safety can be verified.[30] An example of a recipe from *Food for Fifty*[31] that incorporates CCPs and the associated critical limits is illustrated in Exhibit 18–2.

Guidelines for developing HACCP recipes follow[32]:

Exhibit 18–1 Food Flow Considerations[23]

Menu planning	Customer vulnerability Specific menu item safety risks Equipment availability/capability Employee skill level Employee training
Recipe development	Ingredient safety risks Alternative ingredients Advance food preparation procedures Large-volume preparation procedures Satellite operational procedures Written food safety and sanitation recipe procedures
Purchasing	Approved sources HACCP vendor Specifications Delivery schedule Transportation handling practices Product consistency Packaging quality
Receiving	Employee training Packaging condition Temperatures Cross-contamination Seafood/meat tags Product rejection policy
Storage	Cross-contamination Labeling/dating First-in, first-out rotation Temperatures Employee personal hygiene practices
Preparation/cooking	Handwashing Utensil/equipment cleaning/sanitizing Batch preparation procedures Temperatures Final temperature Cooking times Tasting procedures
Serving/holding	Utensil/equipment cleaning/sanitizing Cross-contamination Employee personal hygiene practices Hot food temperatures Cold food temperatures

continues

Exhibit 18–1 continued

Cooling	Rapid cool times/temperatures
	Final temperature
	Cross-contamination
	Recipe instructions
	Utensil/equipment cleaning/sanitizing
	Storage location
	Storage method
	Labeling/dating
Reheating	Rapid heat times/temperatures
	Appropriate equipment
	Final temperature
	Temperature maintenance
	Separation old/new product
	Discard policy

Source: Data from Evelina W. Cross, and J.K. Loken, *The HACCP Food Safety Manual*, pp. 43–45, © 1995, John Wiley & Sons.

- Organize recipes according to type and style of products: thick foods, thin foods, sauces, fruits and vegetables, cold combinations, and hot combinations.
- Incorporate written HACCP procedures into recipes that contain PHFs, are complicated, or contain many preparation steps.
- Address the five stages of food preparation: prepreparation, preparation, chill-store or transport-hold, serving, and leftovers.
- Produce the recipe and prepare a flowchart of procedures through preparation and service.
- Eliminate or streamline unnecessary steps and those creating potential hazards.
- Rewrite the recipe to include the following: ingredients, brand, form of ingredient (fresh, frozen, or canned), cooking temperature, cooling times, thawing and reheating procedures, beginning temperature at center of food, thickest food dimension, container size, whether food is covered, ending temperature at center of food, and completion time in hours and minutes.
- Identify the CCPs and CCP limits.
- Focus attention on CCPs by capitalization, underlining, using color, or bold printing.
- Designate a space for employees to document the completion time of each process.
- Include special instructions for processes such as reconstitution, plating, and leftover food usage.
- Provide a comment section to note irregularities that may guide future revisions.

Step 4: Delineate responsibility of food handlers and managers in making observations and taking temperatures.[33] The purpose of monitoring procedures is to identify potential problems. For example, diligent observation and monitoring of refrigerated storage of raw meat products would determine whether cooked items were stored properly above raw meat products. Observation and monitoring can ascertain whether employees are following appropriate food handling practices that prevent cross-contamination when using cutting boards.[34]

Excessive monitoring requirements will be burdensome to employees. Most CCPs occur during cooking, cooling, holding, and reheat-

Exhibit 18–2 Institutional Recipe Written in HACCP Format with Flowchart

---

MEATLOAF

Oven:	325° F convection	Yield:	50 portions
	350° F conventional		5 loaves, 5 × 9-inch
Bake:	1½ hours		Portion: 4 oz

Ingredients   *Amount*

Ground beef	10 lb
Ground pork	2 lb
Bread crumbs, soft	12 oz
Milk, pasteurized	1 qt
Eggs, pasteurized, frozen	12 (one to 5 oz)
Onions, finely chopped	4 oz
Salt	2 T
Pepper, black	1 t
Cayenne	few grains

Procedures

1. *CCP*: Thaw ground beef, pork, and pasteurized eggs under refrigeration (40° F, 1 day).
2. *CCP*: Clean and rinse onions with cool, running water. Chop onions finely. Use in recipe at once or cover and refrigerate until needed (40° F, maximum of 1 day).
3. Combine all ingredients and mix at low speed until blended, using flat beater of cleaned, sanitized mixer. Do not overmix.
4. Immediately press meat mixture 2 inches deep in five 5- × 9-inch pans, 3 lb 4 oz per pan.
5. Bake uncovered in preheated 350° F conventional (325° F convection) oven for one hour.
6. *CCP*: Internal temperature of cooked meat loaf must register 155° F for a minimum of 15 seconds at end of cooking.
7. Remove from oven. Cool at room temperature for 15 minutes. Place loaves in shallow, 2-inch deep service pans. Slice into 4-oz slices.
8. *CCP*: Cover and hold till service (140° F, maximum of 1 hour).
9. One serving is a 4-oz portion.

Service

1. *CCP*: Hold temperature of meatloaf at 140° F or above throughout service period. Cover when possible. Take and record temperature of unserved product every 30 minutes. Maximum holding time: 4 hours.

Storage

1. *CCP*: Transfer unserved meat loaf into clean, 2-inch deep pans. Quick chill from 140° F to 70° F within 2 hours and then from 70° F to 40° F or below within an additional 4-hour period. Take and record temperatures hourly during chilling.
2. Cover, label, date. Refrigerate at 40° F or lower for up to 10 days or freeze at 0° F for up to 3 months.

Reheating

1. *CCP*: If frozen, thaw meatloaf at 40° F or below.
2. *CCP*: Remove from refrigerator, transfer to 2-inch deep pans and place immediately in a preheated 350° oven, covered. Heat for approximately 30 minutes until the internal temperature reaches 165° F or above. Discard unused product.

continues

Exhibit 18–2 continued

The flowchart that accompanies the recipe is displayed below.

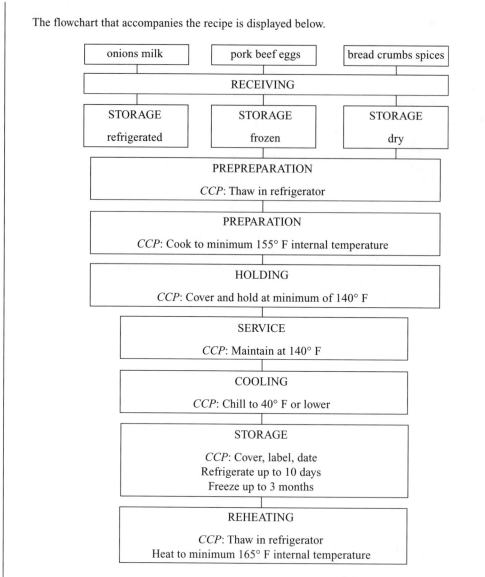

```
┌─────────────────┐  ┌─────────────────┐  ┌──────────────────────┐
│  onions milk    │  │ pork beef eggs  │  │ bread crumbs spices  │
└─────────────────┘  └─────────────────┘  └──────────────────────┘
┌──────────────────────────────────────────────────────────────────┐
│                          RECEIVING                                 │
└──────────────────────────────────────────────────────────────────┘
┌─────────────────┐  ┌─────────────────┐  ┌──────────────────────┐
│    STORAGE      │  │    STORAGE      │  │      STORAGE         │
│  refrigerated   │  │    frozen       │  │        dry           │
└─────────────────┘  └─────────────────┘  └──────────────────────┘
```

PREPREPARATION
CCP: Thaw in refrigerator

PREPARATION
CCP: Cook to minimum 155° F internal temperature

HOLDING
CCP: Cover and hold at minimum of 140° F

SERVICE
CCP: Maintain at 140° F

COOLING
CCP: Chill to 40° F or lower

STORAGE
CCP: Cover, label, date
Refrigerate up to 10 days
Freeze up to 3 months

REHEATING
CCP: Thaw in refrigerator
Heat to minimum 165° F internal temperature

Source: Data from Evelina W. Cross, J.K. Loken, *The HACCP Food Safety Manual*, p. 158, John Wiley & Sons, and G. Shugart and M. Molt, *Food for Fifty, 9th ed.*, pp. 370–371, © 1993, Macmillan Publishing Company.

ing. Key times to monitor can be selected, for example, recording temperatures every 30 minutes to one hour during hot holding or recording temperatures every two hours during chilling. Employees should have access to the tools they need, such as thermometers, writing instruments, easily observable wall clocks, and accessible recording charts. Keeping requirements simple and incorporating them into forms already in use will increase compliance and reduce employee apprehensions.[35]

The suggested critical limits or criteria for the CCPs should be monitored for a specified time period. If monitoring during this time period reveals that the product does not meet the critical limits or criteria consistently, then the product cannot be safely produced and served. This item must be modified, deleted from the menu, or purchased as ready to serve.[36] Formal, documented monitoring of the critical limits for some CCPs may be continued indefinitely, while monitoring of other CCPs may be relaxed or deleted after lengthy (six months or a year) supervision indicates that the critical limits of the CCP are consistently met. New CCPs may be added at any time to improve the entire HACCP process. Typical methods for monitoring include visual observations; observing practices of workers; inspecting raw materials; measuring sensory characteristics such as odors, colors, or texture; chemical measurement for pH or acidity, viscosity, salt content, or water activity; and physical measurements of time and temperature.

Step 5: Take corrective action as needed. This step is implemented when monitoring reveals that critical limits have been exceeded. The degree of potential risk of a food-borne illness will determine the necessary actions.[37] Depending on the problem, the following actions are recommended by the FDA: removing suspect food products from serving and discarding or correcting the situation on the spot, or removing suspect food products from service and chilling/heating according to the HACCP standard. Instances where critical limits have been exceeded should be reviewed at school food and nutrition staff meetings and actions plans that incorporate employee input developed.

Step 6: Keep records and conduct routine reviews of records to ensure that controls work. Record keeping is an essential element of the HACCP system. These records demonstrate that foods and ingredients have been evaluated, handled, and processed appropriately. Records should be easily accessible to allow quick checks of the safety of food preparation processes. These records form the basis for systematic improvement of the HACCP. If records indicate potential problems, the school food and nutrition director should investigate, institute and document corrective actions promptly. Records of the components of the HACCP program that should be kept on file include the following:

- The responsibilities of individuals charged with administering the HACCP program
- Flow diagrams illustrating CCPs
- Hazards associated with each CCP and related preventive measures
- Critical limits for each CCP
- Monitoring system
- Corrective actions plans
- Record keeping procedures
- Verification procedures
- All records created during the operation of the plan, including training records.[38] (Such records may be in the form of product flowcharts, forms, checklists, work sheets, graphs, logs, product specifications, and time temperature logs and graphs.[39])

Step 7: Verify that the HACCP system works. It is essential that school food and nutrition directors are able to verify that hazards have been investigated, risks assessed, and CCPs identified. In addition, effective criteria for control, use of control measures, and realistic and effective monitoring procedures must be confirmed. The verification process should demonstrate that employees are actually implementing control procedures and recording only data actually observed.[40]

Audits should be conducted periodically (possibly at three- or six-month intervals) at each school to ensure the effectiveness of the HACCP system. District management should conduct an annual audit of the entire HACCP system. Audits also should be conducted at each site with the introduction of new products, recipes, or processes, as each demands a new HACCP plan.[41] Guidelines for implementing HACCP in school food and nutrition programs follow:

- Commitment from school food and nutrition program district administrators and directors, site managers and employees, and school principals
- Continuing school food service personnel training that is task specific
- Dedicated, empowered district and site-based teams
- An action plan that has necessary direction, procedures, and responsibility

An effective HACCP system requires planning and cooperation among all district and site personnel involved. School food and nutrition program directors need to provide the rationale and direction for implementing HACCP. Everyone involved needs to understand the importance of HACCP and her or his role in the process. A district school food and nutrition HACCP team is critical to program success and should be formed to conduct the following specific responsibilities:

- Select district team.
- Develop HACCP implementation plan.
- Develop appropriate forms.
- Provide training to school managers and other site-based personnel.
- Implement plan at district and school level.
- Conduct annual audit of program.
- Revise forms and procedures as needed.
- Train and repeat process.

School food and nutrition program directors must educate themselves and their staff about HACCP. Employee cooperation is a key to a successful program. While directors may be responsible for designing the program, it is the employees at each school who conduct the daily activities of an HACCP program. Most employees will be concerned with how HACCP will affect their job. It is important to keep the lines of communications open so that school food service employees understand what is expected of them, feel free to ask questions, and suggest improvements.[41] Training for school food service personnel should em-

phasize monitoring activities such as taking end-product temperatures and completing logs correctly. The information gathered for HACCP will assist in updating the employee training program.[42]

The formation of a strong school food and nutrition HACCP team is critical to success. The district director should select an interested, detail-oriented site-based manager to head the team. Representatives from the transportation, maintenance, and purchasing departments, as well as a county or city sanitarian, should be included. The team is responsible for the ongoing effectiveness of the school food and nutrition HACCP Program. Providing a model of a HACCP program for the team to follow will assist in planning and clarifying procedural issues.[43] The plan should clearly delineate the required tasks and individual responsbilities.

The manager and employees at each school work as a team to implement the school food and nutrition HACCP. Each school food and nutrition manager serves as the link between the school and the district team. The obligations and activities of the school-based team are as follows:

- Identify the school food and nutrition manager as the leader of the site-based team.
- Complete HACCP education and training.
- Implement HACCP program at the school level.
- Conduct periodic review of site procedures and records.
- Forward results and recommendations for improvement/revision to district school food and nutrition HACCP team.

The school food and nutrition director should incorporate preventive measures into the design and planning stages to ensure success. Many factors can render the program ineffective. Such failures may be caused by lack of management commitment, failure to communicate the system and expectations adequately to school food service employees, general resistance to change, failure to fit the program to the financial capabilities of the district, integrating new policies too quickly, resistance to change, and establishing a static rather than a dynamic system.[43] An overview of the planning process for a school-based HACCP program follows.

- Specify who is responsible for the HACCP.
- Identify all regulations that must be met.
- Identify members of the HACCP team.
- Include purchase specifications and microbial testing requirements.
- Note which suppliers have the HACCP.
- Design flowcharts for each food type or recipe.
- Create appropriate recipes based on flow diagrams.
- Include an assessment of CCPs in management, personnel, environment, facility, equipment, materials and supplies, food production, and service.
- Establish monitoring requirements and identify responsibility for monitoring.
- Establish corrective action to be taken if hazards are discovered. State who has what responsibilities.

Summary

The HACCP is a continuous self-inspection process designed to ensure safe food to the school food service customer. It is consistent with the quality improvement philosophy. The basic concepts of quality management are utilized throughout an effective school food and nutrition HACCP. Teamwork at both the district and school level guide and implement the HACCP. School food service processes are continually scrutinized for effectiveness and opportunities for improvement. Identifying the CCPs in the flow of food throughout each school food and nutrition program and monitoring success in meeting critical limits for the CCPs provide the information necessary for setting benchmarks important to the service of safe food to school children.

The site-based HACCP can be integrated easily into the current operational quality management program as it encompasses all components of the school food service system from menu planning through service and final sanitation procedures. The emphasis on teamwork and continual, incremental improvement of processes is common to both quality management and HACCP. The documentation required in an HACCP program serves as verification of effectiveness of both the HACCP and school food and nutrition quality management programs. Food quality is specifically addressed from the perspective of safety and sanitation. These elements are basic goals of all school food and nutrition programs. A successful HACCP program offers proof to school food service customers and other interested parties, such as parents and regulatory bodies, that the needs of the child are the foundation of the school food and nutrition program.

A decision model of the entire process of initiating, planning, implementing, and evaluating the effectiveness of a school food service HACCP program is provided in Figure 18–2. It will assist in establishing a plan that includes all levels of school food and nutrition program management and employees.

**ENERGY CONSERVATION:
A TEAM APPROACH**

Rationale

School food and nutrition operations are energy intensive, using large amounts of electricity, gas, and steam. According to a study by Messersmith et al.,[44] the average energy cost per school meal is $.13. As customer service and quality meals become the target goals of school food and nutrition programs, and resources continue to decline, school food and nutrition program directors need to develop and implement an energy-conservation plan. Energy use should be monitored and controlled to reduce expenses. Savings in energy

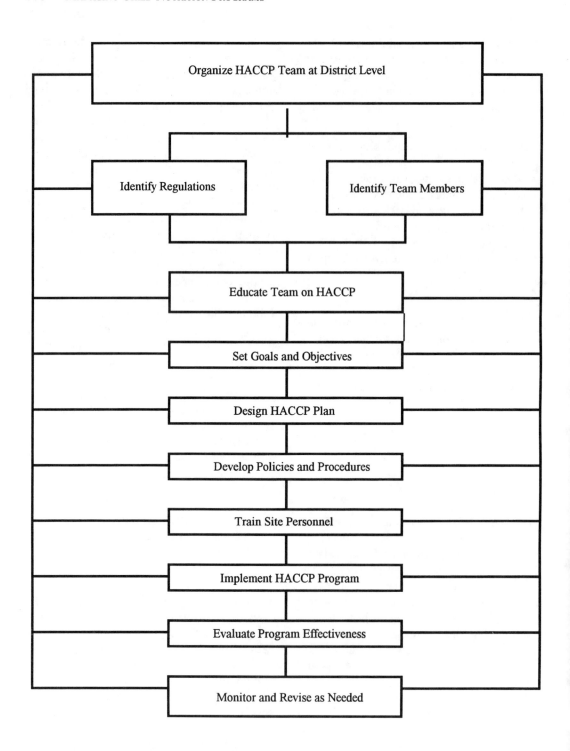

Figure 18–2 HACCP Program Decision Model

costs can be applied directly to the bottom line of the operation. An effective energy management program that maximizes resources assists in meeting program goals. Energy use is a potential hidden cost that can, in subtle ways, reduce funds for goals that relate directly to the customer, such as meal quality, personnel, and marketing. The future will bring changes that school food and nutrition professionals can plan for today. Customers are more informed and desire good-tasting, nutritious, and high-quality food. Environmental concerns about clean air and waste management will intensify. Equipment and communication technology are becoming more sophisticated daily. Energy management plays a role in addressing these issues that impact school food and nutrition programs. Perceptive school food and nutrition professionals can meet the challenge of the twenty-first century by preparing today.

Background

Prior to the 1970s, school food and nutrition program directors were unconcerned with energy costs. Rates were low, and many school districts paid energy expenses from general funds. However, many school districts now are charged with the responsibility for generating revenue to cover their costs, separate from general fund subsidies. During the early 1970s, the oil crisis precipitated inflated prices and concern about energy conservation and the development of alternate sources of energy.[45] Despite legislation and consumer pressure, energy conservation programs did not become a priority among school food and nutrition program directors.

Although the energy crisis of the 1970s is long past, serious energy problems still exist, especially increasing energy costs.[46] Today, there is renewed interest in energy conservation. The Gulf War caused energy prices to increase sharply for a period of time, illustrating that there are no guarantees that oil prices will remain stable. Utility rates have risen with the

inflation rates, and school food and nutrition program directors have increased energy usage during the past several years. A primary cause of this expanded energy use is customer and employee demand for comfort. Air-conditioned dining rooms and kitchens have become the usual environment, and in some cases, an air-conditioned working environment has been a union bargaining position.[47]

Another factor driving renewed interest in energy conservation is the Energy Policy Act of 1992. This act addresses energy conservation in residential and commercial facilities and offers incentives for meeting planned goals for energy conservation. It encourages the development of energy-efficient standards and equipment. Amendments have been made to the law to include low-income weatherization programs at both state and federal levels. In addition, student and community concern for the environment has been a strong factor in the increased interest in energy conservation.[48]

Because school food service is energy intensive and depends on energy-consuming equipment, the impact of rapidly increasing energy cost can be severe.[49] Efforts by school food and nutrition program directors to conserve energy can have a significant impact on the broad efforts to protect the environment and preserve natural resources.[50] Conserving energy through a comprehensive, ongoing, energy-conservation program represents a long-term strategy to ensure customer comfort while minimizing operating costs. It also is responsive to increased environmental consciousness expressed by students, parents, and the community and addresses the requirements of regulatory agencies.[51]

Although an effective energy management program requires the support and commitment of district administration, the school is truly the center for energy management. This is where the many daily actions that affect energy use take place. The food service in the school represents a major energy use center and provides opportunities for the school food and nutrition program director to respond to student and community environmental concerns.

In each school the food service manager must monitor and control energy use and promote energy conservation practices throughout the school food service. Concern for energy use influences menu evaluation, equipment scheduling, employee training, budgeting, and planning for building and remodeling. This frequently is difficult, since many school food service managers must work with equipment purchased and installed prior to the development of more modern energy-saving equipment options and features. The food service department often shares facilities with other energy-using areas such as classrooms, gymnasiums, libraries, restrooms, and heat plants. These areas have differing energy needs and operating schedules, yet often are controlled as one unit.[52] However, knowledge of energy use in school food service can prompt conservation measures that will reduce the cost of operations. This information can assist school food and nutrition program directors in making informed decisions about menu management, remodeling, new construction, and equipment purchases. The savings realized from an effective energy management program can be applied to the functions of the school food service that directly address the goals of high-quality meals served to students in an environment that promotes healthful eating habits.

Energy conservation requires group effort to become an integral, effective part of school food and nutrition programs. The Federal Energy Administration (FEA), and the National Food Service Management Institute (NFSMI), recommend a team approach to the development and implementation of an energy management program.[52] A decision model for initiating, planning, implementing, and evaluating an energy management program for school food service follows (Figure 18–3). Eight steps make up the process for the development, implementation, and continuing operation of an energy management program for school food and nutrition programs.

Steps To Implementing an Energy Management Program

Step 1: Select a district energy management planning team. Members of the district energy management planning team include the school food and nutrition program director, the maintenance/physical plant engineer/supervisor, utility company technical professionals, a school district administrator, and a school food service personnel representative. The district team has the major responsibilities of planning and developing the school food and nutrition energy conservation program.

The school food and nutrition program director serves as leader of the energy management planning team. This group identifies goals and objectives, determines methods for collecting information needed to develop the program, and establishes a time frame for developing and implementing the program.[53] A list of the major responsibilities of the district energy management planning team follows:

- Collects data for program development.
- Determines schedule for planning and implementation.
- Identifies goals and objectives.
- Sets criteria and standards.
- Develops policies and procedures.
- Develops energy management plan.
- Trains and coaches team members and employees.
- Coordinates with school teams.
- Monitors progress.
- Reviews and maintains records.
- Evaluates results.
- Guides revisions.

The energy management planning team collects data that are immediately available, including utility bills, metering records, equipment specifications, customer meal counts, and any past energy-monitoring studies. This information is used to establish baseline energy utilization for the prior 12 months. The data are utilized to determine the amount of energy used to produce and serve a customer

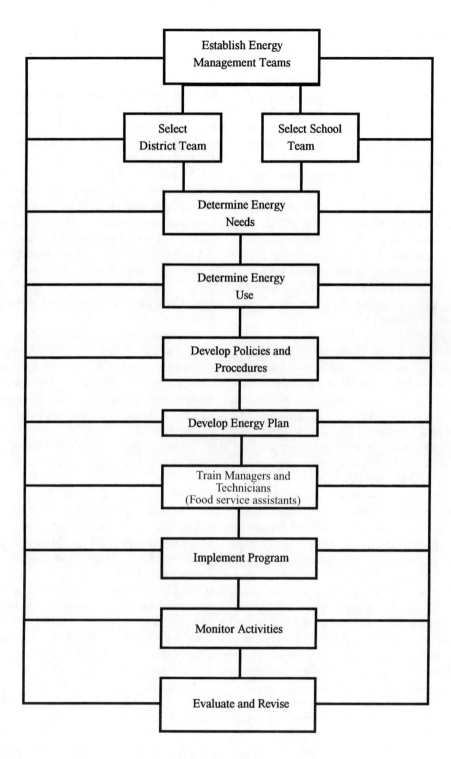

Figure 18–3 Decision Model for Energy Management in School Food and Nutrition Programs

meal. Energy use during the base period is compared with current use to monitor the effectiveness of the program.[54]

Step 2: Select school energy management planning team members. An effective energy-conservation program requires commitment from the school food and nutrition program director and school administrator, but energy must be managed as any food service function, activity, or resource: at the school level by the manager and technicians. The leader of the school energy management planning team is the manager who assumes responsibility for energy conservation. Team members, in addition to the school food service manager, include technicians, a representative from the maintenance/physical plant, and if possible, a representative from the district energy management planning team.

The major responsibility of this team is to implement the energy management plan in all operational functions of the school food service. Energy management is a part of operational functions such as menu development, production scheduling, storage, distribution, and service. Therefore, the district director, head of the energy management planning team, should meet regularly with the school food service managers to ensure the communication and coordination that is essential to implementing and maintaining an effective plan.

Step 3: Determine energy use and requirements. The next step in developing the energy management program is to determine energy use and requirements. This step is begun by initiating a walk-through survey of each school by district energy management planning team members, observing and listing energy-using equipment, operating procedures, and environmental control (heat, light, security systems). Potential energy-loss areas and energy requirements for each piece of equipment should be recorded. Employee practices and work methods related to energy conservation also should be noted. All members of the team will then jointly review and summarize their findings.[55]

A sample energy observation record form that can be used in a walk-through survey is depicted in Exhibit 18–3.

An energy audit should follow the walk-through survey. The audit record form can be compiled based on the details provided on the energy observation records (Exhibit 18–3). An example of an audit record form is provided in Exhibit 18–4.

The purpose of the audit is to examine and review methodically energy use and conservation. This is accomplished by recording current operating costs, specific energy consumption levels, and operating practices in each school. An audit record form can be developed based on the walk-through survey and used for future audits. The district energy management planning team plans and coordinates the energy audit with the school energy conservation teams. Employees in the school actually collect the audit data. A three- to five-day test period should be scheduled so that employees can record equipment operation. Each action performed on every piece of equipment is recorded throughout the work period. All changes, such as temperatures, times, and on/off times, should be noted. This monitoring must be accurate and consistent for the results to be valid. Each piece of equipment then can be analyzed for energy utilization. Several days of data can be evaluated and an average calculated to represent energy use per day. Other information that should be collected includes the meal census, production schedules, and menus. Energy cost determinations are helpful but utilization data provide a standard more consistent and reliable for long-term comparisons.[56]

Step 4: Develop energy management program. Information from the walk-through survey and energy audit provides the basis for developing the energy management plan. The two teams should coordinate to identify long-term goals and objectives. The goals should be realistic and the objectives specific and measurable. The plan should incorporate food service objectives, financial resources, produc-

Exhibit 18–3 Energy Observation Record (an Excerpt)

ENERGY OBSERVATION RECORD

Observer _____   Date _____

Please record energy-using equipment by area.

Area	Energy-Using Equipment and Environment	Comments
Receiving	Hydraulic dock motor	
	Electric tugs	
	Can crusher	
	Box baler	
	Lights on dock (outside)	
	Bug fans	
	Lights in receiving area	

Source: Reprinted with permission from A.M. Messersmith, et al., Energy Monitoring: Organization and Procedures, *Energy Conservation Manual for School Food Service Managers*, p. 7, © 1994, National Food Service Management Institute.

tion requirements, and human resources. Specific strategies and activities should focus on improving employee practices, and the operation and maintenance of equipment should be identified.[57] Information on energy conservation techniques is widely available in the literature, from utility companies, and equipment manufacturers. Table 18–2 illustrates an energy conservation checklist for school food service facilities.[58]

Step 5: Train school food service managers and employees. Training should be conducted by the district energy management planning team for school food service managers and staff. Employees should be trained soon after they begin working in the school food and nutrition program, and ongoing training on new and revised procedures and routines should be implemented at the school level. Specific training in the use of the forms developed for use in collecting energy management information should be included. These records form the basis for district team decisions concerning the energy management program. The records are a

Exhibit 18–4 Audit Record Form

			ACTION			
AREA	EQUIPMENT	COMMENTS	Repair	Replace	No Change	Change Operation
Receiving	Hydraulic dock				x	
	Platform				x	
	Doors				x	
	Lights				x	
	Electric tugs	Plugged in 8 hours instead of 4 hours	x			
	Can crusher				x	
	Box baler				x	
	Outside door	Cold air leak	x			
	Lights on dock	Excessive number		x		
	Bug lights	Not working	x			
Refrigerator	#1 Dairy	Door gasket split on side	x			
	#2 Veg/Fruit	Door stands open				x
	#3 Grain, flour, misc.	Air curtain unavailable		x		

AUDIT RECORD FORM

Recorder _____   Date _____

resource that can be used by administration and managers as a part of decision making related to a broad spectrum of areas such as menu development, equipment procurement and scheduling, training programs, production and service techniques and options, employee scheduling, resource allocation, and financial management.

Energy management is not a separate concept that stands alone. Energy conservation is a concept that is an integral component of processes throughout the entire school food and nutrition program. Thus, all training, especially that relating to production and service, should incorporate energy conservation and re-

Table 18–2 Nontechnical and Low-Cost Enhancement Conservation Checklist and Rationale

Have Done	Will Do	Conservation Action	Rationale
		PLANNING AND SCHEDULING	
		Plan menus to include energy conservation.	A balance of high and low energy consuming equipment will reduce energy demand.
		Operate the equipment at full capacity.	Maximum product to be cooked with the energy used.
		Schedule the preparation and production of menu items to distribute energy use.	Staggering energy consuming equipment use will decrease the total demand at any one time.
		Sub meter the food service to determine energy use.	Provides accurate usage data for energy calculations and conservation records.
		OVENS, STEAMERS, RANGES	
		Do not preheat oven equipment unnecessarily when baking and roasting menu items, i.e., meat loaves, roasts, turkeys, and other large meat items and many breads, cookies, and cakes.	Menu item quality is achieved without preheating the oven with an energy saving of 10–14%.
		Use minimum preheating times for all equipment if preheating is necessary.	Test the food service equipment to determine the preheating time for it to reach expected temperature. Newer equipment will have a short preheat time.
		Schedule nonfood cooking equipment to operate at non cooking time, i.e., refrigerator and freezer defrost to operate "after hours."	The facility engineer can assist in establishing times for nonfood production equipment to operate.
		Establish a cleaning and preventive maintenance schedule for all equipment.	Schedule to clean and maintain equipment at non production hours. This will prevent delays in production and stress of the food service personnel.
		Turn off equipment when it is not in use. (Do not turn on all equipment at the beginning of the work schedule.)	Reduce energy use and peak demand.
		Cook food at the <u>lowest safe</u> temperature that will give satisfactory results.	Lower temperatures use less energy.
		Thaw frozen food in refrigerators unless product characteristics prohibit it.	Less cooking time will be required for thawed food and the refrigerated space will require less energy.
		Adjust gas equipment burners until the flame is entirely blue with a firm center cone.	Routine maintainance of gas equipment will help maintain efficient use of gas.

continues

Table 18–2 continued

Have Done	Will Do	Conservation Action	Rationale
		Recalibrate thermostats on cooking equipment at least once a year. A technical person can be contracted to do this.	To maintain even temperature cooking without excess consumption of energy.
		Load and unload ovens quickly to avoid unnecessary heat loss.	For every second an oven door is open, oven temperatures will drop by approximately 10° F.
		Use lids instead of aluminum foil over products baking or roasting in the oven.	Aluminum foil reduces oven effectiveness and increases the cooking time.
		Schedule microwave and convection ovens at peak demand periods if possible.	Microwave and convection ovens use less energy.
		Turn the steam off for steam kettles when not in use.	Reduces unnecessary heat loss from kettles and steam lines, preheat times are short.
		Plan to use steam cooking as much as possible.	Steam cooking uses less energy because steam transfers heat to food readily.
		Turn off ventilating hood fans over cooking equipment when equipment is not in use.	Hood ventilating systems consume energy needlessly if cooking is not scheduled.
		Group pots and kettles close together on range tops.	Consolidates heat and allows unused sections to be turned off.
		Reduce heat on range as soon as the contents begin to boil.	Lower heat will maintain the cooking temperature (once food boils, excess is lost to the environment).
		Cover pots and kettles with lids.	Retains heat and shortens the cooking time.
		Replace pans if the flat bottoms are no longer flat.	Requires more heat and longer time for range-top cooking.
		REFRIGERATION/FREEZERS	
		Allow hot foods to cool to 140° F before refrigerating or freezing them, except bread and cake items can cool to a lower temperature.	Extremely hot foods will place an extra demand on the cooking units.
		Place cold or frozen food in temperature-controlled storage immediately upon delivery.	Eliminates recooling or freezing warmed food, which uses extra energy and maintains food quality.
		Do not store <u>empty</u> mobile racks in refrigerators or freezers.	Save the energy it takes to cool them.

continues

Table 18–2 continued

Have Done	Will Do	Conservation Action	Rationale
		Consolidate refrigerated and frozen foods where possible. Shut down refrigerators and freezers if not needed.	Full refrigerators and freezers use energy more efficiently.
		Avoid frequent, long opening of freezer and refrigerator doors.	Heat enters the unit, causing energy use to increase.
		Check temperatures on all refrigerated and freezer units.	A check on the operation of the unit and to ensure temperature safety levels.
		Store or pack food to allow air to circulate freely around the food items. Don't block vents.	Maximizes the cooling process.
		Arrange and label food items in the refrigerator or freezer in an orderly system to allow easy and quick placement and removal of food item.	Reduces the time that the door will be open and/or a person is in the refrigerator or freezer.
		Maintain the condenser coils so that they are free of grease and dust.	About once a month, vacuum and remove grease from coils with hot soapy water to maximize energy efficiency.
		Defrost to keep the evaporator free of frost. Set defrost schedule for after peak production hours and defrost for a minimum time to achieve complete defrost.	Frosted/iced evaporator unit will use excess energy to maintain operation.
		Reset defrost time clock (and other time clocks) regularly and after power outages.	Correct timing will better achieve desired results and save energy.
		Compressor should be checked periodically for loss of refrigerant.	Maintain refrigerant levels to maximize efficiency.
		Install "strip curtains" in the entrances of refrigerators and freezers.	Reduces warm air entering when the doors are open.
		Replace cracked or torn door gaskets on all refrigerator and freezer doors.	Reduces the amount of air leakage and conserves energy.
		DISH AND WAREWASHING	
		Use warm or cold water if possible when scraping dishes prior to the wash process.	Hot water uses more energy.
		Do not heat rinse water above 190° F.	Temperatures above 190° F increase evaporation and use more energy.
		Add pressure regulator to adjust water pressure if needed. (Contact a technician.)	Dishes don't wash and rinse well with low pressure and water will be wasted with high pressure.

continues

Table 18–2 continued

Have Done	Will Do	Conservation Action	Rationale
		Turn off the machine and pumps when not in use.	Conserves energy.
		Check water temperatures.	Excessive temperature wastes energy. Thermostats may need to be adjusted.
		Clean rinse arms and nozzles daily.	Dishes will get clean and require less energy use.
		Wash only full racks of dishes.	Uses energy and time effectively.
		Install a wetting agent in the dishwasher.	Eliminates the need for power drying on china dishes and glasses.
		HOT WATER	
		Do not leave faucets running.	Saves water and energy.
		Use cold or warm water whenever possible.	Conserves energy by reducing hot water use.
		Repair leaky faucets.	Saves water and energy.
		Locate the hot water booster heater as close to the dishwasher as possible or insulate pipes.	Eliminates loss of heat being delivered to the dishmachine.
		LIGHTING	
		Rewire lights to multiple switching for different lighting levels and for separate areas.	Allows partial lighting when full lighting is not required.
		Install dimming controls for spaces requiring more than one light level such as dining rooms.	Lights can be dimmed, which reduces energy yet maintains security.
		Rewire ventilation hood lamps to operate separately from the fan.	Some lights and fans are on the same switch. The fans are left on just to provide light.

Source: Reprinted with permission from A.M. Messersmith, et al., Energy Conservation and Improvement, *Energy Conservation Manual for School Food Service Managers*, pp. 28–30, © 1994, National Food Service Management Institute.

sult in effective use of energy. The energy conservation program will be effective only when personnel understand the need for conserving energy, are trained to use correct practices, and incorporate them routinely into their daily tasks.

Step 6: Implement the energy management program. After training, the energy management plan can be implemented. Results of energy management efforts should be reported to district and school team members, and widely shared with school food service employees. It also may be helpful to provide implementation incentives such as awards for improvement of the program. Frequent communication of results and coordination of efforts are key elements to successfully implementing an energy management program. The image of the school food service as responsive to environmental concerns and a center for action may be enhanced by reporting energy conservation actions and results to district and school administrators, principals, students, parents, and the public.

Step 7: Monitor the energy management program. The activities of the energy management program should be monitored regularly. The results should be reported to the district and school teams. This assists in developing a continuous process for improvement. The energy management program is an important component in the overall goal of school food and nutrition programs to meet the food and nutrition-related needs of their customers—the students.

Step 8: Evaluate the effectiveness of the school food and nutrition energy management program. After implementing each activity, the school team should assess the effectiveness of their efforts. The leader of the school energy management team should communicate these results and employee feedback to the district energy management planning team so that modifications can be made as necessary and program goals maintained.

Summary

Energy conservation requires school food and nutrition program directors to plan strategically when choosing the most cost-effective energy-conserving methods. Energy conservation in school food service can serve as a resource for management decisions as a cost management tool, an educational focus, and an environmental contribution, and can provide a strong, positive image for the school food and nutrition program.[58] An effective energy management program benefits the students, the public, and the community. Perceptive managers and directors understand that a comprehensive, ongoing energy conservation program contributes to customer satisfaction and helps preserve the quality of life for everyone.

SOLID WASTE MANAGEMENT PROGRAM: A SYSTEM APPROACH

Introduction

Students become teachers when they challenge school officials by asking, "why aren't we recycling?" Student activists often force school officials to look at recycling and purchasing issues and respond. In some cases, officials are proactive on environmental issues and set policy before the issues are required by the public or the government. A new budget-line item for "waste hauling" has compelled school officials to examine alternatives to landfilling all of the school waste generated. School officials are confronted with both financial and environmental issues that will mandate solid waste management decisions based on the resources available, legal constraints, economic limitations, and environmental pressure. The manual *Environmental Issues Impacting Foodservice Operations*[59] provides food service operators with a complete guide to establishing a cost-effective and environmentally friendly solid waste management school food service program.

The Environmental Protection Agency recommends an integrated waste management hierarchy beginning with source reduction, then recycling, incineration, and finally landfilling.[60] School food and nutrition program directors have the power to make operational decisions for their departments, but must work within the school system framework. The school district's plan for solid waste management is ultimately the responsibility of the school board; however, the *Systems Model for Solid Waste Management in School Food Service*[61] can be adapted for use in the school district (Figure 18–4).

The Decision Model for Solid Waste Management

The decision model[61] will most benefit a school system establishing a solid waste man-

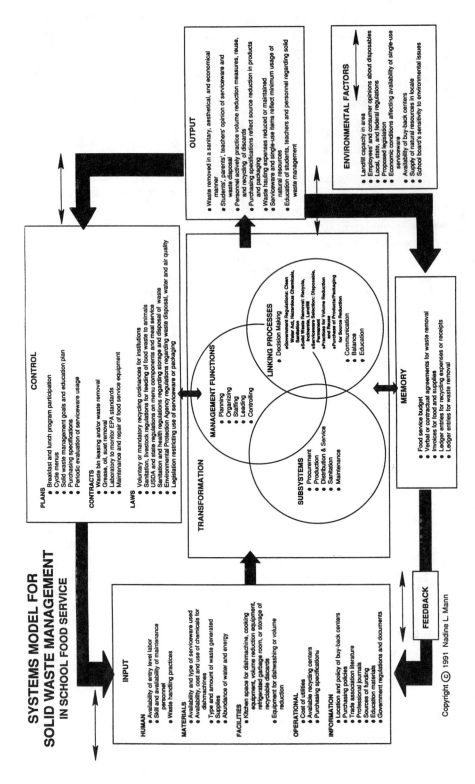

Figure 18–4 Systems Model for Solid Waste Management in School Food Service. Courtesy of Nadine L. Mann, © 1991, Baton Rouge, Louisiana.

agement plan that includes all departments, such as administration, food service, purchasing, transportation, warehousing, custodial services, data processing, graphic arts, and academic services. The model provides solid waste management guidelines for school food and nutrition program directors by expanding five key program components where critical decisions are made that vary district by district. The five key program components for school food service are as follows: government regulations, solid waste removal, serviceware selection, practices for volume reduction and reuse, and purchasing products/packaging for source reduction. Because situations and conditions change within and outside a school system, waste management program components require continual monitoring once initiated (Figure 18–5). Some large school districts have a recycling coordinator who handles the organization, implementation, and evaluation of their solid waste programs; however, the program can be managed by a school board employee with administrative experience if release time from regular duties is allowed.

Step 1: Obtain board approval to organize a solid waste management team. In order for a school systemwide solid waste management program to be effective, the board must require the plan to be implemented in all school, administrative, and warehouse sites owned and operated by the school district. Characteristics of an effective solid waste management program are demonstrated by an objective examination of whether the amount of waste sent to the landfill has been reduced, total cubic yardage of dumpster space has been reduced, labor hours for handling recyclable discards has been maintained or reduced, financial goals for waste removal have been met, students and adults are actively participating in the program, all possible discards are being recycled, and whether the recycler is satisfied with the materials collected for recycling. Changes in solid waste management practices are made to improve customer support and participation, to become more environmentally friendly, or to improve the cost effectiveness of the program.[62,63]

Step 2: Organize a solid waste management task force. Request a meeting of departmental directors to determine solid waste issues in their departments. Solicit a volunteer or designated employee from each administrative department and each school site to act as a team leader to coordinate the operations of the task force. The district school superintendent should appoint a solid waste management task force chairman to oversee this committee. The chairman prepares a proposed time line for each process, from investigating the possibility of recycling and other solid waste options to implementation of the program. The chairman should set up regularly scheduled meetings of the task force in order to move from gathering information to implementation of the program.

Include the school board purchasing agent or the person responsible for writing contracts and bid specifications on the task force. Contact neighboring school districts to look at their contracts and items being recycled and specifically examine pertinent contractual inclusions, such as combined versus separate contracts for solid waste removal and recycling, termination and cost escalation clauses, additional fee paid by the waste hauler for failure to pick up recycle or waste containers, the additional fee paid by the school board for contaminated recycle containers, the school board's ability to change the size and number of dumpsters at sites, and the school board's ability to add additional recyclable material to the contract if a market opens for the product.

Task force members should begin scouting their department or school for potential team members. School site teams should include a teacher who is excited about environmental science, the custodian, the food service manager, and a parent volunteer. The recycling coordinator can generate enthusiasm by informing task force members of solid waste management issues during regularly scheduled meetings. Invite the city or county recycling coordinator to talk to the task force about

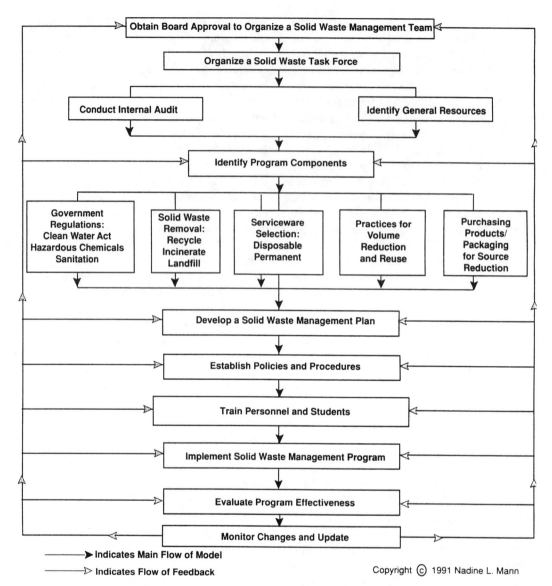

Figure 18–5 Solid Waste Management Decision Model—An Overview. Courtesy of Nadine L. Mann, © 1991, Baton Rouge, Louisiana.

mandatory versus voluntary recycling for institutions, including schools. Additionally, invite representatives from local waste haulers, recycling companies, and/or waste-to-energy companies to speak on current or future recycling or incineration possibilities, and probable cost and logistics for recycling from individual sites

or from a central location. The recycling coordinator is to set up subcommittees to prepare an internal audit and identify external resources.

Step 3: Conduct an internal audit to assess the current status and potential for solid waste management in each department or school.

Task force leaders are to identify each department and/or building where potentially recyclable products are housed, such as food service, graphic arts, warehouse, transportation, maintenance, school sites, and administrative buildings. Each leader must identify ways to minimize packaging waste generated from purchased items. An example from the food service area is the purchase of one-gallon, polyetheylene plastic pouches of catsup instead of individual portion–packaged catsup. Changing packaging waste to minimize discards is called source reduction. Potential recycling possibilities of products at each location are to be explored. The leaders are to identify discards made of materials that have volume-reduction (reducing the volume of the discard, such as collapsing corrugated cardboard boxes or stacking disposable plates), reuse, and/or waste-to-energy potential.

Members of the task force are to identify any volume-reduction practices that are currently being used, discards (items thrown away) that are currently being averted from the landfill, and how the discards are being collected within departments. Determine the amount of discards generated in quantity by examining the amount purchased and/or entering the school system. For instance, school food and nutrition program directors can calculate the number of steel cans that can be recycled by determining the beginning inventory of cans, adding the total number of cans purchased (include commodities), then subtracting the number of cans left at the end of the year. The total number of cans used multiplied by the weight of a no.10 can (about three-fourths pound per can) gives the director an approximate weight of the number of cans discarded last year or the potential weight to be recycled.[64] This is a figure that a waste hauler will ask when a school district wants to recycle steel cans. How much (weight) steel will your district recycle? How much aluminum is generated? Each district is unique. East Baton Rouge School food service recycles 55 tons of steel cans each year.

Determine how the cost or receipt of payment for discards can be handled. Should it be department by department or in the central office? Will the cost be handled differently if the district moves into a contract with a waste hauler or recycler? Some departments, such as data processing, may be selling used computer paper and keeping the revenue for the department. School sites may be collecting aluminum cans or newspaper as a fund-raiser. If the district recycles under one contract, decisions must be made on how to handle some recycling that has been going on for years. Subcommittees should report findings from the internal audit and make an assessment.

Step 4: Identify informational resources by conducting an external audit. The task force leader should get copies of state and/or city regulations/ordinances on recycling; disposal of hazardous chemicals and tires; disposal of cooking grease, oil, or suet; and the Clean Water Act standards. Contact the city recycling coordinator, state and the United States Department of Environmental Protection (EPA), and the FDA to get the mandatory or voluntary waste removal information.[65] Determine state and local regulations regarding the disposal of food waste by contacting the county health department, the state livestock and sanitation board, and the state agency for school food and nutrition. Some states allow swine farmers or owners of dog kennels to pick up food waste for use as animal fodder. If this process is allowed, no food waste is placed in the school dumpster and none goes to the landfill.

Determine all available sources for recycling discards. The local waste hauler should be aware of recyclers in the immediate vicinity. Environmental groups, such as the Sierra Club or Keep America Beautiful, are frequently in contact with recycling agents. Student clubs or organizations, such as the Scouts, 4-H, or science clubs could be involved in a community recycling project. Businesses with in-house recycling, such as a fast-food restaurant that recycles grease from the deep-fat fryers or a pub that recycles glass from liquor bottles, may be willing to share their recycling source. Office-supply stores or copy services could be tapped for printer cartridges and/or office paper recycling sources. Automobile service stations or tire stores could be queried as a potential recycler of automobile tires or motor oil from school buses or school board delivery vehicles. County or state cooperative extension services can be questioned regarding the composting of food waste or paper. Plastics or paper manufacturer representatives, such as Mobil, Amoco, DuPont, or International Paper Company, could be contacted regarding the recycling of disposable serviceware or packaging. Government agencies, such as the United States Environmental Protection Agency or the state department of environmental quality, could be contacted for recycling information. Trade associations or coalitions, such as the Council on Solid Waste Solutions, Foodservice & Packaging Institute, Inc., National Restaurant Association, and National Solid Waste Management Association, can be contacted for information on recycling. There is an abundance of information on recycling and source reduction available, free for the asking. School food and nutrition professionals must be proactive and resourceful when seeking the latest environmental information published.

Determine procurement guidelines for purchasing recyclable materials such as paper towels, napkins, and toilet tissue. Some state agencies require local school districts to purchase a minimum percentage of recycled products. The task force should evaluate the external information and resources to determine the reality of what type of waste disposal methods can be implemented.

Step 5: Identify program components and evaluate to develop policies and procedures.

Government Regulations

Identify and obtain copies of federal, state, and local regulations/ordinances governing solid waste management. Review the EPA reg-ulations and documents, such as Agenda for Action and Clean Water Act standards, that have an impact on solid waste management. Identify current federal, state, and local regulations affecting management of solid waste in institutions, such as schools, and food service operations, such as school food service. Determine answers to the following questions under each topic area.

Clean Water Act Standards. Are the Clean Water Act standards for total suspended solids, biochemical oxygen demand, or ph being monitored by an EPA enforcement agency? If yes, are penalties being assessed if standards are not met? If yes, review or establish a pretreatment plan to reduce the number of food particles entering the sewage system. Take necessary steps to correct the problem, and include the following: repair and clean grease traps regularly; reduce or eliminate use of garbage disposers for plate, production, and leftover food waste; scrape all food particles from plates, pans, and pots prior to washing; use sink strainers in all kitchen sinks to prevent food scraps from entering the sewage line; use pan liners or plastic baking film when baking products; avoid pouring used grease, cooking oil, or suet into grease traps or down sink drains; and dispose of used grease, cooking oil, or suet by placing it in grease barrels destined for a reprocessing plant. If no grease recycling is available, place used grease, cooking oil, or suet with food waste saved for animal fodder. Some city ordinances governing landfills may prohibit placing grease in dumpsters.

Clean Water Act standards for water received (incoming) and water discarded (outgoing waste or effluent water) are being strictly monitored with steep fines for violation of standard levels. Determine which standards, such as total suspended solids or biochemical oxygen demand, are being monitored in the locale. Determine the sampling point for effluent water samples when determinations for "Total Suspended Solids" are being made. Request that samples be taken at the farthest point allowed. Request that three samples be drawn with the clearest one used for the test. Determine the formula used to compute food service water usage when penalty is calculated by contacting local wastewater treatment facility managers to determine local regulations. Determine whether lead and copper are being monitored in the drinking water. Establish policies and procedures to comply with the Clean Water Act.

Hazardous Chemicals. Identify local, state, or federal regulations controlling the use and disposal of chemical agents used in the food service department that are generally considered hazardous. Identify hazardous chemicals used in food service facilities. Determine disposal methods for hazardous chemicals that are in accordance with EPA regulations. Establish policies and procedures to comply with regulations.

Sanitation Impacting Waste Disposal. Do local, state, or federal regulations exist that prohibit or control the methods of final disposal of food waste or leftover edible food? If yes, determine approved methods for final disposal of food waste or leftover edible food. Secure and prepare required documentation. States may allow edible food to be disposed of in one or all of the following ways: saved for swine or dog fodder; given to charity houses (only wholesome, edible food that was never served); ground and flushed into the sewerage system using a garbage disposer; pulverized and strained using a pulper, then sent to landfill; and scraped into garbage bags, then sent to landfill, incinerated, or composted.[66,67] If any of the above practices are allowed, the sanitation board may impose constraints on saving food waste from the production area or from plate waste, including a holding place requirement such as in a refrigerated garbage room or the distance away from kitchen loading dock, holding time regulations, container requirements, and/or frequency of pickups. Establish school board policies and procedures.

Solid Waste Removal: Recycle, Incinerate, Landfill

Decisions to recycle, incinerate, and/or landfill waste generated within a school system are complex and unique to each locale. Many variables must be considered. Choices are always selected based on the most cost-effective methods of disposal that are environmentally and user friendly.[68] Every attempt should be made first to recycle discards, then incinerate, with the decision to landfill made only as the final alternative. Decisions will vary by district, town or city, and state.

If there is mandatory/voluntary state, county, or city recycling, incineration, or landfill usage legislation, either enacted or pending, that affects the school district or school food and nutrition program, then investigate the recycling and composting options first. Determine discards being collected and recycled from institutions in the area. Items that may be recycled or composted in your area include tin cans, corrugated cardboard, glass, plastic (polyethylene terephthalates, such as in plastic bottles; high-density polyethylene, such as in trash cans, bins, pails, drums; low-density polyethylene, such as in garbage liners, milk or juice pouches; polystyrene, such as in disposable plates or other containers), aluminum, office paper (white bond, computer, colored, or ledger), grease or suet, printer cartridges, food waste for animal fodder or composting, motor oil, tires, scrap wood, leaves, limbs, and grass clippings. An internal audit would identify the greatest sources of waste. Refer to the informational resources identified in the external audit to determine potential recyclers in the area.

Estimate the potential volume of weight of discard to be recycled by adding total number of cases/cans/packages purchased for the year (beginning inventory + amount purchased − ending inventory = amount of discard used). Usage formula: amount used multiplied by weight or volume per unit. Refer to the internal audit report. Determine and evaluate cost of discard removal from individual sites or central location, and labor and time involved in storage and transport of discards. Make the following determinations: recycling bin leasing requirements and cost of pickup and whether waste bin number and/or size can be reduced if high-volume discards, such as tin cans and corrugated cardboard, are recycled. Estimate the following: cost of garbage liners; labor cost to separate, handle, and store discards; and savings in loss of time and workers' compensation if lifting injuries are prevented after the recycling program is implemented.

Develop a recycling program for sorting, collecting, holding, and transporting discards with the understanding that a pilot program will precede district-wide implementation. Develop the plan with the involvement of the team leaders and the waste hauler. The plan should provide for

- Selecting the site and method for collecting the recyclables;
- Determining storage procedures and pickup schedule;
- Estimating cost and writing specifications for a contract;
- Preparing flyers describing acceptable items for recycling;
- Communicating the plan to team members, students, teachers, and staff;
- Training employees and answering all questions and address all concerns;
- Communicating the plan to parents and community leaders;
- Piloting the program and making adjustments;
- Establishing a time schedule for full program implementation. If the city/town has a waste incineration plant that burns waste from schools, follow municipal guidelines for incineration, then landfill the remaining waste generated in the school;
- Establish policies and procedures for recycling, incinerating, and landfilling discards.

Selection of Serviceware: Disposable versus Permanent

Use of disposable serviceware that is not being recycled will require more dumpster space, thus increasing waste-hauling costs. Many variables must be examined when making a serviceware selection decision. Determine if there are state or local ordinances that restrict use of polystyrene or plastic single-use serviceware or packaging. Determine whether restrictions apply even though discards are being recycled. If yes, are nonprofit institutions, such as schools, exempt from restrictions? If schools are exempt and disposable serviceware is used and not recycled, volume-reduction practices would minimize the space needed to store the disposables.

Determine which serviceware or packaging currently in use will require changing to comply with the ordinances. For instance, polystyrene, inflated foam, or clear-type serving containers may need to be eliminated and either paper containers or permanent serviceware used. Investigate sources of supplier for alternate types of containers. Determine availability of quality needed and supplier's ability to deliver. Calculate cost of alternates. Evaluate service and marketing implications. Investigate recycling possibilities for alternate types of containers.

- Evaluate serviceware selection, consider the following factors that will affect operations for 20 years when considering changing from disposable to permanent serviceware.
  1. Natural resources, water and energy, to operate dishmachines
  2. Finances to pay wages and benefits for labor to wash permanent serviceware
  3. Labor to operate dishmachine
  4. Capital outlay for initial purchase and replacement cost of dishmachine
  5. Initial purchase and replacement costs of trays, utensils, and chemicals
  6. Finances to remodel kitchens that lack space for dishmachine

7. Availability and cost of in-house maintenance or service contract
8. Marketing implications and expenditures to avoid the "fast-food" image
9. Noise, heat, and moisture causing increased need for ventilation and acoustical protection
10. Natural resources required to manufacture permanent serviceware
- Examine serviceware selection factors when considering changing from permanent serviceware to disposable serviceware.
    1. Savings in water, energy, and labor hours
    2. Reduced pollution from detergents
    3. Sanitation improved by single-use of product
    4. Recycling potential
    5. Cost of disposable serviceware (biodegradable paper products currently cost more than nonbiodegradable polystyrene disposable serviceware)
    6. Supplier reliability
    7. Legislation restricting use of disposable serviceware
    8. Cost of warehousing and transporting single-use plates, trays, and utensils to sites
    9. Cost of holding (garbage liners and bin leasing) and transporting discards to landfill or recycling source
    10. Consumer opinion and marketing image
    11. Natural resources required to manufacture disposable serviceware
- Explore ways to minimize the number of serving containers used to portion items prior to service for à la carte, extra sales, or offer-versus-serve option.
    1. Allow customers to self-serve items directly onto their plate or tray
    2. Use permanent, individual, serving containers if dishwashing equipment, labor, and serviceware are available
    3. Use disposable, individual, serving containers if serviceware is recyclable

Select serviceware that is most cost effective, environmentally safe, and acceptable by customers.[69] Establish policies and procedures on selection and use of various types of serviceware.

Practices for Volume Reduction and Use

Waste haulers generally charge for waste removal based on the size (volume in cubic yards) and number of containers (dumpsters or bins), and the frequency of pickups. When the volume of discards (waste or recyclables) is minimized, fewer containers will be leased, fewer pickups will be required, fewer garbage liners are needed, and employees make a minimal number of trips outside to remove refuse. Practicing volume reduction of discards is both cost saving and time efficient for employees within a facility and is a practical means of controlling the variable expense of waste hauling. The establishment and implementation of policies and procedures for waste volume-reduction practices ensures the most efficient use of manpower, time, and money.

The volume of waste minimized should be minimized prior to removal from facilities. The following waste volume reduction practices can be implemented where appropriate: (1) collapse corrugated cardboard boxes, (2) stack disposable serviceware, (3) sort waste by recyclable items, (4) crush no. 10 food cans, and (5) separate food waste. If the volume of a particular discard is high, the district may consider purchasing one or more pieces of volume-reduction equipment. Small school districts that centrally warehouse food and supplies may consider a baler for cardboard only. Alief Independent School District, Houston, Texas, has a central warehouse and successfully bales and sells corrugated cardboard and polystyrene serviceware from 44 school sites.

Examine the amount of copy paper purchased by the school district. Even if office paper recycling is ongoing, a considerable cost savings is possible if the district has guidelines established to reduce the amount of purchased and disposed office or computer paper used.

The following practices can reduce the amount of office paper used:

- Make two-sided copies when possible.
- Use the blank side of waste paper for notes and scratch pads.
- Reuse manila file folders and large envelopes.
- Use address labels when sending large envelopes; labels can be removed easily and the envelopes reused.
- Use envelopes without plastic windows when possible. Some recyclers will not accept envelopes with plastic windows.
- Print or photocopy drafts or in-house memos using good side of used copy paper.
- Use voice mail, computer networking, and E-mail.
- Circulate one memo rather than making individual copies.

When all volume-reduction measures are in place, an assessment of the number and size of dumpsters at each school, administrative, and warehouse site needs to be prepared. If half-full rather than full dumpsters are being emptied by the waste hauler, then either the number or the size dumpster(s) should be reduced. The waste hauler may conduct an audit using a check-off sheet for the driver to indicate the location, number, and size of each dumpster and the waste volume (full, three-fourths full, half-full, one-fourth full, or empty) at the pick up time. Evaluate the number and size of the dumpsters at each location. The district is leasing empty space if any dumpster is less than three-fourths full at the pickup time. Assess the frequency of waste removal from each facility; the cost of waste bin leasing is generally lower with fewer pickups per week. Lock dumpsters to prevent neighbors from using equipment leased by the school district. Tree limbs and leaves should not be placed in the dumpsters; instead the leaves should be used for mulch in flower beds or placed in a compost pile.

To determine the total cubic yardage of dumpster space needed by school food service, calculate 0.66 gallon of waste per lunch and breakfast participant.[70] Convert waste volume to cubic yards by multiplying the number of gallons times 0.005. Compare the cubic yardage generated with cubic yardage of dumpster space currently located and/or paid for by school food service at each site. Make changes in the number and/or size of dumpsters.

The menu is the driving force behind the amount and kind of waste generated in school food and nutrition programs. Two types of waste are generated: production and service area waste. Production waste consists of food waste generated during meal preparation or leftover food items that must be discarded. Examples include vegetable peelings, bones, fat, or burned/spoiled food items. Packaging waste, generated during food preparation, consists of such items as tin cans, cardboard, glass jars or bottles, plastic one-gallon containers, and five-gallon pails or bags. Service area waste is composed of food waste left on plates, wrappers, milk containers, straws, napkins, paper towels, and items discarded from bag lunches. Convenience foods of the heat-and-serve type have considerably more packaging (production) waste and less food waste than menu items prepared from scratch cooking. Menu items, such as baked chicken and baked potatoes, have a high service area plate waste yield due to bones and peels. Hamburgers and pizza have a very low service area plate waste yield due to popularity and the fact that the entire item is eaten. The menu is a driving force behind the amount and kind of waste generated in school food service. If dumpster space is limited, menus can be planned to balance waste generated during the week.

Purchasing Products/Packaging for Source Reduction

The EPA advocates source reduction as the initial method for reducing waste. Source reduction is a means of packaging items to achieve the least weight or volume of packaging waste. Bulk purchase versus individual packages, plastic milk or juice pouches or K-PAC packaging versus gable-top cartons, concentrated packages of juice and janitorial supplies versus containers of full-strength items, partial versus whole cardboard cases for no. 10 cans, and one-gallon plastic pouches versus no. 10 cans or one-gallon plastic or glass containers are examples of items purchased in food service that have an alternative type of packaging that generates less waste. Evaluate the type and amount of waste generated from the use of individually packaged preportioned purchased items; alternatives include purchasing items in recyclable packages or purchasing condiments in bulk and allowing students to self-serve using squeeze bottles or a dispensing device, or to serve directly onto the plate. Rewrite purchasing specifications to include packaging that yields less waste. If vendors are not able to provide packaging with desired specifications, continue to specify desired options, such as reduced size of labels, decreased corrugated cardboard, recycled packaging materials, or flexible pouch packaging to demonstrate consumer demand for source reduction.

Some states have guidelines on the mandatory purchase of recycled paper or materials such as napkins, paper towels, garbage liners, or toilet tissue. Contact potential vendors to determine the availability of recycled paper and materials and the cost of the items. Have the vendor send samples for testing product acceptability. Determine availability of recycling sources for specified discards. Make changes in packaging specifications as recyclers become available. Collaborate with the school system's purchasing agent to establish policies and procedures for purchasing items and products that produce fewer discards.

Step 6: Develop a solid waste management plan. Each school district will have a unique plan according to the needs of the system. Set financial goals for solid waste management. It is doubtful that the district will profit from recycling, except through a cost avoidance. The task force should collectively prepare a mis-sion statement declaring the school district's position on current and future solid waste management. After the school board approves the mission statement and the financial goals, develop the plan by compiling policies and procedures. Prepare a solid waste management manual by compiling policies and procedures for each program component. Train personnel and students. Change job descriptions to reflect tasks listed in the manual.

Step 7: Train personnel and students. Set up training for team members and leaders. Prepare a poster depicting all office items, such as paper, folders, and printer cartridges, to be recycled. List steps in separating and collecting recyclable materials. Have a display of types of items that can be recycled. Secure and label recycling bins for separating kitchen and food service area waste to be recycled. Train food and nutrition program managers, secretaries, and administrators in office recycling. Train food service employees and custodial staff on waste volume reduction, sorting, holding, and transporting procedures. Using classroom and/or group meetings, train students, teachers, and administrators on waste "separating or sorting" procedures for waste generated in the cafeteria. Be proactive by contacting teachers to ask for a coordination of the students' role in waste reduction throughout class curricula. School administrators, the food service manager, the custodian, and the school recycling team leader should site-visit a successful pilot school recycling program prior to beginning a new recycling program. Then all school personnel should be trained. Continue this process until all school sites have implemented the waste management program. Establish training policies and procedures.

Step 8: Implement solid waste management program. Implement a pilot program at a school where principal, teachers, cafeteria manager, and custodian support environmental science. Meet with the waste hauler representative and team members and leader to establish a time period for the pilot program. Evaluate the effectiveness. Identify and resolve problems associated with the program at the school site or the recyclery. Recognize and publicize success. Add additional sites as soon as training and problems can be resolved. Continue until the entire school district is on the program. (The case study in Chapter 18 describes positive outcomes from a food waste project.)

Step 9: Evaluate program effectiveness. To evaluate the effectiveness of the solid waste management program, begin by comparing the volume of materials collected with the estimated volume generated. Assess the adequacy of the dumpster capacity and recycling container capacity. Look at the frequency of pickups for both solid waste and recycling. Keep a log listing the problem called in by the site location and when it was resolved by the waste hauler. Dumpster needs should decrease as new items are added to the recycling side of the program. Assess sufficiency of labor, supplies, and equipment to handle collection of disposables properly. Examine practices and procedures in departments where labor hours have increased. Calculate income and expenses for recycling and waste removal. Pinpoint program components that cost more than expected. Monitor changes and update.

Look at participation levels at each site. Compare school sites of similar enrollment to see whether more cubic yards of recyclable items are collected at one than the other. Retraining may be necessary. Publicize the waste management program to stimulate interest and enthusiasm. If the recycling bin is being contaminated and the recycler is not satisfied with the product, investigate to determine whether personnel or students are sorting materials correctly. Retrain, if necessary. Are all discards that can be recycled actually being recycled? Continue to look actively for recyclers of discards that are not currently accepted for recycling. Monitor changes and update. As situations and conditions change in the locale, be flexible and open to make necessary program changes.

Since implementing the solid waste management program, have the following characteristics of an effective program been demonstrated:

- Amount of waste sent to the landfill reduced
- Total cubic yards of dumpster space reduced
- Labor hours maintained or reduced when handling recyclable discards
- Financial goals for waste removal being met
- Students and adults actively participating in the program
- All discards that can be recycled in the area are being recycled
- Recycler satisfied with the materials being recycled

To be most effective the solid waste management program should be comprehensive and include all departments and school sites. However, the program can be successful if only implemented in the school food and nutrition program. As this section has described, solid waste management is complex with no set right or wrong answers for every district. Directors must examine resources, legal and political forces, market availability, student and parental opinions, and other criteria to determine the best program possible under the constraints that exist. Districts will not start at the same level or progress at the same rate toward a comprehensive solid waste management program. School food and nutrition program directors or the district solid waste team will determine implementation, training, procedures, monitoring, and evaluation process. By using the information set forth in this section, any school district or any school food authority can set up an outstanding, cost-effective, and environmentally friendly solid waste management program.

SUMMARY

This chapter provides child nutrition program administrators with a preventive approach to food safety through the establishment of an HACCP, a team approach to energy usage and conservation, and finally a system approach to controlling the variable cost of solid waste generation and disposal. A decision model is included in each section to guide the reader through the process of identifying and controlling problem areas at a school site, in a department, or within a school district. Utilization of the concepts presented in this chapter will benefit potential and current school food and nutrition professionals by the identification of the processes, resources, constraints, and expected outcomes that will allow justified decisions on food safety, energy conservation, and solid waste management to move the program toward excellence into the twenty-first century.

The twenty-first century will find school food and nutrition professionals continuing to strive toward excellent management practices. The primary purpose of the school food and nutrition program's existence within a school system is the preparation of acceptable, health-ful food items and service of safe and sanitary nutritionally sound meals to students at an affordable cost. To achieve the goal of serving meals under safe and sanitary conditions and effectively managing resources to protect the environment, the district-level school food and nutrition program directors/supervisors must be competent in the development of sanitation procedures, establishment of safety standards and rules, the maintenance of a system of waste disposal, and implementation of a quality assurance/quality improvement program.[71] The *Keys to Excellence: Standards of Practice for Nutrition Integrity* identifies sanitation, safety, and waste management as a key focus area in the school food service setting.[72] To achieve excellence, a district must maintain an environment for safe and sanitary food production and establish a commitment to responsible solid waste management, energy conservation, and environmental practices in the school community.[72]

CASE STUDY
IMPLEMENTING A COST-EFFECTIVE, ENVIRONMENTALLY FRIENDLY SOLID WASTE MANAGEMENT PLAN

Nadine L. Mann

Challenge: To develop and implement a cost-effective and environmentally friendly solid waste management program in a school district.

Solution: Identify recyclers and recyclable products, plan a program, conduct a pilot study, train all personnel, implement, evaluate, make changes, continue to identify recyclers.

Outcomes: Conservation of local landfill; fewer waste disposal containers on the school campus; improved cost-control and budget management; environmental education of students, parents, and teachers; child nutrition personnel actively participating as school and community team players; improved public image of the school food and nutrition program; and compliance with EPA and local government regarding municipal regulations.

Louisiana's East Baton Rouge Parish School District was forced to address a financial and environmental issue that never before had been a problem in the history of the school system. In 1988, all 101 public schools lost the benefit of free waste-hauling services previously provided by the city/parish government. The local landfill was served notice by the EPA of a forced closure in four years due to noncompliance with federal regulations. When the $150,000 unbudgeted school board expense of districtwide waste-hauling service was awarded, the finance director assigned a 50/50 split of the waste-hauling expense to the general fund budget and the school food service budget. A school food service manager, Melba Hollingsworth, set out to determine through scientific research whether food services could reduce the volume of waste generated by converting the packaging of the 10.5 million half-pints of milk purchased annually for schools

from gable-top cartons to plastic polyethylene milk pouches. The research project demonstrated student acceptance of the milk pouch, a volume and weight reduction of waste sent to the landfill and a reduction (nearly 50 percent) in the amount of school food service waste generated by each school cafeteria. After presenting the results of the research project to the finance committee, Mary Eleanor Cole, Director, Child Nutrition Program, requested and was granted a reduction in the portion of the waste-hauling bill assigned to the school food service budget from 50 percent to 26.5 percent. Additionally, the six schools involved in the research project found that the volume-reduction practice of collapsing corrugated cardboard boxes prior to being placed in the dumpster reduced the amount of dumpster space needed.

The number and size of dumpsters had been arbitrarily assigned to schools by the waste hauler and the school board purchasing agent. At that time principals called the waste hauler and had extra dumpsters delivered to school sites with no regard to cost or need. The researcher examined the number and size of dumpsters and recommended a reduction in the number and volume of dumpsters, taking into account the volume reduction when milk pouches were used districtwide and the practice of collapsing boxes was implemented. An additional cost saving was achieved since fewer garbage liners were used to bag empty pouches versus empty milk cartons.

Municipalities, including Baton Rouge, were mandated to show a 25% reduction in waste going to landfills through source reduction and recycling by 1992. No recycling was available for any Baton Rouge schools until the fall of 1990, when a nationally known waste hauler opened a materials recovery facility (MRF) and agreed to pilot the recycling of tin cans and cardboard from 10 schools. This enabled a procedure to be established prior to implementing the program in the remaining 91 schools. Food service personnel removed labels, rinsed, and collected cans in a large plastic bag until the recycle day (every-other-week pickup). All boxes were collapsed and daily placed in the recycle bin.

Training and implementing the recycling phase was initiated by Dr. Nadine L. Mann, Assistant Director, Child Nutrition Program. Lenny Meadows, Executive Secretary, Physical Plant Services, was the official liaison between the schools and the waste hauler. She worked closely with the waste hauler and custodians to determine placement of recycle bins near the kitchens at all schools. Meadows also arranged for and participated in training of custodians, school food and nutrition managers, and school principals prior to school starting in August of 1991. All of the key players learned how to implement the recycling program at the individual school sites. The timing was right for implementation of a districtwide school recycling program, since the city of Baton Rouge had implemented a curbside recycling program the same year; therefore, school board employees were open and willing to participate in a recycling program. To raise money, school administrators allowed teachers and students to collect and recycle newspaper and aluminum cans at each school location. The district recycling program did not infringe upon individual schools' newspaper and aluminum recycling projects.

An eight-yard recycle bin was placed at each school and administrative site, with pickups scheduled every other week. The weight of the corrugated cardboard and tin cans picked up from school board sites was determined daily. By the end of the school year in 1992, the figures were in—each month the waste hauler consistently picked up an average of 30 tons of cardboard and 5 tons of steel from schools in East Baton Rouge Parish.

In the spring of 1992, an office paper recycling program was piloted at six schools with a plan to implement the program at all school locations in the fall. Flyers depicting types of paper accepted for recycling were developed and distributed to all administrative offices, classrooms, and cafeterias. Again, principals, custodians, and food service personnel were trained prior to implementation. Some principals requested training for teachers during a monthly faculty meeting. A few custodians feared recycling would add to their regular workload. Anxiety diminished when the custodial staff learned that only boxes of paper, labeled RECYCLE and placed outside a classroom, had to be placed in the recycle bin and that no janitor would have to sort classroom trash to separate out paper that was discarded.

District Profile

School District: East Baton Rouge Parish, Baton Rouge, Louisiana

1996 Enrollment: 58,000

Average Daily Participation Lunch: 42,000

Average Daily Participation Breakfast: 15,200

Number of Schools (1996):
65 Elementary 36 Secondary

Source Reduction: Gable-top milk and juice cartons changed to polyethylene milk pouches

Recycling: Corrugated cardboard, tin cans, office paper, computer cartridges, grease, and suet

Type of Serviceware: Permanentware used in 96 percent of the school cafeterias

There was actually less trash to remove from the classrooms than before the recycling program began.

A school board warehouse holding rows and rows of outdated state-mandated forms was discovered and targeted as a potential opportunity for recycling cardboard and white paper. After securing approval from the supervisor of curriculum and instruction and having a 30 yard roll-off dumpster delivered to the warehouse, 30 tons of office paper were purged and sent to the MRF rather than to the landfill.

In the fall of 1992, custodians were surveyed to determine whether a "leaf and limb" disposal problem existed at school sites. Huge oak trees surrounding some school buildings generated vast amounts of leaves and fallen limbs in the fall of the year. The usual custom was to place bags of leaves in the school dumpster (waste disposal container), resulting in little space left in the dumpster for food service or school waste. Calls were coming in to physical plant services to request a second dumpster pickup, resulting in an additional waste hauling charge. As a result of the survey, a policy stating that "no leaves or limbs shall be placed in any school dumpster" was established. A new procedure for removing limbs and leaves from schoolyards was established requiring custodial staff to place the leaves in existing flower beds or in a compost pile away from school buildings. Thirty elementary schools received compost bins donated by the city's Office of Recycling. In some schools with compost bins and vegetable gardens, leaves and vegetable food waste from the cafeteria were mixed into the compost bin. When composted material was used in the classroom garden, vegetables, such as green onions, radishes, turnip greens, and turnips were grown and harvested by the students, cooked and served by cafeteria personnel, and consumed by the students who raised the vegetables.

It was logical that if schools were placing office paper, cardboard, and tin cans into a recycle bin (eight-yard size at each school site), the number and size of dumpsters needed at a school site should decrease, therefore reducing the cost of leasing. School dumpsters were audited to determine how full the dumpsters were at the time the garbage truck emptied it. The results of the audit were useful in observing a pattern of dumpster needs at a school. If the schools used milk pouch packaging; recycled all tin cans, cardboard, and office paper; and avoided placing newspaper, leaves, and limbs in the dumpster, one yard per 100 students enrolled proved to be sufficient dumpster space. The formula was applied to all schools. Dumpster volume and sizes were evaluated, with reductions made at nearly all schools.

The district continues to use the milk pouches and successfully recycle. Grease and suet from school cafeterias have been recycled for at least 25 years. Current recycling efforts center on adding the polyethylene milk pouches to the list of recyclables. As of this writing, the constraint of "holding" the pouches at the MRF until a sufficient weight of the product is collected has not been resolved.

Dr. Nadine L. Mann was the recipient of the Association of School Business Officials International, 1993 Pinnacle of Excellence award for developing and implementing an environmentally friendly and cost-effective solid waste management program in the school district.[73–77]

REFERENCES

1. J.K. Loken, *The HACCP Food Safety Manual* (New York: John Wiley & Sons; 1995).

2. C.W. Shanklin and L. Hoover, "Position of the American Dietetic Association: Natural Resource Conservation and Waste Management, *Journal of the American Dietetic Association* 97 (1997): 425–428.

3. N.L. Mann, "Market Outlook—Recycling," *American Schools and Universities* 67, no. 5 (1995): 32.

4. D.A. Ferris et al., "Solid Waste Management in Foodservice," *Food Technology* 48, no. 3 (1994): 110–113, 115.

5. N.L. Mann and C.W. Shanklin, "Solid Waste Management in School Food Service Facilities: A Critical

Issue for the 1990's," *School Food Service Research Review* 14, no. 2 (1990): 83–85.

6. American School Food Service Association, *Keys to Excellence: Standards of Practice for Nutrition Integrity* (Alexandria,VA: 1995).

7. B.A. Byers et al., *Food Service Manual for Health Care Institutions* (Chicago: American Hospital Association Publishing , Inc., 1994).

8. W.H. Sperber, "The Modern HACCP System," *Good Technology* 45 (1991): 116–120.

9. B.W. LaVella and J. Bostic, *HACCP for Foodservice: Recipe Manual and Guide* (St. Louis, MO: LaVella Food Specialists, 1994).

10. U.S. Public Health Service, *Food Code 1993* (Washington, DC: U.S. Government Printing Office, 1993).

11. B.W. LaVella BW,"HACCP—Not Just Another Dirty Word," *National Culinary Review* 20, no. 2 (1996): 25, 28.

12. Loken, *The HACCP Food Safety Manual.*

13. LaVella, "HACCP—Not Just Another Dirty Word."

14. B. Lorenzini, "Verify the System," *Restaurants and Institutions* 105, no. 26 (1995): 122.

15. Loken, *The HACCP Food Safety Manual.*

16. M. Sherer,"Anticipating Paradigm Shifts," *Food Management* 28 (1993): 93–108.

17. Loken, *The HACCP Food Safety Manual.*

18. Byers et al., *Food Service Manual.*

19. B.J. Elder and K. McMillan, *Hazard Analysis Critical Control Point: Guide for the Development and Implementation of a HACCP Program* (Baton Rouge, LA: Louisiana State University and the Louisiana Meat Industry Association, 1995).

20. Byers et al., *Food Service Manual.*

21. The Education Foundation, *The HACCP Reference Book* (Chicago: National Restaurant Association, 1994).

22. Hospital Food Service Management, "Get Ahead on Pending Regulatory Changes: Implement Hazard Analysis System Now," *Hospital Food Service Management* 1, no. 1 (1993): 33–42.

23. Loken, *The HACCP Food Safety Manual.*

24. Byers et al., *Food Service Manual.*

25. Loken, *The HACCP Food Safety Manual.*

26. The Education Foundation, *The HACCP Reference Book.*

27. Loken, *The HACCP Food Safety Manual.*

28. M. Beasley, "Implement *HACCP* Standards," *Food Management* 30 (1995): 38–40.

29. LaVella, "HACCP—Not Just Another Dirty Word."

30. Hospital Food Service Management, "Document HACCP Plan To Prevent Food Borne Illness, Law-

suits," *Hospital Food Service Management* 1, no. 4 (1993): 49–55.

31. G. Shugart and M. Molt, *Food for Fifty*, 9th ed. (New York: Macmillan Publishing Co., 1993).

32. "Food Management," *Food Management* 30, no. 11 (1995): 66.

33. Hospital Food Service Management, "Document HACCP Plan."

34. Byers et al., *Food Service Manual.*

35. Lorenzini, "Verify the System."

36. Food Management.

37. Byers et al., *Food Service Manual.*

38. Elder and McMillan, *Hazard Analysis Critical Control Point.*

39. Loken, *The HACCP Food Safety Manual.*

40. Byers et al., *Food Service Manual.*

41. Loken, *The HACCP Food Safety Manual.*

42. M. M. Cody and M. Keith, *Food Safety for Professionals: A Reference and Study Guide* (Chicago: American Dietetic Association, 1991).

43. Hospital Food Service Management, "Get Ahead on Pending Regulatory Changes."

44. A.M. Messersmith et al., "Energy Used To Produce Meals in School Food Service," *School Food Service Research Review* 18, no. 1 (1994): 29–26.

45. M.C. Spears, *Foodservice Organizations: A Managerial and Systems Approach* (Englewood Cliffs, NJ: Prentice Hall, 1995).

46. Byers et al., *Food Service Manual.*

47. J. Payne-Palacio et al., *West and Wood's Introduction to Foodservice* (New York: Macmillan Publishing Co., 1997).

48. T. Jones,"The Resurgence of Energy Auditing in Hospitality Operations," *The Bottomline* 10, no. 7 (1995): 23–25.

49. Spears, *Foodservice Organizations.*

50. Payne-Palacio et al., *West and Wood's Introduction to Foodservice.*

51. J.C. Dale and T. Kluga, "Energy Conservation: More Than a Good Idea," *The Cornell H.R.A. Quarterly* 33, no. 6 (1992): 30–35.

52. A.M. Messersmith et al., *Energy Conservation Manual for School Food Service Managers* (Hattiesburg, MS: National Food Service Management Institute, 1994).

53. Byers et al., *Food Service Manual.*

54. Messersmith et al., *Energy Conservation Manual.*

55. Byers et al., *Food Service Manual.*

56. Spears, *Foodservice Organization.*

57. Byers et al., *Food Service Manual.*

58. Messersmith et al., *Energy Conservation Manual.*

59. D.M. Mason and C.W. Shanklin, *Environmental Issues Impacting Foodservice Operations* (Manhattan, KS: Kansas State University, 1996).

60. *Characterization of Municipal Solid Waste in the United States: 1994 Update*. Executive summary. (Washington, DC: Office of Solid Waste and Emergency Response, 1994. US Environmental Protection Agency publication 530-S-94-042).

61. N.L. Mann, *A Decision Model for Solid Waste Management in School Food Service* (Denton, TX: Texas Woman's University, 1991). Dissertation.

62. N.L. Mann et al., "What Are We Doing with Our Waste?" *School Foodservice & Nutrition* 48, no. 7 (1994): 46–50, 78.

63. N.L. Mann et al., "An Assessment of Solid Waste Management Practices Used in School Foodservice Operations," *School Food Service Research Review* 17, no. 2 (1993): 109–114.

64. M.D. Hollingsworth et al., "Waste Stream Analysis in Seven Selected Food Service Operations," *School Food Service Research Review* 19, no. 2 (1995): 81–87.

65. *Guide to Environmental Issues* (Washington, DC: Office of Solid Waste and Emergency Response, 1995. U.S. Environmental Protection Agency publication 520/B-94-001).

66. R.J. Behan, "The Greening of School Food Service," *School Foodservice & Nutrition* 48, no. 7 (1994): 30–34.

67. C. Kunzler and M. Farrell, "Food Services Composting Update," *Biocycle* 37, no. 5 (1996): 48–55.

68. Shanklin and Hoover, "Position of the American Dietetic Association."

69. R. Ghiselli et al., "Reducing School Foodservice Waste through the Choice of Serviceware," *Hospitality Research Journal* 18, no. 3 (1995): 3–11.

70. Hollingsworth et al., "An Assessment of Solid Waste Management."

71. M.B. Gregoire and J. Sneed, "Competencies for District School Nutrition Directors/Supervisors," *School Food Service Research Review* 18 (1994): 89–100.

72. American School Food Service Association, *Keys to Excellence*.

73. Behan, "The Greening of School Food Service."

74. N.I. Hahn, "The Greening of a School District," *Journal of the American Dietetic Association* 97 (1997): 371.

75. C. Braun, "East Baton Rouge Schools Prove Recycling Happens Beyond Curbside," *The Recycling Magnet* 5, no. 2 (1994): 4.

76. N.L. Mann, "Solid Waste Management Practices in EBRP Schools," *School Business Affairs* 60, no. 2 (1994): 36–37.

77. K. Shuster, "School Food Service Recycling Challenges and Solutions," *Food Management* 29 (1994): 60.

HACCP and Solid Waste Management Resources

For more information about HACCP, the following resources are listed:

Resources

American Hotel & Motel Association
The Educational Institute
(800)344-4381

Centers for Disease Control and Prevention
Food Borne Illness Line
(404)332-3497

The Educational Foundation
National Restaurant Association
Technical Education Division
(800)765-2122

Food and Drug Administration
Division of HACCP Programs
(202)646-7077
http://www/fda.gov/fdahomepage.html

U.S. Department of Commerce
National Technical Information Service
(703)487-4650

Hospitality Institute of Technology and
Management
(612)646-7077

U.S. Department of Agriculture
Food Safety and Inspection Service
http://vm.cfsan.fda.gov/~lrd/haccpsub.html

For more information about solid waste management, the following resources are listed:

Resources

Foodservice & Packaging Institute, Inc.
http://www.fpi.org

National Restaurant Association
http://www.restaurant.org

U.S. Environmental Protection Agency
http://www.epa.gov

American Plastics Council
800-243-5790

Council on Packaging in the Environment
(COPE)
(202) 331-0099

National Recycling Coalition
(703) 683-9026

American Paper Institute, Inc.
260 Madison Avenue
New York, NY 10016

Polystyrene Packaging Council, Inc.
http://www.polystyrene.org

Solid Waste Association of North America
http://www.swana.org

Steel Recycling Institute
http://www.recycle-steel.org

Recycler's World
Associations Director
http://www.recycle.net/recycle/assn/index.html

PART V

Communications
and
Marketing

Marketing

Tab Forgac

OUTLINE

INTRODUCTION

Marketing plays a key role in the success of child nutrition programs. There are actually two aspects of marketing—direct marketing and social marketing—that are essential for successful implementation of child nutrition programs. Direct marketing is the process by which one entity influences another entity to act on a behavior. For example, direct marketing might be the actions school food and nutrition program staff take to get children to participate regularly in the School Breakfast Program. Social marketing is the process by which one entity influences the environment in which the marketing efforts exist in order to change the environment to one that is more conducive to the efforts being taken in direct marketing. An example of social marketing as it applies to the School Breakfast Program might be a campaign to reach the general community with messages about the benefits of eating breakfast at school, such as the positive effects of breakfast on the behavior and ability of children to learn. In order to market child nutrition programs effectively, both aspects of marketing must be customer-focused. The ultimate objective of any marketing effort is to influence the behavior of the target audience.

To market child nutrition programs successfully, a well-defined and disciplined marketing plan must be developed and implemented. In developing a marketing plan, a thorough, conscientious, and honest approach must be applied. This chapter focuses on how marketing should be applied to child nutrition programs to meet the demands of the future. This chapter also provides basic information on how to develop a marketing plan in a step-by-step format. Each step is essential to achievement of a successful plan that will meet the needs of the target audience and increase participation in child nutrition programs. Also, this chapter discusses the concepts of social marketing and how social marketing can be used to enhance child nutrition programs. Finally, a case study is provided on how a successful marketing plan has been implemented.

The American School Food Service Association's *Keys to Excellence*[1] identifies three achievement areas related to marketing, which are of concern in child nutrition programs.

- A comprehensive marketing plan promotes a positive image of the school food and nutrition program.
- A team of school food and nutrition personnel, teachers, school administrators, students, and parents provides and promotes quality, nutritious food, and nutrition education.
- The school food and nutrition team promotes policies for nutrition integrity in the school food and nutrition program.

The objectives of this chapter are as follows:

- Provide an overall understanding of marketing.
- Describe the role marketing plays in successful child nutrition programs.
- Demonstrate how to market child nutrition programs.
- Provide resources for further study on successful marketing of child nutrition programs.
- Provide a case study on successful marketing of child nutrition programs.

THE ROLE OF MARKETING IN CHILD NUTRITION PROGRAMS

Marketing may be the most misunderstood concept in business today and is a relatively new competence identified for school food and nutrition program managers and directors. This chapter will assist in developing the competencies needed for developing and implementing a marketing program. Four major competencies[2] are needed in the area of marketing: (1) developing a marketing plan that attracts students, teachers, administrators, support staff, and the community; (2) providing information to encourage and secure support from the school board, administration, faculty, students, and the community for the child nutrition programs; (3) implementing a plan for providing food for special functions consistent with school board policies; and (4) conducting an ongoing evaluation of the marketing plan.

Many people think of marketing as the advertising, promotion, or selling of a commodity—from soup to nuts, or nutcrackers. But marketing is much more than advertising, promotion, or selling. Marketing includes everything from identifying the target market and defining what will be delivered to that target market to evaluating whether the product or service has been delivered to the target market and whether that product or service has helped to achieve an established goal. This chapter will apply basic marketing principles to the successful implementation of child nutrition programs.

In virtually all books on marketing, some mention is made of the four Ps of marketing. It is important to understand the four Ps and how to address them in marketing child nutrition programs. The four P's are

- Product
- Place
- Price
- Promotion

Although each of these elements may seem straightforward, a common understanding is provided here.

- Product is the goods or services that are provided to the customer. For the purposes of child nutrition programs, the product will most often be the food served to the customer. However, if the target market is the working parents of the children in a school district, the product could also be a service—such as the availability of food service during the summer when school meals are not available and the parents are not able to provide a meal at noon. Other products might include nutrition education in the classroom and cafeteria, community services, catering, and other aspects of the services provided by a school food and nutrition program.

- Place is where the product or service is provided. Again, this will most often be a cafeteria within a school if the focus is on school lunch, breakfast, or after-school snacks. But it may also be a community center or park if a program such as summer feeding is being provided.
- Price is the value placed on the product or service being offered. Typically this is stated in terms of currency. However, in providing free or reduced-price meals, there is still a "value" for that product. It is important not to underestimate the value of the product or service being provided. Whether the product or service is provided free or for a fee, there is still a price or value that can be attributed to it.
- Promotion is how the product is sold. Promotion includes all the activities used to influence, increase, or improve the acceptance and/or sale of a product. Promotion may include advertising, publicity, public relations, incentives, displays, merchandising and more.

STEPS TO A SUCCESSFUL MARKETING PLAN

This chapter will cover nine basic steps in the development and implementation of a successful marketing plan. These steps are as follows:

1. Establishment of a goal
2. Identification of the target audience
3. Assessment of strengths and weaknesses
4. Development of messages
5. Refinement of the goal and development of messages
6. Plan for evaluation
7. Development of tactics and budgets
8. Implementation of the marketing plan
9. Evaluation of the marketing plan

Each of these steps is important. In order to achieve success in a marketing plan, even one step cannot be skipped. These steps are not difficult to accomplish. All the tools and information needed are usually readily available within an operation. Applying these nine basic steps will help to develop and achieve the goals set.

Establishment of a Goal

To start, the goal of successful marketing of any child nutrition program is to increase the participation in or support for these programs in order to help students develop healthy eating behaviors and secure their school day food needs. Whether the program is school lunch, school breakfast, summer feeding, or any other child nutrition program, this goal must be applied to the marketing efforts. For example, in the consumer products area, goals are set to increase consumer use of a product. This same concept can be applied to child nutrition programs. Taking the example of Pepsi-Cola, Pepsi wants to increase consumer use of a product—such as caffeine-free Diet Pepsi. In other words, Pepsi wants to gain market share from Coca-Cola by introducing this product targeted at teen girls and taking them away from the competitive Coca-Cola product. Pepsi must develop a marketing plan that targets teen girls and delivers messages that appeal to that audience, such as how it will help them look good and feel great. Then Pepsi must develop a strategy and tactics that reach teen girls—from ads in magazines read by the target to direct mailing of discount coupons or product samples in order to encourage a trial taste of the product.

For example, the goal of school food and nutrition programs is also to gain "market share"—from other sources of lunch, breakfast, or other meals. By increasing the participation in these programs, more customers will consume meals at school food and nutrition programs and thus gain "market share" from competing meal service providers. Not only is there concern that more students purchase meals but also that those who qualify for free or reduced-price meals will choose a school meal. More details about how this can be done will be covered later in this chapter.

Identification of the Target Audience

Although the four Ps are said to be the basic elements of marketing, there is one even more basic element to marketing that cannot be forgotten as a marketing plan is being developed. That element is the target market (or target audience). Identifying the target market or target audience is the most important step in the entire process of marketing. If the target for whom the product is being marketed is not defined, the appropriate strategy and tactics for the market will not be developed and it will be impossible to evaluate whether the goal set was achieved.

Using the Pepsi-Cola/Coca-Cola example, if Pepsi wants to increase its share of the market for a new caffeine-free Diet Pepsi and does not define its target market (e.g., teen girls), the marketing efforts Pepsi develops may not focus on the target market. Their marketing efforts might use tactics that reach young adult men who do not represent a market for the product (e.g., they are not concerned about calories or caffeine). However, if Pepsi did define its target market and developed specific marketing efforts that appealed to teen girls, they may be able to get new customers for their product and thus achieve their goal. (Pepsi might consider marketing a high-caffeine, high-calorie soft drink to young adult men to appeal to their wants and needs.)

So before marketing efforts are initiated, the following questions must be answered in order to identify and analyze the target audiences for the product, that is, child nutrition programs. It is important that this process be completed separately for each individual child nutrition program, since there are different audiences for each program:

- Who is the target audience for the program in which participation is to be increased? The target audience may be not only the actual consumer of the food served, but also all the people that affect child nutrition programs, such as the parents of the consumer, the school administration, the community in which the program operates, and many others. In order to identify the target audience, the following questions should be asked: who decides the budget, who influences whether the consumer eats the meal provided, and who makes decisions that affect the operation of the child nutrition program?

- What is the size or sphere of influence of the target audience? In order to prioritize the efforts made to affect a target audience, the level of influence they might have on the program must be known. For example, there is only one principal per school, but that one principal has tremendous influence on many decisions that affect child nutrition programs. The principal generally decides when lunch is served and how long students have to eat, when the school opens in the morning and whether the cafeteria can be open at that time, or whether teachers can monitor the meal service, or if other foods are available during the school day. So despite the fact that principals are only one person, they have a significant level of influence over school food and nutrition programs and, therefore, probably would be a target audience in any marketing efforts for school meals.
- What does the target audience know about the program in which participation is to be increased? How the target audience feels about the program is essential—are they supportive or are they negative? Do they participate in the program themselves—either as an observer or as an actual participant regularly? What motivates them to be involved in the program? What actions need to be taken to change the target audience's perception of the program? The target audience's perception of the program will have a significant amount of influence on what must be done to "sell" them on the goal of increasing participation in the program.

Target Audiences

Listed below are some of the target audiences who will affect the child nutrition program in which participation might be increased. It is essential to identify all potential targets who can influence the program(s) being marketed.

- School breakfast: students, parents, teachers, principals, school administrators, custodians, bus drivers, school nurses
- School lunch: students, parents, teachers, principals, school administrators, fast-food chains, nurses, school board members
- Summer feeding: children, parents, community leaders, churches, school administrators
- After-school snacks: school administrators, parents, teachers, students

Once target audiences are defined and how they affect the program is understood, it is essential to prioritize them. Prioritization is needed in order to use available resources most effectively on the most important target to achieve the established goal(s). Those target audiences toward which the efforts will be focused must be selected. To do this, the list of target audiences should be reviewed and those with the most influence on increasing participation in the child nutrition program should be selected as the target. There may be any number of target audiences, with a minimum of one. It is important to consider how each target audience will help reach the goal and what must be done to reach them. Careful assessment of the relative importance of each target to reaching the goal is essential, both for achieving the goal and making the most effective use of resources.

Assessment of Strengths and Weaknesses

In developing the marketing plan, a critical look at the program must be taken and an assessment of its strengths and weaknesses made. Through this assessment, the benefits of the program to the target audience(s) will be identified and then used to market the program. The shortcomings of the program will be recognized, and these should be corrected prior to initiation of the marketing efforts. It is important to take a critical look at all aspects of the program. One way to do this is to use the four Ps again.

- Product: Is the product what the customer wants? Does it appeal to the majority of the target? Could it be improved in order to meet the target's wants and needs?
- Place: Does the location provide an atmosphere that is conducive to generating additional participation by the target? Does it compete with the competition in customer service (e.g., do long lines prevent quick service)? Could the location be improved to increase acceptability (e.g., could multiple short lines enhance quick service)?
- Price: Can the target get a similar product at a lower price? Is price the most important factor in selecting the product purchased?
- Promotion: What has been done to increase participation in the program to date? Was that successful? How was success measured?

Once all the strengths and weaknesses of the program have been identified, the next step is to determine whether changes can be made to maximize the strengths and minimize the weaknesses. If weaknesses have been identified that are having a major effect on the participation levels of the program, it is essential that improvements be made in those areas before time and effort are spent in marketing the program. However, depending on what the weaknesses are, it may be possible to include the changes within the marketing plan.

Development of Messages

So far, three very important steps have been discussed about the development of a marketing plan: establishment of the goal, identification of the target audience, and assessment of the strengths and weaknesses of the program. The next step is to develop the appropriate messages for the target audience. These messages will form the basis of the marketing plan. In order to develop appropriate messages, the following questions must be asked:

- What is it that the target audience must do? Examples: eat breakfast at school daily (students); change the bus schedule to get the students to the school ten minutes earlier (principals)
- What information does the target need to support the goal? Examples: breakfast in the cafeteria is a place to meet friends (students); students who eat breakfast at school increase average daily attendance or make better grades (principals)
- What is the goal specifically for the child nutrition program in which the increase in participation is desired (i.e., to add a breakfast program to a school or to increase participation in an existing program)?
- How can the target audience help in the achievement of this goal?

In order to reach the target audience, clear, direct messages that appeal to the needs of the target audience must be developed. For example, if the goal is to increase participation in an existing School Breakfast Program and one of the target audiences is the school business official, the message might be that increasing school breakfast participation will generate additional revenue for the school food and nutrition program and achieve a positive fund balance that can be used to make needed improvements without requiring additional budget from the school's operating funds.

The messages must be developed specifically for the target audience to be reached. The use of the strengths or benefits of the program that were identified may be helpful in developing messages that appeal to those strengths/benefits to the target audience. Using the example again of increasing participation in an existing School Breakfast Program, the following target audiences and these messages may be applicable for them:

- Students: School breakfast is a place to meet friends before school and have a quick meal while catching up on the latest news.
- Parents: School breakfast is an inexpensive alternative to breakfast at home, where trying to get the kids to eat breakfast before they leave for school is a constant battle.
- Principals: School breakfast decreases absenteeism and tardiness and therefore increases average daily attendance.
- Teachers: School breakfast helps students concentrate in class and improves student scores; it also reduces disruptions from hungry kids.
- School nurses: School breakfast reduces the number of students who come to the nurse's office complaining of stomachaches and headaches during the midmorning slump.
- School food service staff: School breakfast can make a difference in students' behavior, and the program helps contribute to the overall learning experience of students.

While developing messages, it is important to keep in mind the weaknesses or shortcomings of the program as well. For example, it is important to know what the competition is doing to attract customers or potential customers to their operation. A comparison of their strengths and weaknesses and those of the child nutrition programs is essential for success. For example, if the competition for school breakfast is fast-food establishments, it is key to consider what they offer as menu items, how quickly students get served, the cost of a meal there, and the atmosphere of the establishment. The answers to these questions must be considered in developing messages and then in developing in the marketing plan.

Refinement of the Goal and Development of Objectives

In the early part of this chapter, the overall goal of the marketing of child nutrition programs was stated to be increasing the participation in child nutrition programs. That goal must be further defined based on the specific programs that are planned to be marketed to the target audiences. Successful marketing plans are based on clear goals and objectives. As goals are refined, it is essential to identify the program on which focus will be placed to increase participation, to determine the desired increase in participation, and set a date by which time this goal will be accomplished. For example, if the School Breakfast Program has been identified as the program in which participation is to be increased, a more specific marketing goal must be defined. The revised goal might be that participation in the School Breakfast Program will be increased by 10 percent over last year's participation level by the end of the current school year. This goal will help clearly define what will be accomplished and will give a specific measure against which performance can be evaluated. Refinement of goals is needed for all the programs that are planned to be marketed to customers. However, it is important that reasonable and achievable goals be set for the program and that goals be set that can be handled by the staff or budget. For example, it is better to tackle the marketing of one program and be successful than to try to market too many and be unsuccessful in some or all of them.

Setting objectives for the goal is the next step. Each objective should be written in action-oriented words and should support the overall goal. For example, if the goal is to increase participation in the School Breakfast Program by 10 percent over last year's level by the end of the school year, some of the objectives for the goal might be

- Decrease negative comments from teachers about the School Breakfast Program.
- Improve the quality of the food served at school breakfast.
- Enhance the perception of school breakfast by the parents.
- Promote breakfast as a "cool" place for students to meet friends.

Objectives should be written to provide a direct action that can then be developed into tactics to achieve them. The tactic would describe action to achieve objective. The objectives should be observable. In other words, it should be possible to observe the target audience in achieving the objective written. For example, using the first objective above, this objective is observed when fewer negative comments are heard from teachers about breakfast or maybe some positive comments are heard about their students' behavior related to their eating breakfast!

Objectives should be written for each target audience that has been identified in the marketing plan. Tailoring the objectives to the interests, wants, and needs of the target is essential. For example, teachers may not care about an objective written with parents in mind (such as, to improve the quality time parents can have with their children in the morning if children can eat breakfast at school). However, teachers might be interested in an objective that focuses on increasing the understanding of the role of breakfast in their students' ability to learn.

Plan for Evaluation

In order to assess honestly whether the marketing plan actually accomplishes the goals and objectives that have been established, a plan must be developed for evaluating the results of the marketing efforts. Without an evaluation component, the marketing plan is incomplete. Also, the information needed to make critical decisions regarding the direction, modifications, and future of the plan will not be available. The results of the evaluation of the plan will help to achieve the following:

- Establish credibility for the program.
- Demonstrate the ability to accomplish goals and objectives with key target audiences, such as the school administration, parents, and the community.
- Provide essential information on what works and what does not work so that

learning from this experience can be applied to future plans.

Evaluation can take many forms, but the key evaluation that needs to be conducted is whether the goal(s) have been achieved. Taking the example of increasing participation in an existing School Breakfast Program, comparisons would need to be made between the participation levels from the current year in which the marketing plan is being conducted and the previous year's participation levels. This can be done relatively simply by obtaining and reviewing the previous year's figures and developing a system for comparing the current year's figures with them. The comparison can be done by month, by quarter, by semester, or by year, whatever is appropriate to the goal. It is important to compare the same measures and for the same time period. For example, if the goal is simply to increase overall participation levels in the School Breakfast Program over the year, then the only data needed are two figures—last year and current year total annual participation levels. If the goal is to increase the number of paid breakfasts, it will be necessary to break down the annual participation levels by type of payment and compare the figures for the paid breakfasts with those of the last year and the current year.

With regard to the objectives, evaluation measures also should be established to ascertain whether the objectives have been achieved as well. If one of the objectives was "improving the quality of the food served at school breakfast," then an objective method to measure whether this objective has been achieved must be set. For example, a survey could be conducted of student reactions to the food at breakfast—before and after the menu was altered. It is essential that baseline information be assessed on students' perceptions prior to the changes in order to assess the level of improvement. Obtaining information from students who regularly participate as well as students who do not participate in the School Breakfast Program may be important as well.

Also, it may be important to obtain information from all appropriate age levels of students. One very important caveat to consider is whether the evaluation measure is more complicated than the objective it is attempting to measure. Try to keep evaluation measures simple and straightforward and not overly time consuming or expensive.

Another aspect of evaluation is market research. Market research is actually evaluation conducted at the beginning stages of development of the marketing plan. The reason market research is conducted at this time is to assess whether the target audience understands the message to be delivered and whether the message is compelling enough to precipitate an action by the target audience. For example, market research is essential in the development of an advertising message about the benefit delivered by a product. A consumer needs to see a reason to buy that product. If students do not see the benefit of eating breakfast in school (e.g., they get to sleep at home 15 minutes later) they will not feel compelled to eat breakfast at school.

Market research can be simple or complex. It can be a short series of "focus" groups among students to find out what they want to see served more often or it can be a comprehensive survey of the community on what the perceived role of the school food and nutrition program is to the community. Whatever form it takes, market research both in the formative and in the evaluative stages of the development and implementation of a marketing plan is essential to the success of the plan.

Development of Tactics and Budgets

Probably the most frequently developed aspect of a marketing plan are the tactics. Often these are developed without going through the entire process of developing a marketing plan and, therefore, the tactics are not connected to a goal or objective and an evaluation measure has not been developed. This results in an incomplete plan that does not achieve desired objectives. It is essential that all previous steps in developing a marketing plan be completed before the tactics and budgets for the plan are started.

Again, the first step is to start with the target audience. For each target audience, specific tactics should be planned based on the messages to be delivered and the goals and objectives to be accomplished. As an example, the goal might be refined for the target audience of the school business official to the statement that school food and nutrition programs will generate a certain income (in dollar amount) that will be used to update the dishwashing equipment that must be replaced within the next school year. The objectives might be to demonstrate how the school food and nutrition program has achieved positive fund balances over the past two years, determine a monthly level of earnings that will ensure a year-end positive fund balance that will cover the cost of the new dishwashing equipment, and increase the number of teachers who eat breakfast at school thus generating new customers who pay full price for the meal. The tactics need to then include the methods by which these objectives will be achieved. For the first objective of demonstrating that the school food and nutrition program has achieved positive fund balances over the past two years, the following tactics might be developed:

- Obtain the last two years' budgets and review them carefully to be certain that a positive fund balance has been achieved in both years.
- Develop a concise presentation (either for written or oral delivery) that demonstrates the positive fund balances have been achieved and includes the projected positive fund balance for the current year based on the increased participation levels in school breakfast.
- Make an appointment with the school business official and present the case.
- Obtain approval to move forward with the plan to increase participation.

- Provide regular reporting (based on the plan) to the school business official on the progress toward the goals and objectives (keep in mind that keeping the report short and simple may be the best way to deliver this information).
- Present the positive fund balance data at the end of the year and the plan to purchase the new dishwashing equipment.

As the specific tactics are being developed for the marketing plan, the budget requirements to accomplish the plan must also be developed. The budget needs to include all costs that will be required—both in terms of items that must be purchased and in terms of staff time spent to implement the tactic. In the example, of the target of the school business official, the majority of the budget would be designated in terms of the time that will be spent reviewing the records, developing the case and presenting it, and preparing a regular reporting mechanism. With other tactics, there may be expenses related to print materials or services purchased, time spent by staff assembling a promotion, or additional food costs for new items requested by customers.

While the tactics and budgets are being developed, the four Ps of marketing—product, place, price, and promotion—should be considered. Each of these elements can influence the tactics and budgets for the marketing plan. A few examples are described below:

- Product is the goods and/or services delivered through the child nutrition programs. In the marketing plan, tactics might include adding a new product (e.g., a student-requested food item once a week to increase student participation). Another potential tactic could be adding a catering service for teachers and parents to provide foods for social events and/or meetings at school or to take home.
- Place is the location where the product is delivered. The marketing plan might include the provision of breakfast items on food carts in the school hallway near the entrance to common gathering areas for students. Another example of place is providing a snack service for the teachers' lounge that would show them the quality of the food provided in the cafeteria.
- Price is the established value set for the product delivered.
- Promotion is the action or process of influencing a customer's behavior. All the activities that are employed to influence, increase, or improve the acceptance and/or sale of a product are considered promotion. Promotions might include the following activities:
  1. Contests
  2. Incentives and/or discounts
  3. New menu items
  4. Posters, billboards
  5. Publicity
  6. Public relations
  7. Specific events
  8. Special services

This list is not exhaustive. There are many other promotion ideas that have been used and are very successful. It is important to identify those promotions that will work for the target audience that has been identified in the marketing plan. Previous experience with a promotion idea is also very valuable information. If the promotion was successful in an elementary school, the same promotion may not work as well at a higher-grade-level school. If a catering service for parents is being considered, it is essential to know that the parents can and will come to the school early enough in the afternoon to pick up their food, or that by extending a staff person's hours to stay late to deliver the food after school hours, the service is still cost effective.

Implementation of the Marketing Plan

The marketing plan that has been developed, including all the steps of the process, is now ready for implementation. The goal has been established, the target audience identified, the goals and objectives refined, the messages developed, the evaluation planned, and the tactics and budgets determined.

Because there is a specific marketing plan, a very thorough, step-by-step approach can be followed to accomplish the goal. Specific tasks can be delegated to other staff, and the help of outside resources can be enlisted where appropriate. The plan should be reviewed on a regular basis to be sure that all steps are being done to accomplish the goal. Feedback—both formal and informal—should be obtained from the target audiences to be sure their needs are being met. As the plan is implemented, it is important to keep in mind that unexpected details of a tactic may need to be dealt with, and it may be necessary to alter a tactic to address a new situation. Using the example of the school business official, there may be a request for the case to be presented to the school board and this was not written into the plan. The plan would need to be adapted as it is implemented to be able to accomplish the goal.

Evaluation of the Plan

The final step to the marketing plan is the evaluation of the plan. As has been discussed previously, it is important that a commitment be made to the ongoing evaluation of the plan as it is implemented. This may take the form of monthly, midproject, and/or year-end reports. However, at the completion of the stated date of achievement of the overall goal, the plan must be evaluated against the stated goal(s).

Consider the example of "increasing participation in an existing School Breakfast Program by 10 percent over the previous year's participation level by the end of the current school year." This would require that a comparison be made of school breakfast participation levels for the two years at the end of the current school year. If the goal has been achieved, a marketing plan should be developed for the future, using the data and information from the evaluation. If the goal has not been achieved, a review must be made of which tactics worked and which did not. Further, a determination must be made of what needs to be significantly refined or revised in the marketing plan in order to move ahead. The evaluation process provides the data and information needed for future planning.

SOCIAL MARKETING

In addition to the use of direct marketing that has been described until now in this chapter, success of child nutrition programs can also be influenced by social marketing. Social marketing can play a very important role in the success of school food and nutrition programs. Historically, social marketing has enhanced the acceptability of these programs to the public at large. The steps of social marketing are essentially the same as those of direct marketing with only slight alterations. The steps are as follows: definition of the problem; setting of goals; identification of target audiences; market research on the consumer and the key influencers; development of strategies and tactics; implementation of the tactics; and, finally, evaluation of the tactics. Effective social marketing depends on following a deliberate step-by-step approach to developing a social marketing plan. One of the keys to successful social marketing is the development of partnerships with individuals and/or organizations with a similar goal. Partnerships not only can extend the reach of the marketing efforts, but they can also bring added credibility to the efforts.

An excellent example of social marketing is the Food Research and Action Center (FRAC) campaign called the Campaign to End Childhood Hunger. For a number of years, FRAC and its many partners have worked to increase the acceptability of the School Breakfast Program. Many different tactics have been used to increase awareness of the programs and their benefits to children, their families, and the community at large. Tactics have included news conferences, published reports, television public service announcements, and community outreach. Participation in the School Breakfast

Program has grown significantly since the initiation of this campaign.

Another social marketing campaign is the campaign by the American School Food Service Association entitled "Take Your Family to Lunch" day. The intent of this campaign is to increase awareness of the availability of quality, nutritious foods at schools. Parents and community leaders were encouraged to participate in the school lunch programs in their communities. A third social marketing example is that of the Milk Mustache ad campaign. This public education campaign is intended to increase awareness among consumers of the healthful aspects of drinking milk. Positioning milk with positive role models, including celebrities and sports leaders, has positively impacted consumer attitudes about milk.

Social marketing, in conjunction with direct marketing, can have a tremendous impact on the target market and the use of the product being marketed. As marketing plans are being developed, both aspects of marketing should be kept in mind. Both direct and social marketing can play integral roles in the success of child nutrition programs.

SUMMARY

Marketing is a key factor in the success of child nutrition programs. Use of direct market-ing and social marketing can effectively enhance the growth and health of child nutrition programs. Thorough, step-by-step measures to increase marketing efforts can lead to increased participation in and increased support for existing programs and opportunities in new, under or unutilized programs. In developing a marketing plan, school food and nutrition directors must keep in mind federal and state program regulations when developing tactics related to price and/or promotions. If in doubt, contact the child nutrition state agency.

An overall understanding of marketing and the role it plays in child nutrition programs is essential to a successful program. The tools needed to market child nutrition programs have been described. A hands-on approach to learning about marketing, the Target Your Market training, is available through the School Food Service Foundation. It is a training workshop that will provide school food and nutrition staff with a step-by-step learning of each of the nine basic steps covered in this chapter. Social marketing plays an integral role in the promotion of child nutrition programs. Specific examples of social marketing have been described. An aggressive marketing plan is essential for child nutrition programs to maintain a competitive advantage in the market place.

CASE STUDY
SEEING WITH YOUR CUSTOMERS' EYES

John Bennett

Before you can have a plan, you have to have a vision. Whether you're running a single, small elementary school cafeteria or managing hundreds of employees in a large urban district, you can't meet your marketing goals unless you're committed to thinking—and *seeing*—in radically new ways.

The marketing case study that follows describes such a "vision." The events took place at a small, sleepy elementary school in a semirural suburb of Annapolis, Maryland. The insights into marketing success that formed this project (and grew out of it) can be applied in marketing plans for school cafeterias and child nutrition programs, large and small, anywhere in the United States.

Get in Line for Marketing Success

Debbie Gill figures that she might not have been as successful in her first school food service job if she hadn't been so short. On a good day, Debbie is *maybe* five feet tall, but she turned that lack of stature to her benefit—and the benefit of her customers—when she took over as manager of the Davidsonville Elementary School Cafeteria in Anne Arundel County, Maryland, in early 1992.

Debbie had been inspired to see herself and her job differently by a Maryland School Food Service Association marketing training seminar she attended in March 1992. She decided on the spot that, from then on, she would see the kids as customers, her cafeteria as a restaurant, and herself as a restaurant manager.

"I knew I wanted to make some changes, and the most important change was in my attitude about myself and my work," Gill said. "Once I committed myself to that change, the next trick was to see what my customers saw. So I literally got out from *behind* the line and

got *in* line instead. Since I'm so little, it was easy for me to assume their perspective!"

She didn't like what she saw. A single choice on the lunch line. Days, whole weeks even, when that one choice just didn't look very appealing. A sterile, colorless, institutional setting. Indifferent service. A boring and lifeless menu going home with the kids. She also observed little sense among the staff that school meals were important or even necessary. Not coincidentally, participation at her school averaged just 125 students out of 400, a pathetic percentage for an elementary school.

Debbie had only just taken over at Davidsonville, but she already had a *vision* of a very different place. She was committed to change. Now, she needed a plan to make that vision come to life, to make that commitment pay off. Her near-term, one-year goal was to raise her participation by at least half. She intended to target parents as well as kids. And she intended to build on the strength of her own new-found perception of her cafeteria as a restaurant, of her students as customers. That new way of seeing would drive every change and govern every decision at her new restaurant.

These were the six guiding strategies of the plan Debbie put into action at her school that spring, as follows:

1. *First, Debbie determined to change her way of thinking: the school cafeteria at Davidsonville Elementary School would henceforth and forever be a restaurant.* Debbie's immediate tactics for enacting this strategy were to select a restaurant-style name for the restaurant and to seek permission to increase the number of daily choices on her line from one (some choice, right? Take it or leave it!) to three. She also regularly visited her

kids' favorite local commercial restaurants, not merely as a customer, but as an observer.

2. *Second, Debbie decided from the outset to create ownership for the new restaurant among her customers. The kids were to be actively involved in the creation and operation of the new enterprise.* The first step in creating ownership for her customers was to let them choose the restaurant's name. They chose "Gator Galley," as a tribute to the school's alligator mascot and its location close to the water (a galley, of course, is a ship's kitchen). She also used kids' own artwork to decorate her serving line; regularly sought customer input on menu selections and brands; and featured games, puzzles, giveaways, and promotions on her monthly menu. "The kids always felt that they had a say in what was happening," Debbie said. "It was as much their restaurant as mine. I'd even ask them what vegetables they wanted me to serve. That involvement was crucial."

3. *Debbie's third strategy was to "communicate and conquer." She told everybody what she was doing and asked lots of people for help.* At the time, I was Community Outreach Coordinator for the Child Nutrition Programs at the Maryland State Department of Education. Debbie asked for my help in communicating in new and innovative ways with her customers (we designed a new monthly take-home menu and a newsletter, "Gator Gab," to keep parents apprised of the changes we were making). She sought permission and support from her district office for menu and décor changes she wanted to put in place. She kept her principal and teachers in the loop concerning the progress of the project, and repeatedly underlined to them that the end purpose of Gator Galley was to make Davidsonville's educators'

jobs easier by making sure that as many kids as possible came to class ready to learn. She asked vendors for promotional support. She even shanghaied her husband into painting a few gators for her! In short, she knew she couldn't execute all of her plans by herself, so she talked up the project to everyone and asked everyone to contribute a piece of their own expertise and resources. This strategy simultaneously lightened her load and got lots of other folks involved in the project—making them much less likely to find fault with or hinder her efforts at change.

4. *Debbie also "revisioned" her menu as a marketing, promotion, and educational tool.* New strategies and new outlooks require fresh approaches to all of the tools in one's marketing arsenal. Debbie took a long, hard look at the menu she sent home each month and decided that it was basically just a literal list of food, with no personality and little marketing appeal. With help, she turned it into a marketing dynamo, with games, promotions, giveaways, and interesting information for parents. She was determined to get that place of honor on her customers' refrigerators and keep those customers (and their parents) interested all month.

5. *In her day-to-day operations, Debbie emphasized quality, service, and choice.* Debbie didn't stop getting in line with her customers after that first trip; she made a *habit* of looking at her operation from the customer's point of view. That habit led to a near-fanatical commitment to customer satisfaction, particularly in the areas of food quality standards, customer service, and selection. By the end of the project, she had added pizza every day as a fourth menu item, a far cry from the single choice her customers had always had before.

6. *A final strategy was to change the way the place appeared. The new restaurant*

demanded a new look. Gator Galley was like a lot of 1940s and 1950s era school cafeterias: bland, institutional, and sterile, with a predominant motif of stainless steel and pale yellow brick. In short: not very hip. Debbie asked her central office for help, and Director Renee Koehler responded with a modest makeover that nonetheless nicely complemented the other changes and reinforced the new restaurant emphasis. Décor changes included a lively green awning for the serving area entrance, a bright red framework over the serving line that enclosed a rotating selection of student artwork, and gators everywhere. Total cost for the changes was around $1,200, so this was by no means a radical redesign of the facility—but the changes were enough to give the attitudinal and operational changes another dimension.

One important caveat here: Debbie cautions that décor changes, no matter how extensive, do not offer a magic bullet for transforming a cafeteria into a restaurant. When people call her for insights into making such changes, Debbie says she advises them that "the cosmetic changes are the most expensive ones, and if you can make those kinds of changes, fine, but that shouldn't be your top priority. First, you need to change your attitude, change the way your people think, offer more choices, offer customers more than they expect, more than they're used to getting from the school cafeteria. That's the heart of any change in our business."

These six strategies formed the basis for Debbie's marketing plan, and the strategies paid off. Within nine months of the beginning of Debbie's restaurant project, participation at Gator Galley was up to 189 students on an average day, a 52 percent increase in that short period of time. Best of all, with this framework for change firmly in place and continuing to guide operations at Gator Galley, participation kept climbing—to 206 a year later, 225 two years later, and (after Debbie had moved on to become manager at a middle school) over 260 six years after Debbie's initial decision to change the way she perceived herself and her cafeteria. Clearly, this kind of innovative thinking and commitment to the customer carried over to future customers and even to future staff at Gator Galley.

Furthermore, this blueprint had effects beyond Davidsonville Elementary school. The food service office in Anne Arundel County used the Gator Galley experience as a model to turn all 70 of the county's elementary schools into what they now call "Galley" schools. And employees all over the country have heard about Debbie's plan for marketing success through customer service training that I've conducted. There's even a "Gator World" at a middle school in Grand Junction, Colorado—*that* could never have happened without Debbie's example.

In the final analysis, what does Debbie see as the most important step in the process of changing a cafeteria into a restaurant? *That first step from behind the line.* "Stepping out and seeing what they see, what they expect, and how we're meeting or not meeting those expectations, that has to come first, last, and during every point in between," Debbie said. "Sometimes it looks entirely different from their point of view than from the back of the house. No matter what school you're in or what grade levels you serve, you can learn a lot from capturing that perspective and reacting to it."

Debbie tried to see with her customers' eyes. She committed herself to expanding the universe of customer choices. She understood the importance of projecting a new and progressive image of her operation. And she began with a vision that was carefully and painstakingly translated into a workable plan. And the most important part? Her plan worked!

REFERENCES

1. American School Food Service Association, *Keys to Excellence: Standards of Practice for Nutrition Integrity* (Alexandria, VA: 1995).

2. D.H. Carr et al., *Competencies, Knowledge, and Skills of Effective District School Nutrition Directors/Supervisors* (University, MS: National Food Service Management Institute, 1996), 99, 145.

SUGGESTED READINGS

Department of Health and Human Services, The National Center on Child Abuse and Neglect. 1997. *Marketing matters: Building an effective communications program.* Washington, DC.

Feltenstein, T. 1992. *Foodservice marketing for the 90's.* New York: John Wiley & Sons, Inc.

McNeal, J. 1987. *Children as consumers: Insights and implications.* New York: Lexington Books.

McNeal, J. 1992. *Kids as customers: A handbook of marketing to children.* New York: Lexington Books.

School Food Service Foundation. 1994. *Target your market: Child nutrition program marketing course.* Alexandria, VA.

Underwood, R. 1988. *Fifty-Two cafeteria promotions that really work.* Gaithersburg, MD: Aspen Publishers, Inc.

CHAPTER 20

Communicating with Students

Tami J. Cline

OUTLINE

- Overview
- Understanding Customer Opinions
    - External Research
    - Internal Research
- Communicating Your Key Messages to Students
    - Tips for Communicating with Students
    - Starting a Nutrition Advisory Council
- Summary
- Case Study: How the San Bernardino City Unified School District Nutrition Services Listened and Responded to the Students
  Mary Kay Meyer

OVERVIEW

Communicating with customers is key to the success of any school food and nutrition program. Since students are the primary customers, good communication results in understanding their opinions, their values, and the degree of satisfaction they have with the program. It means gathering information before waiting to receive a complaint or compliment. It involves a systematic approach to collecting and analyzing data, and identifying what factors influence overall sales and participation.

The purpose of this chapter is to help school food and nutrition program directors better understand their customers by suggesting several methods and tools they can use to gather information on how well their program is meeting student expectations. This chapter also includes a model for enhancing communication with students by forming student nutrition advisory groups, which is a standard in the American School Food Service Association (ASFSA) *Keys to Excellence*.[1(p.31)]

Specific chapter objectives are to enable the reader (1) to recognize why research is a critical first step in the process of communicating with students; (2) to develop strategies for conducting external and internal research to identify customer (student) opinions; (3) to identify tactics for involving students in the process of enhancing communication among school food service staff, students, and the community; (4) to cite examples of the types of tools used to collect student feedback; and (5) to apply communication strategies discussed in this chapter in the development of an action plan to enhance communication with students.

UNDERSTANDING CUSTOMER OPINIONS

Companies that market products to young people recognize that today's students are more sophisticated than ever before. Choices have become the norm. These students have been raised in a society with fast-food restaurants on every corner, food courts in every shopping mall, and caregivers working away from home.[2] Analysts agree that students, just like adults, value convenience, quality service, and speed.[3] How does a school food and nutrition program director find out whether or not students' expectations for convenience, quality service, and speed are met? What other factors influence their decision to participate, or not to participate in the school food and nutrition program? The challenge is to find out how students define quality from their perspective, and what standards will deliver the quality they demand.

Conducting external and internal research is a logical first step. External research means taking a look at what's going on in the environment that has an impact on the school food and nutrition program. It may not be possible to influence or change these forces, but by understanding them, one can better shape a program to meet the changing needs and wants of its customers. Internal research involves directly asking the customers their opinions. Successful school food and nutrition programs employ a variety of techniques to gather customer feedback. Several suggested methods for gathering this information are contained within the chapter.

External Research

Understanding Demographic and Societal Trends

Environmental forces, such as changing demographics and societal and general food service trends, affect school food and nutrition program operations. The menu and all phases of operational planning are influenced by what's happening in society in general. The United States' demographic characteristics have changed dramatically over the past 25 years and will continue to do so well into the future. The population is more mobile and represents growing ethnic diversity and changing household composition. Citizens also are willing to spend more money for convenience, quality service, and speed.[3]

Students today have more money, more responsibilities, and more influence on purchases than they did in the past because of major societal changes. Changing family roles, including two working parents and single-parent families, and the proliferation of child-targeted media are important societal changes affecting students. The average 10-year-old directly makes 250 purchases annually; children control $41.5 billion per year of their own money.[4] Teen spending is staggering—nearly $100 billion a year.[5]

Food Service Trends

Understanding overall food service trends is a basis for predicting the future direction of school food and nutrition programs. Changes within the industry at large influence changes in school food service operations. Trends in college and university food service are frequently predictors of what will occur in school food service. Popular menu ideas, delivery methods, and marketing concepts used in other food service segments are recognized by student customers and must not be ignored.

In recent years, an explosion of menu choices along with variety in serving and packaging methods has been observed in most food service establishments. Sophisticated heating and cooling equipment, point-of-service terminals, and other electronics have affected food preparation, service and sales, and distribution in general. These changes improve a director's ability to meet customer demands without sacrificing accountability or increasing labor costs.

Changes in the types of food and the time of day they are consumed are important trends to follow, too. In general, people of all ages are consuming less at meal periods and more at off hours. Breakfast has become an increasingly important meal for food service chains, quick-service restaurants, and schools alike. The carryout, takeout, and delivery markets have ex-

perienced continual high growth over the past decade. Modified and upgraded packaging to accommodate carryout and delivery of a multitude of food items is widely available.

More companies are targeting students, creating more competition for the students' money and appetite. To gain a competitive advantage, the school food and nutrition program director must appreciate the purchasing power of students and how to influence them to make healthy meal choices at school. Students are not only looking for quality in the meal, but they are looking for value as they perceive it. School food and nutrition leaders need strategies built into their marketing plans to communicate the value of school meals from both a monetary and nutritional viewpoint. Students may not buy into the long-term benefits of healthful foods, but they may buy into foods that give them energy for competing on the football field or foods that contribute to a "peaches and cream" complexion.

Furthermore, students, and in particular teens, have a unique way of evaluating products. The quality of "cool" is of paramount importance, and teens can quickly label products as either "cool" or "uncool."[5] By understanding what makes a product cool, a director is more likely to create a cool quality within the program. Companies spend millions of dollars identifying what brands are cool and why. Taking the time to identify what products, what delivery methods, and what promotions will be labeled as cool among students is a valuable and critical investment in the program.

Students as Customers

Students are sophisticated customers! According to research, teens select quality as the number-one criterion of cool. Next in importance is the perception that it is "for people my age."[5] Teens prefer products and services that are specifically made for them. Newness of a product or brand is often associated with making it cool. Interestingly, celebrity promotions don't do much for creating a cool product; rather, the use of cool celebrities is effective in gaining the attention of students and initially positioning the product.[5] Exhibit 20–1 lists the characteristics of a "cool" brand as identified by students in a survey conducted by Teenage Research Unlimited (TRU).

Research conducted at the National Food Service Management Institute (NFSMI) reveals that students of different ages rank factors differently when asked about their satisfaction with the school food and nutrition program. Middle/junior high students rated food quality, dining ambiance, staff, time, and price factors contributing to satisfaction (Table 20–1). Staff, food quality, nutrition, time/cost, dining ambiance, and diversity were cited by the high school students. This suggests that while many of the factors are the same, it may be necessary to design or use different surveys to collect information from different groups of students. For example, the atmosphere of the school cafeteria was of greater concern to students in grades six to eight than with high school students. NFSMI research also found that satisfaction decreased the longer a student is in a building using a particular food service. This supports the TRU research that reported students relate "new" to "cool."

So, how is it possible to conduct external research on an ongoing basis? Reading popular trade and professional publications, eating out at competitive establishments such as fast-food chains, and collecting menus from a variety of sources are simple and inexpensive means of gathering information to gauge menu and promotion trends within the greater food service environment. Directors must listen to their peers, their competitors, and their customers—the students! Never discount what large, successful companies that market products to students do to get their attention. Remember, it's not necessary to spend a lot of money to conduct external research; rather, it means taking the time to observe and take note of what's happening in the environment.[6] By doing so, the school food and nutrition program capitalizes on forces to strengthen its position as a competitive food service establishment.

Exhibit 20–1 Characteristics of a "Cool" Brand

WHAT MAKES A BRAND A COOL BRAND?

*After quality, the most common description
of what makes a brand cool to teens is that
it is "for people my age."*

(percentage of teens citing characteristics as making a brand cool, 1993)

Quality	66%
If it's for people my age	47%
Advertising	39%
The name of the brand	28%
If cool friends or peers use it	24%
If it's a new brand	18%
It it's a brand that's been around a long time	18%
Packaging	18%
If a cool celebrity uses it	16%

Source: From P. Zollo, *Wise Up to Teens—Insights into Marketing and Advertising to Teenagers*, TRU Teenage Marketing & Lifestyle Study, © 1995. Reprinted with permission from New Strategist Publications, Inc.

Table 20–1 Comparison between Middle/Junior High and High School Students on Factors Related to Satisfaction with School Food and Nutrition Programs

Factors Related to Student Satisfaction with School Food and Nutrition Programs	Student Rankings[a]	
	Grades 6–8	Grades 9–12
Food quality	1	2
Dining ambiance	2	5
Price	5	4[b]
Staff	3	1
Time	4	4[b]
Diversity	Not ranked	6
Nutrition	Not ranked	3

Source: Reprinted with permission from M.K. Meyer et al., *High School Foodservice Survey,* © 1997 and M.K. Meyer, *Middle/Junior High School Survey,* © 1997, National Food Service Management Institute.

[a] Rankings were determined by factor analysis.

[b] Price and time (time/cost) were combined into one factor in the high school study.

Internal Research

Implementing a variety of internal research techniques to gather data about the school food and nutrition program is another strategic step for gathering and understanding customer opinions. From comment cards to formal surveys, from cruising the cafeteria for comments to focus groups, the collection of data must be organized, planned, and implemented on a systematic basis.[6]

Informal Feedback

Where can the school food and nutrition program director start? The simplest way to gather customer feedback is to ask the customer. Observe! Watch them, listen to them, see what they do and how they do it.[7] On-site cafeteria managers should spend a significant amount of time each day mingling with students to gather and observe this vital information. This can be done on an informal basis in the school cafeteria during breakfast and lunch periods. Students are generally quick to respond and answer openly when approached in a nonthreatening manner.[8] This method is an easy way to stay tuned to customer desires, but it lacks a means for collecting solid quantifi-

able data that more closely represent viewpoints of all students. For example, it excludes potential customers who are not in the school cafeteria. There is, therefore, a need to employ additional, more formal methods to gather information from the greater student body.

Roundtable Discussion and Focus Groups

Roundtable discussions or focus groups provide a medium to gather targeted information in a short and controlled amount of time. A focus group is generally composed of 6 to 12 participants. In forming focus groups, include some students who currently participate in the school food and nutrition program, and some who do not.[9] A non-biased and confident facilitator can control and guide the group without pushing for specific or biased responses.[9,10] Some districts hire professional market researchers to conduct focus groups or telephone surveys. One district reports that the use of telephone surveys of its high school students resulted in very positive results. The students liked being asked their opinion about a subject they felt they knew about.[11] Also, the use of outside "experts" can be leveraged to add credibility when reporting findings to students, the school board, or parents.

Written and Formal Surveys

Perhaps the most effective way of measuring student preferences and overall satisfaction is through the use of written surveys. Designing survey instruments can be a difficult task! The development of a reliable and valid tool involves testing and retesting of several versions of the same instrument.[12] The NFSMI has developed and validated two food service surveys to determine student satisfaction with school food and nutrition programs. One survey instrument is for middle/junior high students and another is for high school students. The comprehensive instrument for use with middle/junior high school students is included in Figure 20–1. The survey can be administered using a computerized scan sheet and a separate page for student comments. NFSMI has developed survey guides to assist school food and nutrition program directors with gathering and interpreting data on food service characteristics affecting student satisfaction in grades 6–8 and 9–12.[13,14]

Simpler surveys can be used as a means to gather information more quickly on a broader range of topics. Figure 20–2 illustrates a satisfaction instrument developed and used in the Tulsa, Oklahoma, Public School District.

Another example includes using the questions covering the topics below to design a brief survey. Through statistical analysis, the NFSMI determined which of the survey questions on their high school survey most highly influenced the students' level of satisfaction for students who *had a choice* in whether they ate the school lunch. These questions concerned the following:

- Variety of food offered
- Flavor of food
- Attractiveness of foods on the serving line
- Staff smiling and greeting students
- Quality of food choices
- Ability to meet cultural and ethnic preferences
- Courteousness of staff
- Quality of ingredients

NFSMI found that if high school students were more highly satisfied with these eight questions, they were more highly satisfied overall with school food and nutrition programs. This research points to the fact that students are very concerned with "food quality," but it also suggests that students care about other issues.

Everything that happens to students in the school cafeteria communicates a message. The appearance of the dining area, the way the food looks on the serving line, menus planned to meet cultural and ethnic food preferences, and especially the appearance and manners of the food service personnel all highly influence students' satisfaction with food and nutrition programs.[15]

Before a district develops its own student satisfaction tool, the following questions should be considered:

- How are the questions phrased? Will they naturally prompt negative, positive, or neutral answers?
- Is there a mix of multiple-choice, along with open-ended questions?
- Have students been asked to identify themselves by age, gender, and participant versus non-participant?
- Are there available resources to tabulate and evaluate the information once collected?
- How will the results of the survey be communicated and placed into action plans?

Once the tool has been selected or developed, the next challenge is to find the most effective environment to administer it. Will it reach a broader, more diverse student population if it is presented to students in the cafeteria or in a classroom setting? Will students take the survey more seriously if it is administered by a teacher, other administrator, or a member of the school food and nutrition program staff? How can one be assured that the survey reaches a wide school representation? Regardless of which setting is ultimately selected, it is necessary to secure approval and support from school administrators, teachers, and in some

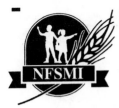

Middle\Junior High School Foodservice Survey

PLEASE ANSWER THE FOLLOWING QUESTIONS ABOUT YOUR SCHOOL FOODSERVICE AND NUTRITION PROGRAM WHETHER YOU EAT SCHOOL LUNCH OR NOT.

COMPLETELY FILL IN THE CIRCLE OF YOUR ANSWER.
USE A #2 PENCIL.

I.D. NUMBER	⓪ ① ② ③ ④ ⑤ ⑥ ⑦ ⑧ ⑨
	⓪ ① ② ③ ④ ⑤ ⑥ ⑦ ⑧ ⑨
	⓪ ① ② ③ ④ ⑤ ⑥ ⑦ ⑧ ⑨
	⓪ ① ② ③ ④ ⑤ ⑥ ⑦ ⑧ ⑨
	⓪ ① ② ③ ④ ⑤ ⑥ ⑦ ⑧ ⑨

Fill in this number as instructed by your teacher.

Are you happy with the school foodservice and nutrition program?

HOW HAPPY ARE YOU WITH THE SCHOOL FOODSERVICE AND NUTRITION PROGRAM? PLEASE FILL IN YOUR ANSWER USING THE FOLLOWING SCALE:

1 = VERY UNHAPPY TO 7 = VERY HAPPY   8 = I DON'T KNOW

① VERY UNHAPPY   ②   ③   ④ NEITHER HAPPY NOR UNHAPPY   ⑤   ⑥   ⑦ VERY HAPPY   ⑧ I DON'T KNOW

1. How happy are you with the foodservice overall?   ① ② ③ ④ ⑤ ⑥ ⑦   ⑧

How would you rate your school foodservice concerning the following?

PLEASE RATE THESE STATEMENTS ABOUT YOUR SCHOOL FOODSERVICE ON A SCALE OF:

1 = STRONGLY DISAGREE TO 7 = STRONGLY AGREE   8 = I DON'T KNOW

① STRONGLY DISAGREE   ②   ③   ④ NEITHER AGREE NOR DISAGREE   ⑤   ⑥   ⑦ STRONGLY AGREE   ⑧ I DON'T KNOW

2. The school menu includes food I like.
3. Main dishes on the serving line (such as spaghetti or chicken) look good.
4. Servers and cashiers are polite.
5. School foodservice prices are OK for what I get.
6. I like how the food smells.
7. Servers and cashiers treat me with respect.
8. The dining area is cheerful/upbeat.
9. The food serving lines are clean.
10. The noise level in the dining area is OK.
11. Spills and trash in the dining area are cleaned quickly.
12. Students are not allowed to misbehave in the dining area.
13. Servers and cashiers listen to the students.
14. I like how the food looks.
15. Tables in the dining area are clean.
16. Servers and cashiers smile and greet me when I am served.
17. Meal prices are reasonable.
18. I like the taste of the food.
19. Vegetables on the serving line look good.
20. I like the quality of the food choices.
21. The time given to eat once seated is OK.
22. The choices of food allow me to pick food like I eat at home.
23. I like the quality of the main dishes (such as spaghetti and chicken).
24. Total time given for meal periods is OK.
25. I like the choices of food offered.
26. I like the quality of the brands offered.

SAMPLE

Turn page →

continues

Figure 20–1 Middle/Junior High School Foodservice Survey. *Source:* Reprinted with permission from M.K. Meyer et al., *High School Foodservice Survey,* © 1997, National Food Service Management Institute.

Figure 20–1 continued

```
┌─────────────────────────────────────────────────────────────┐
│              We want to know about you.                       │
└─────────────────────────────────────────────────────────────┘
```

27. The number one reason I eat school breakfast is:
    (mark only one)

- ◯ The prices are good   ◯ My parents make me
- ◯ The food is good   ◯ The popular kids eat there
- ◯ It is convenient   ◯ I have no other choice
- ◯ My teachers encourage me   ◯ We do not have a breakfast program
- ◯ My friends eat there   ◯ I do not eat breakfast at school

28. The number one reason I eat school lunch is:
    (mark only one)

- ◯ The prices are good   ◯ My parents make me
- ◯ The food is good   ◯ The popular kids eat there
- ◯ It is convenient   ◯ I have no other choice
- ◯ My teachers encourage me   ◯ I do not eat school lunch
- ◯ My friends eat there

29. How many times per week do you eat school breakfast?   ⓪ ① ② ③ ④ ⑤
30. How many times per week do you eat school lunch?   ⓪ ① ② ③ ④ ⑤
31. How many times per week do you bring your lunch?   ⓪ ① ② ③ ④ ⑤

32. What is your grade in school?

- ⓪ 6th grade
- ① 7th grade
- ② 8th grade

33. What is your gender?

- ⓪ Male
- ① Female

34. What is your approximate age:

- ⓪ 10 years
- ① 11 years
- ② 12 years
- ③ 13 years
- ④ 14 years
- ⑤ 15 years or over

National Food Service Management Institute

The University of Mississippi
University, MS 38677-0188
Telephone 1-800-321-3054
Order Number R-33-97

This instrument was designed and validated by the Division of Applied Research located at The University of Southern Mississippi, Hattiesburg.

This project was funded at least in part with federal funds provided to the National Food Service Management Institute at The University of Mississippi from the U.S. Department of Agriculture, Food and Consumer Services under Grant number F33385. The contents of this publication do not necessarily reflect the view or policies of the U.S. Department of Agriculture, nor does mention of trade names, commercial products or organizations imply endorsement by the U.S. government.

LET US HEAR FROM YOU

After all, you're the reason we're here. Our biggest job is making sure you're satisfied with the food and service you get from us. So, if you'll take just a few minutes to fill out this little form, it'll help us serve you better.

Thanks for your time.

You can help us provide the very best in quality food and fast service by taking just a few moments to complete these questions.

	Good	Fair	Un-Satisfactory
1. Food taste	☐	☐	☐
2. Food temperature	☐	☐	☐
3. Promptness of service	☐	☐	☐
4. Courteousness of service	☐	☐	☐
5. Cleanliness	☐	☐	☐
6. Other suggestions			

Date _____   Time_____

Figure 20–2 Satisfaction Survey Developed and Used in the Tulsa, Oklahoma, Public Schools. Courtesy of Tulsa Public Schools, Child Nutrition Services, 1997, Tulsa, Oklahoma.

---

cases, parents.[16,17] Directors must plan for time to follow up with students after the survey has been conducted. There may be additional questions that need answering to clarify the results. This stage of the process should be completed while the original survey is fresh in the students' minds. The NFSMI has published survey guides to assist school food and nutrition directors with gathering data in school settings.[18]

Conducting an annual student survey is an excellent tactic for monitoring the school food and nutrition program. Consideration should be given to the month, day, and even time of day the survey is administered. It is also important to survey students more frequently as program enhancements are made. This can be done using one of the informal methods suggested in the tips for gathering information from and communicating with students, given

later. A school food and nutrition program director must not minimize the importance of surveying students, or the amount of time it takes.

School districts may not have the equipment to scan computer surveys or the support available to assist with data tabulation and analysis. The University of Southern Mississippi in collaboration with the Applied Research Division at NFSMI has instituted the Food Service Analysis and Benchmarking Service (FABS), a management tool to be used by school food and nutrition program directors. The first component developed as a part of this service includes the scoring and statistical analysis of survey questionnaires, comparisons with similar schools within a geographical area or nationally, and the identification of factors and questions most highly correlated with overall student satisfaction.[19]

Menu Item Evaluation

On a more frequent basis, school food and nutrition program directors are required to evaluate new or modified menu items. Why can't they rely solely on food service staff to determine the quality and acceptance of these products? Research shows that the ratings of menu items by school food service personnel are generally higher than the ratings given by students. This suggests that the school food service staff alone may not be able to predict the degree to which students prefer food items. Therefore, there is a need to develop tactics for including students in the process of evaluating new or modified menu items. This can be done simply by offering complimentary samples during regular mealtimes along with the rating forms, pencils, and collection boxes for gathering feedback. For information on student involvement in the selection of foods to be purchased, see Chapter 13. It may be more effective in some instances to convene formal

panels as a part of student nutrition advisory committee activities. In the latter situation, a controlled environment can be created, and it is possible to evaluate several new products during a given session. (Information on starting a student nutrition advisory group is given later in this chapter.)

Tools designed for elementary or younger students to evaluate food products are usually simple and pictorial in nature. Younger students may require the assistance of cafeteria monitors or teachers to complete the survey. A survey example from the Portland Public Schools uses "smiling" versus sad faces (Figure 20–3).

Tools used with older students may contain more evaluative factors and quantitative parameters. A tool for evaluating new recipes or menu items using five qualitative factors (flavor, texture, color, presentation, and nutrient value) and a four-point quantitative scale is included in Exhibit 20–2. In using a more com-

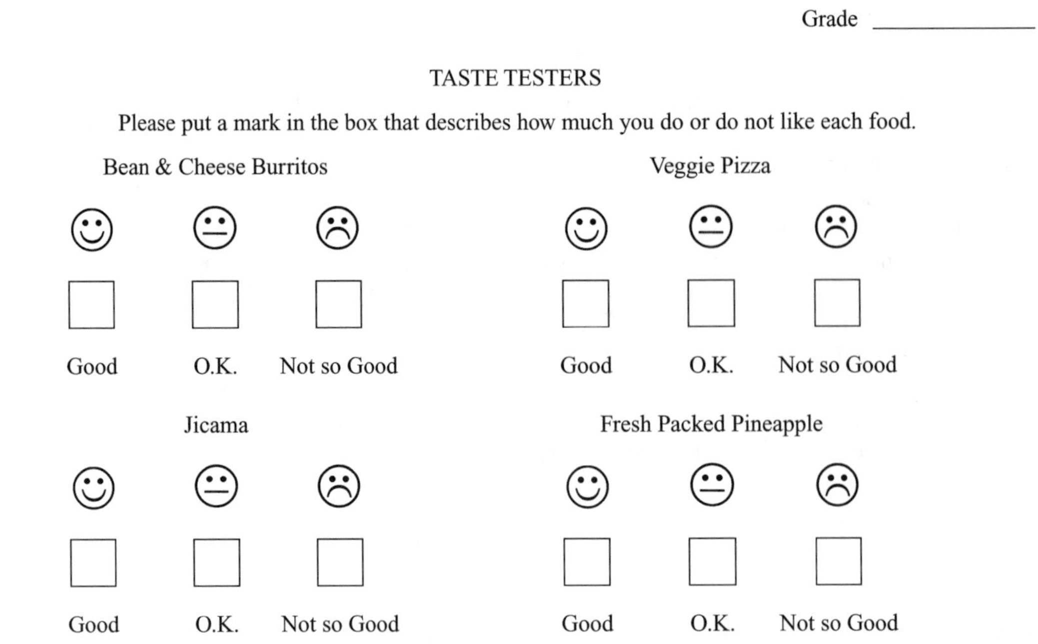

Grade _____

TASTE TESTERS

Please put a mark in the box that describes how much you do or do not like each food.

Bean & Cheese Burritos   Veggie Pizza

Good   O.K.   Not so Good   Good   O.K.   Not so Good

Jicama   Fresh Packed Pineapple

Good   O.K.   Not so Good   Good   O.K.   Not so Good

Figure 20–3 Satisfaction Survey from the Portland Public Schools. Courtesy of Portland Public Schools, Nutrition Services Department, 1998, Portland, Oregon.

plicated rating form, students may require training to clarify what constitutes qualitative differences within in each factor.

COMMUNICATING YOUR KEY MESSAGES TO STUDENTS

After collecting external and internal information about the program, the school food and nutrition program director needs to initiate an action plan for improvement. According to ASFSA's *Keys to Excellence: Standards of Practice for Nutrition Integrity*, the organization of "a school nutrition team which includes the school food service and nutrition personnel" is critical in the development of an improvement plan.[20(p.32)] The director should establish a school food and nutrition team to share in the development of an improvement plan and to secure the cooperation of staff in making lasting changes. This team can discuss the information collected both formally and informally and offer suggestions to maintain areas of success and make plans for improvement. Their commitment to change and their involvement in the process are critical to success.

Next, the proposed plans and strategies should be communicated to students. It is equally important to secure their buy-in to reinforce the goals of the school food and nutrition program. With all this in hand, a director is armed with the information necessary to develop and implement an action plan. Successful plans are based upon a solid assessment of the situation, clear goals and objectives, a defined audience, action steps, and means for evaluation. Refer to the tools and the nine steps outlined in Chapter 19 on marketing in order to put together a successful plan. It is important for students to observe program changes that result from their involvement and suggestions.

Tips for Communicating with Students

The following tips are helpful in developing tactics for communicating with students.

Student Talk

Encourage on-site cafeteria managers and other food service staff to develop relationships with students on a day-to-day basis by being visible in the dining room and being seen at student events. Some of the best information is gleaned informally by meeting with students as they are receiving and eating their meals. While easy to implement, one is generally restricted to those who frequent the school cafeteria. Getting to know student names is important. If that seems like an impossibility, assign school food service employees as "moms" to classes. The cafeteria "moms" can learn all the students' names in their assigned class.

The Menu

Use menus to communicate important information, such as new promotions or nutrient analysis, or to gather feedback from students and parents. This method broadens the reach beyond the school cafeteria.

School Newsletter/Newspaper

Offer information about the school food and nutrition program to the editors of the school newsletter or local newspaper. Invite the editorial staff to tour the kitchen and get to know about the program and its goals. Find out the publication's schedule for production, including deadlines for submitting information, the length of articles generally accepted, and the format most helpful to the editors. Do they need a camera-ready article, or do they prefer an electronic computer file in a specified software format? Build rapport with the editorial staff so they will be coming to the manager for information on a regular basis. A newsletter published by the school food and nutrition program is an excellent means by which to communicate goals, concerns, and proposed changes to identified target audiences.

Student Nutrition Advisory Councils

Consider developing an organized group of students that meet on a regular basis to provide

Exhibit 20–2 Recipe Evaluation Form: Baked Items

Rating System: 1-Poor   2-Fair   3-Good   4-Excellent

ITEM NAME	FLAVOR	TEXTURE	COLOR	PRESENTATION	NUTRIENT VALUE	TOTAL
1. Chocolate Cake						
2. Gingerbread						
3. Fruit Crisp						
4. Peanut Butter Bars						
5. Oatmeal Raisin Cookies						
6. Chocolate Chip Cookies						

Overall Evaluation/General Comments: _____

_____

Evaluator's Name: _____   Date: _____

Courtesy of California Prune Board, 1997, San Francisco, California.

feedback on menus, new products, new promotions, and methods for communicating with other students about important nutrition education lessons. Once vested, these students often serve as ambassadors for the school food and nutrition program.

Comment Cards/Feedback Forms

Solicit information on simple comment cards, an easy method to gauge feedback on new menu items, promotions, or overall suggestions or comments. By creating a means for students to post their opinions and comments, students will know that there is a serious intent to address their concerns and acknowledge their compliments.

Formal Survey

Gather objective information on student satisfaction at least annually, to gauge students' opinions about the school food and nutrition program. Consider using a variety of techniques to implement this method, from a written survey with computerized scan sheet to an on-line response mechanism on a World Wide Web home page.

Home Page

Use technology to grab students' attention. In today's rapidly changing technological environment, don't overlook the value of a home page to communicate with students. Student surveys, menus, meal applications, and promotions are easy to format, update, and place on-line. The World Wide Web is a medium to which students readily relate. The school computer or information services department, or an outside vendor, may be available to assist in the design and maintenance of a home page. With a relatively small investment, the school food and nutrition program is positioned to communicate and market the program to a much wider audience.

Starting a Nutrition Advisory Council

A student Nutrition Advisory Council can strengthen the ability to communicate with students. An organized council is an excellent communication link among students, and among students and school food and nutrition personnel, faculty, administrators, and the community. Not only is a council a vehicle by which to spread the word about the program's goals and the important role good nutrition plays in health, it provides important feedback from students on what they like—or don't like—about the school food and nutrition program.

What is a Nutrition Advisory Council? Nutrition Advisory Councils (NAC) are sponsored by the ASFSA, a national group of school food service and nutrition professionals who promote the importance of sound child nutrition practices. An NAC is similar to other school clubs and organizations. It brings students together to learn and spread the word about the importance of good nutrition, physical fitness, and the role that healthful school meals contribute to overall health and academic performance. By involving students, an NAC reinforces the premise that the school food and nutrition program is planned for them.

The activities of the NAC are limited only to the imagination of the students and the school food and nutrition program staff. One young person who was a member of an NAC in Arizona attended the World Food Conference in Rome because his group was interested in world hunger. NACs can provide opportunities for students to learn about careers in the food and nutrition industry as well as become involved in issues such as hunger, elderly nutrition, coaching their peers, and mentoring younger students. Ways to use students to promote good nutrition and improve the program include having an NAC do the following:

- Participate in taste testing of new food products.
- Survey peers about food preferences and the overall quality of the school food and nutrition program.
- Write a nutrition column for the school newspaper.

- Promote the importance of exercise and diet during a health fair.
- Develop fund-raising ideas for other student groups that do not compete with the school food and nutrition program.
- Tour school kitchens and food preparation areas.
- Present skits, plays, or games about nutrition, hunger, or other topics of interest in classrooms to younger students.[21] (Note: for more information on starting an NAC, contact the American School Food Service Association.)

The student nutrition advisory group can be formal or informal. A member of the food service staff may serve as the advisor, or teachers and other educators may assume a leadership role. One thing is for certain, the program will reap the benefits of involving its primary customers—the students—in meaningful ways to promote healthy food behaviors.

SUMMARY

This chapter has provided an overview of how to better communicate with students by better understanding their opinions of the school food and nutrition program. The need for conducting external and internal research was described as essential to remaining competitive in the eyes of the students. Of particular importance to competent performance as a school food and nutrition program director is the ability to collect information on customer preferences and food acceptability to use in menu planning and communicating to school boards.[22] Several tools for assessing student satisfaction were included, along with a model for starting a student advisory group.

CASE STUDY
HOW THE SAN BERNARDINO CITY UNIFIED SCHOOL DISTRICT NUTRITION SERVICES LISTENED AND RESPONDED TO THE STUDENTS

Mary Kay Meyer

The Problem

In the fall of 1997, the staff of the Nutrition Services Center of the San Bernardino City Unified School District realized that students' wants and needs were not being met, as evidenced by low participation rates. San Bernardino is a relatively poor area with pockets of higher income. The percentage of students eligible for free and reduced meals varied within the four high schools. The participation rate ranged from 23 to 35 percent. However, many students purchased individual items such as fries, nachos, and soft drinks from the snack bar, which would not be represented in the participation figures.

The San Bernardino nutrition services administrators recognized that as the students moved up in grades, they ate less frequently in the food service. Although the campuses were closed, students were not choosing to eat in the food service areas provided. Students were looking for something new, different, and fun with foods they liked to eat. The San Bernardino Nutrition Services administrators also recognized the uniqueness in their market, and that trends often start in California. One of the popular trends in California's school food services is self-branding. School food and nutrition professionals in California recognize that students are more sophisticated and are exposed to a variety of foods and service styles and that adolescents seek the unique and are not apprehensive about trying new things if they are marketed correctly. They also know that students use outside experiences for comparison and that school food service is competing with brand-name fast foods for students' purchasing power. In order to increase participation, the nutrition services administrators

recognized the need for input from the students to determine what would meet their wants and needs. As a result, the San Bernardino Nutrition Services Center hired a marketing firm to assist it with developing a self-branded concept that would be fun and attractive to the students.

The marketing firm developed 15 separate concepts based on interviews previously conducted with students in this age range. The San Bernardino Nutrition Services Center thought that 15 concepts represented too many choices to give the students for voting. To narrow the choices, focus groups were held with the food service staff in each school. The staff were asked to consider feasibility and student characteristics when making their recommendations. Following these focus groups, students in each of the schools were then given the opportunity to vote for their favorite concept.

Even though the students had selected the concepts, Nutrition Services needed to validate that these concepts would accomplish their goals of increasing student satisfaction and participation. Gathering baseline data would help them fine-tune their concepts and help them further understand the wants and needs of the students. After researching the alternatives for gathering these baseline data, the Nutrition Services Center selected the High School Food Service Survey developed by the Applied Research Division of the National Food Service Management Institute (NFSMI).[23] Using this survey would reduce the time needed to implement a solution. This survey had been tested and was valid and reliable. A year would not have to be spent developing and validating a survey. Money was needed for improvements and the school board would have to be involved. The nutrition services administrators also knew the school board members would want concrete data to show that these concepts would meet students' wants and needs. They had to move fast. An improvement plan had to be in place by summer 1998 so that work could be done prior to schools'opening in 1998. They did not know exactly what the changes would be, but they knew that changes were needed and they needed the students to guide their decision.

Actions

In early spring 1998, under the supervision of Adriane Robles, three of the four district high schools conducted the survey. The NFSMI survey was easy to use, and a guidebook was available to explain all the steps needed to conduct the survey. It was a turnkey process and could be conducted easily. The survey was composed of two parts, a standardized computer Scantron sheet and a separate comment sheet with two open-ended comments. The comment sheets allowed the students to give additional information that would help clarify responses to the survey. NFSMI Applied Research also offered a Food Service Analysis and Benchmarking Service (FABS), in collaboration with The University of Southern Mississippi, to analyze the data and give recommendations for continuous improvement. These recommendations would be used in developing the concepts.

The NFSMI survey provided interesting insight into the wants and needs of the students. FABS provided a complete report, including averages for each question, comparison with national averages, and graphs showing their results. Figures 20–4, 20–5, and 20–6 show some of the information provided by FABS. Results showed that students were less satisfied than the national average as established by FABS in two schools and slightly more satisfied in the third school.

A statistical analysis, multiple regression, was also conducted for the district to determine the relationship between satisfaction and the attributes of the program. By using this statistical procedure, questions that predict student satisfaction can be identified. When specific questions can be determined to predict satisfaction, then they are important to the students.

Results

For the district, seven survey questions were identified as important to the students. They are listed here with the corresponding question number taken from the actual survey.

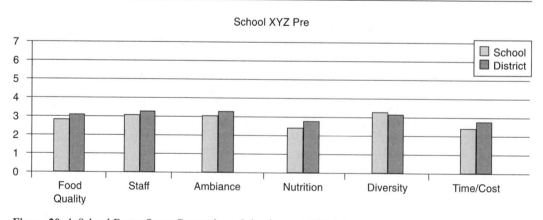

Figure 20–4 School Factor Score Comparison: School versus District.

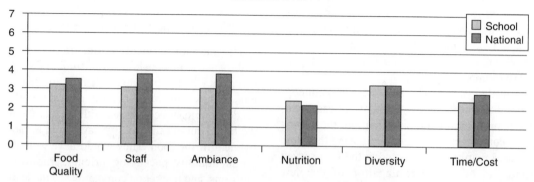

Figure 20–5 School Factor Score Comparison: School versus National.

1. Foods on the serving line are attractively presented (2)
2. The flavor of the food is (26)
3. The quality of the brands of food offered is (24)
4. Theme days/special events are offered (12)
5. The choices of food allow me to meet my ethnic and cultural choices (6)
6. The appearance of the food service staff is (27)
7. School food service prices are reasonable for the amount of food I get (9)

Using the information from the high school survey results and the recommendations from FABS, the district fine-tuned the self-branding concepts and again asked students for feedback. The same classes that participated in the first survey participated in this step. Each class was given an explanation of all the changes that would occur in the food service program. Students were shown the proposed self-branding logos developed by the marketing firm and drawings of the newly remodeled food service, and all student questions were answered. This occurred in two of the three schools. In the third school, because of scheduling, it was not possible to talk with students in the same classes in which the survey was originally taken. Instead, the concept was shown and explained to the students in a

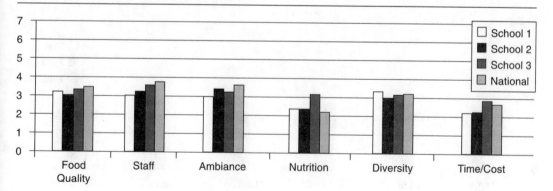

Figure 20–6 School Factor Score Comparison: District Schools versus National.

large group in the school auditorium. The same information and presentation format was used. In the auditorium setting, it was difficult to gain the students' focused attention and answer all questions as had been done in the classroom setting.

To determine whether the new concept would meet the district goals of increased student satisfaction and participation, the survey was conducted the second time using the same classes that had participated in the first survey and had heard the explanation of the new branding concept. This would validate whether the new concepts would increase their satisfaction scores. Results showed that the new self-branding would increase satisfaction in two of the schools. In the third school, satisfaction was not affected. This was attributed to the setting in which the new concept was explained to the students and the lack of focus they gave to the presentation. Figure 20–7 shows the students' perceived satisfaction with the self-branded concepts compared with their original satisfaction scores. Multiple regression using the second data set showed that the important questions to the students changed. The students were now concerned with

- Theme days/special events are offered (12)
- The appearance of the food service staff is (27)

- School food service prices are reasonable for the amount of food I get (9)
- The quality of the brands offered is (24)

The nutrition services administrators knew that, because of the shift in the students' concerns, they had to pay close attention to the details to make this new branding concept work. Students were still concerned with the quality of the brand but not the variety, flavor, and attractiveness of the food. They would have to have product quality, packaging, pricing, employee uniforms, and marketing comparable to those of nationally branded fast foods to be competitive.

Future Plans

Armed with this information, the nutrition services administration was ready to present its proposal to the school board for funding. They were asking for approximately $70,000 to $100,000 per school. They proposed to begin with one school. This school would have a 1950s theme. Their plan was to remodel the food service and have it ready for the students beginning in the fall of 1998. In the spring of 1999, the district administration would again survey the students to see whether they were successfully accomplishing their goals.

Special thanks go to Adrian Robles, Assistant Director of Nutrition Services, San Bernardino City Unified School District, for sharing her thoughts, which were essential for the development of this case.

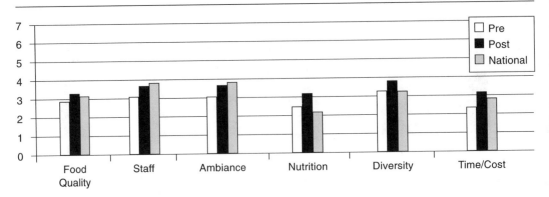

Figure 20–7 School Factor Score Comparison: Pre versus Post.

REFERENCES

1. American School Food Service Association (ASFSA), *Keys to Excellence: Standards of Practice for Nutrition Integrity* (Alexandria, VA: 1995), 31, 32. (To obtain more information about standards, call the American School Food Service Association at 800/877-8822.)

2. M.K. Meyer and B. Sackin, "Does Your Branding Program Work? Ask Your Students," *School Foodservice & Nutrition* (February 1997): 32–36.

3. American School Food Service Association, *School Food Service Industry External Environmental Scan* (Alexandria, VA: 1997), 1.

4. S. Guber and J. Berry, *Marketing to and through Kids* (New York: McGraw-Hill, 1993).

5. Zollo, P. *Wise Up to Teens* (Ithaca, NY: New Strategist Publications, Inc., 1995).

6. J. Cornyn and J. Coons-Fasano, *Noncommercial Food-service–An Administrator's Handbook* (New York: John Wiley & Sons, 1995).

7. Zollo, *Wise Up to Teens.*

8. Meyer and Sackin, "Does Your Branding Program Work?"

9. Cornyn and Coons-Fasono, *Noncommercial Foodservice.*

10. Meyer and Sackin, "Does Your Branding Program Work?"

11. K. Schuster, "How To Find Out What Your Customers Really Want," *Food Management Magazine,* December 1996.

12. Meyer and Sackin; "Does Your Branding Program Work?"

13. National Food Service Management Institute, *Middle/Junior High School Food Service Survey* (University, MS: 1997).

14. National Food Service Management Institute (NFSMI), *High School Food Service Survey* (University, MS: 1996). (To obtain more information about the surveys, call the National Food Service Management Institute at 800/321–3054.)

15. M.K. Meyer, "High School Food Service Survey: A Continuous Improvement Tool," *NFSMI Insight,* No. 8, 1997.

16. M.K. Meyer et al., *Child Nutrition Program Director/Supervisor's Survey Guide: High School Food Service Survey* (University, MS: National Food Service Management Institute, 1997).

17. M.K. Meyer, *Child Nutrition Program Director/Supervisor's Survey Guide: Middle/Junior High School Food Service Survey* (University, MS: National Food Service Management Institute, 1997). (To obtain more information about the survey guides, call the National Food Service Management Institute at 800/321–3054.)

18. Meyer et al., *Child Nutrition Program Director/Supervisor's Survey Guide: High School.*

19. K. Schuster, "Benchmarking: How Do You Measure Up?" *Food Management Magazine,* August 1997, 42–49.

20. ASFSA, *Keys to Excellence.*

21. American School Food Service Association, *How To Start a Nutrition Advisory Council in Your School* (Alexandria, VA: 1995). Brochure. (To obtain more information about NACs, call the American School Food Service Association at 800/877-8822.)

22. D.H. Carr et al., *Competencies, Knowledge and Skills of Effective District School Nutrition Directors/Supervisors* (University, MS: National Food Service Management Institute, 1996), 99, 145.

23. NFSMI, *High School Food Service Survey.*

CHAPTER 21

Communicating with School Officials

Martha T. Conklin

OUTLINE

INTRODUCTION

School food and nutrition program directors are middle managers in school organizations, although they are essentially the chief administrators of child nutrition programs (CNPs). As noted in Chapter 1, the food and nutrition program is a subsystem of the educational system, and as such, the school food and nutrition program director is a middle manager in this environment. Middle managers accomplish goals largely by managing relationships. Managing relationships at this level requires individuals to act as a subordinate, an equal, and a superior. This triple set of relationships is demanding, and for school food and nutrition program directors who also have to juggle many other duties, the task may seem overwhelming.[1]

Effective communications skills are very crucial to middle managers. The American School Food Service Association's (ASFSA) *Keys to Excellence* notes several areas where excellent communication skills are important to effective CNPs.[2] The competencies for school nutrition directors/supervisors developed by the National Food Service Management Institute also underscore the importance of directors' developing an ongoing system for informing CNP personnel and school administrators of current information on the program.[3] Although communication skills are important equally in relating down and across levels in CNPs and school organizations, this chapter will concentrate on upward communication to school officials. Specific objectives are to discuss strategies for managing relationships with the boss or bosses, relate how research can be used to communicate effectively to school officials, and suggest methods to persuasively communicate with school boards.

MANAGING THE BOSS OR BOSSES

To many the phrase of *managing the boss* sounds odd because school food and nutrition program directors may think only about managing subordinates. Effective directors, however, take the time and effort to manage not only employees but their bosses as well. The phrase does not mean political stroking. It refers to the process of consciously working with superiors to obtain the best possible results for the CNP, school officials, and the students. Many professionals in organizational structures of the new century report to more than one boss. Managing all bosses in a manner tailored to each of their specific personalities, goals, and objectives is very important to the long-term success of CNP directors.

Managing the boss or bosses means that food and nutrition professionals gain an understanding of bosses and their needs. At a minimum, appreciating the boss's goals, pressures, strengths, and weaknesses is important. What are the bosses' organizational and personal objectives? Were they educated as businesspeople or as school administrators? What is the jargon or language with which they feel most comfortable? What journals do they read, and what are the issues of concern identified by their professional association? What are the pressures on them from school boards? What are the bosses' specific strengths and weaknesses? What did they do before they were superintendents, school business officials, or directors of support services? Were they successful at what they did before? Directors can predict current performance and biases of bosses by knowing about their past. Remember that people tend to perform in ways that were successful in the past even though circumstances now dictate another approach.

Effective CNP directors seek out information about bosses' goals, problems, and pressures. They are alert for opportunities to question their superiors and others around them to test their assumptions. They read the same journals as their bosses and read minutes from school board meetings and other meetings that disclose goals and objectives of the school system. Successful directors think win-win. They strategize how the CNP can help bosses achieve goals that are important to them while at the same time supporting important objectives of the CNP. They may even use informal means such as making friends with bosses' secretaries or using the power of a cup of coffee to gain more insight into the work pressures and priorities of their bosses.

School food and nutrition program directors should be sensitive to the work style of directors of support services, school business officials, and superintendents. Style means "a particular, distinctive, or characteristic mode of action or manner of action"[4(p.1890)] as distinguished from its substance. Are they formal or informal in their approach to people? Do they prefer to read background information before entering into discussion or making a decision, or do they prefer to think on their feet and bat ideas around in person?[5] How do they deal with conflict? Do they sidestep potential disagreements and uphold the motto, "Not to decide is to decide?" Are they prone to compromise and splitting the difference, or do they believe in collaboration to find a new solution and create a win for everyone?[6] Being sensitive to issues of style is crucial to good working relations with bosses.[7]

Analyzing the boss's style will only be effective if, in turn, school food and nutrition program directors become conscious of their own styles. They should be aware of personal traits that facilitate or deter working with superiors and take actions to make relationships more constructive. For example, by reflecting over experiences, Margaret Toliver, CNP director, learned that she was not very good at dealing with emotional or confrontational issues where people were concerned. Because her instinctive responses to such issues were often disastrous for Margaret and her employees, she developed a habit of first talking to her boss, the director of support services, before taking action. Their discussions always unearthed approaches Margaret had not considered. In many cases, they even identified specific actions her boss could take to help situations.

A subordinate's reaction to authority may be a hindrance to effective communication. Constantly bridling against authority of superiors

and always caving in even when bosses are wrong are both nonproductive behaviors showing that directors hold unrealistic views of their bosses' authority. These views ignore that most bosses, like everyone else, are imperfect. They do not have unlimited time, knowledge, or extrasensory perception. They have their own pressures and deadlines to meet that are sometimes at odds with the wishes of subordinates, and rightfully so.[7] The scope of their responsibilities is much broader than those of school food and nutrition program directors.

Managing the boss is an acquired skill that is necessary for optimizing the goals and objectives of school food and nutrition programs. If one were to develop a set of rules for managing bosses, they would pertain to the following:

- A good working relationship must accommodate differences in work style. If in a meeting, bosses push their chairs back from the desk, cross their arms, or play with their pens, these are clues that they are uncomfortable with the discussion. School food and nutrition program directors should defer decisions until a later date to give them time to reflect and possibly talk with others before they make a decision. If bosses fidget and look distracted every time subordinates go into lengthy detail during meetings, directors should become more succinct and direct. They should develop brief agendas to use as a guide for meetings with the boss, and whenever digressions are necessary, they should explain why. These small changes will make meetings more effective and less frustrating for all.
- School food and nutrition program directors should adjust their styles to match their bosses' preferred method for receiving information. Some bosses like to read information ahead of time so they can think about their responses. Others work better with information and reports communicated in person so they can ask questions immediately. People who prefer

reading are easy to uncover because they become very uncomfortable when asked to think on their feet and usually defer decisions until later. When they do decide, more than likely they will respond in writing. If the boss is a reader, school food and nutrition program directors should cover important items or proposals in memos, E-mails, or reports, then discuss them. If the boss is a listener, they should brief the boss in person, and then follow up with a memo to document the discussion.

- When writing, directors also need to be aware of the bosses' preferred style of writing. Writing style is made up of particular words selected to express ideas and the types of sentences and paragraphs used to convey ideas. Words carry connotations, and it is the feelings and images associated with words that give style to writing because they produce emotional reactions in readers. Tone comes from what people read into the words and sentences writers use. The tone of writing can be forceful or passive, personal or nonpersonal, colorful or less colorful. Table 21–1 charts the style options available to business writers. Style should be matched to the style of the boss, the position of the writer, and the intended purpose of the document.

    Scrutiny of Table 21–1 might lead one to conclude that reports and memos to bosses should always be written in a passive, impersonal style that is tactful and devoid of colorful language.[8] Whereas that would be the safest strategy, depending on the boss, it may not be the most appropriate. A question to answer is, Does the boss tend to want straightforward facts or a lot of interpretation? The answer to this question should be determined from the boss ahead of time. If interpretation and recommendations are required, how assured is the director writing the report? Is personal opinion okay? The boss should

tell the director whether opinions and recommendations are desired.[9] Style cannot be separated from the situation and must be altered to suit the circumstances. Writing style also must be discussed with the boss as an option available to aid their mutual communication.[10]

- Consideration should be given to bosses' decision-making styles. Some prefer to be involved in decisions as they arise. It is better to involve this type of boss at a time convenient to the school food and nutrition program director rather than at the discretion of the boss. Wise directors control the circumstances surrounding bosses's input into their agenda. Other bosses prefer to delegate and do not like to be involved. They only want to know about major problems or impending changes that are important to the program. Even in these circumstances it is important to give these bosses enough information so that they can respond knowledgeably if issues related to the CNP arise in the community. The old adage of CYB, "cover your backside," should be extended to CYBB, or "cover your bosses' backsides" and never let them get caught looking like uninformed administrators.

- Bosses and subordinates should draw upon the strengths of each and compensate for each other's weaknesses. If school food and nutrition program directors are better at technical reports detailing statistics, they could help the boss pull together the language necessary for a report to the school board. Conversely, if bosses know their school food and nutrition program directors are weak in the area of maintenance of equipment, they can make sure that the maintenance or engineering department implements a preventive maintenance system in the school kitchens.

- CNP directors need to take the responsibility to determine bosses' expectations. Some superiors will explain what they want very explicitly, but most will not. Getting

Table 21–1 Writing for Effect

Factors to Consider	Forceful Style	Passive Style	Personal Style	Impersonal Style	Colorful Style	Less Colorful Style
Appropriate business situations	Use when writer has power and when giving orders or saying no firmly to a subordinate.	Use in negative situations and when writer is in a lower position than the reader.	Use for good-news and persuasive action-request situations.	Use for negative and information-conveying situations.	Use for good-news and in highly persuasive writing.	Use in ordinary business writing.
Voice	Active: Create sentences that do something to people or objects.	Passive: Subordinate the subject to the end of sentences or bury entirely.	Active: Put the writer at the front of the sentences.	Passive: Have writer conveniently disappear when desirable.	Active: Blend personal style with active voice.	Passive: Blend impersonal style with passive voice.
Sentence structure	Write sentences in subject-verb-object order. Do not use qualifying phrases. Do not relegate the point or action to subordinate clauses.	Avoid the imperative by never giving an order. Avoid taking responsibility for negative statements by attributing them to others.	Use short sentences that capture the cadence of ordinary conversation. Direct questions to the reader.	Make sentences complex and paragraphs long. Avoid brisk, direct, simple-sentence structure.	Use straightforward sentences with highly emotional language and figures of speech.	Write longer sentences. Avoid emotional language and figures of speech.
Word usage	Avoid weasel words like possible, maybe, perhaps.	Use weasel words, especially if the reader is in a high-power position and may not like what is said.	Use persons' names instead of titles. Use personal pronouns, especially *you* and *I.* Use contractions to sound informal.	Do not use persons' names; refer to them by job title. Do not use personal pronouns, especially *you* and *I.*	Use adjectives, adverbs, and metaphors frequently.	Avoid witty, lively, picturesque, flamboyant, and vigorous words.

Source: Adapted and reprinted by permission of *Harvard Business Review.* From *What Do You Mean You Don't Like My Style?* By J.S. Fielden, May–June 1982. Copyright © 1982 by the President and Fellows of Harvard College, all rights reserved.

bosses to express these expectations can be difficult but not impossible for effective directors. Some directors may draft a detailed memo covering key aspects of their work and then send it to their bosses for approval. They follow this with a discussion at which all items are addressed. This discussion often uncovers virtually all of the bosses' relevant expectations. Another way to handle it is to establish an ongoing series of informal discussions with bosses about "good management" in relation to program objectives. Others find out information more indirectly through former employees of bosses or by watching bosses work with others such as other department heads, faculty, and the school board. School food and nutrition program directors need to communicate their own expectations to their superiors to find out if they are realistic and to influence them to accept the ones that are important to directors.

• Effective school food and nutrition program directors know they may underestimate what bosses need to know, and they make sure they find ways to keep them informed through a process that fits their style. Even bosses who only seem to want the good news need to be apprised of problems. Some directors deal with this by establishing a management information system and letting the numbers do the talking so there is no messenger to kill. Others inform bosses of potential problems so bosses are never blindsided with either good or bad news.

Setting aside time each week or month to communicate with the boss helps keep school food and nutrition concerns visible. This routine communication may be oral or written. Sharing an item of good news about the food and nutrition program or a research article related to nutrition and learning is an easy way to keep bosses informed. One local director sends a news item to her boss each week for the in-house newsletter; another sends a summary at the end of the month highlighting financial and program status. Another method to keep the bosses involved is to make sure their names are on all the lists for invitations to school food and nutrition program events such as National School Lunch Week, School Breakfast Week, and National Nutrition Month.

Regular communication with the boss from the school food and nutrition program director also serves as a reminder to the boss to share information with the director. Items of interest to the director would be exhibits viewed by the boss at professional meetings, sales and marketing people in the food or food service contract industry who have made calls or sent information, and positive feedback received from the board or community. Regular communication provides talking points when the subject of school food and nutrition arises. Nurturing open communications on an ongoing basis makes it easier to deal with issues that emerge, and issues do evolve. Open communications with the boss pays dividends in return.

• To solidify communications with bosses, school food and nutrition program directors must at all times be honest and dependable. Although no one is intentionally undependable, directors may become so due to an oversight or uncertainty about the boss's priorities. Dishonesty may happen if the truth is shaded and potential problems are downplayed. Without a basic feeling of trust, bosses feel they must check all subordinates' decisions, which limits directors' opportunities for decisive action.

Competent directors of school food and nutrition programs recognize that managing the boss or bosses is a legitimate task in administering their programs. Astute performance in this area will simplify directors' jobs by eliminating potentially severe problems and resulting job turnover. Successful directors know they are ultimately responsible for all they achieve, and these responsibilities include the managing of relationships with everyone on whom they depend, especially bosses.[11]

USING RESEARCH TO SUPPORT REQUESTS TO SCHOOL ADMINISTRATION

Everyone knows the old adage, "Statistics don't lie, but you can lie with statistics." Even though this is an accepted truth and should indicate caution, school officials and others in positions of decision making are swayed by numbers in print. They are particularly influenced by numbers or statistics collected by objective methods that ensure the validity and reliability of the information. That's what research is all about. The use of research, conducted either by others or by directors of school food and nutrition programs, to support intended actions will get the attention of superiors. Maybe it is because superiors were trained to revere and conduct research in their doctoral or business degrees or maybe it is just the mystique associated with numbers—regardless, it works.

Validity and Reliability

When using research conducted by others or when school food and nutrition program directors design studies in their own programs, they need to be concerned about validity and reliability or they just might be unintentionally "lying with statistics." Validity means you measure what you intend to measure. A study with internal validity is free from nonrandom error or bias. This bias might be introduced by how subjects are chosen or assigned to groups, maturation or naturally occurring changes in subjects unrelated to the study, historical events that can affect the study results, imprecise instruments or training of raters, and loss of data or subjects because sometimes people who fail to complete a study have different characteristics than people who do. External validity means a study's results correctly apply to the target population. Risks to external validity are most often associated with the way in which subjects are selected and assigned. They may become alert to the kinds of behaviors expected or answer questions in a certain manner just because they are being studied—the Hawthorne effect.[12]

Reliability refers to how relatively free from measurement error the study's data collection methods are. Consistency and repeatability are key principles associated with reliability. Reliability is measured in three ways. First, internal consistency examines whether the items on a questionnaire are all interrelated. If items are highly interrelated, they are measuring the same construct or topic. Second, stability or reliability over time means that test scores separated by time are highly correlated. This is sometimes referred to as test-retest reliability. Finally, when raters are used in a study methodology, rater drift or inconsistent ratings by different raters may occur. Checking to ensure consistency in raters is referred to as interrater reliability.[12,13]

When considering the validity and reliability of research, several questions need to be answered by the authors or the intended researchers. Those questions are listed in Exhibit 21–1, and directors should find satisfactory answers to these questions before feeling confident in the study's results. Research needs to be reliable to be valid.[13] The converse is not true, but it is necessary for quality research. William Tell knew that both validity and reliability were necessary prerequisites for effective performance. He would not have shot the arrow at the apple on his son's head if he had not been confident that he could hit the apple (validity), and that he could do it every time (reliability).

Published Research

Directors of school food and nutrition programs can use published literature to document points they wish to make to school officials, es-

Exhibit 21–1 Questions on Validity and Reliability

- *Are data collection methods described adequately?* Researchers should define all key variables and provide information on the type of test or survey used. If a measure is given more than one time, check to see that the length of time between administrations is explained and the effect on test-retest reliability is discussed.
- *Is the test or survey instrument reliable?* Watch for evidence that instruments have internal consistency (alpha-levels) or test-retest reliability. Look for data on interrater or intrarater reliability where pertinent to the study design. If surveys ask demographic questions such as age, sex, income, and education, check to see whether questions have been shaped to diminish inaccuracies and bias given the reading level and background of the respondents.
- *Is the measure valid?* If an instrument was specifically developed for the study, was it pilot tested? What facts do the researchers provide about the instrument's accurately measuring the variables of concern? If the instrument is adapted from another study, do the researchers offer proof that the current study population is similar to the validation population in important areas such as background, knowledge, or health condition?
- *Do the researchers explain the consequences of using measures with less than optimum reliability and validity?* Without information on the validity and reliability of a study's measures, a reader cannot tell if the findings are likely to be true or false. Do the researchers justify their confidence in their findings by comparing their results with other studies with similar populations? How convincing are they?

Source: Adapted with permission from A. Fink, *Conducting Research Literature Reviews* pp. 116–117, © 1998; Sage Publications, Inc.

---

pecially about procedures and practices tested in other CNP settings. Research findings from refereed journals will provide information that has passed the scrutiny of peers. These journals, by definition, use a panel of fellow professionals to review the quality of articles and to make suggestions for improvement. The questions listed in Exhibit 21–1 were more than likely answered to the satisfaction of the editors and reviewers prior to publication of the research findings in a refereed journal. Examples of these journals are the *Journal of Child Nutrition & Management* and the *Journal of The American Dietetic Association.*

Refereed journals are not the only place to find published research. Trade magazines are publications furnished gratis to the profession or trade. They make their income selling advertisements. Embedded among the ads, however, are articles of interest to the profession. Many times these articles will report on surveys conducted on current issues. This is a wonderful source for trends and topical sub-

jects that have yet to be studied through formal research projects. Articles are approved by the editor, but not peer reviewed. The validity and reliability of instruments are rarely discussed in the articles, and often the source of information is purely anecdotal, but they still have value. As long as directors know how these articles were developed and their findings are placed in the proper context when communicating to school officials, they can be used very effectively. Examples of useful trade magazines are *School Foodservice & Nutrition, The Foodservice Director,* and *Food Management.*

Conducting Research in CNPs

When making points with school officials, the most effective strategy is to compare and contrast published information with data collected at home. This means that school food and nutrition program directors must systematically collect data in their own programs; they must engage in research. Directors can answer many questions about their school food and nutrition programs by doing small studies. Detailed experiments can be conducted, but the most likely types of research to be used in CNPs are descriptive studies using some sort of survey instrument or focus group. Once information has been obtained from either a survey or focus group, the results can be compared with other data to benchmark or conduct cost-effectiveness analyses.

Surveys

The first step in developing a survey is to consider the information desired and the people who can provide that information. Students, parents, teachers, and school administrators are all CNP customers who could provide valuable information to the director of school food and nutrition programs. The procedure for accessing this information also has to be decided. Will this be a written survey distributed in classes or faculty lounges? Will it be a written survey sent home with the students for parents to complete? Will it be a short survey published in the hometown newspaper? Or will telephone calls be made to parents in the evening? Any of these strategies may work, and how the actual instrument is created will be dictated by the distribution decision, which, in turn, is dictated by where the people to be surveyed are most easily accessed.

Once these questions have been addressed, the next step is to develop the instrument itself. An important tip is to avoid reinventing the wheel, if possible. Developing a survey is hard, tedious work. If a survey developed for the same or similar purposes already exists, it should be used as is or adapted. This is particularly true if information on the instrument's validity and reliability is available. For example, the middle/junior high and high school student satisfaction surveys were mentioned in Chapter 20. Researchers at the Applied Research Division of the National Food Service Management Institute (NFSMI) developed and validated these for use by directors across the nation. Di-

rectors should consider using them if their goal is to survey students about the school food and nutrition program. Even if there are specific questions that are not covered by the NFSMI surveys, they can be added on an additional paper for students to complete.

If the entire survey cannot be used, directors may be able to use some of the questions. For example, a survey developed to determine math curriculum needs might be adapted to ask teachers about similar curriculum needs in nutrition education. If directors decide to write questionnaires from scratch, there are resources to help them with the process,[14–17] or they may solicit the aid of someone in the school district or neighboring college with this expertise. Important steps are to maximize the validity and reliability of instruments and to conduct a pilot test before actually using them in studies.

When conducting a survey, Meyer points out other items to consider.[18] School food and nutrition program directors must follow procedures in the school district to obtain approval from all levels of the school community. In some districts requests have to be reviewed by the school board. Parental permission to involve students in a study is another factor that must be considered in some school districts. The best day of the week, time of day, and place to conduct the survey have to be decided, as well as what time in the school year or semester will elicit the most meaningful information. Attitudes of school administrators, teachers, and students vary, depending on the time of the year and the pressures of the academic calendar. Where to access the study participants also has to be determined. Students might take a survey about the school food and nutrition program more seriously if they fill it out in an academic class rather than on the run in the cafeteria. A lot of time is required to make decisions and coordinate the process of designing and conducting a survey. Exhibit 21–2 gives a sample time line for the survey process.[18]

Once the survey has been administered data must be analyzed. First, completed survey

Exhibit 21–2 Time Line for Conducting a Survey in Schools

✓	Time	Date	TASK
	One to two months prior to survey		Gain necessary approvals.
	One month prior to survey		Discuss survey process with CNP managers.
	One month prior to survey		Schedule a date for the survey with the school principal and CNP manager.
	One month prior to survey		Order the surveys and pencils.
	One month prior to survey		Arrange for data analysis
	Two weeks prior to survey		Remind the principal of the survey date.
	Two weeks prior to survey		Discuss survey details with CNP managers.
	One week prior to survey		Confirm with CNP manager that students for random method or teachers for the classroom method have been reminded of the survey.
	Two to three days prior to survey		Distribute surveys, comment sheets, and pencils to the survey coordinator at each school.
	Survey day		Discuss any last-minute details with the CNP managers.
	Day after survey		Obtain surveys from the survey coordinator at each school.
	Day or two after survey		Send surveys for analysis. Have comments typed and organized.

Source: Adapted with permission from M.K. Meyer, Why Should CNP Professionals Ask Students for Their Written Opinions? in M. Conklin et al., eds., *Recipes for Practical Research in Child Nutrition Programs*, pp. 2–10, © 1998, National Food Service Management Institute.

forms must be scrutinized for accuracy and completeness. Directors should watch for forms that are filled out in nonrandom fashion. For example, students might choose the "a" response for all the questions or routinely mark in order "a" through "d" all down the page. Patterns such as these indicate students were not taking the survey process seriously, and these questionnaires should be discarded.

Results could be entered by the CNP secretary or clerk on a spreadsheet, and simple averages could be calculated by either a manual calculator or a computer. A more sophisticated approach would be to calculate frequencies, means, and standard deviations using a statistical package. Regardless of the method, directors will want the range of scores and the average score associated with each question. They also will not want to fall victim to overstating their results simply because a computer did the calculations. For example, a computer will calculate a mean to five or six decimal places but the calibration of a typical, written survey does not warrant this degree of specificity. If participants rated a characteristic of CNPs on a hedonic scale of *strongly disagree* (1) to *strongly agree* (5), it would not be logical to use all four decimal places with the average score. The precision of the scale warrants rounding the mean to only one decimal place. Thus, reporting of results has to be consistent with the method by which the results were obtained. *Modesty* is the watchword. Directors do not want to overstate their findings, nor should they draw conclusions unwarranted by the data.

Focus Groups

Surveys yield numbers that can be "crunched" and they are considered quantitative. Focus groups gather data from people, too, but the results are not reduced to neat little numbers. This type of research is considered to be qualitative. Depending on the objectives of the study, both approaches have merit. Qualitative research methods are appropriate to use when researchers are just beginning to explore a subject, when context and depth in a subject matter are desired, or when interpretation of a complex issue is necessary.[19] Just because numbers are not generated does not mean that research using focus groups is ill conceived and inconsistently executed.

Focus groups use group discussions to learn about a topic. They are a way of listening to people and learning from them. Research with focus groups uses a three-stage process:

1. The research team decides what issues they want addressed among participants.
2. The focus group moderators create a conversation among the participants around those issues.
3. The research team summarizes what they have learned from the participants.

Communications are a two-way proposition; thus focus groups work best when participants are as interested in the issues as the researchers. In quality focus groups, the moderators asks questions that produce lively discussions addressing issues about which school food and nutrition program directors want to learn. Not all groups of people talking about issues are focus groups. True focus groups must be convened for the purpose of collecting qualitative data. They must be carefully planned so the right participants are asked the right questions through a carefully orchestrated moderating style. Exhibit 21–3 is a checklist for determining whether focus groups are a match to the purpose of the study.[19]

Before beginning focus group research, school food and nutrition program directors need to invest the time to clearly formulate the purpose, expectations, and anticipated outcomes of the project. A question they should answer is whether there are better ways to collect the information needed other than bringing a group together because this type of research can be expensive when compared with other methods.[19] An important fact to recall is that the purpose of a focus group is not to arrive at consensuses or decisions but simply to gather information for a research study.[20]

When developing focus groups, the school food and nutrition program director should plan on an optimum of seven to ten partici-

---

Exhibit 21–3 Focus Group Checklist

Use focus groups when:
✓ Your goal is to listen to and learn from others.
✓ You can obtain in-depth knowledge by listening.
✓ You can effectively explore research topics through conversations among participants.
✓ You can pursue questions about "how and why" through group discussion.
✓ Your purpose is to identify problems to be addressed.
✓ Your purpose is to plan for programs, survey questionnaires, or quality service.
✓ Your purpose is to improve program implementation.
✓ Your purpose is to determine the outcome of a project or service.

Source: Adapted with permission from D.L. Morgan, *The Focus Group Guidebook,* pp. 97–98, © 1998, Sage Publications, Inc.

pants in each session. A minimum of three sessions should be held, each with a set of different participants that match the same criteria for participation. The participants should be chosen carefully. Factors to consider when using student participants are listed in Exhibit 21–4.[21] When convening adult participants, they should be matched to their level within organizations because subordinates might defer to bosses. Adults also like to be informed of the objectives of the focus group and how the data will be used. School food and nutrition program directors should make modest claims and take care to avoid making promises on program changes that cannot be delivered.[21,22]

Questions for the focus group session should be carefully constructed and pilot-tested. Questions should be created as though moderators were having a friendly discussion about the topic in their living rooms. Different types of questions are used at different times during the focus group, but mostly open-ended questions are designed to encourage participants to talk. There are five categories of questions, and the optimum length of time to cover the questions is no more than 90 minutes. If the participants are students, the time

should even be shorter to fit into a typical class period.

After the moderator introduces himself or herself and explains the purpose of the focus group, participants are asked the opening question, which is an easy question that everyone can answer. It helps people get acquainted and feel comfortable talking before the group. Experience has shown that the longer people wait to speak before a group the less likely they are to want to speak at all. For a focus group with parents of elementary children, an opening question might be, "Please tell us your name, the grade your child is in, and tell us one thing you remember about school lunch when you were a child?" Introductory questions begin discussion of the topic. An introductory question could be, "Describe an ideal school lunch for elementary students?" Transition questions move the conversation smoothly and seamlessly into key questions. A transition question could be, "What comes to mind when you think about your child's experience with the school lunch program?"

Key questions are structured to obtain insight on the main areas of interest for the study. These two to five questions drive the study. The moderator needs to allow sufficient

---

Exhibit 21–4 Using Students as Participants in Focus Groups

- Students in each group should be relatively close in age and should eat in the same cafeteria.
- All approvals for involving students in research should be obtained.
- Questions should be carefully constructed, keeping in mind the age group and being careful not to stereotype students.
- Students will act and respond differently than adults.
- Students who "hang out" together should not be asked to participate because the friends will defer to the dominate person in the group.
- A nonthreatening, comfortable environment should be planned to allow students to express positive and negative feelings.
- Food always helps ease conversation, especially pizza.
- Extra incentives like water bottles are a nice gesture.
- A letter to students and their parents should be sent to confirm participation in the study.

Source: Adapted with permission from J. Cater and L. Lambert, Focus Groups, in M. Conklin et al, eds., *Recipes for Practical Research in Child Nutrition Programs*, p. 4–12, © 1998, National Food Service Management Institute.

time for a full discussion of these questions. Key questions may need as much as 10 to 15 minutes each. The moderator also will need to use pauses and probes to determine the exact meaning of comments. Such probes might be, "Can you say more about that?" or "Can you give me an example from your experiences?" A key question with this same focus group of elementary school parents could be, "What actions should be taken to make the current school lunch program match your ideal?" or "What changes can be made to the school lunch program so your child will be encouraged to eat school lunch every day?"

Ending questions bring closure and emphasis to the discussion. There are three types of ending questions. One allows participants to state their final position. This could be, "If you could change only one thing about the school lunch program, what would it be?" This type of question helps analysis because trivial concerns might be talked about a lot, and it's a serious mistake to assume that frequency reflects importance. Summary questions occur after the moderator or assistant moderator has given a short oral summary of the discussion on the key questions and the big ideas. A summary question asks, "Did I accurately reflect what has been said?" The final type of ending question is one to ensure that critical aspects have not be overlooked. The question begins with a short overview of the purpose of the study. The moderator then asks, "Is there an important issue we missed?" This question works only if there is sufficient time to pursue the answers. It is best to have at least 10 minutes remaining before the promised adjournment time.[23] All questions need to be pilot-tested before the actual focus group session. A good strategy is to have the research team ask the questions aloud to each other. If they do not flow in logical sequence, or they are not easily stated and understood, the research team should revise and retest.

A misconception about focus group research is that one must use a professional moderator. School food and nutrition program directors should decide whether a professional moderator is needed by considering all the roles that person might play in the project. Commonly, professional moderators are actively engaged in writing interview questions, moderating the groups, analyzing data, and writing the report for school officials. If the CNP research team can accomplish all these tasks, a moderator is probably not required. If not, then it may well be worth the expense to have a professional involved. A different version of this myth implies that professionals are necessary to produce the best data. The amount of experience is not what matters most, but rather the moderator's experience as it directly relates to the topics discussed and the participants in the study. Sometimes a less experienced moderator who has more contact with the key issues will produce better data than a professional who has never worked in this area.

So can directors or members of the school food and nutrition program staff be moderators? The answer is a definite "maybe." There are two caveats. Moderators must be able to orchestrate discussions without becoming part of them. They must remain free of emotion and body language that discloses their reactions to statements made. Participants, especially students, also have to perceive moderators as neutral; otherwise they will not talk because they won't want to hurt feelings or incur the moderator's wrath by honest comments. If school food and nutrition program directors or members of their staff cannot respond in this way or if participants will not feel free to comment candidly with staff in the room, they should not moderate the session.[24] Short of hiring an outside professional, however, there may be individuals within the school district who have the skills to serve as objective, neutral moderators. They at least would be familiar with the school system and the school food and nutrition program.

In addition to ensuring an open flow of communication in the group, moderators should exercise control over the group while at the same time establishing a climate of trust so that members feel free to comment openly. They should be able to convey to the groups that all members have knowledge about the subject and all comments are legitimate. Many times the moderator will have an assistant who plays a very special role. The assistant takes notes, operates the tape recorder, arranges the room to ensure everyone's comfort, and doesn't speak unless spoken to. The assistant is another set of unbiased eyes and ears in the room. After the session is over, both the moderator and the assistant reflect on the discussions and the assistant helps in assembling and writing the report.[25,26]

Once the responses of participants in all the focus group sessions have been recorded, the task of analyzing the results begins. The main characteristics of focus group analysis are disciplined and systematic processes. Disciplined analysis starts by going back to the intent of the study. Material should be organized by major points of discussion according to themes or focus group topics. A systematic process to follow is the coding of data by attaching a label whenever a researcher comes across a pertinent idea. When the idea appears again a similar label is attached. Later, the researcher can selectively retrieve information pertaining to specific labels or codes.[27]

A written report serves three basic functions: to report the results, to assist the researcher in developing a description of the investigation, and to provide a record of the findings. Focus group reports can be oral, written, or a combination. The report should be targeted to the audience and appropriate for the purpose of the research. A report should include a discussion of the topic and why it is important to study, a description of the method (number of focus groups, where held, and when), the study findings (major points), and recommendations for action and for further study.[26,27]

Benchmarking

Benchmarking is a word derived from a land surveyor's term for a distinctive mark made on a rock, wall, or building. In general, a benchmark was originally a sighting point from which measurements could be made or a standard against which others could be measured. In today's business world, benchmarking is the ongoing search for best practices that produce superior performance when adapted to one's organization. On the other hand, benchmarks are measurements to gauge the performance of a function, operation, or business relative to others. The underlying causes of operating differences cannot be discerned from benchmarks alone. They are like divining rods that lead organizations to hidden opportunities to innovate and improve performance. Benchmarking is the actual process of investigation and discovery that emphasizes successful operating procedures. Best practices benchmarking is the process of seeking out and studying the best internal and external practices that produce superior results. This performance is measured through various financial and nonfinancial performance indicators, or benchmarks.[28] In school food and nutrition programs, these performance measures might be plate cost per meal, percentage food and labor costs, percentage participation, and scores on student satisfaction surveys.

Benchmarking helps create a powerful tool for organizational change. It helps build organizations in which all employees accelerate improvement processes by shamelessly borrowing or adapting the best ideas from other successful companies.[28] The first rule for choosing benchmarking partners is to take a look at the core processes in school food and nutrition programs that support customer satisfaction and then look for partners that have the same or similar core processes. School food and nutrition program directors should not only think about other CNPs, but they should think generically. Other segments of the food service industry might be a place to find best practices. Even other departments in the school district might have best practices with regard to core processes. For example, the orientation program for faculty might be adapted for the school food and nutrition program.

Finding a benchmarking partner takes extensive research, but some sources may be close at hand. School food and nutrition program directors could ask vendors and suppliers to recommend other CNPs that appear to be good at a particular process. They also could ask their employees, especially those who come from other food service jobs. Professional associations, state child nutrition agencies, and the United States Department of Agriculture (USDA) often highlight CNPs who demonstrate exceptional performance in a given area of operations. Trade magazines also have "show and tell" articles about successful CNP processes. Another source of information is professional conferences such as the Annual National Conference of the American School Food Service Association. Experts suggest that directors use site visits sparingly at the research stage because of the time and expense involved. Site visits should be scheduled later in the process, when the best in practice program(s) have been identified and then only to help with implementation.

A benchmarking study has four phases: planning, data collection, data analysis, and adapting the change. When planning, school food and nutrition program directors should identify an area in their operations for improvement. Mrs. Swift, a school food and nutrition program director, conducted the middle school NFSMI student satisfaction survey and the surveys were analyzed by FABS, a Food Service Analysis and Benchmarking Service (see Meyer's Case Study in Chapter 20). Findings showed that her school food and nutrition program scores on food quality were below the national average. Upon further investigation through student focus groups, she determined that the main problem was presentation of food on the cafeteria line. Her benchmarking goal would be to partner with another CNP who is best in practice in merchandising and food presentation.

The second step for Mrs. Swift is to locate school food and nutrition programs in middle schools that excel in food presentation and merchandising. If others in her state have used the NFSMI survey, she could ask other directors to share their scores on food presentation. If the state CNP agency sponsored the use of the surveys in middle schools throughout the state, she could ask state staff to give her the names of directors whose schools had been rated highly by students in this area. Investigation may uncover 20 programs that are good at the process. The next step is to ask all these program directors to fill out a questionnaire and agree to a site visit if they become finalists. The questionnaire should ask for detailed process information and process results measures. Mail questionnaires should be limited to 20 minutes for completion, using closed-ended questions. Mrs. Swift should save the open-ended questions for phone and personal interviews with programs that seem to be meaningful benchmarking partners. She also should plan to visit one or two of the programs at a later date to go into detail about their food presentation and merchandising practices.

The next step is for Mrs. Swift to analyze the data to determine short- and long-range improvement goals and set priorities for implementation. At this point, she should know the gaps between her processes and those of the benchmarking partner. Adaptation and improvement are the last stage. Mrs. Swift reviews the funds needed to implement the change and develops a plan that fits within financial resources. Part of the plan should be a tracking process and a test to see whether change has been effective. In this example, the director would want to resurvey middle school students once changes have been fully implemented.[29]

Benchmarking means learning from others. Directors should "hitch their wagons to the stars" and only compare their programs with the best, or at least with those who are substantially better. Benchmarking skills are really the skills of networking. Benchmarking takes informal networking skills and turns them into a science for fast, vicarious learning. Benchmarking adds structure, quantitative muscle, research rigor, and implementation focus.[30]

Cost-Effectiveness Analysis

Benchmarking is a comparative process, and so is cost-effectiveness analysis. When someone states that a program is cost-effective, the very first question one should ask is, "Compared to what?" Cost-effectiveness analysis is a form of economic analysis whereby decision makers determine the least money an organization must pay to produce a given outcome or the greatest outcome possible for a given cost. Issues of cost effectiveness are among the last issues addressed when a program or project is evaluated. The questions of evaluation should be addressed in sequence as shown in Exhibit 21–5.[31] If a program, intervention, or project is found to be ineffective, decision makers should stop at that point. No program is worth funding if it is not meeting its objectives.[32] In cost-effectiveness analysis, efficacious programs with similar goals are evaluated and their costs compared to determine the "biggest bang for the buck."

Cost-effectiveness comes from a simple equation:

> Costs associated with producing outcomes ÷
> Outcomes expressed by an objective measure

For example, the cost effectiveness of distributing free textbooks to intercity children could be expressed as $500 for increasing reading scores by an average of one grade. When figuring costs one must calculate from a consistent accounting perspective. The three most common perspectives are those of the target population (student or client), the organization delivering the program or service, and society.[33] School food and nutrition program directors would most often take the perspective of the CNP program that commits resources to deliver the service.

Table 21–2 shows results from a hypothetical study[34] to compare three techniques to train food service employees in sanitary food-handling techniques. The three methods used were a standard lecture format using a professor from a local college who held classes in the evening, computer-assisted instruction (CAI), and tutoring by expert peers from the work unit. Employees were paid for training in each instance. The average costs per student are shown in the table. Costs were calculated from the viewpoint of the school food and nutrition program and included labor costs of the supervisors, trainer, and employees, purchased or rental equipment, and materials such as computer software, notebooks, and transparencies, and even snacks if they were served. These

---

Exhibit 21–5 Systematic Questions of Evaluation Research

- What are the nature and scope of the problem?
- What interventions are likely to lessen or fix the problem significantly?
- Are there specific target groups for an intervention?
- Is the intervention reaching the target group?
- Is the intervention or project being implemented as planned?
- Does it work; is it effective?
- How much does it cost?
- What are its costs in relation to its effectiveness?
- Are there other interventions or projects that are as effective but cost less?

Source: Adapted with permission from P.H. Rossi and H.E. Freeman, *Evaluation: A Systematic Approach, 5th ed.*, p. 5, © 1993, Sage Publications, Inc.

Table 21–2 Hypothetical Results of Three Techniques to Train Food Service Employees in Sanitary Food Handling

Method	Cost/Student	Effectiveness (Points Gained in Posttest Scores)	C/E Results
Lecture	$100	10	$10
CAI	$100	20	$ 5
Peer tutoring	$ 56	8	$ 7

Source: Adapted with permission of H.M. Levin, *Cost-Effectiveness: A Primer*, p. 20, © 1983; Sage Publications.

costs were then divided by the number of students trained. CAI may seem expensive but because of the many employees who were able to take advantage of this technique during work hours, the cost per student was the same as that of using a professional trainer. The cost of using peer tutors was the least expensive. The effectiveness measure was the average number of points per student gained on the posttest above the score on the pretest. After the effectiveness measure was divided into the costs, the results showed that CAI was the most cost effective. This method resulted in the least cost per point gained on the posttest.

This was a hypothetical example to illustrate the power of this type of analysis. Directors gain additional knowledge by using a cost-effectiveness approach rather than simply considering costs. In this example, the lecture and CAI methods cost the same per student and the peer tutoring was the least expensive. The picture becomes clearer when costs are divided by the points gained in the posttest. If a decision were made strictly on cost the wisest decision would not be made. Directors of school food and nutrition programs should think carefully about using this method. They could use it to compare the old method of achieving objectives with newer methods. They could use cost-effectiveness analysis to evaluate potential changes in their programs and to convince school officials of the wisdom of certain strategies even though the best alternative is not the lowest in cost.

MAKING PRESENTATIONS TO THE SCHOOL BOARD

Speaking before the school board is usually a command performance. Either the director of the school food and nutrition program has asked the superintendent for an opportunity to speak to the school board, or the superintendent has requested the director to make a presentation. Regardless of who initiates the interaction, these occasions are tension-filled for directors because they require a presentation that informs and persuades. To persuade, one has to arouse the school board members' emotions as well as present facts.[35]

The single biggest factor in persuasion is credibility of the speaker. Experts in persuasive presentations suggest that speakers include messages designed to enhance their credibility in the presentation. Credible speakers should answer the audience's implicit questions, "Why is the director telling me this . . . and what is her motivation?" Directors want members of the school board to believe that if they follow the directors' plans or approve their proposals, members or their constituencies will benefit. When audiences believe speakers have high credibility they listen more intently and for longer periods of time.

There are several aspects to credibility. The first is expertise. School food and nutrition program directors demonstrate expertise through the speed, accuracy, and facility with which they use terminology, and how well they translate technical terms for lay people. Expertise is demonstrated through the job title, advanced educational degrees, and certification. In educational settings where degrees are the outcome of the business, advanced degrees are the "coins of the realm." Educational degrees also serve as evidence of self-discipline and therefore trustworthiness.

A second aspect of credibility is trustworthiness. Trustworthiness might be honor, truth, and ethics. It could also mean showing up at the right time for the meeting and completing a project by the deadline. Trustworthiness takes time to build, so it will not happen on the first meeting. Directors must build a track record before trustworthiness is established, and gaining personal recommendations from superiors and fellow professionals could certainly hurry the process along.

Credibility means goodwill toward the audience. This is the only aspect speakers can and should control during the actual presentation. Speakers have to feel it; it cannot be faked. In planning the speech, directors should think how this information will affect the listeners. They should think win-win for the CNP and the school board. Directors must find something they admire about their listeners before they can project goodwill. There has to be at least one member of the school board who is sympathetic to the school food and nutrition program. When planning and delivering the speech, directors should think only of that person in the audience, so genuine respect and admiration come across.

The last aspect of credibility is dynamism. People are persuaded by dynamic communicators. This does not mean that one should be flamboyant or cute. To be dynamic, all directors of school food and nutrition programs have to do is care about whether listeners get the point of their speech. Dynamic speakers are well prepared and practiced so that during the speech they can talk freely and let words flow from their minds unedited. They know it is okay to search for the right word and to let audiences see them struggle for an expression.

It shows they care whether or not the audience gets the message.

Written communication skills were emphasized at the beginning of this chapter, and the ability to create solid reports using objective data is indispensable to successful communication with school officials. Oral communication, however, is more effective when trying to persuade. Speaking allows school food and nutrition program directors to build their credibility and become more persuasive.[35] Words are but a part of the power of speeches. In fact, research has shown that 93 percent of the information audiences receive comes from the tone of voice and what they see.[36] Their voice, the way directors move, their inflections, emphasis, tone, and pauses all convey meaning to listeners. The way directors look during the speech, their personal grooming, and their dress are nonverbal signals the audience sees. Exhibit 21–6 lists factors to consider in effective verbal and nonverbal communications.[37]

In designing an effective speech, opening the presentation and making the right impression are critical. Three things have to happen. The speaker must capture the audience's attention, take control of the meeting and the room, and build a good feeling of rapport with the audience.[37] Directors of school food and nutrition programs should introduce themselves and give the purpose of their presentation. They should give a taste of the bottom line or give a verbal executive summary to whet the audience's appetite. For example, a director might say, "The superintendent and I believe we can increase parent and student satisfaction and increase participation by 10 percent if we renovate the high school dining areas. And now to show you why we believe this . . ."

The body of the speech should contain information and supporting details. Attributes of a director's proposal that would be viewed favorably by the school board are the following:

- Plan a short time line to implementation. The shorter the time period for solving the problem, the better or more willing the group will be to support it, especially if it will be finished near a school board election.

- The more the plan or project can be adapted to changing circumstances the more comfortable people will feel about endorsing it.
- Plans or projects should keep disruptions in the normal operations of the school district to a minimum.
- If the proposal can meet both short- and long-term needs of the district, it will have added value.
- The more the project can be shown to fit within the defined vision, mission, strategic priorities, and directions of the school district, the more it will be seen as timely and appropriate.
- The shorter the payback period, the greater the return on investment, and the more cost savings or revenue generation

shown, the more attractive the project or proposal will be perceived.

- The proposal should concentrate on positive outcomes or tangible benefits such as increased productivity or customer satisfaction. Also the intangible benefits such as improved morale and motivation or greater prestige for the school district should be mentioned.
- The speech should always establish how members of the school board or their constituents will directly or indirectly benefit from supporting this program or proposal.

Directors should always prepare more information than they give to leave room for fielding questions.[38] The ending of the speech also needs careful thought. A good strategy is to summarize briefly the points of the speech by reducing them to two. These should be either two points for the audience to take home or

---

Exhibit 21–6 Effective Verbal and Nonverbal Communication

✓ Tone of voice is closely related to facial expressions. If you want to sound happy, try smiling. Smiling conveys power, love, and confidence.

✓ When you first stand, you want to stand upright and lean slightly toward the audience. Do not drape or lean on the podium because it impedes movement. You should be able to move around when you speak; the added dynamism from the movement will translate into more effectiveness.

✓ Your attitude will control your vocal tone, facial expressions, and body language. A great attitude is feeling powerful and centered. You don't have to be perfect and know every word by heart; as a matter of fact, a slightly flawed presentation is preferred by audiences and is more credible.

✓ Enthusiasm will move your audience better than any other emotion. When you speak with enthusiasm you are more animated and dynamic, and you communicate belief and honesty. Enthusiasm is transmitted by vocal variety, excitement about the subject matter, and body language.

✓ Your voice needs to sound relaxed. To prepare for a speech, hum slowly and quietly beforehand. Choose a gospel hymn that has lots of high and low notes. This allows your vocal cords to stretch and relax. Also stretch your facial muscles by opening your mouth as wide as you can, and while stretching your eyes wide, raise your eyebrows up high. Take about ten deep breaths, slowly letting the air out with a hiss; however, watch that you do not hyperventilate. It would be wise to perform all this activity in private.

✓ Establish rapport with the audience during the first few minutes of your speech. Be interested in them as people, be good-natured, be direct and straightforward, use humor, and use common experiences to establish common ground.

Source: Adapted with permission of D.J. Whalen, *I See What You Mean: Persuasive Business Communication*, pp. 12–35, 71–96, and 117–137, © 1996, Sage Publications.

two thoughts before making their decision, but in all likelihood they will remember and act on these two points.[39]

SUMMARY

School food and nutrition program directors are middle managers in the school district who need to communicate effectively with subordinates, peers, and superiors. This chapter concentrated on factors associated with communicating to school officials. As pointed out in Chapter 5, communication skills are critical to competent job performance for anyone. School food and nutrition program directors are no exception. Effective performance occurs when directors match their speaking and writing styles to expectations of bosses, be they super-

intendents, directors of support services, or school business officials. Part of effective writing is the ability to assemble technical reports using research conducted by others or school food and nutrition program directors. Some research methods available to directors are written surveys, focus groups, benchmarking, and cost-effectiveness analysis. The closer the data are to home and the specific needs of the school district, the more impact they will have on decision making. Making speeches is a necessary part of directors' jobs, and they potentially have more impact on school board decisions than written reports. Good speeches, delivered persuasively, focus on both substance and style. Good communication skills separate mediocre from highly effective school food and nutrition program directors.

CASE STUDY
BUILDING A SUCCESSFUL PROGRAM BEGINS WITH BUILDING BRIDGES

John Bennett

Sometimes foresight can be a particularly useful kind of vision. Just ask Mary Klatko, Food and Nutrition Services Administrator for Howard County Schools in Maryland. Mary traces one of the key elements of her marketing plan for boosting business at her schools to a specific oversight power she asked for (and got) in 1987 when she took her job. That simple act of communication symbolizes Mary's approach to working with school administrators—and good communications were never more important than when Mary set out to plan and build the food service facility at the new Wilde Lake High School in Columbia, Maryland.

Howard County is one of the nation's wealthiest and fastest-growing jurisdictions. Mary took over a 40-school operation in 1987, but she knew it wouldn't stay that size for long; indeed, she now has 65 schools, with two more on the drawing board. For the long term, Mary knew that control over design and construction of her portion of those multiplying school buildings would be good for the child nutrition department, good for her customers, and good for education in her county.

"One of the things I noticed about construction that had been done before was that substitutions were being made in all areas—equipment, materials, décor, finishing work—so that contractors could make their budgets," Mary said. "Since I've been here, the contractors building our kitchens and cafeterias don't get paid until I sign off on their invoice and send it over for payment. And I don't do that until I'm completely satisfied with their work."

"I work with a kitchen consultant to write the specifications, and we follow everything through, right down to the electrical and plumbing connections. I'm right there on site for the whole thing, so I can really hold the contractors accountable until everything's done—and done right."

The foresight to request that level of control has paid off handsomely for Mary in the 25 kitchen construction projects she's overseen in the last 12 years, and never more so than at Wilde Lake High. Because, at Wilde Lake, Mary had a vision that differed significantly from the other three high school building projects she had undertaken. Indeed, the design of the serving area was an integral piece of her marketing plan, and that design had to be executed to the letter of her instructions. Without ongoing, effective communications with her bosses and officials at the school, Mary never could have wielded the authority to realize that plan effectively.

Howard County sends a high percentage of its graduates on to college, and the educational philosophy in the county schools is very much geared to college prep. Mary reasoned that the nutrition program should adopt that emphasis, too; and, significantly, the administrators in her county readily agreed with her—*because Mary took pains to make her food service objectives dovetail perfectly with the system's overall objective of preparing kids for college.* So when she began planning for the September 1996 opening of the new Wilde Lake High School cafeteria, Mary proceeded from the outset as if she were building a college eatery.

That meant lots of food choices and a high degree of customer control over how and where those choices are made. Her marketing plan included a scatter system with eight to ten free-standing stations, each providing several choices. The result was a service area that looked nothing like a traditional school cafeteria line. Mary was confident that the kids would catch on right away, but she knew that she'd have to convince administrators, teachers, and staff at the school that a radically different system wouldn't mean more work for them. It's hard enough keeping order in an old-style cafeteria; how could they keep problems from cropping up when kids had so many different stations to choose from?

One of Mary's answers was to convince school staff that kids who were treated like adults and who were happy with their meals would automatically behave better. Who wouldn't be happy with all these choices? One station features prepackaged salads, yogurt, three daily soup choices, and pasta entrées. Another features subs and cold sandwiches. A third offers three or four hot sandwich choices, with sandwiches prewrapped in fast-food restaurant-style foil wrappers. Several pizza choices and french fries are available at another station. Two featured hot choices (on the day of my visit, lasagna and chicken hoagies) are served at yet another. A fixings station is available for any and all of the items chosen at the other areas. Another station holds self-serve side salad mix, fresh fruit, veggies, and milk. À la carte choices are available at the three registers where all customers eventually check out with their meals.

The kitchen itself is virtually out of sight—the customer's entire experience takes place in the scatter area. Indeed, the staff presence is incredibly unobtrusive and low key, so kids really have the sense that they're in charge of their own food choices. Restocking and cleanup take place mostly between serving periods, unless a station runs out of an item or a bigger-than-usual spill happens.

So given all of the entrée choices at the stations and the various combinations kids can create (soup, for example, can be taken as a vegetable choice with any entrée), customers have 15 or more center-of-the-plate choices and literally hundreds of different possible meal combinations to choose from every single day. The day's choices are posted on a large back-lighted menu sign, and individual signs are displayed at each station, too. The sense among Wilde Lake customers, though, is that

you don't even need to know what's on the menu when you walk in. With so many choices, all you need to do is look around to find something that strikes your fancy—kind of like the college commons, which is, of course, exactly the intention.

And when customers look around they'll also see an environment carefully designed to create a pleasing, "grown-up" feeling. No bright primary colors or hand-painted murals here, but rather a soothing pastel color scheme coordinated right down to the equipment. The artwork is small scale and inspirational, and tasteful floral displays crown many of the serving stations. There's plenty of room to maneuver, and none of the claustrophobic "cattle-chute" feeling of old. The message to the students is subtle but consistent: we consider you to be adults.

This approach to the customer also pays off with the school staff. Not only have teachers' order-keeping functions not increased, they've diminished. Indeed, the only teachers in evidence in the large service area are the many teachers who enthusiastically queue up with the kids to buy lunch!

Because she offers so many self-branded choices, Mary doesn't need to provide selections from any outside commercial vendors—not that she would anyway. Mary is one of America's preeminent and most passionate advocates of self-operation and self-sufficiency for child nutrition programs, and that philosophy is also very much a part of her marketing plan at Wilde Lake. "Our program has its own identity and needs to keep it," she says. "I think we can do it better than vendors from commercial restaurants can anyway."

Who needs outside vendors? The many food options give Wilde Lake's customers—kids and teachers alike—tremendous freedom to "design" their own meals, much like the range of choices the kids will find when they get to college, maybe even better. "Our school system is composed of highly motivated educators and highly motivated kids," Mary said. "If we really believe that nutrition promotes health, that nutrition promotes learning—and in Howard County, we really do believe that—then we have to do something to make that philosophy work, and that means giving the kids choices and allowing them to act like adults in a college-like environment. That's where they're headed, so let's get them prepped for it, even in the lunchroom."

Of course, *some* limits need to be imposed on behavior—Mary strives to treat all of the students at Wilde Lake like adults, but, after all, they *are* teenagers. Theft, eating on the line, and line-cutting are the major behavior problems that can plague a scatter system. The trick to avoiding these problems, Mary says, is to build deterrence of these behaviors into the concept—and to work closely with building administrators so that such behaviors are discouraged without the need to resort to heavy-handed discipline. Thus, her customers at Wilde Lake are allowed into the service area in staggered groups of no more than about 50; as the current group moves to the registers, the next group is allowed to enter. No bookbags or jackets are allowed. All students in the service area must carry a tray. And all à la carte items are behind the cash registers. On the rare occasions when theft is spotted, the employee does not confront the offender, but turns the matter over to the principal, with whom Mary has established clear lines of responsibility for enforcement. These protocols deter negative behavior without requiring Mary's staff to act as cops.

The staff consists of eight employees, who not only prepare and serve all of the meals at Wilde Lake, but at three satellite schools as well. Actually, there is a ninth employee—Mary herself, whose office is close by and who serves as the "permanent substitute" at Wilde Lake. Her willingness to pitch in gives her crucial credibility with the staff and high visibility with the students. Her regular presence there also allows her to monitor the progress of her prized scatter system concept. And perhaps most crucially, she knows (and communicates regularly with) everyone else in the building, too—from the principal right down to the custodians.

So far, Mary's painstaking communications habits have helped deliver substantial bottom-line results at Wilde Lake. The Maryland counties that serve as bedroom communities for Washington, D.C.—in particular, Howard and Montgomery counties—are notoriously hard nuts to crack when it comes to high school participation. The kids are as sophisticated as anywhere in the country; they're largely well off, and they have exceptionally refined and experienced palates for high-schoolers. Many traditional area high school cafeterias languish at 20 to 30 percent participation, and the old Wilde Lake school (which the new school replaced) was no exception, serving barely 300 of its 1,300-plus students on an average day, or about 22 percent. The new scatter system, by contrast, is attracting 550 full-meal customers a day, better than 40 percent of the total enrollment, and 83 percent more than in the old building. That's just below the statewide participation average for all schools, elementary and secondary.

Mary's approach at Wilde Lake had to be every bit as sophisticated as her customers. She applied her college-eatery concept to every phase of her marketing plan for the new cafeteria, and her commitment to that concept and that plan has paid off dramatically. But Mary and her food service operation could never have realized this level of success—at Wilde Lake or elsewhere in Howard County—if Mary had not understood, from the outset, the need for good communication with her administrators. She made her vision for Wilde Lake an organic part of her administration's vision for the county's educational system as a whole, and she made sure that the building staff at Wilde Lake appreciated the advantages that the new system would provide to *them*, with the result that she was allowed to design and execute her plans the way she wanted to, with a minimum of nay-saying from above or opposition from staff at the building.

REFERENCES

1. H.E.R., Uyterhoeven, "General Managers in the Middle." *Harvard Business Review.* 50, no. 2 (1972): 75–85.

2. American School Food Service Association, *Keys to Excellence: Standards of Practice for Nutrition Integrity* (Alexandria, VA: 1995).

3. D. H. Carr et al., *Competencies, Knowledge and Skills of Effective District School Nutrition Directors/Supervisors* (University, MS: National Food Service Management Institute, 1996).

4. *Random House Dictionary of the English Language,* 2nd ed. unabridged (New York: Random House, 1987).

5. J.J. Gabarro, and J.P. Kotter, "Managing Your Boss," *Harvard Business Review 58,* no. 1 (1980): 92–100.

6. T. Simons, "Executive Conflict Management: Keys to Excellent Decision and Smooth Implementation," *Cornell Hotel & Restaurant Administration Quarterly,* December 1996, 34–41.

7. Gabaro and Kotter, "Managing Your Boss."

8. J.S. Fielden, "What Do You Mean You Don't Like My Style?," in *People: Managing Your Most Important Asset* (Boston: Harvard Business Review,1986).

9. J. Fielden, "What Do You Mean I Can't Write?," in *Business Classics: Fifteen Key Concepts for Managerial Success* (Boston: Harvard Business Review, 1986).

10. Fielden, "What Do You Mean You Don't Like My Style?"

11. Gabarro and Carter; "Managing Your Boss."

12. A. Fink, *Conducting Research Literature Reviews* (Thousand Oaks, CA: Sage Publications, 1998).

13. J.T. Johnson, "Statistical Measures: You Can't Measure Your Weight with a Yardstick," in *Recipes for Practical Research in Child Nutrition Programs,* ed. M. Conklin et al. (University, MS: National Food Service Management Institute, 1998).

14. M.K. Meyer, "Why Should CNP Professionals Ask Students for Their Written Opinions?," in *Recipes for Practical Research in Child Nutrition Programs,* ed. M. Conklin et al. (University, MS: National Food Service Management Institute; 1998).

15. D.A. Dillman, *"Mail and Telephone Surveys: The Total Design Method"* (New York: John Wiley & Sons, 1978).

16. A. Fink, *The Survey Handbook* (Thousand Oaks, CA: Sage Publications, 1995).

17. F.F. Fowler, *Survey Research Methods* (Thousand Oaks, CA: Sage Publications, 1993).

18. Meyer, "Why Should CNP Professionals Ask Students?"

19. D.L. Morgan, *The Focus Group Guidebook* (Thousand Oaks, CA: Sage Publications,1998).

20. R.A. Kreuger, *Focus Groups* (Thousand Oaks, CA: Sage Publications, 1994).

21. J. Cater and L. Lambert, "Focus Groups," In *Recipes for Practical Research in Child Nutrition Programs,* ed. M. Conklin et al. (University, MS: National Food Service Management Institute, 1998).

22. D.L. Morgan, *Planning Focus Groups* (Thousand Oaks, CA: Sage Publications, 1998).

23. R.A. Krueger, *Developing Questions for Focus Groups* (Thousand Oaks, CA: Sage Publications, 1998).

24. Morgan, *The Focus Group Guidebook.*

25. R.A. Krueger, *Moderating Focus Groups* (Thousand Oaks, CA: Sage Publications, 1998).

26. Carter and Lambert, "Focus Groups."

27. R.A. Krueger, *Analyzing and Reporting Focus Group Results* (Thousand Oaks, CA: Sage Publications, 1998).

28. C.E. Bogan and M.J. English, *Benchmarking for Best Practices: Winning through Innovative Adaptation* (New York: McGraw-Hill, 1994).

29. H.K. Brelin, "Benchmarking: The Change Agent," *Marketing Management* 2, no. 3 (1993): 32–43.

30 Bogan and English, *Benchmarking for Best Practices.*

31. P.H. Rossi and H.E. Freeman, *Evaluation: A Systematic Approach,* 5th ed. (Newbury Park, CA: Sage Publications, 1993).

32. M.T. Conklin, "Productivity and Cost-Effectiveness in Nutrition Services, *Nutrition Assessment: A Comprehensive Guide for Planning Intervention,* 2nd ed., (Gaithersburg, MD: Aspen Publishers, Inc., 1995).

33. Rossi and Freeman, *Evaluation.*

34. H.M. Levin, *Cost-Effectiveness: A Primer* (Beverly Hills, CA: Sage Publications, 1983).

35. D.J. Whalen, *I See What You Mean: Persuasive Business Communication* (Thousand Oaks, CA: Sage Publications, 1996).

36. E. Raudsepp, "Body Language Speaks Louder," *Machine Design* 65 (1993): 85–88.

37. Whalen, *I See What You Mean.*

38. R. Anthony, *Talking to the Top: Executive's Guide for Career-Making Presentations* (Englewood Cliffs, NJ: Prentice Hall, 1995.)

39. Whalen, *I See What You Mean.*

CHAPTER 22

Community Relations

Ruth W. Gordon

OUTLINE

INTRODUCTION

To paraphrase the quote, "It takes a village to raise a child," it takes a community to help a school food and nutrition program meet its goal of helping children develop healthy lifelong eating habits. Positive community relations is the result of open communications and is crucial to effective marketing of the school food and nutrition program. Child nutrition programs do not operate in a vacuum. Don Barr has been quoted as saying that establishing "power with" relationships, with community collaborators and the families we seek to serve, versus a "power over" relationship is critical to developing successful community relations.[1(p.55)]

Parents, industry, allied health groups, extension leaders, physicians, and dietitians in the community are interested in the decisions made to provide services for children. They feel some ownership of the program since the health and education of children in their community are affected. By funding the program these stakeholders also have taken a financial risk. They want to know how the program is being operated and contribute to decisions that are being made.

Key processes in proactive community relations include communicating, networking, marketing, involving stakeholders, and resolving potential conflicts. To have the support necessary for a profitable, successful program, school food and nutrition personnel must establish close working relationships with numerous groups within the community. Community advocates who recognize the benefits of the program and "speak out" for the school food and nutrition program become even more important as threats of budget cuts and privatization become greater. This chapter will focus on networking with community stakeholders and involving parents. Possible ways to extend the school food and nutrition program into the community will also be introduced. Specific objectives of this chapter are to accomplish the following:

- Define selected terms related to community relations.
- Identify people, groups, and organizations that are most likely to be community stakeholders in the school food and nutrition program.
- Explain why the school food and nutrition program must address community relations and parent involvement.
- List the risks and benefits of networking with other groups to achieve the school food and nutrition program's mission.
- Identify appropriate steps to take and strategies to use to involve parents and the community in the school food and nutrition program.
- Solicit support for the school food and nutrition program by extending the program into the community.
- Describe the role of the school food and nutrition program during a disaster.
- Evaluate the community relations aspect of a school food and nutrition program by applying a checklist of indicators.

Definitions

- *Coalitions* are groups of people or organizations that have joined together for a specific purpose.
- *Collaboration* is a mutually beneficial and well-defined relationship entered into by two or more organizations to achieve common goals.
- *Community relations* are dealings between people who live in a particular area or district and the school or school food and nutrition program.
- *Networking* in educational settings involves creating a linkage structure deliberately to help participants solve identified problems.
- *Partnerships* are relationships with other people or groups participating in a particular effort or team.
- *Stakeholder* is anyone who has a vested interest in an organization or program.

NETWORKING WITH COMMUNITY STAKEHOLDERS

Who Are Community Stakeholders?

To identify community stakeholders of the school food and nutrition program, reflect on its history. The program was established to serve a health and military need experienced by the nation. Many agricultural and industry groups such as the Peanut Commission or Dairy Council have supported the school food and nutrition program throughout its more than 50 years of existence. Schools have provided a market for excess commodities so that the federal government can stabilize the price of selected agricultural items for farmers while providing nutritious foods for children. Manufacturers and distributors of foods, equipment, and paper and cleaning supplies have also been supportive. These individuals and groups are stakeholders in the program.

Taxpayers fund the program through the votes of legislators, so they are also stakeholders. When they pay for the program, taxpayers expect positive results. They expect the program to offer healthful, low-cost meals that enable students to achieve academically and grow and develop physically. Throughout the program's existence taxpayers have increased their expectations. The interpretation of "protecting the health and well-being of the nation's children" has changed from preventing malnutrition to preventing overconsumption and promoting a healthy lifestyle.[2(p4)] Civic organizations and churches are stakeholders of the program because of their common interest in serving the needy. The school food and nutrition program serves as a safety net to prevent hunger and malnutrition for our nation's neediest children. When concern about fraud and abuse of government programs became widespread, the school food and nutrition program withstood the taxpayers' scrutiny.

As the impact of eating habits on the medical needs and health care costs of this nation has been recognized, the school food and nutri-

tion program has gained increased attention from allied health groups. The publication by the Centers for Disease Control and Prevention (CDC), *Guidelines for School Health Programs to Promote Lifelong Healthy Eating,* issued in 1996, states that "School-based programs can play an important role in promoting lifelong healthy eating. Because dietary factors 'contribute substantially to the burden of preventable illness and premature death in the United States,' the national health promotion and disease prevention objectives encourage schools to provide nutrition education from preschool through 12th grade."[3(p.1)] Stakeholders committed to the program for this reason might include members of coordinated school health committees and local chapters of organizations such as the American Cancer Society and the American Heart Association.

A stakeholder is anyone with a vested interest in the program who will suffer if the program fails. Compare these stakeholders with stockholders of a corporation. Losses and gains affect both stockholders and stakeholders. Other stakeholders include physicians and dietitians, home economists, public health nutritionists, and extension agents. Educators, parents, and members of the community at large are also stakeholders. Teachers, especially health and physical education teachers, and educational administrators have much to lose if children are hungry and unable to concentrate on content being taught in the classroom. The establishment of collaborative networks between all of these stakeholders who are committed to the best possible future for children in this nation can benefit the program. Networking for successful community relations requires conceptual, organizational, and communication skills.

Rationale for Networking with Community Stakeholders

Community relations is not a new concept for child nutrition programs. From the very beginning, school food and nutrition leaders realized that child nutrition problems could not be solved alone. In 1938 Mary DeGarmo Bryan wrote about the relationship between the cafeteria and the community and reported that attempts to carry the educational benefits of the cafeteria into the community were meeting with success. She described many activities that are still being conducted today, such as inviting parents to eat with their children, sending menus home or publishing them in the local newspaper, and urging mothers to attend lectures and exhibits. Mary DeGarmo Bryan projected that the lessons learned at school would carry over into improved feeding at home.[4]

During the 1990s resources and governmental budgets cuts played a significant role in the formation of coalitions, collaborations, partnerships, and networking for the purposes of survival and continuing services. Partnerships and collaborations help organizations fulfill their public responsibilities, achieve mutual benefits, obtain customer feedback, improve the quality of programs and services, and increase effectiveness.[5] Although coordination and collaboration is important to improving the quality of the school food and nutrition program, studies have shown that program collaboration is higher at the state and district level but drops at the school level.[6]

Benefits of Networking

Fulfill Public Responsibility

Each citizen has some responsibility for the environment in which he or she lives. Today's society expects citizens to actively shape public affairs. Interest in volunteerism is growing. The federal government has initiated a grant program, Learn and Serve America, to support this effort in schools. Schools are incorporating civic responsibility and community service into the curricula. If citizens fulfill this role, then school food and nutrition program directors and managers must possess an openness and a willingness to involve them as partners

in the program and its activities. In fact, the program belongs to them. School food and nutrition personnel's obligation is to operate the program in accordance with the laws and regulations legislated by their representatives. The coveted Malcolm Baldrige National Quality Award assesses public responsibility as one criterion when businesses are judged for this award. They ask companies to determine how their policies and procedures address health, safety, and environmental issues. If companies encourage employees to promote quality in the community to external organizations, they earn more points during this evaluation. Likewise, if school food and nutrition programs are to be quality programs they must address the needs of the environment outside the school and the effect the program has on the public's health, safety, and environment.

Achieve Mutual Benefit

Competition rather than cooperation reigns throughout American society. The fourth habit in Stephen Covey's book, The 7 Habits of Highly Effective People, is "Think Win-Win" to seek mutual benefit.[7] When working in cooperation with others, it must be as important for our partners to achieve their goals as it is to reach the program's goals. Do not approach relationships with a fear of scarcity and a mindset that says, since there are so few resources for so many demands, when a partner gets something the school food and nutrition program loses. Covey's sixth habit is "Synergize" for creative cooperation. This habit explains how the whole can be greater than the sum of its parts. Synergy means that working together in networks or partnerships achieves greater outcomes than if each partner worked alone and the outcomes were added together.

Covey's 1991 book, Principle-Centered Leadership asserts that organizations such as schools or school food and nutrition programs are ecological systems.[8] The systems view of organizations recognizes that all parts of the organization, including the people and the networks, affect all the other parts. Each entity makes a unique contribution. In many situations, school food and nutrition personnel have tried to manage without "bothering" school administrators, superintendents, or board members. When doing so, they have not been aware of how program decisions, such as the number of menu choices, affect the rest of the educational setting. Conversely, educational administrators have not been aware of how decisions, such as scheduling or fundraising, affect the goal and mission of the school food and nutrition program. As pointed out in Chapter 1, looking at the school as a system helps staff recognize that their actions affect another person's or program's goals (see Exhibit 22–1).

Systems need a way to collect information from all stakeholders. By participating in a collaborative network, school food and nutrition personnel can observe the people involved in the network, and learn more about their perceptions, motivations, values, and habits. They can learn more about the formal organization, including the structure, policies and procedures, physical environment, and the technology used to manage the services provided. Also they can see the informal organization or culture emerging from the interaction between the school food and nutrition program and the other members of the network or community. When the staff has this information, they should be able to see a more balanced picture and make better decisions.

Commitment to quality pertains not only to the products and services but also to the quality of networks and relationships established. For example, the Children's Nutrition Network is a group of partners from the public, private, corporate, health, and education segments of society that can help any organization in Canada interested in establishing a nutrition program for children. School food and nutrition leaders must continually build good will and negotiate in good faith. Directors, managers, and assistants must make deposits into the "emotional bank accounts" of others. Depending on personality type and leadership style, some people might have to work harder at this than others. When groups or departments break down barriers, interpersonal effectiveness improves and partnerships evolve to address the needs and wants of customers. When this happens, expectations of stakeholders are ultimately addressed. This type of communication requires a level of trust.

Obtain Customer Feedback

Covey advises readers to "Seek first to understand before being understood."[9] Quality begins with understanding stakeholders' needs and expectations. Peters and Waterman in *In Search of Excellence* revealed that one of the eight attributes of America's most successful companies was their ability to stay close to the customer.[10] They defined excellent companies as better listeners. School food and nutrition personnel can get others to understand their needs if they care enough to try to understand those of stakeholders first. Once they understand their needs and expectations employees must work to meet or exceed those expectations.

The desire to provide service and quality through innovative problem solving in order to serve customers effectively demands an external focus. When an organization or school food and nutrition program focuses on the needs of stakeholders from the external environment, it is more likely to adapt to the community's needs than competitors who do not address the external environment. School food and nutrition leaders do not necessarily have to conceptualize innovative ideas for customer satisfaction. Many innovations in excellent companies come from suggestions to improve products or services already existing in the market. Listen to stakeholders and use or modify ideas introduced by competitors to beat them at their own game. A school food and nutrition program director in south Georgia received recognition for supporting the educational goals of the school by modifying a business model to offer incentives to elementary students for reading books.

Exhibit 22–1 The Educator's Checklist

Educators can facilitate nutrition education and help students develop good eating habits by taking some of the following actions to support the efforts of the school food and nutrition program. See how many ways you actively embrace the school food and nutrition program. Do you:

Eat the meals served in the cafeteria?
Try new foods occasionally?
Try familiar foods prepared in new ways?
Eat with your students?
Balance your food selections to be sure that they include a wide variety of foods in the Food Guide Pyramid?
Avoid eating too many salty foods, fried and fatty foods, and sweets?
Encourage administration to develop policies that prohibit or limit other foods from being sold before or during meal periods?
Make positive comments about the cafeteria, the food, and the staff?
Know the policies that affect what types, the amounts, and the times that foods are served in the cafeteria?
Encourage your peers to be positive about the food in the cafeteria and the staff?
Consider nutrition when planning student parties, snacks, and refreshments for meetings?
Avoid using food to reward or bribe children?
Post cafeteria menus in your classroom?
Make sure that students and parents know what foods are being served in the cafeteria?
Use examples from the cafeteria as ways to illustrate concepts being taught in the classroom?
Know if the students in your class eat lunch or what they bring from home?
Arrange for students to discover the health risks of skipping meals and having poor eating habits, as part of your class?
Know the members of the cafeteria staff?
Invite the manager to present information related to meal preparation as it is relevant to educational concepts taught in the classroom?
Invite family members to eat with their students in the cafeteria?
Assist the manager by preparing bulletin boards, table tents, or other needed items for special events and promotions?

In a previous era, businesses operated from the concept that one size fits all. Given today's circumstances, this approach no longer works. Futurists predict that tomorrow's successful corporations and businesses will customize their products and services to meet the individual needs of customers even more than they do today. School food and nutrition programs striving to excel must further identify ways to individualize their products or services. Many schools are already offering a multitude of menu choices. One program marketed its ability to cater birthday parties for customers!

The prestigious Malcolm Baldridge National Quality Award recognizes the significance of customer focus and satisfaction by assigning more weight to this area than any other.[11] Businesses applying for this award must assess how they manage their relationships with customers. To remain competitive school organizations and structures must recognize students and their parents as customers. Meeting customers' wants as well as their needs is critical if the program is going to be successful. Managing relationships with customers is equally important to effective school food and nutrition programs. For more information on communicating with students, refer to Chapter 20.

Improve Total Quality

Unleash the power of collaborative efforts and partnerships to improve the quality of services the school food and nutrition program provides. School food and nutrition programs should adopt the slogan of a popular retail store, "Quality you want, prices you need." Schools are under tremendous pressure to improve students' academic performance. School food and nutrition programs can make a definite contribution to help meet this challenge. Interagency and intra-agency relationships can have an important bearing upon customers. These relationships may have to be formed, nurtured, or improved to facilitate the service necessary for customer satisfaction.

How can a school food and nutrition program director know if schools in a district are operating excellent or mediocre programs? The director may apply standards for program assessment and improvement. Organizations such as the U.S. Department of Agriculture (USDA), the American School Food Service Association (ASFSA), state school food service associations, and state departments of education have developed standards for this purpose. USDA has established national program standards that include nutrient standards legislated as part of the Healthy School Meals Initiative. The ASFSA has published *Keys to Excellence* to serve as national standards. [12] State agencies could set standards at the state level. The Georgia Department of Education's School and Community Nutrition Program released *Quality Measures for Georgia's School Nutrition Program* as nonbinding characteristics of quality in 1997.[13] Many times standards set at federal or state levels are minimal because the needs of local districts are so varied. School food and nutrition program directors and school administrators should review existing standards and propose the ones that they want to adopt to their local school board.

Standards adopted represent the desired level of quality. Each school or school system will need to set a goal of where it wants to rank on the continuum of implementation. For example, if the standard is to post sanitation scores in a predominant location, the local school or school system will have to decide whether to meet this standard at the lowest or optimal level. Is it acceptable to tape the sanitation report up on the wall in the kitchen or should it be framed and hung attractively so that it can be seen by the customers waiting in line? Some directors might determine standards in isolation, but community support will be much greater if they seek input from managers, assistants, parents, faculty, and other members of the community. This collaborative effort might take longer but it will pay off in the long run.

Another way to improve the quality of the program is to network with community stakeholders in the development of product specifications. Stakeholders can help determine which branded products to purchase and offer on menus. One school system invites educators and parent leaders to an afternoon tasting session to complete an evaluation form on each product that might be introduced into the school menu. What a wonderful way for a school food and nutrition program director to communicate to citizens in the community that their expectations about the quality of the food served at school will be considered!

Sometimes school food and nutrition personnel avoid involving others or gathering data about performance because they care too much or are too vulnerable to criticism of their work, service, or product. It's no secret that people often prefer to live in a protected niche where they can function with an acceptable error margin. To compete in today's society, improvement of performance must be continual. As competitors increase their quality and service, school food and nutrition personnel must take similar actions. In an atmosphere of continuous quality improvement, quality continues to spiral upward. Protecting egos of those involved in directing, managing, and implementing the program is not adequate justification for jeopardizing the program's future existence.

Communities will be much more powerful when they reflect a coordinated approach to schooling their children. The 1994 reauthorization of the Elementary and Secondary Education Act called for the strengthening of parental involvement in order to address Goals 2000.[14] *Turning Points,* the Carnegie Foundations' report on improving middle school performance indicates that parents should be involved in meaningful ways in the educational program. School food and nutrition programs will become a part of this movement when the community feels ownership of the program and are involved in meaningful ways. Proactive school food and nutrition leaders involve potential partners and stakeholders in program decisions. They reach out to the community and tell others of the need for support and assistance.

Increase Effectiveness

Networking intensifies efforts to achieve the school food and nutrition program's mission in cost-effective, efficient ways. Sharing the program's resources with more people usually results in having access to a greater range of resources. For example, the 5 A Day campaign is stronger because retail grocers, food stamp offices, public health nutritionists, schools, and extension agents worked together to coordinate the message and the timing of its delivery. Networking facilitates a more effective use of available staff time from the collaborating organizations on innovative projects. Networking can help identify inconsistency of efforts and prevent unnecessary duplication of services. Coalitions of service providers have even increased opportunities to play increasingly larger roles in developing policies and programs affecting youth. Materials funded by the Nutrition Education and Training (NET) Program might be appropriate for preschoolers waiting in Women, Infants and Children (WIC)

clinics or for children of food stamp recipients. When program managers coordinate efforts to meet local needs, they can have a greater effect on the populations served. Networking can help facilitate further research into areas such as child health or nutrition education and can result in consolidated reporting to funding sources.

Opening schools to communities facilitates a dynamic exchange of resources and information when functional networks or coalitions are created. For example, partnerships with local businesses have provided increased resources to schools. School food and nutrition programs that investigate ways to benefit from school and business partnerships flourish instead of letting these partnerships impinge on the program's operations. Increased social complexity and the demand for immediate decisions in the midst of insecurity and conflicting values have contributed to the decentralization being experienced in today's schools as site-based management. Expansion of school site-based management makes the establishment of functional networks at the school level even more important and critical to a successful school food and nutrition program.

Risks of Networking

Networking with other groups and organizations is not without the drawbacks and risks, as follows:

- More time is required from each partner for coordination and communication. Time is needed to place phone calls, send E-mail messages, type and distribute memoranda or meeting minutes, and attend meetings.
- Partners might have different standards of success or failure. The cooperating agencies might not be able to support fully some of the decisions made by the coalition. Participation in the network implies endorsement and approval of all outcomes.

• Partners might fear loss of control of the project. Losing control of decision making or control of one's own data is a major obstacle to networking.

• There is always the potential development of conflicts whenever a decision is being made. Each partner has specific reasons for choosing to be part of the network or coalition. Sometimes these reasons may be in opposition with others'.

• Motivations of some members of the network may be questionable. There may be interpersonal conflicts based on the personality types involved. This may be especially true if one member is domineering, commands all of the meeting time, or tries to claim credit for the work being done by the coalition members.

Steps in Networking

1. Choose partners with a similar vision. Partnerships work best when members share common beliefs and interests. Developing a shared vision or mission helps build commitment to the collaborative effort. Without a common mission and values there is nothing to motivate people beyond self-interest. Ford Motor Company had a vision of public transportation for the masses. Polaroid had the vision of instant photography. What might be a common vision for a group of organizations that are health based? What might this vision be if they are education based? According to Peter Senge in *The Fifth Discipline*, developing this shared vision begins to create a sense of trust that comes from sharing our highest aspirations or picture of the future.[15] A shared vision undermines the internal politics of the group.

2. State needs and expectations to determine a common mission. Conduct a needs assessment of the customers and stakeholders. Determine the problem or goal to be addressed. Share the results of the needs assessment. Let representatives from the groups involved share in the decision making to address identified needs.

3. Delineate distinct roles and functions. Successful networks have established positive administrative support, especially in the lead organizations involved. Be flexible. Don't be too concerned about who gets the credit for the activities of the coalition. Activities within collaborative efforts might be parallel, cooperative, or integrated.

4. Establish open, clear communication channels. Decrease the use of jargon. Encourage participation and openness. Nothing undermines openness more than members of the groups' being too sure of themselves. Members of the group must be willing to look inward, challenge their own thinking, and realize that their ideas are always subject to error and improvement.

5. Commit to group decisions. Commitment by all members of the network to decisions made is critical to the proper functioning of the group. Attitudes toward other agencies are most important. Establish a culture for the group. Build a sense of community.

6. Plan and implement realistic projects. Integrate planning. Match existing resources to identified needs. Empower the network with permission, time, and capabilities to create change.

7. Evaluate the results and improve future endeavors. During the planning stages determine how to evaluate the results. Share the results with all involved groups and their decision makers. Debrief all involved members and document changes to use the next time a similar effort is undertaken.

Networking Strategies

Only time and imagination limit opportunities and ways to network with others. Remember that organizations or, in this case, programs exist to fulfill external needs. There is no way to learn how stakeholders define these needs without asking them. Needs assessment is a natural place to begin networking. Involving stakeholders can help to learn more about the changing demographics of the community. Surveys and focus groups open doors for networking on future activities. Networking might also be particularly helpful for information retrieval and dissemination, program evaluation, and nutrition education and training.

Networking strategies do not necessarily have to be original. In fact, many times successful corporations learn and benefit from the successes and failures of their competitors. What networking ideas can be gleaned from competitors? What is innovative in one school or school system may have been in place for years at another location. Innovative approaches include the establishment of advisory groups and the use of focus groups. A school health coordinating committee might advise a local school system on the development of policies governing the selling of competitive foods or scheduling of meal periods.[16]

Participating in networking opportunities facilitates telling others in the community about the benefits of the school food and nutrition program and its services. School decentralization, sometimes referred to as site-based management, provides additional networking opportunities with local school and community leaders.

Partners might help identify ways to increase participation in the lunch program or assist with special events such as National Nutrition Month. Should the school food and nutrition program have a customer satisfaction guarantee? Involve stakeholders in measuring the program's share of the market and evaluating the quality of products and services provided by the program. Track trends over a period of years. Cooperative extension service may be a helpful partner when addressing nutrition education, training, and technical assistance for students, teachers, parents, or even

staff. Members of the network might conduct taste tests with students or present sessions about the program to a local civic organization. They might volunteer to teach employees about a job-related subject or suggest how to obtain free or low-cost resources that will reinforce employee training.

During the mid-1990s USDA led a national Team Nutrition initiative by creating innovative public and private partnerships to improve food choices of children that involved the media, schools, families, and the community. Schools signed up to indicate that they were making an effort to comply with the Dietary Guidelines for Americans. Nutrition education kits were developed and sold by Scholastic, and the services of Disney were solicited to produce public service announcements. USDA distributed a *Community Nutrition Action Kit* to support community institutions in their efforts to create and sustain a healthful environment to influence children's attitudes and behaviors about food.[17]

It is important to have an open door policy. Be available to members of the community to receive comments. Do not become defensive. Be willing to listen to suggestions. One school district in Georgia used NET Program grant funds to pilot a phone hotline. Parents and members of the community could call for the week's menus or facts on selected nutrition topics or to leave suggestions for program improvement. Another local school food and nutrition program director tells about a parent who demanded that her child's favorite menu item be served in the cafeteria. She invited the mother to submit the recipe and to be present the day it was prepared, just to be sure the recipe was prepared correctly. The parent was appalled to learn that the children in the school did not choose the food item, nor did those children who chose it eat it. She became much more supportive of the employees in the cafeteria after having this experience.

Consider other strategies such as the development and use of a mascot, such as Rudy the Raccoon or Crunchy Critter. These mascots make appearances at school carnivals and ride on floats in community parades. In the mid-1990s USDA, through Team Nutrition funds, negotiated an arrangement with Walt Disney to use two of the characters from the hit movie, *The Lion King,* to promote good nutrition. Messages such as "School Meals Build Healthy Student Bodies" have been posted on billboards throughout the state of Alabama. County fairs, health fairs, mall exhibits, and special community events offer even more opportunities to network with community stakeholders and result in improving the program's image.

PARENT INVOLVEMENT

Rationale

Parent involvement has always been an important part of the National School Lunch Program. Under the direction of the Committee on Hygiene of the Home and School Association, an elementary school in Boston served the first school luncheon in 1910. In 1938 Mary De-Garmo Bryan wrote that a great variety of persons was responsible for the development of school lunches including Parent-Teacher Associations (PTAs). She went on to write that menu planners should consider the meals apt to be served at home. The dietary habits of the community must be taken into account. "This is usually a simple matter providing that the manager is in close touch as she should be, with the mothers of the children in the school."[18(p205)] This seems to coincide with Peters and Waterman's more recent research to stay close to the customer. Federal regulations governing the child nutrition programs (7 C.F.R. 210.12) require a student, parent, and community involvement component.[19]

When a parent or the child's primary caregiver takes an active role in the child's education, it makes a difference in academic success. According to Pat Henry, a former national PTA president, more than 50 studies demonstrate that the more a parent participates in a child's education, the higher the child's achievement will be. Nationally, the Household Education Survey includes information on parent involvement.[20] The results of this survey revealed that parent involvement varies by the age of the child. Parents get more involved when the children are in elementary school. Parent involvement is also greater among parents with higher education and income levels. Increasing rates of poverty, divorce, single parenting, teen pregnancy, family mobility and instability, and employment by women outside the home have made parent involvement in schools more difficult while the need is even greater.

Parents are busy and may be hard to reach. A study done in 1989 in North Dakota reported that the parents of fourth graders considered nutrition important. They wanted children to read and understand labels, make choices in restaurants, read a recipe, make their own lunch, and choose their own snacks. They preferred nutrition interventions, such as nutrition information sheets to post on the refrigerator, which could be used in their homes, instead of attending evening meetings.[21]

Additional research has shown that parents affect the health behaviors of children. Children learn what is important by listening and watching adults. There is a more formal "what we say" method of teaching children and a less formal "what we do" method.[22] In order to help children develop healthy eating habits that will last a lifetime, messages about healthful foods must be consistent. It's important to remember that people are working toward the same goal: they want to do what is best for the children they serve. Sometimes they don't agree on how to progress toward the goal. With good communication, they can begin to see each other's perspective (see Exhibit 22–2).

Child nutrition programs should welcome parent involvement at any one of three levels. Parents or caregivers can become involved in education through directly assisting with school management and by being present in

Exhibit 22–2 The Parents' Checklist

Parents' attitudes about school meals can influence how students perceive their school food and nutrition program. As a parent, do you:

Know what menus are being served at your child's school?
Know how the foods are prepared (i.e., french fries may be baked rather than fried)?
Know what foods your child selected?
Know how much of the food the child left on his or her tray?
Know why they may not be buying or eating the school meals?
Express your interest in nutrition to the teacher and school principal?
Volunteer to serve on menu-planning committees or to help in the cafeteria during promotions or
   special events?
Set a positive example by eating a wide variety of foods from the Food Guide Pyramid yourself?
Serve healthful meals at home?
Avoid using foods as a reward or a bribe?
Make positive comments about the school food and nutrition program?
Visit the cafeteria and eat meals with your child?
Know if there is adequate adult supervision of students in the cafeteria during meal periods to help
   open packages, especially when children are very young?
Know what time the meals are served and why?
Know how long students have to eat their meals and why?
Discuss the food choices with your child?
Encourage your child to make low-fat, healthy food selections, including fruits and vegetables?
Send healthful low-fat snacks to school with your child?
Encourage your child to try new foods prepared in new ways?
Support policies that limit or prohibit the sales of foods that compete for your child's appetite?
Coordinate menus served at home with those served at school to avoid needless repetition?
Know the school food and nutrition manager and the cafeteria staff?

the school, through participation in special parenting training programs, and through family resource and support programs. Many schools have solicited parent support in menu planning and in selecting foods to be purchased. These are management decisions. When the school food and nutrition program manager or director makes a presentation at a parent meeting about how the menus are planned, the parent is being trained, as suggested by the second level. Working with children who medically require special dietary modifications might be considered the third family support level.

Principles of Parent Involvement

- Parent involvement is most effective when it is comprehensive and well planned.

Identify a multitude of ways parents can participate and let them choose a way. Never assume that parents know how to be involved or that they feel comfortable in doing so. See Exhibit 22–3 for an outline of organizational procedures.[23]
- Reach a common understanding about the form parent involvement will take. Parent involvement should be developmental and preventive, rather than remedial (see Exhibit 22–4).
- Develop ways to let involved parents represent others (see Exhibit 22–5).
- Parents should participate K–12, not just during the early years of education (see Exhibit 22–6).
- Include all parents, including those parents who are hardest to reach. Parents do

Exhibit 22–3 Organizational Procedures

A nutrition volunteer program should not just evolve. There should be careful planning to set policy, establish objectives, and develop monitoring procedures. A planning committee should be established to provide direction to and supervision of the program.

Any one of the following people could initiate a program:

- Principal/Assistant Principal
- Volunteer Coordinator, District/School
- PTA Representative
- Elementary/Secondary Curriculum Director
- Nutrition Education Teaching Coordinator
- Nutrition Advisory Council
- School Advisory Committee
- School Food and Nutrition Program District Director
- Administrator/School Manager

The steps listed below should be considered when starting or complementing a nutrition volunteer program:

Step 1: Research the existence of any nutrition programs in the school or district. Coordinate efforts through a comprehensive school health committee. Any new developments should enhance these nutrition programs.

Step 2: Develop an organizational committee. The people listed above would be potential members.

Step 3: Secure approval from the school administrator before proceeding.

Step 4: Select a volunteer coordinator to provide guidance and daily direction to the volunteers.

Step 5: Formulate a startup plan.

Source: Reprinted with permission from Georgia Parent Teachers Association and Georgia Nutrition Education and Training Program, *Nutrition Education: A Comprehensive Guide for Better Student Health*, p. 6, © 1995, Georgia Department of Education.

not have to be well educated or financially independent to make a difference. Respect cultural diversity.

- Recognize parents as the child's first teacher. Establish opportunities for parents to learn the value of role modeling. Stress that what they do will be more important than what they say. Try giving them a self-assessment to let them check themselves to see if they are being supportive.
- Establish open, democratic, participatory functional relationships with parents. Begin conversations with use of "I" in sentences to convey feelings, instead of "you" words that make the other person defensive.
- Ensure that there is a two-way exchange of information.
- Listen more than talk.

Strategies for Parent Involvement

- Learn what parents need and expect from the school's food and nutrition program.
- Communicate the vision of the program to them. Explain why and how the staff keep meal costs so reasonable.
- Use networking skills to make nutrition an integral part of all parent meetings, fundraising events, and school-related activities. For example, refreshments served at meetings should be nutritious. Help plan the menus for parent dinners or the school carnival. Pretzels or popcorn might be healthier offerings than chips!
- Post the menus. Get menus published in the school or local newspaper and send them home to parents.

Exhibit 22–4 Introduction to Planning the Program

The ultimate success of any volunteer program depends upon the foundation on which it is built. The foundation for a nutrition volunteer program is formed during the planning process. A solid plan establishes direction, clarifies expectations, provides a blueprint, focuses needs, and helps to target costs. The following planning categories are offered as suggested steps. As a plan to start a program is developed, or if it is built on one that already exists, the list below may be beneficial.

Planning the Program

Beginning

- Write program goals and objectives.
- Design volunteer job descriptions.
- Coordinate schedules.
- Set policies and procedures.

Recruitment

- Target the potential volunteers.
- Develop recruitment materials and procedures.
- Contact groups, i.e., hospital dietitians, county health department personnel and extension agents.

Interviewing and Placement

- Design application.
- Conduct interviews.
- Screen volunteers.
- Place volunteers in appropriate jobs.

Orientation and Training

- Develop an orientation and training plan.
- Provide materials and resources.
- Conduct in-service training.

Supervision

- Provide adequate supervision.
- Write standards for volunteer performance.
- Monitor compliance of standards.

Motivation and Recognition

- Provide adequate recognition.
- Enable volunteers to provide feedback.
- Promote communication between volunteers.
- Recognize schools and students as well as volunteers.
- Record keeping.
- Maintain records on each volunteer.
- Gather data on number of students reached.
- Develop a regular reporting system.
- Develop a budget to cover expenses.

Source: Reprinted with permission from Georgia Parent Teachers Association and Georgia Nutrition Education and Training Program, *Nutrition Education: A Comprehensive Guide for Better Student Health*, pp. 6–7, © 1995, Georgia Department of Education.

Exhibit 22–5 Selecting Volunteers

Volunteers for this program are similar to other volunteers who donate their time on a regular basis to work with students and make presentations in a school. Volunteers in a nutrition program can provide presentations on the value of a balanced diet. In selecting volunteers for this program, consideration should be given to people with knowledge or interest in nutrition.

Volunteers for this program should know:

- Basic nutrition principles.
- Basic information about vitamins and minerals.
- Importance of nutrition on lifelong health.
- Value of proper, balanced nutrition.
- State and local agencies offering nutritional services.
- Basic guidelines of Child Nutrition Programs.
- How to relate with students.
- How to use creative activities.
- Importance of a caring attitude toward students.
- Importance of enthusiasm and resourcefulness.

Training Volunteers

The volunteers in the nutrition volunteer program should receive an orientation to the school. They need to be familiar with the standards and procedures within the school setting and know what to do if problems arise. After an orientation to the volunteer program, ongoing training in nutrition should include these following items as its initial focus and then should progress into other areas:

- Nutrition education for primary or secondary students.
- Methods for teaching nutrition.
- Nutritional services provided by the school food service.
- Community nutrition resources.
- Audiovisual materials and software for nutrition education.
- Methods for feedback from other volunteers.
- Methods for reaching exceptional students.

Source: Reprinted with permission from Georgia Parent Teachers Association and Georgia Nutrition Education and Training Program, *Nutrition Education: A Comprehensive Guide for Better Student Health*, pp. 7–8, © 1995, Georgia Department of Education.

- Ask for parental support to get equipment or items that the cafeteria might need, such as silk plants or awnings for the serving line. Let parents help make and keep the dining area an interesting and attractive environment for students.
- Organize student and parent advisory councils. Solicit help in decorating the cafeteria for special events, posting nutrition information on bulletin boards, and reading nutritional announcements on the PA system during morning announcements. Some schools have scheduled students to read menus on local radio or television stations. Ask for help preparing and posting signs with nutrition messages or flyers for parents telling how the money they pay for the school meal is used. Post sanitation ratings and list of precautions taken to be sure food is safe to eat.
- Conduct plate waste studies to learn which foods students are not eating. Survey stu-

Exhibit 22–6 Suggested Nutrition Topics

Many possibilities exist for practical topics dealing with nutrition at each grade level. Health or nutrition fairs, nutrition exhibits in the cafeteria, nutrition awareness campaigns, or food customs of other cultures are exciting ways to teach nutrition and can be offered to students and the community. The following topics are suggestions that volunteers can use for the various grade levels:

Primary

- Foods and Growth
- Foods and Energy
- Foods and Health
- Food Guide Pyramid
- Food Tasting

Elementary

- Foods in America
- Food Processing and Transportation
- Food Labeling
- Vitamins from Foods
- Foods to Eat

Middle School

- Food Choices
- Nutrition and Sport Performance
- Appearance and Diet
- Cultural Influences on Foods
- Fast Food Facts
- Sports Nutrition

High School

- Dieting Drugs and Nutrition
- Controversial Nutrition Issues and Myths
- Planning Meals and Shopping
- Consumer Issues

Source: Reprinted with permission from Georgia Parent Teachers Association and Georgia Nutrition Education and Training Program, *Nutrition Education: A Comprehensive Guide for Better Student Health*, p. 8, © 1995, Georgia Department of Education.

dents to find out why they are not eating specific foods and then work to "fix" the problem.

- Invite parents to the cafeteria to taste and experience meals firsthand. Schedule kitchen tours and exhibits during open houses and school registration periods.

EXTENDING THE PROGRAM INTO THE COMMUNITY

School-Related Opportunities

It is not necessary to limit meals served at school to breakfast and lunch. Many schools offer extended-day or after-school programs when children need snacks. School boards, administrators, and teachers may want luncheons catered during planning sessions or meetings of professional associations. School food and nutrition program directors should embrace these opportunities to showcase the skills of the school food and nutrition staff. Extra working hours provide an opportunity for staff to earn additional dollars needed for the holidays or to offset the cost of district school food service activities, such as a trip to a national conference. Establish and follow policies and procedures so that no federal and state regulations and guidelines are violated.

Well-trained staff members also serve as excellent ambassadors for the program. Are employees proud of the meals they prepare and serve? It's surprising to learn the number of taxpayers just one employee reaches! Think of the opportunities that one might have to share opinions while at church, the hairdresser's, or the grocery store. Does Sheila talk about how the students love the food or about how students just waste the food and how she can't wait to get those monsters out of the cafeteria? Training helps employees to answer questions about the program and gives them a sense of self-assurance about the contributions they are making. It is easy to feel intimidated in an environment where the emphasis is on degrees and education. Training helps to empower the school food and nutrition staff when they are relating to other members of the school staff. Training enables them to command the respect they deserve for a job well done.

Other Programs

School food and nutrition programs aren't confined to school campuses. There are many government-funded feeding opportunities that can provide more hours of employment for staff and maximize the use of equipment and facilities. By networking with others in the community involved in nutrition and food service, opportunities such as bidding on meals for prisoners, preschool children, or the elderly are more likely to arise. During the summer, camps and recreation centers may need meals for the Summer Food Service Program. Contracting these meals can improve the image of the program in the community. It can offset some of the costs of program operation and provide funds for improvements that might not otherwise be affordable.

Special Projects

Special projects can further extend the child nutrition programs into the community. For example, a middle school in an Atlanta suburb sponsors an annual project to feed the homeless in a nearby shelter. The school food and nutrition manager works with interested seventh graders to make sandwiches and other foods needed for the meal in the school kitchen. PTA volunteers assist. Students and their parents transport the food to the homeless shelter and serve it. What a great opportunity for the students to develop insight, on a small scale, about what the school food and nutrition employees do daily! This award-winning project fulfills a community service need and provides an opportunity for parents and students to interact with the school food and nutrition manager on a meaningful project. It teaches the students civic responsibility, promotes their appreciation for services provided to them and establishes a positive public image for the school, the PTA, and the school food and nutrition program. Everyone involved in this project comes out a winner!

Activities and projects sponsored by local and district school food service associations can also affect community relations and the image of the school food and nutrition program. During the summer Olympic games in Atlanta in 1996 many school food and nutrition employees helped feed hungry visitors and athletes by working temporary jobs. Imagine the response from students and faculty when they learned that a member of their school food and nutrition staff helped feed leading athletes and political leaders from other nations! If a district association sold fresh, seasonal citrus fruits as a fund-raiser would parents and the community stakeholders perceive the program differently than if a bake sale was sponsored?

DISASTER FEEDING

School food and nutrition programs have an opportunity to demonstrate how they can benefit their communities when natural disasters strike. Beth Hanna, director of school food service in West Des Moines, Iowa, had an opportunity to do just that during the summer of 1993 when the Mississippi River and its tributary rivers flooded. So did Linda Stoll, director of Matanuska-Susitna Borough School District during 1996 when Alaska had the worst wildfire in its history.[24] (See Exhibit 22–7.)

Use of USDA Commodity Foods

Congregate feeding might be needed in the community during disasters such as hurricanes, tornadoes, and floods. According to the *Code of Federal Regulations* (7 C.F.R. 250.8), commodity foods that the USDA provides can be used for disaster feedings.[25] The state's director of commodity distribution is responsible for directing the distribution of these foods within the state during emergencies. USDA does not specifically designate foods for this purpose. Therefore, the community must depend on foods in state warehouses, foods that are being stored by commercial distributors for the schools, and those foods stored by local school food authorities.

Foods can be provided to any recognized disaster-relief agency, such as the American Red Cross, the Salvation Army, Civil Defense,

---

Exhibit 22–7 Disaster Dos and Don'ts

DO

Cooperate.
Get permission to use federal commodities.
Remember who you are doing this for —your neighbors.
Keep records as best you can for food used and meals served.
Have someone answer the phone and log all phone calls.
Log all accidents with the name, address, and phone number of the victim, as well as details of what happened.
Have volunteers sign in, record name, address and phone number; these are good for Red Cross records as well as thank-you notes.
Be flexible; counts may go up and down quickly.
Be specific.
Be willing to make decisions quickly.
Be tactful and diplomatic.

DON'T

Turn over your kitchen to an outside organization.
Be afraid to ask for help.
Forget sanitation.
Be afraid to stand your ground and insist on important issues.

Source: Reprinted with permission from P.L. Fitzgerald, Ed., When Nature Turns Nasty, *School Foodservice & Nutrition*, No. 51, p. 44, © 1997, American School Foodservice Association.

and many religious denominations, civic organizations, and unions. USDA must issue prior approval before food is used for disaster feeding.

Disaster Planning

Preparedness is the key to successful delivery of services during an emergency situation. See Exhibit 22–8 for a checklist of commonalties that should be addressed during planning. A response team in each community should develop a written emergency plan. Procedures should be developed and followed for keeping this plan current. Include food service as a part of the local board of education, city, and/or county plans. Since schools frequently serve as emergency sites, local school food and nutrition program directors should serve on food preparedness committees.

Keep an updated list of state and local contacts. (See Exhibit 22–9.) Know which specific schools in the school system are designated as emergency shelters. Generally, do not select a school with an all-electric kitchen to be an emergency shelter. Determine how to identify, secure, and distribute foods for use. Take steps to maintain sanitary conditions during distribution, storage, and preparation of the foods. Establish procedures for transferring foods to other schools or sites and returning unused products, if necessary. Be sure that workers have written policies and procedures to follow. (See Exhibit 22–10.) Integrate disaster feeding plans with the rest of the disaster plan for the community.

The emergency agency responsible for the site can provide a trained site manager and personnel to operate the feeding operation. Directors who have experienced disasters in their communities recommend refraining from turning the kitchen over to an outside agency.[26] If local school food and nutrition personnel are needed, determine whether funds are available from local, state, and federal disaster organizations to pay them. Determine who is responsible if equipment is broken or misplaced. Find out how the school system will be reimbursed for commercially purchased foods that are utilized. Clarify these issues in advance of the emergency. Offer training annually to staff members who will be involved if an emergency occurs. Exhibit 22–11 provides training suggestions from a school system in Wisconsin.[27]

Exhibit 22–8 Disaster Planning

Can you really plan for a disaster? Beth Hanna, food service director for the West Des Moines, Iowa, school district, notes that while each crisis is different, there are commonalties you can plan for.

What Must Be Planned?

Menus	They should be simple but filling, easy to eat, two to three meals per day. Keep in mind hot or cold, preparation techniques (canned versus scratch) and special diets.
Supplies	Don't forget the little things, like spices, condiments, utensils, pens, paper, masking tape, name tags.
Staffing	Review volunteers versus paid staff.
Distribution	Can you get the food to where it needs to go? How? Can you receive items in a timely manner? How?
Cleaning	Schedule lots of help; it's something no one likes to do and everyone is tired when it needs to be done. Remember that your volunteers don't know sanitation and will need to be trained. Use instant sani-solutions when possible.
Repairs	Your equipment will be used hard; expect repairs for the next year.

Source: Reprinted with permission from P.L. Fitzgerald, Ed., When Nature Turns Nasty, *School Foodservice & Nutrition*, No. 51, p. 48, © 1997, American School Foodservice Association.

Exhibit 22–9 Players & Partners

Victims	School district administrators	Donors
Salvation Army	School board	Distributors
National Guard	City officials	Media
Red Cross	Volunteers	Government
	Health inspector	

Source: Reprinted with permission from P.L. Fitzgerald, Ed., When Nature Turns Nasty, *School Foodservice & Nutrition*, No. 51, p. 48, © 1997, American School Foodservice Association.

Importance of Record Keeping

The school food authority must keep accurate records of all foods used or provided during emergency situations. If foods are transferred to disaster feeding organizations, obtain signed receipts. The state's director of food distribution will ask for the approximate numbers of meals and people fed, the number of days, and the types and amounts of foods used if the school food and nutrition program had to assume feeding on an immediate basis. Feeding of volunteers or similar support personnel with USDA commodity foods is not authorized. Prompt reporting of required information to the state agency involved is essential. If possible, USDA will either obtain replacement value for some of the foods used or replace foods with other desirable foods. (See Exhibit 22–12 for suggested menus to be used in emergency situations.)

APPLICATION

School food and nutrition personnel often want some way to evaluate their community relations to see if they are doing a good job in this area. The following checklist (Exhibit 22–13) identifies characteristics of a school food and nutrition program that has good community relations.[28] Apply the following indicators to a specific school or school system. After completing the evaluation, collaborate with members of the community to develop a plan to work on problem areas.

Establishing successful community relations can enhance the morale and working environment for school food and nutrition personnel. While networking with community groups and involving parents in the program, remember the following tips for success:

Exhibit 22–10 Supply Reminders

The following are critical foodservice-related supplies.

+ Styrofoam cups	+ Napkins
+ Dish soap	+ Plastic wrap
+ Bleach	+ Foil
+ Dishwasher supplies	+ Towels
+ Disposable gloves	+ Bar mops
+ Disposable aprons	+ Garbage bags
+ Hair nets	

Source: Reprinted with permission from M. Hurt, An Ounce of Prevention, *School Foodservice & Nutrition*, No. 51, p. 55, © 1997, American School Foodservice Association.

Exhibit 22–11 Top 10 Training Tips

The Red Cross training offered so much valuable information. Here are the top 10 most valuable lessons learned in La Crosse, Wis.:

1. Determine if your school has a partnership agreement with the Red Cross to serve as a mass care shelter during a disaster.
2. Call the Red Cross and offer to serve as a volunteer during an emergency; note your department's food service expertise.
3. Recruit staff and colleagues to become volunteers and take required training.
4. Participate in a disaster drill.
5. Establish a contact person for the Red Cross to call during an emergency.
6. Develop a calling-tree within your department to notify trained volunteers.
7. Prepare menus in advance.
8. Organize a list of supplies and a "to do" list.
9. Clearly define the different roles of the Red Cross and the school during the emergency, particularly as to how food and supplies are paid for and other administrative details.
10. Share with the superintendent, the school board, and the community what good stewards of the community are working in their school kitchens!

Source: Reprinted with permission from M. Hurt, An Ounce of Prevention, *School Foodservice & Nutrition*, No. 51, p. 54, © 1997, American School Foodservice Association.

- Show enthusiasm.
- Be proactive.
- Stick with the program's mission.
- Don't be concerned about who gets the credit.
- Don't burn bridges because your paths may cross again.
- Be persistent.
- Involve all members of the school food and nutrition staff.
- Give employees recognition and credit.
- Compromise, if necessary but more important, create win-win situations.
- Relax and have fun!

SUMMARY

Leading professional nutrition organizations, including The American Dietetic Association, recognize that school-based nutrition programs should be designed to have a parental and community involvement component.[29] Janet Bantly, a past president of the American School Food Service Association, acknowledged the need to work with partners and allied groups at the national, state, and local levels to achieve the association's vision of having healthful school meals and nutrition education available to all children as an integral part of education.[30] This aspect of the program is addressed in federal regulations governing the program. It has meaning only when caring, committed school food and nutrition professionals find innovative ways to involve parents and community stakeholders. An effective community relations program is based on communication, networking, marketing, involvement, and resolution of actual or potential conflicts.[31] In order to successfully accomplish this goal, school food and nutrition personnel must be prepared to facilitate these key processes.

Exhibit 22–12

Best Eats   The La Crosse, Wisconsin, school district suggests the following menus and food offerings. Mix and match or add your own local favorites.

Menus

I. Sloppy Joes/Buns
Chips and Pickles
Fruit (Grapes or Apples)
Corn
Pie or Prepackaged Cookies
Milk (white and
   chocolate)
Coffee and Water

**II. Spaghetti Meat
Sauce**
Spaghetti Pasta
French Bread
Tossed Salad
Dressings
Fresh Fruit
Ice Cream Bars
   or Pudding
Milk (white and
   chocolate)
Coffee and water

**III. Goulash or
Beef-a-roni-type
product**
French Bread
Green Beans
Fresh Vegetables
Dessert
Milk (white and
   chocolate)
Coffee and Water

IV. Chicken Noodle Soup
Cold-cut Sandwiches
Peanut Butter Crackers
Fresh Vegetables
Fruit
Dessert
Milk (white and
   chocolate)
Coffee and Water

V. Cold/HotCereal
Juices/Fruit
Toast and/or
   Coffee Cake
Milk and Coffee

Food Ideas
Entrees
Sloppy Joes
Spaghetti & Meat/
   Marinara Sauce
Goulash
Chicken Noodle Soup
   and Sandwich
Grilled cheese
   Sandwich
Pizza (cheese and
   other varieties)
Macaroni and Cheese
Vegetarian Lasagna
   (pre-made)
Meat Lasagna
Hot Dogs
Hamburgers
Chicken Salad Sandwich
Cheese Dunkers
Broiled Fish/Fish Patties
Tuna Sandwich
Cold-cut Sandwiches
Meatballs/Gravy

Snacks
Cheese/Crackers
String Cheese
Fresh Fruit
Granola Bars
Raisins
Beef Sticks
Veggie Sticks/Dip
Bagels/Cream Cheese
Large, soft Pretzels
Rice Krispie® Bars

Desserts
Prepackaged Cookies
Ice Cream Bars
Rice Krispie® Bars
Pudding
Raspberry Sherbet
Fruit
Brownies
Frozen Pies
Muffins
Dessert Treats
Granola Bar

Breakfast
Boiled Eggs
Bagels/Cream Cheese
English Muffins
Cinnamon Rolls
Ham-n-Cheese
Grilled Cheese
Oven French Toast
Caramel Rolls
Fruit Juice Cups
Peanut Butter & Jelly
Pancakes on a stick
Waffles/Syrup
Muffins

Source: Reprinted with permission from M. Hurt, An Ounce of Prevention, *School Foodservice & Nutrition*, No. 51, p. 53, © 1997, American School Foodservice Association.

Exhibit 22–13 Checklist of Characteristics for Schools with Successful Community Relations Programs

Successful Programs:

1. Announce menu options and food choices available and the prices to the community through local newspapers, radio, and television stations.
2. Use menu boards and signs to clearly communicate the number and types of menu items included in the price.
3. Provide information about the nutrients provided, the menu planning option being used, and offer vs serve.
4. Serve foods and menu items advertised during all serving periods.
5. Encourage employees on the serving line to smile, show that they are caring, courteous and friendly, and treat everyone equitably.
6. Train employees to respond appropriately during emergency situations.
7. Ensure that the kitchen and cafeteria are free of insects and rodents and that employees practice good personal hygiene and adhere to recommended sanitation procedures.
8. Provide an adequate number of lines so that a steady flow of students is served during each meal period and customers spend no more than ten minutes waiting for meals.
9. Respond positively to customer calls and complaints and handle potential community relations problems proactively.
10 Keep self-serve bars and serving lines well supplied with foods and check frequently for both neatness and proper temperatures.
11. Develop and implement a marketing plan that targets students, faculty, staff, administrators, school board members, and the community.
12. Track public perceptions about the program over a period of years and incorporate the results of public perception data into the annual plan of operations and marketing plans.
13. Encourage students, parents, faculty, program staff, and allied health organization representatives to participate in an advisory committee that directs program activities, including menu planning, purchasing, and promotions.
14. Post sanitation scores in a predominant location and share them with the community.
15. Attractively display and garnish foods that are nutritious and safe to eat.
16. Serve the quality of food items that meets the customers' expectations.
17. Season food items to appeal to the customers' taste rather than the school food and nutrition employee's taste.
18. Serve school meals at convenient times and locations, and at prices affordable to the customer and below those of competitors.
19. Use colorful signage, awnings, wall hangings, panels, and dividers to make the environment more quiet, appealing, and attractive.
20. Establish procedures for meal payments that are convenient for students and their families and share with shareholders information about how the school nutrition dollar is spent.
21. Solicit feedback from students, faculty, staff, administrators, school board members, and the community on food quality and service, and use suggestions for program improvement.
22. Encourage students to participate in planned taste-testing activities for various purposes, such as introducing new foods or new recipes for student acceptance.
23. Encourage students and parents to participate in writing and producing program materials, such as videos, posters, or brochures.
24. Involve customers in contests such as guessing the number of peanuts in a jar or developing a theme for the cafeteria or in touring the kitchen.
25. At a minimum, invite parents, local leaders, and policy makers annually to eat school meals.

continues

Exhibit 22–13 continued

26. At a minimum distribute attractive, accurate, printed information on the program or on nutrition to parents or students monthly that contributes to a positive image of the program.
27. Encourage staff to serve on related committees of allied health organizations and serve as a nutrition resource to the community.
28. Encourage staff to make presentations to faculty and local parent and community groups about the program's mission, goals, and accomplishments annually.
29. Invite local media to provide coverage for promotions and special events.
30. Annually issue several press releases about program-related events.
31. Annually train employees about the importance of maintaining positive working relationships with stakeholders in the community.
32. Use innovative outlets such as Internet sites, closed-circuit or cable television, and homework hotlines to deliver program information to the community.
33. Fulfill requests to cater special school and community events consistent with established local policies.
34. Cooperate with local allied health organizations to implement special promotions and celebrate special events, such as community health fairs or National Nutrition Month.
35. Respond to the community's nutrition needs by participating in programs such as elderly feeding, summer feeding, after-school care, and disaster feeding.
36. Schedule staff to participate in school registration events and open houses held by the school to promote school meals.
37. Communicate quality of commodity foods and the brands or brand equivalents of products used through displays, menus, newsletters, or other means.
38. Use point-of-choice materials, bulletin boards, signage, and other nutrition awareness exhibits in the serving area to communicate information that is accurate and scientifically valid.
39. Include promotions for holidays and special occasions that currently appeal to customers and that support the educational goals of the community.
40. Deliver nutrition messages on milk cartons, promotional items, and disposable items such as sandwich wraps, table tents, or napkins, when they are used.

Source: Reprinted with permission from A. Bomar, *Quality Measures for Georgia's School Nutrition Programs,* School and Community Nutrition, © 1997, Georgia Department of Education.

CASE STUDY
PARTICIPATION AT STATESBORO HIGH

The Challenge

JemmeBeth Winskie has been the school food and nutrition program director in Bulloch County for the past 15 years. Throughout this period she has worked to have the program recognized as a school food and nutrition program, not just a feeding program. At the beginning of her tenure, she had the foresight to develop a competitive food policy that was approved by her local board of education. During the past two or three years JemmeBeth has noted that student participation at Statesboro High School has continued to drop. This quiet, rural area was changing rapidly. Fast-food restaurants continued to be built and it seemed as if families were eating out more often. Approximately 56 percent of the 1,500 students who attended the high school from Statesboro, a community of about 30,000, and the surrounding county were eating school lunches. This percentage of students did not meet JemmeBeth's expectations for the program. She knew that it was important for all the students to be eating lunch every day. They needed to serve foods enjoyed by the students while ensuring that the meals met the new federal nutrient standards.

Actions

Last year JemmeBeth and her coordinator, Kathy Szotkiewicz, attended a training session that advocated a more systematic approach to managing their program. They decided to implement this approach. First, JemmeBeth called together the high school and middle school managers and explained to them what she had in mind. She asked the managers to decide what types of lines they wanted to offer.

This same group went on to meet regularly to plan the cycle menus and the work schedules, which specified how these menus would be prepared. JemmeBeth took this opportunity to shift some of the managers from one school to another. She placed Ann Thompson at Statesboro High School. Ann had 14 years of work experience in the school food and nutrition program, with about seven of these years working as a manager. She had good organizational skills and supervised the production of good-quality food, and the employees she supervised seemed to have a good attitude. JemmeBeth wanted her at the high school because she felt that she could relate well to students of this age.

Before this group went too far in their planning, she surveyed the high school students to determine whether they would be willing to pay more if they had more choices. Overwhelmingly, the students approved an increase in sales price if they could have more choices. The group of managers decided to offer a five-day cycle menu on five types of lines. Before they had offered three lines that included a fast-food line, a hot food line, and a salad line. Now they were going to offer a grill line, a pizza line, a sub sandwich line, a salad line, and a mama's cooking line. They modified recipes such as macaroni and cheese to reduce the fat content. They put more seasonal fresh fruit on the menu. They substituted desserts with a cobbler topping for items such as pie, and reduced the serving size of some items, such as potato chips. At breakfast, in order to meet the nutrient standards, they reduced the number of times that eggs were served. To keep the fat content low, hash browns had to be removed from the menu. They did offer both a hot line and a cold line at breakfast, though.

Source: Reprinted with permission from Bulloch County Schools, Bulloch County Case Study, © 1997, Nutrition Education and Training Program, *School & Community Nutrition,* Georgia Department of Education.

To make life even more interesting, Statesboro High School had a new principal this year. Daryl Dean, the principal, seemed to make a difference in the attitude of the school food and nutrition program. He was more involved. He was in the lunchroom every day, and it seemed to be operating in a more organized fashion. The program had also made a decision to switch to disposable serviceware so that one person in the dishroom could be relieved to help assist with the extra choices.

Outcomes

This year JemmeBeth was tracking participation figures closely to determine what impact these changes had made. The coach had asked just last week about working with the school food and nutrition program to serve pregame meals, and she hoped that was a good sign. At the end of September, JemmeBeth was pleased to see that participation for lunch at Statesboro High had jumped from a low of 46 percent to 63 percent and at breakfast from 30 percent to 34 percent.

The *Statesboro Herald* included an article on the updated program in its back-to-school section of the paper. The manager had written a letter to the faculty explaining the changes in the program. JemmeBeth had even personally written a letter to parents and sent it home to them through the students.

JemmeBeth wondered which of these changes contributed the most to the improved participation. She thought that perhaps most of all the participation increase was due to the commitment that the managers had to making these new menus work. It was obvious that they had ownership of the changes that had been made. Surveying the students in advance was also critical to this improved participation. Very few of these changes actually cost the system a great deal of money. Their public image had improved because they had customized menus for the high school situation.

CASE STUDY
DISASTER FEEDING DURING THE FLOOD OF 1994

The Challenge

Jackie Harrell, the school food and nutrition program director in Decatur County, had looked forward for weeks to going on a cruise with her husband. On a Thursday in July when they began their drive to Florida to the cruise ship, the banks of the Flint River in their hometown of Bainbridge, Georgia, were beginning to overflow. When the cruise ship returned to shore on Monday, Mr. And Mrs. Harrell learned that the water levels in Bainbridge had not been that high for 100 years. Their home was being threatened and their college-age son was on his way to the house with a semi-truck to move the furniture. Approximately 500 people had been evacuated from 150 homes. One nursing home in the city had been totally flooded and had to be evacuated. All the projections indicated that the water levels were going to be at flood stage for at least two weeks. No one was even willing to discuss when people were going to be able to get back to their homes. Transportation to some parts of the city had been cut off and these areas had become islands. Jackie and her husband had to find an alternate route home because the highway leading to their home was covered with water.

When Jackie got home she found out that the National Guard had been called to help. The Red Cross and the Salvation Army each had set up an emergency shelter in one of the local schools. The kitchens in these two schools were being used to feed the temporary residents. The superintendent had directed the warehouse manager to dispense needed food. There seemed to be mass confusion about who was doing what. Jackie understood that the commodity foods that she had in storage for

the summer needed to be used during this disaster. She was concerned however, about the volunteers from these organizations using the equipment in her school kitchens, without any supervision or training. Who was going to be responsible if the equipment was broken? Were sanitation and safety rules being followed? How did she know if they were even using purchased foods? What condition would the kitchens be in when they left?

Actions

She called many of the managers and employees who normally worked in the kitchens and asked them if they were willing to volunteer to help. She even offered to pay them for some of the time from school food and nutrition program funds. Jackie was really pleased to learn that Sandra Mauldin, a volunteer in charge of one of the kitchens, was a school food and nutrition manager from Oconee County in north Georgia. Jackie knew that she could count on Sandra to help document the food that was being used in at least one of the kitchens. She began to coordinate efforts with numerous national, state, and local agencies. These included USDA; the American Red Cross; the Federal Emergency Management Agency (FEMA); the Salvation Army; the state fire marshal; Georgia Emergency Management Agency (GEMA); the National Guard; the Georgia Department of Education, since they were the state distributing agency for commodity foods; the local WIC nutritionist; and several church representatives in the area.

The slough, a low-lying area outside of town, saved Bainbridge and kept the flooding from being as bad as had been predicted. In the

Source: Reprinted with permission from Decatur County Schools, Case Study, Disaster Feeding during the Flood of 1994, © 1997, Nutrition Education and Training Program, *School & Community Nutrition*, Georgia Department of Education.

end, Jackie ended up with more USDA commodities than needed. USDA sent in approximately 700 cases each of peanut butter, raisins, and cheese. Inexperienced but well-meaning volunteers had ordered more than was actually needed. Jackie even recalled the fresh chicken that had been delivered. It could not be prepared because of the lack of electricity, so the chicken spoiled while it was being stored in the truck that delivered it. A set of preplanned menus, along with a list of foods to order, would have been helpful. Menus that were planned in advance could give more consideration to the nutritional needs of such a diverse group of people and to the shelf life of foods that needed to be stored for such emergencies. Preplanned menus would also incorporate items normally thought of as comfort foods. Jackie would never have dreamed that they would have to deal with so many special diets! Just about every one of the nursing home patients needed something special.

Outcomes

When the immediate crisis was over, Jackie realized that the community needed to develop a written disaster plan in order to reduce the confusion and problems that she would encounter if a similar situation should ever occur. The superintendent and the school food and nutrition program director needed to be involved in the development of this plan. Schools needed to be selected as emergency shelters based on their location outside the flood plain and their use of gas, rather than electricity. A contact person for each relief agency as well as an alternate person needed to

be named. These contacts needed to be trained on the procedures being established and existing regulations that must be followed. She noted that they must include in the plan an agreement about whether a relief organization would be given the authority and responsibility to manage school kitchens and, if so, which one. They needed to establish procedures to order foods and dispense food from the food storage warehouse. They needed to specify who would be held responsible for the condition of the equipment and address liability issues. Jackie had vivid memories of the volunteer who had tried to repair the fryer without disconnecting the electricity. Also, she knew that she must insist when they wrote the plan that either she or one of the managers that she designated would be assigned to each kitchen to help the person assigned the responsibility for managing it during the crisis to ensure that it was being left in good condition. Procedures must also be developed to ensure that accurate records were kept regarding the food and supplies received and used by the shelter. The number of people served, their reason for being there (victim, volunteer, etc.), and the amount of food prepared must be recorded.

Reflecting on the situation later, Jackie wished that she had been able to get more press coverage for the contribution that she, Sandra Mauldin, and the school food and nutrition employees in her system had made. She knew that the volunteers who had prepared and served food during the flood better understood their daily contributions now. Maybe their ability to help the community in this way could affect how parents, students, and community leaders perceive the school meals they served daily.

REFERENCES

1. A. Gillespie, "President's Message," *Journal of Nutrition Education* 29 (1997): 55–56.

2. *Code of Federal Regulations, Agriculture,* Parts 210 to 299 (Washington, DC: Office of Federal Register, National Archives and Records Administration, revised January 1, 1996).

3. Centers for Disease Control and Prevention (CDC), "Guidelines for School Health Programs To Promote Lifelong Healthy Eating," *Morbidity and Mortality Weekly Report* 45 (1996):1–41.

4. M.D. Bryan, *The School Cafeteria* (New York: F.S. Crofts & Co., 1938).

5. S.R. Covey, *Principle-Centered Leadership* (New York: Summit Books, 1991).

6. B.C. Pateman et al., "School Food Service," *Journal of School Health.* 65:8:327–332.

7. S.R. Covey, *The 7 Habits of Highly Effective People* (New York: Simon & Schuster, Fireside Books, 1989).

8. Covey, *Principle-Centered Leadership.*

9. Covey, *The 7 Habits.*

10. T.J. Peters and R.H. Waterman Jr., *In Search of Excellence* (New York: Harper & Row, 1982).

11. D.C. Fischer, *The Simplified Baldridge Award Organization Assessment* (New York: Lincoln-Bradley, 1993).

12. *American School Food Service Association, Keys to Excellence* (Arlington, VA: 1995).

13. Georgia Department of Education, *Quality Measures for Georgia's School Nutrition Programs* (Atlanta: 1997).

14. M. Binswanger, "Federal Partnerships for Total Education," *School Foodservice & Nutrition* 48 (1994): 53–54, 56, 59, 107.

15. P.M. Senge, *The Fifth Discipline* (New York: Doubleday, 1990).

16. CDC, "Guidelines for School Health Programs."

17. U.S. Department of Agriculture, *Team Nutrition Community Action Kit: For People Where They Live, Learn and Play* (Washington, DC: 1996).

18. Bryan, *The School Cafeteria.*

19. *Code of Federal Regulations, Agriculture.*

20. Georgia Policy Council for Children and Families, *Aiming For Results: A Guide to Georgia's Benchmarks for Children and Families* (Atlanta: 1996).

21. S.J. Crockett et al., "Nutrition Intervention Strategies Preferred by Parents: Results of a Marketing Survey," *Journal of Nutrition Education* 21 (1989): 90–94.

22. J.C. Berryman and K.W. Breighner, *Modeling Healthy Behavior—Actions and Attitudes in Schools* (Santa Cruz, CA: ETR Associates, 1994).

23. Georgia PTA and Georgia Nutrition Education and Training Program, Georgia Department of Education, *Nutrition Education Handbook* (Atlanta, 1995).

24. P.L. Fitzgerald "When Nature Turns Nasty," *School Foodservice & Nutrition* 51 (1997): 42–50.

25. *Code of Federal Regulations, Agriculture.*

26. Fitzgerald, "When Nature Turns Nasty."

27. M. Hurt, "An Ounce of Prevention," *School Foodservice & Nutrition* 51 (1997): 52–55.

28. Georgia Department of Education, *Quality Measures.*

29. "Position of the American Dietetic Association: Child and Adolescent Food and Nutrition Programs," *Journal of the American Dietetic Association* 96 (1996): 913–917.

30. J.H. Bantley, "Strength in Numbers," *School Foodservice & Nutrition,* April 1997; 6.

31. "Position of the American Dietetic Association."

PART VI

Anticipating the Future in Child Nutrition Programs

CHAPTER 23

Dreams and Deeds for the Millennium

Josephine Martin and Martha T. Conklin

You see things, and you say, "why." But I dream dreams that never were, and I say, "Why not?"

—George B. Shaw

OUTLINE

- Introduction
- Sweet Dreams
    Professional Profile
    Learning Organization
    Delivery on Demand
    Business Savvy
    Meal Deals
    Safe at the Plate
    Customers at the Wheel
    Nutri-Cuisine
    Reading, Writing, and Life
    Food and Nutrition Network
    Respect
    Bridges to the Future
- Clicking of Heels
    The Strategic Task Force
    Environmental Scan
    Strengths and Weaknesses
    Mission and Vision
    Values and Beliefs
    Strategic Outcomes
- Leadership for Excellence
- Case Study: Being Involved as a Partner in Promoting Health and Education in the Independence Community
    Melanie Moentmann

INTRODUCTION

Why not dream? As children we have frequent fantasies, and it is only when we reach "adulthood" that we are told that dreams must be put away for more mundane aspirations. Senator Thad Cochran, long an ardent supporter of child nutrition programs, recently said that a man's list of memories should never be longer than his list of dreams.[1] Child nutrition programs (CNPs) will prevail and flourish into the next century and beyond. This is a reality, not a dream. Children are needed to perpetuate humanity, and children need sustenance and nurturing. The exact type of nurturing may change with conventional wisdom, but unquestionably children need food to sustain their bodies and minds for the serious business of learning and growing into adults who contribute to society. The provision of nutritious food for children at school and in other settings will continue to be one area on which politicians, statesmen, and community leaders agree. CNPs will be on the front row when the nation turns its spotlight on children in the new millennium.

So if we were to dream about CNPs, what would they be like? *Managing Child Nutrition Programs*[2] tells much about dreams and hopes for CNPs. If ideas can exist long enough to be chronicled in a book, surely they can become a reality. In fact, portions of the dream exist in schools today. This chapter describes a vision for *all* child nutrition programs and addresses strategic planning and leadership issues necessary to make the dream come true.

SWEET DREAMS

Our vision for CNPs really is no different from those expressed in the 1920s and 1930s; the only difference is that we dream that "ideal" programs will be the norm in the twenty-first century. In this vision, CNPs are considered as necessary to excellence in education as teachers, technology, and transportation. All children are served nutritious, appealing meals by compassionate and competent people in pleasant surroundings whenever they are under the care of schools or other child-centered institutions. School administrators consider mealtime as important to the learning process as time for math and science. Food choices are available in all menu categories. These choices are attractively presented and prepared to maximize nutrient content. Students are knowledgeable in nutrition and food composition and are motivated to make healthy choices in the school setting, at home, and in the community. Parents or other caregivers reinforce food and nutrition learning in the home, just as they support other instructional areas where homework is required. Community alliances guarantee the sustainability of CNPs through support for continual improvement and coordination whenever it requires resources. Complete nutritional security is a national priority, and seamless programs create a safety net against childhood hunger.

Professional Profile

Converting the dream into reality begins with the education and training of food and nutrition professionals. Even as long ago as the Great Depression,[3] the passage of the National School Lunch Act,[4] and the beginning of the American School Food Service Association,[5] leaders recognized the importance of formal education. They believed that people directing CNPs at all levels should be professionally trained and hold, at a minimum, a four-year degree in a field related to nutrition and food management. They also said that the CNP professional should continue formal education to reach at least a master's degree.

Decision makers who recognize the essential link between nutritional well-being of children and their readiness to learn endorse a requirement for professionally prepared directors of CNPs. They realize the importance of qualified personnel in delivering cost-effective, nutritious meals that children will eat. Certification of professionals is approved by state and national certifying agencies founded on research-based competencies for persons employed in various levels of school food and nutrition program management. Research-based competencies are used at the federal, state, and local level to establish qualifications for personnel. Staffing needs at all levels are established to ensure an adequate type and quantity of labor to support effective delivery of meals and nutrition education to all children.

Competence is the foundation of the profile for food and nutrition professionals involved in CNP management. The next layer of the profile reflects the personal attributes. Turning the dream for CNPs into reality requires professionals who have a commitment for making it come true. Professional and personal integrity radiate in all actions taken by individuals managing CNPs because they see nutritional and fiscal integrity as cornerstones of the program. Working with and through all stakeholders is the standard way goals are accomplished. CNP directors place value on research as the basis for examining and renewing programs and for using technology as a basic support system to achieve goals. Strategic planning, setting priorities, organizing tasks, and delegating responsibilities are keys to program effectiveness.

School food and nutrition professionals wear many hats and play many roles. They are nutrition educators, food and nutrition program directors, marketing specialists, financial experts, entrepreneurs, and CNP advocates. Managing to keep these roles in harmony is an essential attribute food and nutrition professionals display in the new century.

Learning Organization

As excellence one day can become mediocrity the next, CNP directors recognize that every person on the team must engage in constructive learning, and programs must be constantly renewed to maintain their excellence. In our dream, school food and nutrition professionals actively support a learning organiza-tion. They realize that a learning organization will grow only if people are not held accountable for mistake-free performance, but for learning from their mistakes. A system of training, coaching, and immediate feedback is the safety net allowing this to happen. A sense of teamwork and sharing is vital to the growth and maintenance of a learning organization. The reward and recognition system provides clear benefits for employees who help others succeed, and team incentives exist.

School food and nutrition professionals within the national professional association and the federal, state, and local levels of management promulgate the vision of new leadership required by learning organizations. To create and maintain a learning organization, leaders are champions of the people. These leaders take less and less control, make fewer unilateral decisions, and effectively alter their role from "all knowing" to "group learning facilitator." This mind-set of the next millennium requires a different approach to the preparation of leaders and different criteria for selection and recruitment of management-level personnel.

The need for change is consistently and passionately embraced throughout the learning organization. Support systems are in place to help employees cope with the pace of change. Systems help people through rapid change and reinforce the message that change is the status quo in an organization that learns. The fear of living in flux has been replaced with a shared anticipation of future possibilities. This was accomplished by expelling the fear of failure. Leaders of learning organizations know that they are nurturing values, not programs. Their success will be measured by the extent these values form the foundation for an organizational culture that is supportive of learning and change.[6]

Delivery on Demand

All students in preschool and K–12 grades are provided two or three meals each day along with nutritious snacks. As the school calendar is expanded to 12 months to optimize space and curriculum priorities, children have access to year-round school meals. Coordinated health services, including nutrition education, are available at all times. Children are served nutritious meals and snacks wherever they are located in classrooms, halls, patios, walkways, dining rooms, gymnasiums, and even on buses. Meals also are provided in child-care facilities and other remote locations in the community.

Business Savvy

The dream for an effective CNP includes meeting nutritional goals within financial constraints. Directing the program with business savvy is reflected in the school food and nutrition professionals' conceptual approach to managing the program. Management begins with a clear set of objectives, necessary resources, defined controls (including identified standards for each facet of the program), essential linkages with people, and a process for the effective use of data and information to facilitate activities. School food and nutrition professionals understand that achieving nutritional integrity is equally as important as achieving fiscal integrity. CNPs are a business functioning within school walls and beyond, and they must remain viable to exist.

A financial management information system (FMIS) based on consistently followed, uniform standards is essential to fiscal integrity. This system is automated and aggregates school-level data into district reports. The financial positions of all school- and district-level CNPs are calculated at least monthly to provide managers and directors with information on demand regarding program status. This tracking system allows directors to make modifications as needed to keep the program's financial operations in a positive position. The FMIS yields data that can be benchmarked with other programs of similar demographics because performance indicators are calculated

consistently from one CNP to the next. Benchmarking allows districts to identify best practices in financial management and to learn from others' successes. While the two objectives of fiscal integrity and nutritional integrity are independent, the success of one is dependent on the success of the other.

Competence in the area of directing a school food and nutrition business requires professional training, and it requires thinking like a chief executive officer (CEO). CEOs ask questions such as: How will this decision impact product quality? . . . customer service? . . . employee satisfaction? . . . company profit? . . . stockholder support? CEOs expect the team to establish effective procedures because problems most often occur when processes fail. It is less expensive to fix the process than to blame employees for actions gone wrong. CEOs look for ways to meet customer needs and provide service that results in customer and employee retention. They know this combination results in meeting company goals. In spite of new organizational designs where decisions are made at the lowest possible level and involve teams, there will always be someone at the top with final authority and responsibility. Understanding administrators and looking at the CNP from their perspective are essential ingredients for productive relationships. Being savvy is knowing what to do and implementing a management system to accomplish objectives within the organization. Being business savvy is being proactive in establishing processes and strategies that assure a program with fiscal integrity.

Meal Deals

Remember the trite saying, "the proof of the pudding is in the eating"? Turning this dream into reality requires transforming school meal service into a part of the school day that everyone anticipates. The creation of exciting customer-friendly, nutritious meal packages occurs on a regular basis. Everyone gets a little bored with eating in the same place and seeing the same menu week after week. In the new century, school food and nutrition professionals outlaw boredom with school food. Concern for making nutritious meals appealing is a priority for school food and nutrition professionals. Employees are trained in every process that influences meal quality, from buying the best-quality food for the recipe, to using culinary techniques that produce food at the peak of freshness, to the actual presentation and service of meals at appropriate temperatures. Nutrition messages and multiple food choices are available to children at all grade levels. Directors have a collaborative relationship with suppliers that ensures the availability of student-acceptable products within the CNP budget. These new products will be incorporated into meal packages and available to all children, not just those who have extra money to supplement the school meal or those who choose only food items rather than the entire meal. Funds generated by successful programs are not siphoned off to support other school activities, but are used to keep the program invigorated.

Determining student needs and wants by using an extensive array of processes gives school food and nutrition professionals information needed to renew menu combinations, packaging, and delivery frequently during the school year. The way food is packaged and presented is considered as important as preparing the food. Continuing into the new century, customers "eat with their eyes" before they choose to try new meals. School food and nutrition professionals are tuned in to trends in the food service industry. The school food and nutrition team, including some students, visits other food operations in the community on a regular basis to comparison shop. They observe food offerings, marketing strategies, dining décor, and customer service details. They find out what students select when they visit these food service outlets. All this information is shared by the team, and plans are made to incorporate appropriate ideas into the school food and nutrition program.

Safe at the Plate

"Safe at the plate" is a phrase often used when talking about food that is microbiologically safe as well as pleasing and tasty to the customer. As we dream into the next century, food safety continues to be a top priority of food and nutritional professionals. All food service staff are skilled in sanitary food-handling techniques that include hazard analysis critical control point (HACCP) procedures. Temperatures of food routinely are monitored and tracked by "smart" labels and computerized thermometers from the loading dock at manufacturers and distributors to local CNPs. Within local CNPs, food temperatures are monitored at the receiving docks, storage areas, preparation, serving line, and finally to storage as leftovers. Internal temperatures of food commonly are monitored during cooking by electronically sophisticated production equipment. These records are stored for documentation of HACCP procedures. Recipes are encoded with specific HACCP tips to alert employees to potentially hazardous food-handling practices and critical control points that need to be monitored during food production. Food specifications are tightly written to include acceptable temperatures during transit, and they allow or require irradiation for meat, milk, and fruits and vegetables. CNP professionals encourage and lobby for strong sanitation standards and controls for imported food by the U.S. Department of Agriculture (USDA) and the U.S. Public Health Service.

Customers at the Wheel

School food and nutrition programs are customer driven. Program requirements continue whether they come from Washington, the state capitol, the local school board, or an accrediting agency. Within that framework of requirements and standards, school food and nutrition professionals develop and perpetuate customer-driven programs. Directors have the buy-in from school administrators and school teams. With the commitment of stakeholders, necessary resources and time are allocated. In the new millennium, the distinction between quality and service will be obsolete. Customers' perception of quality embrace the service received, including the time standing in line, interaction with personnel, appearance and cleanliness of the facility, and choices of meals offered and their presentation.

National Food Service Management Institute (NFSMI) research conducted on customer satisfaction in high and middle schools found that the most important factors related to the students' general satisfaction with food served at school were quality and variety of food choices, food attractively presented for service, flavor of food, and politeness of the cafeteria staff.[7,8] Students may change their ideas about what food is "good," for example, tacos versus wraps versus sonic burgers, but their feelings about what are important attributes of school food service probably have and will not change. In other words, school food and nutrition professionals in the new century focus on total customer value, which Albrecht describes as a combination of all the tangible and intangibles experienced by the customer.[9]

The primary focus of school food and nutrition programs is to meet the needs and wants of student customers. The basic nutrition needs of customers are defined by research and policy. However, the student customer's wants are affected by a number of factors, including age, peers, culture, economic status, food knowledge, and sophistication. The goal is to have a system that brings needs and wants as closely together as possible. Maintaining a current approach to the wants of children is best achieved by formulating valid and reliable procedures within CNPs. This may include the formation of an active nutrition advisory committee, customer satisfaction surveys conducted on a periodic and regular basis, comment cards in the cafeteria, focus groups, use of the Internet, and student membership on menu-planning and food evaluation task forces.

Keeping students engaged in the process is an integral part of the school food and nutrition program directors' plans for meeting student wants. School food and nutrition professionals carefully identify students who would be early adopters of new ideas. Armed with this information, they select students from the early adopter group to help implement innovative ideas. Students' wants are in a constant state of change. Generation.coms, the current generation in school, are not like generation X'ers any more than they are like the flower children of the 1960s. Integral to the learning organization, school food and nutrition professionals encourage all members of the program team to feel the pulse and stay attuned to expectations of the current generation.

School food and nutrition professionals recognize the value of media advocacy and marketing as essential to the achievement of program objectives and getting clear and consistent messages to all customers. Directors are skilled in using social marketing theories to develop a plan to communicate program values, benefits, issues, and opportunities. The marketing plan, based on market research, includes a mix of strategies designed to reach internal and external customers, the media, and the community overall. Marketing is systematic and involves reaching a variety of groups with appropriate messages about the program. Evaluation of the marketing plan is conducted annually to ensure that services are targeted correctly to internal and external customers. Retooling of products and messages occurs as necessary.

Nutri-Cuisine

In our dream, school meal programs are the Nutri-Cuisine Centers. This means that all food and meals offered in the center are nutritious and reflect a style and quality that ensures food that tastes good and is appealing to the customers. The Nutri-Cuisine Center sets standards for all foods offered during the school day to make sure that they contribute to meeting the child's nutritional needs. School food and nutrition professionals recognize that a breakdown in meeting this goal can occur within the CNP or in other places at the school site that offers food. A nutrition integrity policy in the school district and quality controls are established to ensure that any food the child secures on the school site contributes to meeting nutritional objectives.

A comprehensive plan for evaluating food quality is in place. School food and nutrition professionals institute product evaluation as an essential component of the quality control program and provide for evaluation at four stages: purchasing, receiving, production, and service. Regardless of the form in which food is purchased, quality measures are used to select foods that meet nutrient and microbiological standards and ensure customer acceptability. Using a quality score card, food service assistants evaluate each item before placing it on the serving line, and finally a variety of methods is used to determine student acceptance.

The Nutri-Center is driven by the menu. Building a cohesive team for each food service subsystem helps to ensure appropriate coordination between the parts. Standards for the Nutri-Cuisine are not too different from those of the meals offered in the 1990s. What will be different is the form in which the school district receives, prepares, and delivers food. With the changing labor market and the advances in food processing and technology, a greater amount of food will be purchased in the ready-to-heat or partially prepared state from fewer vendors whose business is targeted to meeting the needs of CNPs. With changes in the delivery of education, including distance education, the packaging of frozen meals for delivery to some students at home or other sites is routinely provided.

Reading, Writing, and Life

Our dream includes school food and nutrition professionals' collaborating with curriculum makers to have life skills, including nutri-tion education, incorporated into the core curriculum. The coordinated health program supports nutrition education and the provision of appropriate nutrition services, including assessments by qualified professionals. There is a direct link among the cafeteria, the classroom, and the community. While students at all grade levels are engaged in active learning about food and nutrition, the cafeteria-classroom is used as a laboratory where students connect that learning with practice by selecting nutritious meals and learning to eat a variety of food.

Teachers and food and nutrition professionals collaborate to provide consistent nutrition messages. A multidisciplinary approach to teaching nutrition is reflected in course objectives and lesson plans. The core objectives approved by the board of education include nutrition objectives integrated into a variety of courses, and these objectives are reflected in written and practical tests students complete. The dream reflects that nutrition education is an integral part of all teacher-preparation programs. Teachers completing their initial training prior to this requirement are allowed to meet this through continuing education.

Food and Nutrition Network

Our dream has school food and nutrition programs functioning as active partners in a community food and nutrition network. This network supports collaboration among all agencies in the state or local communities providing nutrition services to children and families. Such a network serves three important purposes: to ensure a consistent nutrition message communicated to children and their families, to reinforce nutrition messages heard in different settings, and to create advocacy for child nutrition programs. The case at the end of this chapter exemplifies how one school food and nutrition program has made a difference in the community.

The school is the center for community activities that promote health and citizenship, and the school food and nutrition program is at the hub of this activity. Full-service schools provide prevention, treatment, and support services for children and families that are high quality and built on interagency partnerships.[10] CNPs serve meals to community groups of all ages, but particularly to the young, old, and disenfranchised. Meals are served in the school cafeteria but also are distributed to remote locations in the community. In small-town America and in urban centers, the food and nutrition program located at the school is considered a viable option for families and groups to obtain meals for sustenance and celebration.

Respect

Our dream for CNPs is that they are respected as an essential component of quality education. Respect emerges as a byproduct of personal and professional competence, business savvy, accepting some ownership for educational objectives, and sharing ownership of the school food and nutrition program with other stakeholders. Having equivalent education and credentialing brings respect to professionals. Most of all, school food and nutrition professionals who act as leaders in the school and community bring respect to the position. Initiating collaboration with other members of the education team as well as with health, social service, and even business enhances respect for CNPs and for professionals charged with directing the programs. School food and nutrition program directors are recognized as food and nutrition experts by the community.

Bridges to the Future

As the dream becomes reality, child nutrition programs are considered in every way to be an essential part of the child's education day. However, in a dynamic environment where social, economic, and political forces impact program policy, funding, and operation, it is essential for school food and nutrition pro-

fessionals to recognize that the program does not operate in a vacuum. Programs are constantly being modified by internal and external forces.

Changing technology alters the relationship between politicians and the governed for the better in the new century.[11] Sophisticated communication systems make information even more readily accessible. Lobbying politicians is universal through electronic mail, and voting from home through electronic media as an alternative to the polls is now commonplace. These changes are a boon to child nutrition advocates who directly reach the parents and grandparents of children receiving their services to ask for their endorsement of legislation that underscores the safety net against childhood hunger.

Collaboration between citizens and professional groups will be the mode for shaping public policy in the future. Wherever policies are needed to ensure that all children are effectively reached with nutritious food and nutrition education, they are made. This may be in Congress, the state legislature, the state school board, local school board, or the school site. School food and nutrition professionals cultivate alliances with people who share mutual interests in children's health and well-being. In building and maintaining this bridge, CNP directors keep members informed of events, issues, and program concerns at the national and state level. Members of the alliance become CNP advocates. Viable food and nutrition programs will be abetted by influencing and gaining commitment from partners and allies who share the goal that nutritional security is provided to all children.

Alone we can do so little,
together we can do so much.

—Helen Keller

CLICKING OF HEELS

As Glenda, the good witch, told Dorothy, "You've had the answer with you all along, just click your heels and you'll be there." Dorothy had a goal and worked very hard to reach it, even encountering personal perils along the way. At the end of her journey, when all else had failed, she was reminded that the secret to her success had been with her all along. The secrets to success were a clear vision and focus, a belief in what she was doing, and faith in her capabilities. These same secrets apply to success in leading child nutrition programs in the twenty-first century. Just as with Dorothy, success lies within food and nutrition program professionals, the people who make meals magically appear for children and adults on at least 180 days per year in every state in the nation.

Dreams do not happen in real life unless a lot of thought and effort are expended to make them come true. Hamel and Prahalad used a quote from William Jennings Bryan to illustrate the effort involved in thinking strategically to accomplish goals: "Destiny is no matter of chance. It is a matter of choice. It is not a thing to be waited for, it is a thing to be achieved."[12(pxii)]

A strategic process can be used by food and nutrition program directors to begin to stretch for an ideal and to stimulate staff development and problem-solving skills.[13] Strategic planning is a management process and considers decisions on broad technological and competitive aspects of the organization, the allocation of resources over time, and the eventual integration of the organization within the environment. A strategic plan concentrates on decision making, and it is hard work. Food and nutrition program directors must understand the forces that shape the future and evaluate alternative strategies resulting from anticipated changes in CNPs.[14] The future is not what will happen; the future is what is happening. The present and the future are intertwined. The long term is not what happens someday; it is what every CNP is building or forfeiting by its myriad daily decisions.[15]

The Strategic Task Force

The planning process begins with assembling a task force. Data about the present program on the national, state, or local level need to be assembled and made available to the task force, such as participation and enrollment records, student satisfaction data, anticipated growth, payroll and staffing records, and current literature related to CNP trends.[16] The people assembled on the task force should be the key players in the program and the broader community who will take responsibility for implementing the plan to position CNPs in the next century. When all stakeholders are involved, the best thinking of all concerned is brought to the table.[17]

Strategic planning task forces could be established at the national, state, or local CNP level. Many of their deliberations will be the same; only the scope of their actions will differ. When forming a task force at the local level, members might be school administrators, parents, students, school board members, and vendors in addition to employees and CNP management personnel. All task forces should contain thinkers who like to look at the big picture, those who like to deal in details, and those who will take risks and "push the envelope." The task force can then form smaller teams given the charge to go out into professional or local communities to ask specific questions. As many people as possible should be involved in the process because people don't change unless they have ownership in the change.[17]

Environmental Scan

A first step in strategic planning is to conduct an environmental scan to determine demographic, political, social, and economic forces outside the food and nutrition program that will impact its operation. As a federal program with funds flowing through state departments of education, sociopolitical forces at all levels impact CNPs greatly. Expenditures for food and labor are affected by economics. Strategic planning often begins with noting "what is" rather than "what could be."[18] One of the exercises that can be performed to focus on probabilities is to play "what if." The rules are to visualize an event and then discuss how it would impinge on CNPs. The following are scenarios that could be used in this sort of exercise:

- What would happen to CNPs if the USDA were abolished? Child nutrition programs would still be a priority of the country, but where would they be housed in the government? Would CNP administration go to the Department of Education (DOE) or the Department of Health and Human Services (DHHS)? Either might be problematic because the Department of Education has been targeted for demolition by some political groups for years, and alignment with DHHS might reinforce the view that CNPs are strictly a welfare program. A better solution would be to create a separate Department of Food and Nutrition. If the latter were to happen, what alliances would need to be formed so this type of department is created? Who would be the congressional constituency to support the new department? Would the agriculture constituency still be there? How would this affect state and local child nutrition programs, if at all? What would happen to the commodity distribution program?

- What if an educational voucher system becomes law and/or charter schools, privatization, and home schooling gain popularity? School districts may be planning to meet the needs of the baby boomlet by building new schools, but what will happen if the anticipated growth fails to appear because of public school alternatives? How will CNPs adapt to meet the food and nutrition needs of children regardless of school setting?

- What if telecommuting creates reverse migration of workers from cities and suburbs into rural areas? Telecommuters are young and will likely have preschool or school-age children. How will small, rural school systems meet increasing demand for pub-

lic education? Or will these children also telecommute to school using videoconferencing, computers, and faxes at home? If a telecommuting student is considered in attendance at school and he or she wishes to participate in the school food and nutrition program, should home meals be distributed? How might that affect the food production and delivery systems required by CNPs?

- What if the school day is divided into two sessions, a morning and an afternoon, to maximize school facilities? In this scenario, a formal meal service is not scheduled into the school day. How will CNPs face this change? How would CNPs justify their existence?

- What if a comprehensive health education curriculum is mandated by the state, and nutrition education is one of the cornerstones of this curriculum? How would the local food and nutrition program director meet the needs of teachers for effective nutrition education materials? Who in the district would be available to work with teachers in the classrooms or in curriculum-planning task forces?

- What if an incidence of food-borne illness occurred in the nation, the state, or in a closeby town? How would a local CNP respond to the resulting distrust of food prepared away from home? If food safety issues arise in a local CNP, what actions should be taken to work with the local health department and media? What if HACCP procedures were mandated by the state health department?

- What if a contract management company targets school food and nutrition services as the next big area for expansion? How should a local CNP respond when the school board has issued requests for proposals for privatizing the school food and nutrition program?

- What if grocery store chains began preparing and marketing nutritious lunches packed in high tech, insulated bags? How would CNPs respond to this competition? Would microwaves need to be installed in dining areas to allow students to reheat food?

By looking at all the issues in the external environment and thinking creatively about the "what if" and the "what could be," CNP professionals at the state and local level benefit by broadening their attention to all factors that could affect their programs. By developing this wide-angle vision, they may not be able to avoid whiplash, but it can be greatly reduced by learning how to see the future sooner.[19]

Strengths and Weaknesses

Internal strengths and weaknesses should be identified by the planning task force. During this process brutal honesty is the best policy as long as an element of trust has been established with the task force. Competent staff and new facilities might be strengths, and constraints on time to eat and student participation levels might be weaknesses of a CNP program.[20] The important aspect is to address maximizing strengths and minimizing or ameliorating weaknesses in the strategic plan.

Mission and Vision

Once the task force has looked at the external environment and the program's strengths and weaknesses, it is ready to determine the mission and vision of the program. Statements of mission and vision must be clear, concise, discriminating, and inspirational. They must direct attitudes, thinking, standards, and actions. They must help people differentiate between what is okay to do and what is not okay. CNP staff should be able to state the compelling purpose of the program in their own words from memory and with enthusiasm, or it doesn't exist in practice.[21] If a mission and vision already exist, then the task force needs to evaluate whether they are still current in the present climate of the program. The overall

mission of child nutrition programs is detailed in legislation, and the beginning part of this chapter addresses a universal vision for all programs in the next century. Each state or local CNP, however, needs to conceive of their mission and vision specifically as related to the mission of the state department of education or the school district.

Values and Beliefs

It is important for the task force to articulate common values and beliefs of the program. Goals, objectives, and strategies must be in concert with shared values and beliefs to be effective. Values and beliefs dictate not only what is achieved in an organization, but also how work is accomplished. They provide a backboard off which program strategies should be evaluated. Any plans should create meaning for employees as much as establish direction for the organization.[22]

Strategic Outcomes

Strategic alignment occurs when the program structure, policies, procedures, and practices totally support the program's vision of the future. Values, missions, visions, and planned outcomes without actions have the shelf life of ripe brie. They must immediately become part of all significant decision and actions, or the plan simply collects mold. Goals, objectives, and strategies are devised to achieve the mission and vision of the CNP. Directors should use the strategic plan as they prepare agendas for meetings. They should use it when they communicate with colleagues, and they should use it as they decide who gets which resources. All program structure, policies, and procedures must be adjusted to the mission and vision. Change leaders need to be effective role models. Staff needs to know that leaders value the new vision, will stand for it, and will take risks to support it because people don't change unless their leaders show they are serious about the intended change.[23]

Alignment of the plan with actions of those who are part of the CNP is a critical step in creating real and lasting change. Such alignment is fostered through supervision. Every supervisor and manager is a link. If parts of planned strategic actions become optional to any one of these, anyone who reports to them also will think it is optional. All staff members should understand and be able to articulate their role in implementing the strategic plan. All should identify the action steps they must do to achieve the changes indicated. People are unlikely to change unless they have a real-life picture of what that change will look like for them personally.[23] The intent is to do the right thing as well as do things right.[24]

Careful planning will help all food and nutrition professionals achieve their visions of a quality program. The vision described in the beginning of this chapter may seem too far away and unreal for serious consideration, but dreams are necessary for innovative action. There may be a piece of the vision that can be realized relatively quickly through strategic planning. In Dorothy's case the strategic goal was returning home. In the case of CNPs, strategic planning or the "clicking of heels" should not entail a return to what is simply familiar and comfortable. We should never forget the roots of CNPs, but to remain viable we need to change and grow. The future belongs not to those who possess a crystal ball, but to those willing to actively challenge conventional wisdom. The future belongs more to movement than to the starry-eyed.[25] Standing idle on the right track still may get a person hit by a train. That's why each year strategic plans are reevaluated in light of new information, both internal and external. The process evolves into one of continuous strategic thinking about positioning the CNP to achieve the vision of quality and cost-effective food and nutrition services for all children.

LEADERSHIP FOR EXCELLENCE

"While politics may be the art of the possible, leadership is the art of making the impossible come true."[25(p259)] The skills that enable the school food and nutrition professional to shape the future effectively are those of networking, team building, collaborating, advocating, and leading. The future success of programs will depend upon how willing CNP professionals are to share ownership with other stakeholders in the program; how skilled they are in building consensus around issues that can either divide or separate; how much they value being a part of coalitions sharing common goals; and how much they are willing to delegate to others or to technology as a means of freeing professional time to maintain focus on policy issues. As stated by Brown, quality depends on four "Ls": linking to the world, listening through those linkages, learning from and pondering those listenings, and then leading.[26(pxii)]

As school food and nutrition leaders look to the future and their roles in shaping that future, there are essential premises to keep in mind:

- All children who are away from their caregivers during a major portion of the day have special food requirements to meet their physical, social, and emotional needs.
- Every community in America has the same challenge to meet children's needs, but resources vary among communities.
- It is incumbent upon the institutions and professions serving children to endorse and support sound nutrition programs and practices for children.
- There must be a concerted effort to ensure that children have consistent nutrition messages and services as a means of helping them develop healthy food habits for a lifetime.[27]

To ensure the well-being of children at every level and in every part of the country requires a vision and plan to turn that vision into reality. Shirley Watkins described it this way, "We are in the midst of a journey, perhaps the most important journey that America can take, leading us to the universal assurance that every child in this country will have complete nutritional security. As we paint this picture of nutritional security, you will be the artists . . . the painters of this picture . . . and our children will serve as the models of this landscape . . . and it's going to be a wonderful treasure that we will all create together."[28] Being a part of this journey is a commitment, not only for those presently being served, but for those who are to come. It is part of building sustainable programs and the promise of leaving a legacy for the future. When Alice asked the Cheshire Cat, "Where do I go from here?" he calmly replied, "It depends on where you want to go." The dreams for child nutrition programs must be a shared vision, and they must extend in two directions embodying the wisdom and values from the past as well as hopes and dreams for the future.[29]

CASE STUDY
BEING INVOLVED AS A PARTNER IN PROMOTING HEALTH AND EDUCATION IN THE INDEPENDENCE COMMUNITY

Melanie Moentmann

Background

Independence School District is a suburban school district located in the metropolitan Kansas City area. The district enrollment is approximately 12,000 students. The average meals served per day are as follows: 2300 breakfasts, 7600 lunches and 3000 a la carte equivalents. In addition to traditional K–12 curriculum, the district also provides services at two alternative schools, one Head Start facility, and one Special Education GED/Even Start facility. The district has Day Care centers in all elementary buildings for both before and after school care as well as preschool programs. These programs operate 12 months. Independence is primarily a blue-collar community and has approximately 38% economically disadvantaged students.

The Child Nutrition Department offers both breakfast and lunch at all facilities each day. Snacks are available for after school programs, as well. During the summer, the department has worked with outside agencies to provide meals for the Summer Food Service Program in addition to the National School Lunch and Breakfast meals and snacks offered in our own programs.

Independence School District's Child Nutrition Program is fortunate to have wonderful support from the Board of Education as well as central office administration. The district's philosophy is to do what's best for the children in the community, hence the many, many opportunities outside the scope of traditional K–12 schools.

The Challenge: Finding ways to integrate nutrition services into the non-traditional opportunities in the community

The Child Nutrition Program's challenge has been integrating our services into non-traditional opportunities available in our community. The department has been fortunate to be asked to participate in several local task forces and committees. These groups vary in scope from small local groups focused on one or two main tasks, to larger more diverse groups who look at countywide or even statewide programs and outcomes. As a department, even though these meetings involve a time and staff commitment, our participation in them has allowed our program to benefit in many ways. Most important, we are also able to increase our service to our children and their families as a result of our involvement.

Actions

One of the task forces we are involved with is coordinated by FRAC (Food Research and Action Center). It is composed of not only the local school districts in the area, but the City of Kansas City, and many other local agencies concerned with increasing the achievement and development of the children in the area. One of the focuses of this group is to inform local, state and federal officials about our programs, and offer suggestions to eliminate barriers that prevent us from serving the community. We also work with community leaders to increase the awareness of the services available so more participants can take advantage of the programs available to them.

The Child Nutrition Department has used our communication tools, like monthly menus, to inform families of services available, not only at school, but during the summer and out in the community at large. We have also taken the opportunity to provide nutrition education to the families at meetings and other gatherings.

The Child Nutrition Department takes an active role to support the local programs in our district. We serve on advisory boards for the Head Start and Even Start programs, and on a committee to produce a newsletter specifically for Head Start and day care teachers. The newsletter incorporates nutrition and food into all curriculum areas for pre-school. The newsletter has a parent component and basic information for the teachers on nutrition. The activities in the newsletter give the teachers a range of choices to use as they teach their classes about nutrition and begin good food habits. The newsletter gives us another opportunity to inform the community about the opportunities available, such as the Summer Food Service Program, and to use information generated as part of the Missouri Nutrition Network campaigns. Nutrition education for the parents is also provided.

As a support program for the district's 21st century child care programs, the Child Nutrition Department provides information to their staff about current topics in nutrition to be shared not only with the child care providers, but also the parents through their monthly newsletters. We also provide training in food safety and sanitation to their staff, and general food service management information to those staff attending classes in childcare management. Much of the information from the task forces and committees is also shared with this group.

Collaborative efforts from several groups have allowed us to increase the effectiveness of other programs. For example, Missouri's Governor's Council on Fitness, along with several cosponsors, developed a larger than life exhibit of the human body called Body Walk, for elementary students to use as an activity to learn about nutrition and health. A local coalition of agencies formed a task force to increase the effectiveness of this activity. The group holds training for the sponsor schools and encourages them to study nutrition and health in the classroom before and after the Body Walk comes to their schools. We share information and resources to help them incorporate nutrition into the building curriculum.

The Missouri Nutrition Network and Jackson County Nutrition Networks are other groups in which the department participates. Both these networks are interested in providing consistent messages about nutrition to the general public, especially lower income families. A campaign was developed with targeted messages for families about eating more fruits and vegetables, eating more grains, and using lower fat methods of cooking meats. The campaign materials including recipes and handout materials have been used in many ways, and a successful supermarket festival was also held.

Outcomes

Improving test scores, academic performance, and attendance are all district wide goals. The connection between school breakfast participation and all three of these areas has been well documented in recent research. The district has actively encouraged breakfast participation to continue to improve in these areas. As a result of a Nutrition Education and Training grant, the department was able to secure several nutrition education materials for preschool and lower elementary grades.

Looking ahead

One of our greatest challenges is being able to share resource materials as often as we would like with community groups. One department goal is to hire additional staff to provide more nutrition education to the students and staff. Additionally, we are continuing to look for materials to be shared in the classroom for middle and secondary students, to continue our efforts for students of all ages. Another goal is to increase participation in the school meals program so the children can benefit from good nutrition, and the district and community in general, will benefit from their increased academic performance.

When President Harry Truman signed the National School Lunch Act in 1946, he did so "as a measure of national security, to safeguard the health and well-being of the nation's children." The directors of the child nutrition programs in Independence have continued to work to provide the best service to the children and families of our community, including work outside the scope of feeding children. Our work to educate the families and other providers will have a lasting impact on choices they will make for the rest of their lives. We choose to nourish their minds as well as their bodies, knowing that children are our future.

REFERENCES

1. T. Cochran, Remarks at the NFSMI building groundbreaking ceremony. The University of Mississippi, Oxford, MS, March 27, 1998.

2. *Managing Child Nutrition Programs*

3. M. Bryan, *The School Cafeteria* (New York: F.S. Crofts & Co., 1936).

4. Public Law 79-396. Stat. 281. 1946.

5. J. Caton, *The History of the American School Food Service Association: A Pinch of Love* (Arlington, VA: American School Food Service Association, 1990).

6. F. Hoffmann and B. Withers, "Shared Values: Nutrients for Learning," in *Learning Organizations: Developing Cultures for Tomorrow's Workplace,* S. Chawla and J. Renesch, eds (Portland, OR: Productivity Press, 1995).

7. M.K. Meyer et al., *High School Student Satisfaction Survey.* Technical report. (University, MS: National Food Service Management Institute, 1997).

8. M.K. Meyer, *Middle/Junior High School Student Satisfaction Survey.* Technical report. (University, MS: National Food Service Management Institute, 1998).

9. K. Albrecht, *The Only Thing That Matters* (New York: HarperCollins, 1992).

10. H. Raham, "Full-Service Schools," *School Business Affairs,* June 1998, 24–28.

11. F. Cairncross, *The Death of Distance: How the Communications Revolution Will Change Our Lives* (Boston: Harvard Business School Press, 1997).

12. G. Hamel and C.K. Prahalad, *Competing for the Future* (Boston: Harvard Business School Press, 1994).

13. D. Caldwell, "Clear Vision Leads to Success: Foodservice strategic planning," *School Business Affairs* 60, no. 11 (1994):19–22.

14. M.C. Spears, *Foodservice Organizations: A Managerial and Systems Approach,* 3rd ed. (Englewood Cliffs, NJ: Prentice Hall, 1995).

15. Hamel and Prahalad, *Competing for the Future.*

16. Caldwell, "Clear Vision Leads to Success."

17. C. Schwahn and W. Spady, "Why Change Doesn't Happen and How To Make Sure It Does," *Educational Leadership* 55, no. 7 (1998):45–47.

18. Hamel and Prahalad, *Competing for the Future.*

19. W. Burkan, "Developing Your Wide-Angle Vision," *Futurist* 32, no. 2 (1998):35–38.

20. Caldwell, "Clear Vision Leads to Success."

21. Schwahn and Spady, "Why Change Doesn't Happen."

22. Hamel and Prahalad: *Competing for the Future.*

23. Schwahn and Spady, "Why Change Doesn't Happen."

24. Caldwell, "Clear Vision Leads to Success."

25. Hamel and Prahalad, *Competing for the Future.*

26. J.S. Brown, *Seeing Differently: Insights on Innovation* (Boston: Harvard Business School Press, 1997).

27. J. Martin, "The National School Lunch Program—A Continuing Commitment," *Journal of the American Dietetic Association* 96, no. 9 (1996):857–858.

28. S. Watkins, *Carl Perkins Memorial Lecture.* Presentation at the American School Food Service Association Annual Conference, New Orleans, July 14, 1998.

29. R. Kanter, "Managing for Long-Term Success," *Futurist* 32, no. 6 (1998):43–45.

Epilogue

The vision of tomorrow is in the imagination of today. While visions of tomorrow may not always come true, what's remarkable is how often they do. And we must never forget that renewal (or creativity) and innovation will cease without a sense of what tomorrow will bring.

More than a half century ago, in the 1930s, when the United States was preoccupied with coming out of the Great Depression, the National School Lunch Program was founded . . . based on a vision of what tomorrow would bring. What the country wanted then, and now, was an intervention in the lives of children that would result in better health, greater achievement in the classroom, and greater consumption of nutritious and healthful food. They wanted a place in the educational program to make sure that these things could happen. They wanted more productive citizenry, then as now.

This vision was not heralded with fanfare or celebration. But the vision was just what Congress needed to start a simple one-meal-a-day nutrition program for all children that would benefit them and agriculture and the education program. It was a program that could be added to time and again until a full-blown food and nutrition program was made available for all children all day, all year, all time . . . a program that would tie the eating of nutritious food at school to the serving of nutritious food in the home to the learning ability of children. That vision was just what we required.

Today, child nutrition programs are a reality, but there is more to do to reach the vision that was reflected in the congressional debates of the 1930s and 1940s. There will be more to do to keep these programs fresh and consistent with tomorrow's needs for children, education, and our economy. And as so often happens, having the right sense of what tomorrow will bring comes from your *leadership for excellence* for programs for all children. It is the greatness in you!

Josephine Martin
Martha T. Conklin

About the Authors

Josephine M. Martin, PhD, RD, LD, is President of The Josephine Martin Group and an Adjunct Professor of Nutrition at Georgia State University, Atlanta. Dr. Martin earned her PhD at Georgia State University, Master's Degree at Teachers College, Columbia University, New York, and completed a dietetic internship at Duke University. She served as the first Executive Director of the National Food Service Management Institute, University of Mississippi. She began her professional career as an administrative hospital dietitian and quickly moved into the school nutrition program in its infancy. She has extensive experience in child nutrition programs having been an area school nutrition consultant, state director of child nutrition, and an USDA regional nutritionist. Prior to her retirement from the Georgia Department of Education in 1991, she was an Associate State Superintendent of Schools. Martin is recognized as one of Georgia's outstanding educators. Her commitment to professional growth and education has been recognized through leadership in ASFSA, where she served as President, the Association of School Business Officials, the American Dietetic Association and the Society of Nutrition Education. Dr. Martin has published a number of articles and monographs related to child nutrition. She is widely recognized as an inspiring speaker, strategic planner, visionary and historian in child nutrition programs. Her contribution to the development of child nutrition program legislation and public policy is reflected in the current authorizations and funding provisions which form the framework for child nutrition programs. She has made numerous professional presentations in national and state associations and organizations. Dr. Martin has received the ADA Medallion; IFMA's Silver Plate in School Food Service, the Tom O'Hearn Legislative Award and the John Stalker Award for Distinguished Service in Child Nutrition.

Martha T. Conklin, PhD, RD, is Senior Research Professor of Nutrition and Food Systems and Director of Applied Research, National Food Service Management Institute at The University of Southern Mississippi, Hattiesburg. Dr. Conklin earned her PhD from New York University and her MS and BS degrees from the University of Missouri, Columbia. She has extensive teaching experience in food service management at several universities in the Northeast and Midwest and, most recently, in the PhD program in nutrition and food systems at The University of Southern Mississippi. She has served as director of food and nutrition services for a large geriatric center, senior management consultant with a company selling food service management software, and administrative dietitian for residence halls at a large Midwestern university. Dr. Conklin has published several research articles and book chapters and made numerous professional presentations. In 1996 and 1997, she received the Kathleen Stitt Best Paper Award given by the American School Food Service Association for an article published in the *School Food Service Research Review*.

Index